Professional Nursing Practice

Concepts and Perspectives

4th Edition

Kathleen Koenig Blais, RN, Ed.D

Janice S. Hayes, RN, Ph.D

Barbara Kozier, RN, MN

Glenora Erb, RN, BSN

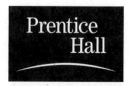

Upper Saddle River, New Jersey 07458

Library of Congress Cataloging-in-Publication Data

Professional nursing practice: concepts and perspectives / Kathleen Blais . . . [et al.].—4th ed.
   p. cm.
  Includes bibliographical references and index.
  ISBN 0-13-028288-X
   1. Nursing—Philosophy. I. Blais, Kathleen.
  RT84.5 .K69 2002
  610.73—dc21   2001051033

Publisher: Julie Levin Alexander
Executive Assistant & Supervisor: Regina Bruno
Executive Editor: Maura Connor
Acquisitions Editor: Nancy Anselment
Editorial Assistant: Sarah Caffrey
Director of Manufacturing and Production: Bruce Johnson
Managing Editor: Patrick Walsh
Production Management: Lisa Garboski/Bookworks
Manufacturing Manager: Ilene Sanford
Manufacturing Buyer: Pat Brown
Creative Director: Cheryl Asherman
Design Coordinator: Maria Guglielmo-Walsh
Composition: Peirce Graphic Services
Electronic Art Creation: Electra Graphics, Inc.
Marketing Manager: Nicole Benson
Marketing Assistant: Claudia Fernandez
Product Information Manager: Rachele Triano
Printer/Binder: Courier, Westford MA
Copy Editor: Linda Thompson
Proofreader: Wayne Beatty
Cover Design: Christopher Weigand
Cover Printer: Phoenix Color

Care has been taken to confirm the accuracy of information presented in this book. The authors, editors, and the publisher, however, cannot accept any responsibility for errors or omissions or for consequences from application of the information in this book and make no warranty, express or implied, with respect to its contents.

The authors and publisher have exerted every effort to ensure that drug selections and dosages set forth in this text are in accord with current recommendations and practice at time of publication. However, in view of ongoing research, changes in government regulations, and the constant flow of information relating to drug therapy and drug reactions, the reader is urged to check the package inserts of all drugs for any change in indications of dosage and for added warnings and precautions. This is particularly important when the recommended agent is a new and/or infrequently employed drug.

Pearson Education LTD.
Pearson Education Australia PTY, Limited
Pearson Education Singapore, Pte. Ltd
Pearson Education North Asia Ltd
Pearson Education Canada, Ltd
Pearson Educación de Mexico, S.A. de C.V.
Pearson Education—Japan
Pearson Education Malaysia, Pte. Ltd

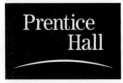

10 9 8 7 6 5 4 3 2 1
ISBN 0-13-028288-X

To Barb and Glen who taught me how, by guiding and assisting with patience, trust, and humor.

K. B.

To my children, Meredith and Matthew, and my loving mother, Bessie Hougland, who have taught me to believe in what can be.

J. S. H.

Brief Contents

Contents

PREFACE

To meet the demands of a dramatically changing health care system, nurses must change and grow. Skills in communication and interpersonal relations are needed for nurses to become effective members of a collaborative health care team. Nurses need to think critically and be creative in implementing nursing strategies with clients of diverse cultural and spiritual backgrounds in increasingly diverse settings. They need skills in teaching, collaborating, leading, managing, advocacy, political involvement, and analyzing and applying theory and research findings to practice. Nurses must be prepared to provide care not only in hospitals, but also in client homes and other community-based settings, including clinics, schools, occupational sites, faith-based communities, homeless shelters, and prisons. Their unique role demands a blend of nurturance, compassion, sensitivity, caring, empathy, commitment, courage, competence, and skill based on broad knowledge of the arts, humanities, biological and social sciences, and nursing science. In addition, an understanding of holistic healing modalities and complementary therapies is becoming more essential. In this book we address concepts on which nurses can build their repertoire of professional nursing knowledge. These concepts include, but are not limited to, wellness, health promotion, and disease prevention; holistic care; multiculturalism; nursing history; technology and informatics; nursing theories and conceptual frameworks; nursing research; and professional empowerment and politics.

Professional Nursing Practice: Concepts and Perspectives, 4th edition, is intended as a text for registered nurses who are in transition or bridge programs to pursue a baccalaureate degree in nursing. It may also be used in generic nursing programs or in transition or bridge programs for vocational nurses (LPNs or LVNs) to complete the professional nursing baccalaureate degree. This text has been revised extensively to reflect the additional areas of knowledge that practicing nurses require to be effective in the changing health care system. A new organization in the text emphasizes the foundational knowledge related to professional nursing, including nursing history, nursing theory, ethics, and legal aspects; the processes guiding nursing, including communication, group, change, and technology and informatics; nursing in a changing health care–delivery system, including health care economics, cultural and spiritual dimensions of nursing care, nursing in a culture of violence; and nursing in the new millennium, which discusses advanced nursing education and practice and visions for the future of nursing.

NEW TO THIS EDITION

There are eight new chapters, one new feature, and a new website created for the fourth edition of *Professional Nursing Practice: Concepts and Perspectives.*

- New chapters focus on important topics and concepts for today's nurse. They include Chapter 1, "Beginning the Transition: Journey to Professionalism," Chapter 3, "Historical Foundations of Professional Nursing," Chapter 11, "The Nurse as Advocate," Chapter 12, "The Nurse as Colleague and Collaborator," and Chapter 13, "Communication," Chapter 16, "Technology and Informatics," Chapter 17, "Nursing in an Evolving Health Care Delivery System," and Chapter 18, "Health Care Economics."
- Nurse Connect logos in each chapter. The web address will take the reader to a website created to support, enhance, and update chapter content. The website has links to nursing, health care, and other sites that provide current information related to the profession and health care. www.prenhall.com/blais

HALLMARK FEATURES

The fourth edition of *Professional Nursing Practice: Concepts and Perspectives* retains several of the features that have been well received by faculty and students who have used previous editions:

- Updated nursing research notes in each chapter describe relevant studies and relate them to clinical practice.
- Bookshelf boxes provide additional readings from popular and professional literature that enhance understanding of chapter content. The readings were chosen to pique student interest in exploring additional literary sources outside the classroom. For example, the readings in Chapter 21, "Nursing in a Culturally and Spiritually Diverse World," provide first-person accounts of the personal experiences of people of diverse cultural backgrounds.

Practicing nurse profiles occur in two chapters, Chapter 19 "Providing Care in the Home and Community," and Chapter 22, "Advanced Nursing Education and Practice." The profiles include information about why these practitioners chose their specific practice areas, what qualities they think are necessary to be a nurse in this setting, what their job entails, and what encouragement they would offer a nurse considering practice in this setting. The profiles provide useful first-person perspectives for readers.

"Consider . . ." sections occur in each chapter. This feature presents questions or ideas for readers to reflect upon and discuss. Items are related to the content presented and are intended to stimulate critical thinking. In most cases, the Consider questions encourage readers to apply the chapter content to their own areas of practice, be it a clinical specialty, a geographic area, or a personal belief about practice. These sections can be used as a basis for group discussions in a classroom setting, bulletin board or chat-room discussions for web-based courses, or independent learning.

All chapters retained from the previous edition have been completely updated.

ORGANIZATION

This edition is organized into five units, with an introductory chapter preceding the first unit. Units and chapters can be used independently or in any sequence.

Chapter 1, "Beginning the Transition: Journey to Professionalism," was created to assist registered nurses as they return to school. It provides information regarding factors influencing nurses' return to school for baccalaureate and higher degrees and overcoming barriers that may interfere with student success.

Unit 1, "Foundations of Professional Nursing Practice," focuses on the concepts of professional and professionalism, historical influences on nursing, ethical and legal issues, and nursing theories and conceptual frameworks for nursing.

Unit 2, "Professional Nursing Roles," includes information related to the professional roles of health promoter and care provider, learner and teacher, leader and manager, research consumer, advocate, and colleague and collaborator.

Unit 3, "Processes Guiding Professional Practice," focuses on processes used in professional nursing practice, including communication process, change process, group process, and the use of technology and informatics.

Unit 4, "Professional Nursing in a Changing Health Care Delivery System," includes chapters devoted to nursing in an evolving health care delivery system, health care economics, providing care in the home and community, nursing in a culture of violence, and nursing in a culturally and spiritually diverse world.

Unit 5, "Into the New Millennium," looks at the future of nurses and nursing. It includes chapters on advanced nursing education and practice, and visions for the future of nursing.

We hope this book helps learners from diverse backgrounds appreciate the proud heritage of professional nursing, understand what is meant by *professional*, view nursing as a profession, and develop knowledge and abilities that will contribute to the advancement of the profession. In addition, we hope the knowledge gained will help nurses provide quality care in a constantly changing health care system.

ACKNOWEDGMENTS

We extend our sincere thanks to the many talented and committed people who assisted in the birthing of this book:

The contributors whose expertise has broadened both the scope and depth of the text: Dr. Sally Weiss for Chapter 5, "Legal Foundations of Professional Nursing," Dr Janice Sandiford for Chapter 8, "The Nurse as Learner and Teacher," Dr. Diane Whitehead for Chapter 9, "The Nurse as Leader and Manager," and Dr. Barbara Happ for Chapter 16, "Technology and Informatics."

All the reviewers, who provided many discerning comments and suggestions that expanded our thinking and writing. Please see page xv for a list of the reviewers.

Nancy Anselment, senior editor, whose commitment to the manuscript, understanding of writing demands, and flexibility in rearranging schedules contributed positively to this revision. Her questions, challenges, and support stimulated the process during the development of this edition.

Mary Beth Ruitenberg, editorial assistant, for her gracious, capable assistance whenever it was needed.

Sarah Caffrey, editorial assistant, who came late in the process but who jumped right in to provide assistance when called upon.

Lisa Garboski, production manager, for her support and technical assistance during the production phase of this edition. Her timely attention to the details of production helped us to meet final schedules.

Linda Thompson, copyeditor, for her contributions to writing style and syntax. She helped make our words and ideas more meaningful.

Donna Nickitas, R.N.C., Ph.D., who created the website to accompany this text. Her work provides a contemporary dimension to readers' use of the fourth edition.

Most importantly, our many students who have challenged and taught us, and in doing so have helped to guide the direction of this book.

Contributors

Dianne Whitehead, Ed.D., RN
Chairperson
Broward Community College
School of Nursing

Janice Sandiford, Ed.D., RN
Associate Professor
Florida International University

Sally Weiss, Ed.D., RN
Broward Community College
School of Nursing

Donna Nickitas, R.N.C., Ph.D.
Hunter College
Old Greenwich, Connecticut

Barbara A. Happ Ph.D., RN
Associate Professor
University of Maryland
Adelphi, Maryland
    And
Kellogg Distinguished Professor
Hampton University
Hampton, Virginia

Reviewers

Nadine Mason MSN, CRNP
Faculty, Clinical Instructor
St. Luke's Hospital School of Nursing

Shirlee Newberry RN, M.S., DNSc (candidate)
Winona State University
Winona, Minnesota

Debra Leners, RN, Ph.D., CPNP
Professor
University of Northern Colorado
School of Nursing
Greeley, Colorado

Karen S. Saewert MS, RN, CPHQ
RN Programs Coordinator
Arizona State University
College of Nursing
Tempe, Arizona

Katherine B. Dougherty Ed.D., RN
Director of BSN Degree Completion Program
    for Registered Nurses
The University of Texas at Brownsville
Brownsville, Texas

Tara N. Fedric
Adjunct Clinical Professor
Texas Women's University
Dallas, Texas

Barbara J. Holtzclaw, Ph.D., RN, FAAN
Professor Emeritus
University of Texas Health Science Center
    at San Antonio
School of Nursing
San Antonio, Texas

Dianne Reed, MSN, Post Masters Family Nurse
    Practitioner
APRN, BC, Associate Professor
Texarkana College
Texarkana, Texas

Nancy D. Rubino Ed.D., RNC
Associate Professor of Nursing
Associate Degree Nursing Program Director
Wesley College Division of Nursing
Dover, Delaware

Lucille C. Gambardella, Ph.D., RN, CS, APN
Chair, Professor, Division of Nursing
Wesley College
Dover, Delaware

Jacqueline Hatlevig, RNC
Professor of Nursing
Winona State University
Winona, Minnesota

Ellen M. Moore, RN, MHSN, CS-FNP
Associate Professor of Nursing
Purdue University, Calumet
Hammond, Indiana

June Alberto, DNS, RN
Associate Professor and RN-BSN Program Director
Georgia Southern University
Statesboro, Georgia

Corrine Jurgens MS, RN-CS, ANP
Clinical Assistance Professor
State University Professor of New York
    at Stonybrook
School of Nursing
Stony Brook, New York

Beginning the Transition:
Journey to Professionalism

Objectives

- Examine changes in society that promote the nurse's return to school and further education.
- Apply models of professionalism to nursing.
- Identify strategies that will assist the nurse in returning to an educational setting.
- Identify helpful approaches to academic success.

NURSE CONNECT

Additional online resources for this chapter can be found on the companion web site at www.prenhall.com/blais.

The evolution of nursing has been dramatic in recent history. Most of the changes in nursing are in response to changes in society and in the health care system. There are also changes that are solely related to the evolution of the profession. The reciprocal relationship between nursing and society requires that nursing must change as society changes.

FACTORS IN SOCIETY THAT PROMOTE THE NURSE'S RETURN TO SCHOOL

Changes in society place new demands on nurses. An aging population results in older patients with more complex health problems. Changing reimbursement practices result in patients being discharged more quickly from hospitals, even though they still need skilled nursing care either in long-term care facilities or in their homes. A more diverse population requires nurses to be more knowledgeable about cultural and social influences on health. New technology and scientific discoveries require nurses to continually update their knowledge and skills. New diseases related to social and environmental problems require nurses to have a greater, integrated knowledge from the biological, psychological, and social sciences to promote health, to prevent illness or injury, and to care for those who are already ill or injured. Many of these societal changes are discussed in more detail in later chapters.

Changing Perceptions of Nursing as a Profession

Changing views of men's and women's roles are at the foundation of some of the profession's internal changes. Historically, nursing was considered a woman's occupation; however, that has gradually changed over the past decades. As more men entered nursing, the image of the profession changed. Use of traditional identifying symbols of nursing, such as caps and white uniforms, declined. There has also been less acceptance of the passive behaviors associated with the historical "handmaiden" role. Within health care institutions and in interactions with other health care disciplines, nurses are expected to be more accountable and responsible for their work. This requires a more assertive and proactive role for the contemporary professional nurse as she or he participates in a more collaborative health care system.

Other factors have also accounted for changes in the role of the professional nurse. The average age of working registered nurses has increased. Nurses are entering school and pursuing nursing degrees at more mature ages and are working longer, thus bringing more life experiences to the role. In the past, a nurse may have been more likely to work until having children and then stop working or work only part time or short term when additional income was needed. Now about 72% (ANA, 2000) of registered nurses are married and more than half have children living at home. About one-third of nurses employed full-time have children.

The education required for entry into the profession has changed over time. This has also influenced professional identity. Hospital-based diploma training was the mainstay of nursing education until the mid-twentieth century, when nursing programs in institutions of higher education proliferated and more nurses

were educated at the associate-degree and baccalaureate-degree level. Educational preparation in institutions of higher learning socialized nurses to formal education and even to the idea of continuing their career development through graduate education.

The practice of nursing has shifted from primarily acute care in the hospital to a more community- and primary-care focus. This has given nurses more autonomy in institutions with less rigid organizational structure and hierarchy. Many of these positions require a minimum of a baccalaureate degree for employment.

Specialty certification for nurses created rewards in terms of both recognition by employers and peers and self-fulfillment for the nurse. In recent years, the requirement for taking many specialty certification exams has included having a baccalaureate degree.

The result of all these changes has been a dramatic increase in the number of nurses returning to school. Between 1975 and 1998, the number of RNs graduating from BSN programs rose from about 3700 per year to more than 11,000 annually. In 1980, just over half of all registered nurses held hospital diplomas as their highest level of nursing preparation and about 22% held a BSN. By 1996, 31% had earned a baccalaureate degree (AACN, 2001).

In 1996, the American Association of Colleges of Nursing issued a position statement recognizing the bachelor of science degree in nursing as the minimum educational requirement for professional nursing practice. (See the box on page 3.) It is seen as critical for a career in professional nursing. The BSN nurse is prepared for a broader role; increasingly, the bachelor's degree is required for employment in many health care settings such as community health, case management, and supervisory positions. The BSN curriculum includes a broad spectrum of scientific, critical-thinking, humanistic, communication, and leadership skills (AACN, 2001).

Throughout this book is a feature titled "Consider." Use this feature to reflect on the content of the book as it relates to practice. There are no right or wrong answers. The answers may come from professional texts, commercial literature, personal and professional experience, or simply each student's own thoughts, beliefs, or values.

Consider . . .

■ the changes occurring in your professional life that require a return to school.
■ the changes occurring in your community that require new knowledge about nursing and health care.

American Association of Colleges of Nursing Position Statement: The Baccalaureate Degree in Nursing as Minimal Preparation for Professional Practice

Rapidly expanding clinical knowledge and mounting complexities in health care mandate that professional nurses possess educational preparation commensurate with the diversified responsibilities required of them. As health care shifts from hospital-centered, inpatient care to more primary and preventive care throughout the community, the health system requires registered nurses who can practice across multiple settings—both within and beyond management—providing direct bedside care, supervising unlicensed aides and other support personnel, guiding patients through the maze of health care resources, and educating patients on treatment regimens and adoptions of healthy lifestyles. In particular, preparation of the entry-level professional nurse requires a greater orientation to community-based primary health care, and an emphasis on health promotion, maintenance, and cost-effective coordinated care.

Accordingly, the American Association of Colleges of Nursing (AACN) recognizes the bachelor of science degree in nursing as the minimum educational requirement for professional nursing practice.

American Association of Colleges of Nursing, approved by the Board of Directors, July 20, 1996.

Pavalko's Occupation-Profession Continuum Model

Changes in nursing roles represent a shift in the view of nursing from an occupation to a profession with a commitment to the role. There are numerous conceptualizations of requirements for professional status, and many have debated whether nursing has yet achieved the status of a profession. Pavalko (1971) identified eight categories in his occupation-profession continuum model that serve as criteria to determine whether an occupation is a profession (see Table 1–1).

1. THEORY. The work group is judged on the extent to which its work is based on a systematic body of knowledge. This knowledge is developed through research. As a profession, nursing is establishing a well-defined body of knowledge and expertise. A number of nursing conceptual frameworks contribute to the knowledge base of nursing and give direction to nursing practice, education, and ongoing research.

2. RELEVANCE TO SOCIAL VALUES. This category suggests that a profession justifies its existence by close association with values that society as a whole embraces, such as life and happiness. Since its inception, nursing has had a history of altruism; that is, it has existed to serve others. In the early history of nursing, nurses were expected to devote most of their lives to nursing. Contemporary nursing still emphasizes service to others, but today's nurses expect adequate compensation and recognition as well as a life separate from nursing.

3. TRAINING (EDUCATION) PERIOD. Training or education is the third characteristic in Pavalko's model. This category has four subdivisions: educational content, length of education, use of symbolic and ideational processes, and degree of specialization that is related to practice.

According to Florence Nightingale, nursing education should involve theory and practice. Over the years, nursing has evolved to include both these dimensions. However, the length of study required for entry to practice is still an issue of controversy.

Historically, nurses were educated in hospitals. However, the education of nurses has now shifted to colleges and universities. The standard for undergraduate nursing curriculum includes education in the liberal arts, the biological and social sciences, and the nursing discipline. The Standards for Professional Nursing Education developed by the American Nurses Association (ANA, 1984, p. 1) states that the "education for those preparing to become nurses as well as those already licensed to practice nursing should take place in institutions of higher education." In 1983 the National League for Nursing (NLN) voted to retain the baccalaureate degree as the minimal academic preparation for the professional nurse (Lewis 1983). Education for advanced nursing practice is dis-

Table 1–1 Position of Nursing on the Occupation–Profession Continuum

Category	Occupation	Profession	Nursing
1. Theory	Absent	Present	Beginning stages
2. Relevance to social values	Not relevant	Relevant	Relevant
3. Training period	Short, not specialized	Long and specialized	Varied in length; some specialization
4. Motivation	Self-interest	Service	Service, but varies
5. Autonomy	Absent	Complete	Incomplete
6. Commitment	Short-term	Long-term	Varies; relatively short
7. Sense of community	Low	High	Developing
8. Code of ethics	Underdeveloped	Highly developed	Highly developed

Source: Adapted from *Sociology of Occupations and Professions* by R. M. Pavalko, 1971, Itasca, Ill.: F. E. Peacock, p. 26. Reprinted by permission of the publisher, *Professionalization of Nursing Current Issues and Trends* by M. M. Moloney, 1986, Philadelphia: Lippincott, p. 27. Reprinted with permission.

cussed in Chapter 22, "Advanced Nursing Education and Practice."

4. MOTIVATION. Motivation to work is Pavalko's fourth category. In this instance, Pavalko refers not to the motivation of the individual but to the group as a whole.

Motivation means the extent to which the nursing group emphasizes caring for individuals, families, groups, and communities through direct care or through advocacy. Advocacy may include political activism through memberships in professional and political organizations or individual involvement in health policy at local, regional, state, or national levels.

5. AUTONOMY. Pavalko's fifth category is autonomy: the freedom of the group to regulate and control its own work behavior. Styles wrote that many sociologists view autonomy as the sole differentiating characteristic of a profession (Styles, 1982). A profession is autonomous if it regulates itself and sets standards for its members. If nursing is to have professional status, it must function autonomously in the formation of policy and in the control of its activity. To be autonomous, a professional group must be granted legal authority to define the scope of its practice, describe its particular functions and roles, and determine its goals and responsibilities in delivery of its services. The amount of autonomy a professional group possesses depends on

its effectiveness at governance. Governance is the establishment and maintenance of social, political, and economic arrangements by which practitioners control their practice, their self-discipline, their working conditions, and their professional affairs.

6. COMMITMENT. Pavalko's sixth category is commitment toward work. In this context, people who are committed to their work view it as more than a stepping-stone to another type of work or as intermittent work. For people who engage in an occupation, commitment tends to be absent; professionals, in contrast, tend to commit to their work for a lifetime or long period of time.

Nurses, most of whom are women, often have conflicting obligations, such as family, which may affect their commitment to the profession. However, in recent years, nurses have tended to remain in the workforce instead of leaving to raise families, as many did in the past. Career-oriented nurses value commitment to people and continued education to broaden their own and nursing's power base; job-oriented nurses, in contrast, chiefly value the income they earn from the job. Increasingly, more nurses are becoming committed to nursing, thus moving nursing toward professional status.

7. SENSE OF COMMUNITY. A sense of community means that members of a group share a common identity and destiny and possess a distinctive subculture. In the past, nursing has been identified by many symbols, including the cap, white uniform, and pin. Although many of these symbols have disappeared, nurses do have a strong sense of identity. One way nurses can develop a sense of community is to join professional associations and groups.

8. CODE OF ETHICS. The existence of a code of ethics is the final category in Pavalko's model. Occupations are not likely to have a written code of ethics that sets forth standards of behavior and relationships between its members and the public they serve. Established professions, in contrast, do have formal codes of ethics. Nurses have traditionally placed a high value on the worth and dignity of others. The nursing profession requires integrity of its members; that is, a member is expected to do what is considered right regardless of the personal cost. Nurses must respect the professional judgment of others and must develop nursing standards and establish mechanisms for identifying and dealing with unethical behavior. The International Council of Nurses (ICN), the ANA, the Canadian Nurses Association (CNA), and other national nursing associations have codes of ethics.

An examination of nursing in relation to Pavalko's eight criteria shows that nursing is an emerging profession. Gains are being made, but nursing must continue to develop its professional standing.

FACTORS IN THE PROFESSION THAT PROMOTE THE NURSE'S RETURN TO SCHOOL

Credentialing Requirements

As knowledge and technology increase and nurses are more likely to specialize in specific practice areas, there is an increasing demand to obtain national certification either to obtain jobs in a specialty or to advance in the specialty. Most national certifications now require the baccalaureate degree in nursing (BSN) to sit for the certification examination; for example, the American Nurses Credentialing Center (ANCC) requires the baccalaureate degree as a minimum requirement for specialty certification. Those organizations that do not require the baccalaureate degree at the present time, e.g., the Association of Operating Room Nurses (AORN), may have future plans to require the BSN for certification.

Research Box

Oheln, J., and Segesten, K. 1998. The professional identity of the nurse: Concept analysis and development. *Journal of Advanced Nursing* 28(4): 720–727.

The purpose of this qualitative study was to describe the concept of registered nurses' professional identity. Eight Australian registered nurses were interviewed using a semistructured format. Results indicated that the professional and personal indentities of the nurse are integrated, consisting of feelings and experience of self as a nurse (subjective part) and other people's image of the nurse (objective part). These identities appear on a maturity continuum, with the opposite poles of strong and weak professional identity. The development takes place in a sociohistorical context through intersubjective processes of growth, maturity, and socialization, where interpersonal relations are important and attained maturity of the nurse influences further growth.

Research Box

Coulon, L., Mok, M., Krause, K., and Anderson, M. 1996. The pursuit of excellence in nursing care: What does it mean? *Journal of Advanced Nursing* 24: 817–826.

The purpose of this study was to determine the meaning of excellence in nursing care. The qualitative study collected open-ended questionnaire responses from 156 undergraduate and postgraduate nursing students. Four major themes emerged: (1) professionalism, (2) holistic care, (3) practice, and (4) humanism. The findings suggest that the client is the central focus of excellent nursing care at all times. Nurses who deliver excellent nursing care implement nursing in a professional and competent manner; demonstrate a holistic approach to caring; possess certain personal qualities that enhance practice; and relate to patients, families, peers, hospital administrators and community members in a competent manner. The comparison of students to registered nurses in higher-degree programs suggests stages of transition through which nurses pass in their quest for excellence.

Bookshelf

Benner, P. 1984. *From novice to expert: excellence and power in clinical nursing practice.* **Menlo Park, Calif.: Addison-Wesley.**

This classic work describes the transition to expert nurse by the new graduate or the experienced nurse who changes to a new nurse-practice setting. It describes the roles of nurses in their various stages of development and the challenges they face.

Hudacek, S. 2000. *Making a difference: Stories from the point of care.* **Indianapolis, Ind.: Sigma Theta Tau International.**

The author discusses the nursing values of caring, courage, comfort, competence, critical thinking, and creativity using nurses' stories to illustrate these values in practice.

WHAT WILL IT TAKE TO GET THERE: OVERCOMING BARRIERS

Returning to school provides the professional advancement that nurses seek. It represents a commitment to goals of both professional and personal growth. Meeting those goals requires lifestyle and role changes. Many nurses returning to school have been away from a formal education setting for some time and are anxious about becoming a student again. Fitting into academe represents a substantial transition from the practice role; because many returning students continue to work, the nurse must become comfortable about fitting into both worlds. Concerns about academic skills, such as library searches, scholarly writing, and test taking, are often a source of stress. Blending the student role with the work role and the family-member role represents great challenges. Learning to deal effectively with the stressors that create barriers to success is important. Some of those barriers include managing time effectively to meet the commitments of family, work, and school; finding the financial resources to pay for tuition, books, and educational supplies; finding and maintaining effective social support systems, including family, work colleagues, and student colleagues; learning to work with faculty who require academic excellence in spite of the many demands on the nurse/student's time; and developing effective study skills.

Time Management

Time-management skills are a necessary tool for survival and success. Organizing, planning, and setting of priorities are keys. Procrastination creates a domino effect when there are multiple tasks related to multiple roles. The ability to handle interruptions goes hand in hand with time-management techniques. Setting limits allows one to be goal-focused and keep the load realistic. Keeping balance among roles and expectations is essential and requires clear priorities. This kind of clear focus allows the streamlining of things to be done. Nurse/students who are assuming multiple roles with high expectations of their performance in each of these roles often forget to maintain one of their major resources—their health. Adequate sleep, good nutrition, and diversion are necessary to keeping the energy level and motivation to succeed.

Consider . . .

■ the activities you enjoy that can serve as a break. Which of those could be used as a short-term break to refresh a tired body and mind? Which of these activities are long-term fixes requiring greater planning? Devise a schedule that allows you to take advantages of these.

Money

For students returning to school, money to pay tuition and fees and to purchase textbooks and other supplies is often a concern. Many employers provide tuition reimbursement as a benefit of employment. Information can be obtained from human resources or personnel departments. Many civic groups and nursing organizations provide scholarships. There are also various state and federal loan opportunities; some may have forgiveness programs if the nurse works in a specific location or specialty for a period of time after graduation. The university or college financial aid office can provide information on scholarships and other forms of tuition assistance.

Social Supports

Although students can be successful on their own, the support of others can make things go more smoothly. The people who can contribute to the success of students include their families and friends, their classmates, and their faculty.

Family and friends might be considered the first level of support and may provide assistance in a variety of ways. This assistance may include financial help, babysitting, cooking meals, typing papers, proofreading papers, being a sounding board for ideas, and helping to study for exams. Some nurses are concerned about whether they can continue to meet the needs of their family, especially young children, when they return to school. The change will require some adjustment on each family member's part, but often the result is positive in ways that were unexpected. For instance, children may learn about the importance of study habits and continuing one's education in the future.

An advantage of returning to school is meeting colleagues from other areas of practice and other health care organizations. This can provide opportunities to broaden perspectives on health care and nursing as well as to establish important networks. The new colleagues may challenge thinking during discussions of ideas, and they may be the "experts" to consult. This new network can become an informal network for obtaining new jobs based on experience and new knowledge.

Working with Faculty

The faculty is an important resource in increasing knowledge, expanding ways of thinking, and enhancing professional capabilities. According to Twiname and Boyd (1999, 27), faculty "are not the enemy. . . . They are there to help you graduate." It's important to use faculty to the fullest while remembering that they are also people. Their suggestions for working with faculty are shown in the accompanying box.

Additionally, *don't expect faculty to be mind readers.* When having difficulties either personally or related to your coursework, discuss them with the faculty. They may be able to suggest solutions, recommend resources in the college/university, or assist with learning. Sometimes personal circumstances occur that necessitate dropping out of a class before the end of the semester or term. There are usually procedures that must be followed so that there is no negative impact on the student's progression or grade.

Study Skills

Study skills may need to be reviewed and enhanced. Unlike many noncredit continuing education activities, there are graded assignments, exams, and grades in college courses. Students need to plan well to balance the many obligations they have. Some suggestions to enhance study skills are found in the accompanying box.

Suggestions for Dealing with Faculty

1. *Show your faculty respect.* When you show faculty respect, they will respect you in turn. Respect and courtesy go hand in hand. Find out your faculty's office hours. When you make an appointment, keep it; if you can't, then call to cancel. Don't be afraid to speak up and let your teacher know what you need to meet your goals.

2. *Remember, as human beings, your instructors will have good days and bad days.* Faculty members experience the same life problems as students. Although most of the time faculty will be fully there for students, there may be times when other things, either work-related or personal, may take precedence. Before dropping in for a visit, confirm that it is a convenient time for both you and the faculty member. This will ensure that the faculty member is fully there for you.

3. *Respect your instructor's privacy.* Don't call your instructor at home unless she or he has given you permission to do so. Visit faculty during posted office hours. Faculty have many responsibilities related to teaching, including course preparation, committee work, and grading student assignments. Recognize that faculty members often schedule office time to complete work-related activities, during which they wish not to be disturbed.

4. *Instructors have many different personalities.* Some will be very tough and demanding, whereas others will be very casual. Students will need to learn from a variety of teachers with different teaching styles. Being exposed to a diversity of instructors prepares students for interacting with the various people they will meet in their professional life.

Source: Adapted from *Student Nurse Handbook: Difficult Concepts Made Easy,* by B. G. Twiname and S. M. Boyd, Stamford, Conn.: Appleton and Lange, 1999.

Suggestions for Study-Skills Enhancement

1. *Decide where you will study.* Most people prefer to study in quiet, whereas others find that background noise is helpful. Determine where you will study. Be sure that there is adequate lighting, comfortable seating, and the supplies you need so that you can study without interruption.

2. *Avoid marathon study sessions.* Plan ahead and keep up with readings and other assignments so that you need only to review for exams.

3. *Be prepared for classes.* Read the reading assignments *before* class and make notes or outline the material. Use class time to clarify information, to ask questions, and to participate in discussion. Don't expect faculty to read the textbook to you. They may assign readings as a foundation and then lec-ture from other resources to enhance the as-signed readings.

4. *Review notes as soon after class as possible.* Make sure you understand your notes. Check your notes against the textbook to determine if there are any discrepancies. Don't wait until the exam to clarify inconsistencies.

5. *Learn how to use the library and how to use computers.* The library is not just a building, it is a collection that is available by computer as well as hard copy. At any time of the day or night, there is access to hundreds of databases where students can locate information related to the area of study. Information from gov-ernmental and private organizations 24 h a day is available by simply going online and using a search engine.

Source: Adapted from *Student Nurse Handbook: Difficult Concepts Made Easy,* by B. G. Twiname and S. M. Boyd, Stamford, Conn.: Appleton and Lange, 1999, and *How to Study,* by R. Fry, New York: Career Press, 1994.

The challenge of returning to school, represented by the changes in lifestyle and the demands upon time and intellect, can be stimulating and satisfying. Many opportunities will be available for personal and pro-fessional growth. New career possibilities will be avail-able and new perspectives on old ones. The journey is an important one to each student and to nursing as a profession.

REFERENCES

American Association of Colleges of Nursing (AACN). 2001. *Your nursing career: A look at the facts.* www.aacn.nche.edu/education/Career.htm.

American Nurses Association (ANA). 1984. *Standards for professional nursing education.* Washington, D.C.: ANA.

American Nurses Association (ANA). 2000. *Nursing facts.* www.ana.org/readroom/fsdemogr.htm.

Coulon, L., Mok, M., Krause, K., and Anderson, M. 1996. The pursuit of excellence in nursing care: What does it mean? *Journal of Advanced Nursing,* **24:** 817–826.

Fry, R. 1994. *How to study,* 3d ed. New York: Career Press.

Lewis, E. P. 1983. News outlook: The issue that won't go away. A report on the 1983 NLN convention. *Nursing Outlook* **31:** 246–247.

Ohlen, J., and Segesten, K. 1998. The professional identity of the nurse: Concept analysis and develop-ment, *Journal of Advanced Nursing* **28**(4): 720–727.

Pavalko, R. M. 1971. *Sociology of occupations and profes-sions.* Itasca, Ill.: Peacock.

Styles, M. 1982. *On nursing: Toward a new endowment.* St. Louis: Mosby.

Twiname, B. G., and Boyd, S. M. 1999. *Student nurse handbook: Difficult concepts made easy.* Stamford, Conn.: Appleton and Lange.

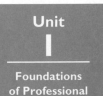

Unit

I

Foundations of Professional Nursing Practice

CHAPTER 2

Socialization to Professional Nursing Roles

Outline

Objectives

- Discuss professionalism and nursing.
- Describe socialization to professional nursing.
- Analyze elements and boundaries of nursing roles.
- Compare socialization models of Simpson, Hinshaw, and Davis.
- Discuss ways to manage role stress and strain while enhancing professional identity.

N U R S E   C O N N E C T

Additional online resources for this chapter can be found on the companion web site at www.prenhall.com/blais.

Professional socialization is associated with the specialized knowledge, skills, attitudes, values, and norms needed to perform the professional role. There is debate as to whether this socialization is a process or an outcome. When described as a process, it is characterized as "a complex and variable form of learning, highly collaborative in nature" (Weedman, 1998, p. 1). It transmits values, norms, and ways of seeing that are unique to the profession and provides a common ground that shapes the ways in which work is conducted and allows members of the profession to communicate effectively. As an outcome, it is the formation of an individual's professional identity, the self-view as a member of a profession with the requisite knowledge and responsibilities. Socialization as a process or an outcome is interactive, because the knowledge, skills, and values of a profession are passed along to new members.

A profession is generally distinguished from other kinds of occupations by (1) its requirement of prolonged, specialized training to acquire a body of knowledge pertinent to the role to be performed and (2) an orientation of the individual toward service, either to a community or to an organization. The standards of education and practice for the profession are determined by the members of the profession rather than by outsiders. The education of the professional involves a complete socialization process, more far-reaching in its social and attitudinal aspects and its technical features than usually required in other kinds of occupations.

There is debate about whether nursing is a profession or has yet to reach that status. Traditionally, only medicine, law, and theology were considered professions, but nursing has been called a profession for many years. The social sciences have developed criteria against which an occupation can be judged to ascertain its professional status. (See the accompanying box.)

CHALLENGES AND OPPORTUNITIES

Level of entry. Professional role socialization has been impeded by nursing's multiple levels of entry into the field and the lack of agreement about role differences at these different levels. Nursing is the only major discipline that does not require its members to hold at least a baccalaureate degree in order to be licensed. Associate degree programs continue to maintain high enrollment and graduate large numbers of individuals (Catalano, 2000). Role socialization depends upon the way the role is conceptualized, and nurses prepared at multiple levels may not have common language, values, etc. Thus, nurses may not be in accord with regard to professional practice and may have different perspectives relative to professional practice.

Criteria of a Profession

FLEXNER (1915)

Professional activity is basically intellectual.

Activities are practical, not theoretical.

Work can be learned because it is based on a body of knowledge.

Techniques can be taught.

A strong organization is in place.

Work is motivated by altruism.

BIXLER AND BIXLER (1945)

Body of knowledge is specialized.

Body of knowledge is increasing.

New knowledge is developed to improve education and practice.

Practice is autonomous.

Education takes place in higher institutions.

Service is considered to be more important than personal gain.

Compensation comes through freedom to act, continuing professional growth, and economic security.

BARBER (1965)

A vast amount of systematic general knowledge.

Oriented primarily to community interest rather than self-interest.

Strong behavioral self-control supported by codes of ethics and internalized through work socialization and through organizing and conducting voluntary associations operated by work specialists.

A system of rewards: monetary and honorary.

PAVALKO (1971)

Work is based on a systematic body of theory and abstract knowledge.

Work has social value.

Work is a service to the public.

Education is required for specialization.

Autonomy.

Commitment to the profession.

Group identity and subculture.

A code of ethics.

Gaps between education and practice. Adding to the quandary is the lack of agreement between educators and employers of nurses regarding expectations of graduates entering the field. Educators in the professional curriculum provide initial socialization, and they make decisions based upon their conception of a beginning-level professional. Employers are looking for graduates who can function independently, require little retraining or orientation, and can supervise a variety of less educated and unlicensed employees. Role incongruity is often experienced in the practice setting.

Professional identity: job versus career. There is little commitment to a job other than going to work, doing what is expected, and collecting a paycheck. A career, on the other hand, is viewed as a person's life work, which develops over time. There is planning for the future and direction with a career that requires commitment. The practice of nursing is not viewed as a career by all nurses.

Consider . . .

- how distance learning and online courses may affect the amount and type of personal contact the student experiences. How might that impact socialization of nurses during the educational programs? How might nursing assure common ground in role conceptualization and expectations about nursing practice?
- autonomy in your practice setting. How autonomous are the nurses? Should the practice be more autonomous? If so, how could more autonomy be achieved?
- Flexner's criterion that in a profession, "work is motivated by altruism." What are your thoughts about this criterion?
- Barber's criterion that a profession is "oriented primarily to community interest rather than self-interest." What do you think of this criterion?

PROFESSIONALISM

Nursing as a Discipline and Profession

Unlike other professions, nursing has three educational routes leading to eligibility for the licensing exam and becoming a registered nurse. This has created controversy within the profession and confusion for the public. The earliest type of nursing education in the United States took place within hospital-based training schools and awarded a diploma in nursing at the conclusion. Baccalaureate nursing education started at the University of Minnesota in 1909 and exists in four-year institutions of higher education. Associate degree nursing (ADN) programs began in 1952 in response to a nursing shortage and developed within community colleges. As nursing education began moving into institutions of higher education, the diploma programs began affiliating with nearby colleges and universities.

Associate degree programs focused on preparing bedside nurses and drew large numbers of students. They helped to solve subsequent nursing shortages in the 1960s and 1980s. Baccalaureate degree programs provide a broader background of knowledge from the sciences and liberal arts than the other two programs and prepare the graduates for a greater variety of roles. These roles include community nursing and leadership. Table 2–1 compares the educational opportunities of the three major routes to becoming a registered nurse.

In 1965, the American Nurses Association published a position paper on educational preparation of nurses that differentiated nurses with baccalaureate degrees and nurses with associate degrees as professional and technical nurses. This issue has been a source of great controversy between those who see all nurses as professional and those who believe professionals should have a minimum of a bachelor's degree. Many changes have occurred since the inception of these programs, allowing for articulation of the programs and making it easier for the ADN graduate to continue for a BSN. RN-BSN transition programs are common today, and many students enter associate degree programs with the intent of continuing for a BSN degree.

At the core of the controversy over level of entry into professional nursing is the definition of profession. Four different conceptualizations of the criteria for a profession are shown in the accompanying box. (Chapter 1, "Beginning the Transition: Journey to Professionalism," discussed Pavalko's criteria.) Educational preparation at the baccalaureate level provides a broader education to better address the body of knowledge. Although nursing meets each of the criteria to some extent, some are more adequately addressed than others. The autonomous practice of nursing has been a source of political activism on behalf of nurses. Whether nursing has a sufficiently developed, unique body of knowledge is also in dispute. It may be concluded that nursing has not yet achieved full professional status but is emerging as a profession.

Nursing as a discipline is less controversial. A discipline is "characterized by a unique perspective, a distinct way of viewing all phenomena, which ultimately defines the limits and nature of its inquiry" (Donald-

Table 2–1 Educational Opportunities for Registered Nurses: A Comparison

	Diploma	Associate Degree	Baccalaureate
Location	Is usually conducted by and based in a hospital	Most often conducted in junior or community colleges, occasionally in senior colleges and universities	Located in senior colleges and universities
Length of Study	Requires generally 24–30 months but may require 3 academic years	Requires usually 2 academic or sometimes 2 calendar years	Requires 4 academic years
Requirements for Admission	Requires graduation from high school or its equivalent, satisfactory general academic achievement, and successful completion of certain prerequisite courses	Requires that applicants meet entrance requirements of college as well as of program	Requires that applicants meet entrance requirements of the college or university as well as those of program
Program of Learning	Includes courses in theory and practice of nursing and in biologic, physical, and behavioral sciences. May require that certain courses in the physical and social sciences be taken at a local college or university	Combines a balance of nursing courses and college courses in the basic natural and social sciences with courses in general education and the humanities	Frequently concentrates on courses in the theory and practice of nursing in the junior and senior years. Provides education in the theory and practice of nursing and courses in the liberal arts as well as the behavioral and physical sciences
Clinical Component	Provides early and substantial clinical learning experiences in the hospital and a variety of community agencies; these focus on an understanding of the hospital environment and the interrelationship of other health disciplines	Requires as a significant part of the program supervised clinical instruction in hospitals and other community health agencies	Provides clinical laboratory courses in a variety of settings where health and nursing care are given
Opportunity for Educational Advancement	Little or no transferability of courses unless affiliated with a community college or university	Is structured so that some credits may be applied to baccalaureate degree	Provides the basic academic preparation for advancement to higher positions in nursing and to master's degree
Competency on Graduation	Graduate is prepared to plan for the care of patients with other members of the health care team, to develop and carry out plans for the care of individuals or groups of patients, and to direct selected members of the nursing team. Has an under-	Graduate is prepared to plan and give direct patient care in hospitals, nursing homes, or similar health care agencies and to participate with other members of the health care team, such as licensed practical nurses, nurses aides, physicians, and other registered nurses, in rendering care to patients.	Graduate is prepared to plan and give direct care to individuals and families, whether sick or well, to assume responsibility for directing other members of the health care team, and to take on beginning leadership positions. Practices in a variety of set-

Continued

Table 2–1 Educational Opportunities for Registered Nurses: A Comparison (Cont.)

	Diploma	Associate Degree	Baccalaureate
	standing of the hospital climate and the community health resources necessary for the extended care of patients		tings and emphasizes comprehensive health care, including preventive and rehabilitative services, health counseling and education, and care in acute and long-term illnesses. Has necessary education for graduate study toward a master's degree and may move rapidly to specialized leadership positions in nursing as teacher, administrator, clinical specialist, nurse practitioner, and nurse researcher
Licensure	Must successfully complete state licensing examination	Must successfully complete state licensing examination	Must successfully complete state licensing examination

Source: Used by permission: J. R. Ellis and C. L. Hartley, *Nursing in Today's World,* 7th ed., Philadelphia: Lippincott, 2000, pp. 217–218.

son and Crowley, 1978). Disciplines reflect distinctions among bodies of knowledge; in other words, human knowledge is divided into disciplines. Nursing as a discipline is defined by the essence of nursing.

Disciplines are divided into academic disciplines and professional disciplines. Academic disciplines, such as physics and mathematics, use descriptive theories and do basic and applied research. Professional disciplines are directed toward practical aims using both descriptive and prescriptive theories and add clinical research along with basic and applied research. The practice of academic disciplines is research and education, whereas the practice of professional disciplines adds a component of clinical practice. Thus, nursing has a better fit as a professional discipline.

Standards of Clinical Nursing Practice

Establishing and implementing standards of practice are major functions of a professional organization. The purpose of **standards of clinical nursing practice** is to describe the responsibilities for which nurses are accountable. The standards (1) reflect the values and priorities of the nursing profession, (2) provide direction for professional nursing practice, (3) provide a framework for the evaluation of nursing practice, and (4) define the profession's accountability to the public

and the client outcomes for which nurses are responsible (ANA, 1998, p. 1). In 1991, the ANA developed standards of clinical nursing practice that are generic in nature and provide for the practice of nursing regardless of area of specialization. The ANA and various specialty nursing organizations have further developed specific standards of nursing practice related to the practice of nursing in a specialty area.

The profession's responsibilities inherent in establishing and implementing standards of practice include (1) to establish, maintain, and improve standards, (2) to hold members accountable for using standards, (3) to educate the public to appreciate the standards, (4) to protect the public from individuals who have not attained the standards or willfully do not follow them, and (5) to protect individual members of the profession from each other (Phaneuf and Lang, 1985, p. 2).

Nursing standards clearly reflect the specific functions and activities that nurses provide, as opposed to the functions of other health workers. The ANA's standards of clinical nursing practice consist of both standards of care and standards of professional performance. *Standards of professional performance* describe the competence level of professional role behaviors. These standards are shown in the box on page 14.

When standards of professional practice are im-

ANA Standards of Professional Performance

I. Quality of Care
The nurse systematically evaluates the quality and effectiveness of nursing practice.

II. Performance Appraisal
The nurse evaluates his or her own nursing practice in relation to professional practice standards and relevant statutes and regulations.

III. Education
The nurse acquires and maintains current knowledge and competency in nursing practice.

IV. Collegiality
The nurse interacts with, and contributes to the professional development of, peers and other health care providers as colleagues.

V. Ethics
The nurse's decisions and actions on behalf of patients are determined in an ethical manner.

VI. Collaboration
The nurse collaborates with the patient, family, and other health care providers in providing patient care.

VII. Research
The nurse uses research findings in practice.

VIII. Resource Utilization
The nurse considers factors related to safety, effectiveness, and cost in planning and delivering patient care.

Source: American Nurses Association, *Standards of Clinical Nursing Practice,* Washington, D.C.: ANA, 1998. Used with permission.

plemented, they serve as yardsticks for the measurements used in licensure, certification, accreditation, quality assurance, peer review, and public policy.

PROFESSIONAL SOCIALIZATION

Socialization can be defined simply as the process by which people (1) learn to become members of groups and society and (2) learn the social rules defining relationships into which they will enter. Socialization involves learning to behave, feel, and see the world in a similar manner as other persons occupying the same role as oneself (Hardy and Conway, 1988, p. 261). The goal of professional socialization is to instill in individuals the norms, values, attitudes, and behaviors deemed essential for the survival of the profession.

An intrinsic aspect of the socialization process is *social control*—the capacity of a social group to regulate itself through conformity and adherence to group norms to maintain the group's social order and organization. Sanctions are used to enforce norms. Positive sanctions reward conformity to norms; negative sanctions punish nonconformity. Sanctions may be either externally employed by a source outside the individual (e.g., disciplinary action by a committee) or internally employed from within the individual (e.g., self-congratulations for a job well done). Socialization implies that the individual is induced to conform *willingly* to the ways of the group.

Norms therefore become internalized standards. Professions require both a relatively long period of formal schooling and an informal, internalized system of ethics that guides practice of the professional role.

Professional socialization involves exposure to multiple agents of socialization. Agents of socialization are the people who initiate the socialization process, such as family members, teachers, child-care workers, peers, and the mass media. For children, the primary agents of socialization are the family, teachers, peers, and the mass media. In one-parent families, surrogate parents, such as child-care workers and baby-sitters, may also be major socialization agents. For adults, the influence of these agents continues but other agents arise, such as superiors and subordinates in the workplace, peers, and people in various other kinds of social groups. Socialization agents that nursing students encounter include clients, faculty, professional colleagues, other health care professionals, family (e.g., a nurse relative) and friends who occupy roles within or outside the formal institutional structure. The degree of congruence between the expectations of these multiple agents may either facilitate or hinder socialization. (See the box on page 15.)

One of the most powerful mechanisms of professional socialization is interaction with fellow students (Hardy and Conway, 1988, p. 267). Within this student culture, students collectively set the level and direction

Factors That Facilitate the Socialization Process

- Clarity and consensus with which the occupants and aspirants (learners) perceive the roles and positions.
- Degree of compatibility of expectations within role sets—that is, all others who are involved with the learner, such as staff nurses, nurse managers, physicians, clients, and their families or significant others.
- Learning that has occurred before an entry to a position.

- Capability of socialization agents to manage the socialization process.
- Role models who demonstrate the desired characteristics and can enhance internalization of admired qualities.
- A well-developed and extended orientation or internship program that may include preceptors (people who act as teachers).
- Group support from others new to the position to share concerns.

Sources: Adapted from *Role Transition to Patient Care Management* by M. K. Strader and P. J. Decker, Norwalk, Conn.: Appleton and Lange, 1995, pp. 64–66, and *Role Theory: Perspectives for Health Professionals,* 2d ed., by M. E. Hardy and M. E. Conway, Norwalk, Conn.: Appleton and Lange, 1988, p. 262.

of their scholastic efforts, develop perspectives about the situation in which they are involved, the goals they are trying to achieve, kinds of activities that are expedient and proper, and a set of practices congruent with all of these. Students become bound together by feelings of mutual cooperation, support, and solidarity.

Consider . . .

- the agents of professional socialization in your own experience. How have other nurses influenced your development as a nurse?
- the sources of sanctions for the professional nurse. What legal, institutional, societal, and professional sanctions (positive and negative) exist for nursing, both in your own practice and in the larger profession? How might these sanctions differ based on specialty area, geographic area, or level of practice?

Critical Values of Professional Nursing

It is within the nursing educational program that the nurse develops, clarifies, and internalizes professional values. Specific professional nursing values are stated in nursing codes of ethics (see Chapter 4, "Values, Ethics, and Advocacy"), in standards of nursing practice, and in the legal system itself (see Chapter 5, "Legal Foundations of Professional Nursing"). Watson (1981, 20–21) outlines four values critical for the profession of nursing:

1. A strong commitment to the service that nursing provides for the public

2. Belief in the dignity and worth of each person

3. A commitment to education

4. Autonomy

The first value, a strong commitment to the service that nursing provides for the public, is considered essential. Nursing is a helping, humanistic service directed to the health needs of individuals, families, and communities. The nurse's role is therefore focused on *health* and *care*. Nurses, being responsible for assessing and promoting the health status of all humans, need to value their contribution to the health and well-being of people. Because "care and caring is the central core and essence of nursing" (Watson, 1979), nurses also need to value the caring aspect of nursing.

The second value—the dignity and worth of each person—is based on Judeo-Christian philosophy of the sacredness of human life and the worth of the individual. Because nursing is a person-oriented profession, a basic belief in the worth of each person regardless of nationality, race, creed, color, age, sex, politics, social class, and health status is basic to nursing. Applied to nursing practice, this value means that the nurse always acts in the best interest of the client.

Commitment to education, the third value, reflects the lifelong value of learning. In terms of professional nursing, graduates need continuous education to maintain and expand their level of competencies to meet professional criteria, to anticipate the role of the nurse in the future, and to expand the body of professional knowledge. Nurses need to question nursing knowledge and practice critically, to contribute to nursing's theoretical base, and to test theories in nursing practice.

The fourth value—autonomy—is the right of self-determination as a profession. Watson (1981, 21) states that "nurses must have freedom to use their knowledge and skills for human betterment and the authority and ability to see that nursing service is delivered safely and effectively." A future challenge for nurses is to become more assertive in promoting nursing care and to develop the ability for independent behavior.

Consider . . .

■ Watson's four values of professional nursing. Identify behaviors that represent these values. What nurses in your experience embody these values? How do these nurses influence your own professional socialization?
■ whether socialization is an outcome or a process.

The Initial Process of Professional Socialization

Professional socialization is the means of developing a professional identity. It is a lifelong process. Registered nurses who return to school for baccalaureate nursing education experience professional resocialization. Their personal characteristics are diverse and affect resocialization in complex ways. Often they need to over-

come prejudices about and resistance to an educational program that may require them to shed habitual ways of thinking. "Baccalaureate education for RNs provides educational resocialization experiences made more complex by the diversity, psychological needs, and multiple roles of adult learners" (Leddy and Pepper, 1998). Although professional organizations adhere to the belief that baccalaureate education is the minimum education for professional nursing, there is an absence of agreement within the ranks of practicing nurses. Furthermore, there are others who promote the idea that the graduate level should be the professional level of entry.

Initial socialization prepares the student for the work setting. Several models have been developed to explain the initial process of socialization into professional roles. The models described here include those of Simpson, Davis, and Hinshaw. Each model outlines a sequential set of phases or "chain of events" beginning at the role of a layperson and ending at the role of a professional. Table 2–2 summarizes each model.

Simpson Model

Ida Harper Simpson (1967) outlines three distinct phases of professional socialization. In the first phase, the person concentrates on becoming proficient in specific work tasks. In the second phase, the person

Table 2–2 Models of Initial Socialization into Professional Roles

Simpson (1967) Model	Hinshaw (1986) Model	Davis (1966) Doctrinal Conversion Model	
Stage 1 Proficiency in specific work tasks	*Phase I* Transition of anticipated role expectations to the role expectations of societal group	*Stage 1* Initial innocence	
		Stage 2 Labeled recognition of incongruity	
Stage 2 Attachment to significant others in the work environment	*Phase II* Attachment to significant others/labeling incongruencies	*Stage 3* "Psyching out" and role simulation	
		Stage 4 Increasing role simulation	
		Stage 5 Provisional internalization	
Stage 3 Internalization of the values of the professional group and adoption of the behaviors it prescribes	*Phase III* Internalization of role values/behaviors	*Stage 6* Stable internalization	

Sources: Adapted from "Patterns of Socialization into Professions: The Case of Student Nurses" by I. H. Simpson, *Sociological Inquiry,* 37, pp. 47–54, Winter 1967, "Socialization and Resocialization of Nurses for Professional Nursing Practice" by A. S. Hinshaw, in E. C. Hein and M. J. Nicholson, Eds., *Contemporary Leadership Behavior: Selected Readings,* 2d ed., Boston: Little, Brown 1986; and "Professional Socialization as Subjective Experiences: The Process of Doctrinal Conversion among Student Nurses" by F. Davis, Evian, France: Sixth World Congress of Sociology, September 1966.

becomes attached to significant others in the work or reference group. In the third and final phase, the person internalizes the values of the professional group and adopts the prescribed behaviors.

Hinshaw Model

Ada Sue Hinshaw (1986) provides a three-phase general model of socialization that is an adaptation of Simpson's model. During the *first* phase, individuals change their images of the role from anticipated concepts to the expectations of the persons who are setting the standards for them. Hinshaw states that (a) adults entering a profession have already learned a number of roles and values that help them to evaluate new roles and (b) these individuals are actively involved in the socialization process, having chosen to learn the new role expectations and enter the socialization process.

The *second* phase has two components: (1) learners attach themselves to significant others in the system, and at the same time (2) they label situations that are incongruent between their anticipated roles and those presented by the significant others. In the initial professional socialization, significant others are usually a group of faculty; in the work setting, they are selected colleagues or immediate supervisors. Hinshaw emphasizes the importance of appropriate role models in both educational programs and work settings. At this stage, individuals are able to verbalize that the expected role behaviors are not what they anticipated. It is a stage that often involves strong emotional reactions to conflicting sets of expectations. Successful resolution of conflicts depends on the existence of role models who demonstrate appropriate behaviors and who show how conflicting systems of standards and values can be integrated.

In the *third* phase, the student internalizes the values and standards of the new role. The degree to which values and standards are internalized and the extent to which incongruencies in role expectations are resolved is variable.

Kelman (1961, 57) defines three levels of value orientation. Individuals may demonstrate one or a blend of three levels:

- *Compliance.* The person demonstrates the expected behavior to get positive reactions from others but has not internalized the values. Compliance behavior can be dismissed when it no longer elicits positive responses.
- *Identification.* The person selectively adopts specific role behaviors that are acceptable to that person. The person may accept only expected behaviors rather than values. Identification behavior usually changes as role models change.

- *Internalization.* The person believes in and accepts the standards of the new role. The standards are a part of the person's own value system.

Davis Model

Fred Davis (1966) describes a six-stage doctrinal conversion process among nursing students.

STAGE 1: INITIAL INNOCENCE When students enter a professional program, they have an image of what they expect to become and how they should act or behave. Nursing students usually enter a nursing program with a service orientation and expect to look after sick people. However, educational experiences often differ from what the students expect. During this phase, students may express disappointment and frustration at the experiences they undergo and may question their value.

STAGE 2: LABELED RECOGNITION OF INCONGRUITY In this phase students begin to identify, articulate, and share their concerns. They learn that they are not alone in their value incongruencies: Peers share the same concerns.

STAGES 3 AND 4: "PSYCHING OUT" AND ROLE SIMULATION At this point, the basic cognitive framework for the internalization of professional nursing values begins to take shape. Students begin to identify the behaviors they are expected to demonstrate and through role modeling begin to practice the behaviors. In Davis's terms, this process becomes a matter of "psyching out" the faculty. The more effectively the role simulation is done, the more authentic the person believes the behavior to be, and it becomes part of the person. However, students may feel they are "playing a game" and are being "untrue to oneself," resulting in feelings of guilt and estrangement.

STAGE 5: PROVISIONAL INTERNALIZATION In stage 5, students vacillate between commitment to their former image of nursing and performance of new behaviors attached to the professional image. Factors that enhance the students' new image are an increasing ability to use professional language and an increasing identification with professional role models, such as nursing faculty.

STAGE 6: STABLE INTERNALIZATION During stage 6, the student's behavior reflects the educationally and professionally approved model. However, preparation of the student for the work setting is only the initial process in socialization. New values and behaviors continue to be formed in the work setting.

Various factors facilitate the socialization process. Absence of these factors interferes with it. See the accompanying box.

Ongoing Professional Socialization and Resocialization

The process of socialization does not terminate with graduation from a program of study. It continues as the graduate begins a professional career and, in fact, continues throughout life. In school, the nursing student assimilates a central core of values emphasized by the faculty and the profession. In the work setting, the nurse faces the need to put the values of the profession into operation. The transition of the graduate to a full-fledged professional is facilitated if there is congruence between the norms, values, and expectations of the educational program and the realities of the work setting. However, practice settings are often bureaucratic and may be nonsupportive of professional career development. Three models of career stages or development—those of Kramer (1974); Dalton, Thompson, and Price (1977); and Benner (1984)—follow.

Kramer's Postgraduate Resocialization Model

Kramer (1974) introduced the concept of *reality shock* to explain discrepancies that arise between the behavioral expectations and values of the educational setting and those of the work setting. Reality shock results when the new graduate is unprepared (ineffectively socialized) to function effectively in the workplace. Kramer describes a four-stage postgraduate resocialization model for the transition of graduates from educational setting to work setting. See the accompanying box.

Dalton's Career Stages Model

Dalton, Thompson, and Price describe a four-stage model that emphasizes the development of competence derived from experience. As the individual's career progresses throughout each stage, activities, relationships, and psychological issues change in focus. For example, the individual's *major activities* progress from healing, learning, and following directions (stage 1) to shaping direction of the organization (stage 4). The *primary relationships* progress from that of an apprentice (stage 1) to that of sponsor (stage 4). The *major psychological issues* progress from a feeling of dependence (stage 1) to a feeling of comfort in exercising power (stage 4). These four stages are summarized in Table 2–3. Only a small percentage of nurses achieve the fourth stage because there are few stage-4 positions available.

Benner's Stages from Novice to Expert

Benner (1984) describes five levels of proficiency in nursing based on the Dreyfus model of skill acquisition derived from a study of chess players and airline pilots (Dreyfus and Dreyfus, 1980). The five stages, which have implications for teaching and learning, are novice, advanced beginner, competent, proficient, and expert.

Kramer's Postgraduate Resocialization Model

STAGE I   SKILL AND ROUTINE MASTERY
The nurse focuses on developing technical expertise and mastering specific skills to overcome feelings of frustration and inadequacy. May not focus on other important aspects of nursing care.

STAGE II   SOCIAL INTEGRATION
The nurse's major concern is having peers recognize the nurse's competence and accept the nurse into the group.

STAGE III   MORAL OUTRAGE
The nurse recognizes incongruities between conceptions of the *bureaucratic* role, which is associated with the rules and regulations and loyalty to agency administration; the *professional* role, which is committed to continued learning and loyalty to the profession; and the *service* role, which is concerned with compassion and loyalty to the client as a person.

STAGE IV   CONFLICT RESOLUTION
The nurse resolves conflicts of stage III by surrendering behaviors and/or values or by learning to use both the values and behaviors of the professional and bureaucratic system in a politically astute manner.

Source: Reality Shock: Why Nurses Leave Nursing, by M. Kramer, St. Louis: Mosby, 1974.

Table 2–3 Dalton, Thompson, and Price Career Stages

Stages	Central Activity	Primary Relationship	Major Psychologic Issue
Stage I	Helping and learning: performs fairly routine duties under the direction of a mentor	Apprentice, subordinate	Dependence
Stage II	Works independently as a competent peer	Colleague	Independence
Stage III	Influences, guides, directs, and helps others to develop	Informal mentor, role model	Assuming responsibility for others
Stage IV	Influences the direction of the organization or a segment of it; has one of three roles: manager, internal entrepreneur, or idea innovator	Sponsor	Exercising power

Sources: Adapted from "The Four Stages of Professional Careers—A New Look at Performance by Professionals" by G. W. Dalton, P. H. Thompson, and R. L. Price, Summer 1977, *Organizational Dynamics*, 19–42.

Benner's Stages of Nursing Expertise

STAGE I   NOVICE
No experience (e.g., nursing student). Performance is limited, inflexible, and governed by context-free rules and regulations rather than experience.

STAGE II   ADVANCED BEGINNER
Demonstrates marginally accepted performance. Recognizes the meaningful "aspects" of a real situation. Has experienced enough real situations to make judgments about them.

STAGE III   COMPETENT PRACTITIONER
Has 2 or 3 years of experience. Demonstrates organizational and planning abilities. Differentiates important factors from less important aspects of care. Coordinates multiple complex care demands.

STAGE IV   PROFICIENT PRACTITIONER
Has 3 to 5 years of experience. Perceives situations as wholes rather than in terms of parts, as in stage II. Uses maxims as guides for what to consider in a situation. Has holistic understanding of the client, which improves decision making. Focuses on long-term goals.

STAGE V   EXPERT PRACTITIONER
Performance is fluid, flexible, and highly proficient; no longer requires rules, guidelines, or maxims to connect an understanding of the situation to appropriate action. Demonstrates highly skilled intuitive and analytic ability in new situations. Is inclined to take a certain action because "it felt right."

Source: From Novice to Expert: Excellence and Power in Clinical Nursing Practice, by P. Benner, Menlo Park, Calif.: Addison-Wesley Nursing, 1984, pp. 21–34. Reprinted with permission.

Benner believes that experience is essential for the development of professional expertise. See the box on page 19.

Consider . . .

- Benner's stages from novice to expert. Where are you on Benner's continuum in relation to your current area of practice? During your nursing career, what have you experienced as you have moved along Benner's continuum? How might you assist a novice nurse to progress successfully to higher levels of practice?

- issues influencing the socialization process of RNs who return to school for baccalaureate education in nursing. What factors influenced your own decision to return to school?

ROLE THEORY

Professional socialization has been based upon role theory, which emerged from the field of sociology. It involves preparation for particular job expectations or roles. A **role** is a set of expectations associated with a position in society. In order to understand socialization to a professional role, it is necessary to have an understanding of role theory. What is it that defines a role and how does one make a transition into that role?

Elements of Roles

Any role has three elements: the ideal role, the perceived role, and the performed role.

The *ideal role* refers to the socially prescribed or agreed-upon rights and responsibilities associated with the role. Persons who assume a certain role are provided with sets of expectations and obligations or norms that can be identified and used as criteria to judge the adequacy of performance in the role. The

Bookshelf

Nicolson, P. 1996. *Gender, power, and organization: A psychological perspective.* **Westport, Conn: Routledge.**
This book looks at the professional socialization of women to the business world.
Goodman-Draper, J. 1995. *Health care's forgotten majority: Nurses and their frayed white collars.* **New York: Greenwood Publishing.**
This book is a class analysis of nurses within the white-collar workforce.

ideal role concept provides a relatively stable view of roles and role requirements, because the society at large is assumed to have the same or similar expectations about the pattern of behaviors that a person in a particular role should carry out. Although changes may occur in the prescribed rights and responsibilities associated with the ideal role, this ideal role tends to support a static view of role behaviors.

Role expectations are the norms specific to a position that identify the attitudes, cognitions, and behaviors required and anticipated of a person in a particular role. Ideal role expectations may also be determined by culture and education.

The *perceived role* refers to how a role incumbent (a person who assumes the role) believes he or she should behave in the role. A role incumbent's perceptions of the expected patterns of behavior may differ from the conventional ideal role expectations: Not every person may accept all the norms about a role or perceive them in the same way.

The *performed role* refers to what the role incumbent actually does. **Role performance** is defined as the behaviors of or actions taken by a person in relation to the expected behaviors of a particular position. **Role mastery** is the term used to indicate that a person demonstrates behaviors that meet the societal or cultural expectations associated with the specific role.

The person's perceptions and beliefs about what ought to be done is not the only factor influencing role performance. Other factors include health status, personal and professional values, needs of the client and support persons, and politics of the employing agency. A healthy nurse, for example, may provide care associated with prescribed and perceived roles more effectively than an unhealthy nurse. A nurse who values the client's right to participate in care planning will elicit the client's thoughts and feelings before planning care. A nurse who must work in a situation in which several of the staff are absent may be required to defer basic aspects of care (e.g., bath, changing bed linen) for some clients in order to meet more critical needs of other clients.

Role transition is a process by which a person assumes or develops a new role. There are two components associated with role behaviors: norms and values. Norms are the general expectations that support the behaviors, and values justify the behaviors and help the nurse conform to the norms (Strader and Decker 1995). In the new role, the person moves to a new set of responsibilities and, often, to new values as well. Role transition is influenced by many factors, such as the individual, interpersonal factors, and organizational factors. A model of role transition is shown in Figure 2–1.

Figure 2–1

Role Transition

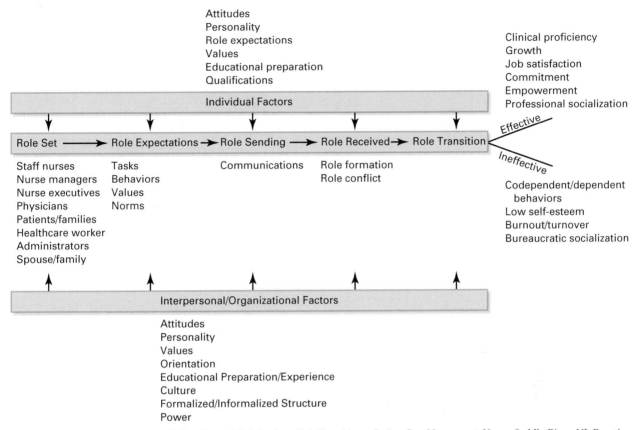

Source: Used by permission from M. K. Strader and P. J. Decker, *Role Transition to Patient Care Management,* Upper Saddle River, NJ: Prentice-Hall. 1995, p. 60.

According to this model, the process begins by determining the **role set,** composed of individuals involved who hold beliefs and attitudes about what should or should not be done in that role, or **role expectations. Role sending** involves the members of the role set communicating role expectations, and it is at this step that problems may develop. After the role is sent, the next phase is **role received,** but what is sent may not be received without misunderstanding or distortion. Role formation is affected by such factors as personality, attitudes, qualifications, educational preparation, and clarity of communication. Role conflict may develop when role expectations of the various people involved are incompatible. The actual **role transition** occurs as the nurse learns role behaviors based upon the role received, resulting in two possible outcomes: effective or ineffective. Effective role transitions have associated behaviors within the norms; these can lead to clinical proficiency, personal growth, job satisfaction, organizational commitment, empowerment, and professional socialization. When

there is a great deal of role conflict, ineffective role transition is likely to be the outcome, resulting in low self-esteem, a low level of confidence, and burnout.

Transition shock or reality shock may happen when the perceived role comes into conflict with the performed role. Many new graduates experience this as cognitive dissonance; that is, they know what they *should* do and how they *should* do it, but circumstances do not allow them to perform the role in that way. The result of this is increased anxiety, which, if not resolved, can result in burnout. Preceptorships, internships, and externships are approaches often found to be helpful in a successful role transition.

Consider . . .

■ the multiple roles you assume and the satisfactions you experience in relation to each. How does your role as a nurse relate to your other roles? In what ways does your choice of nursing as a career enhance or interfere with your other life roles?

■ your perceived roles of the nurse. What is the basis for your beliefs about the nursing role?

Boundaries for Nursing Roles

Five determinants currently form the boundaries for nursing roles:

1. Theoretical and conceptual frameworks identify the concepts of nursing and specify the relationships among them. Conceptual frameworks provide the nurse with an understanding of the recipient of nursing care, what constitutes health and environment, and how these influence nursing goals and actions. (See Chapter 6, "Theoretical Foundations of Professional Nursing.")

2. The *nursing process,* or standard scientific problem-solving method that nurses use in the clinical setting. The nursing process determines nursing actions appropriate for each client. The nursing process consists of five components: assessing, diagnosing, planning, implementing, and evaluating.

3. Standards of nursing practice established by the nursing profession. Standards of practice outline nursing functions and the level of excellence required of the nurse. These standards also define the nurse's ethical and legal obligations to clients and their support persons, to employers, and to society.

4. Nurse practice acts or nursing licensure laws of the specific jurisdiction that legally define the scope of nursing practice. Although nurse practice acts differ in various jurisdictions, they all have a common purpose: to protect the public (see Chapter 5, "Legal Foundations of Professional Nursing").

5. National and international codes of ethics for nurses are fundamental to the practice of nursing. Codes of ethics describe the nurse's relationships to clients, support persons, colleagues, employers, and society (see Chapter 4, "Values, Ethics, and Advocacy").

Consider . . .

■ how nursing models, the nursing process, standards of nursing practice, nurse practice acts, and nursing codes of ethics delineate the roles of nursing.

ROLE STRESS AND ROLE STRAIN

Role stress is probably more prevalent now than ever before because of prevailing social conditions, such as inadequate adult socialization, rapid organizational change, and accelerated technology (Hardy and Hardy, 1988, p. 170). **Role stress** occurs when role obligations are unrealistic, vague, conflicting, or irritating. It is generated by the social structure or system; the source is primarily external to the person. Role stress may create **role strain,** an emotional reaction accompanied by psychologic responses, such as anxiety, tension, irritation, resentment, and depression; physiologic responses, such as diaphoresis, increased heart rate, increased blood pressure, increased rate and depth of respirations, and increased muscle tension; and social responses, such as withdrawal from interaction, job dissatisfaction, and reduced involvement with colleagues and organizations (Hardy and Hardy 1988, 190). Common role stress problems and descriptions are shown in the accompanying box.

Role ambiguity is a characteristic of all positions occupied by professionals who often deal with uncer-

Role Stress Problems

ROLE AMBIGUITY
Unclear role expectations.

ROLE CONFLICT
Incompatible, competing role expectations within a single role or multiple roles.

ROLE INCONGRUITY
Values are incompatible with role expectations.

ROLE OVERLOAD OR UNDERLOAD
Too much is expected in the time available, or the role is too complex (overload); minimal role expectations that do not use the abilities of the role incumbent (underload).

ROLE OVERQUALIFICATION OR UNDERQUALIFICATION
Nurse's abilities and motivation exceed those required (overqualification); nurse lacks necessary resources (underqualification).

tainty, the unexpected, and unpredictable activities and behavior (Hardy and Hardy, 1988, p. 201). Nurses in particular often experience role ambiguity because of the diversity of their role partners and multiple subroles of the nursing role. (In contrast, a technician's role expectations are explicit, and work can often be routinized.) Ambiguity can significantly affect a person's role performance, satisfaction, and commitment.

Role conflict is a widely discussed concept in current literature. The primary consequence of role conflict is role stress. If unreconciled, role stress and role strain lead to *burnout,* a syndrome of mental and physical exhaustion involving negative self-concept, negative job attitude, and loss of concern for clients.

Shead (1991, 737) discusses four major causes of role conflict for nurses. A widely discussed causative factor is professional-bureaucratic work conflict. Nurses who are prepared to provide independent practice and use professional judgment experience conflict in bureaucracies that are more concerned about getting routine tasks completed. The organization's reward systems may contribute to conflict between nurses, who identify with their profession, and supervisors, who identify with the organization. Disproportionate power also creates stress. Increased professionalism often means increased conflict and stress, unless the bureaucratic structure is flexible enough to deal with the professional modality.

A second cause of role conflict arises from different views concerning what nursing is and should be. Role value orientations vary considerably among practitioners; some nurses have a more traditional view of the nurse's role than new managers or new professionals have. The role of the professional nurse continues to change; nurses are becoming increasingly involved in planning and organizing health care activities and are becoming more responsible for delivering total client care services. The nurse's role is becoming one of managing client care activities in general. In this new role, nurses have greater responsibility and accountability and may experience increased stress as a result.

A third cause of conflict is a discrepancy between the nursing and medical view of what the nurse's role should be. Physicians may view the caring ideology of nurses as secondary in importance to their own, idealize curing aspects of care, and view the nurse as a handmaiden. Nurses use behavioral science and communication skills to develop their professional relationship with clients; physicians have traditionally employed a clinical, biologic approach. This variance can create role strain if (1) the physician expects the nurse to handle the client as the physician does and (2) the physician does not listen to the nurse's concerns and suggestions about the client.

A fourth source of conflict arises from the public image of nursing. Personal expectations and self-image may conflict with perceived public expectations. The public may regard the ideal nurse as a dedicated angel of mercy, whereas the media often malign the image by portraying the nurse as a sex symbol or other negative stereotype.

Consider . . .

■ role conflicts in your professional experience. What are the sources of your role conflicts? Are there role conflicts that are unique to your practice setting? Do other nursing colleagues experience the same role conflicts? What attitudes or behaviors do you or your colleagues manifest as a result of role conflicts? How do these attitudes or behaviors affect client care?

Enhancing Professional Self-Concept and Role Image

Nurses who seek to maintain or improve both their personal and professional selves are more effective in caring for their clients. They are also more effective in communicating with other health professionals and in promoting a positive image of nursing in the community. Strasen (1992, 2) defines *professional self-concept* as the set of beliefs and images held to be true as a result of specific professional socialization. The development of professional self-concept is based on one's personal self-concept. An individual's personal self-concept and professional self-concept affect one another. The characteristics of a person who has a positive self-concept include the following (Strader and Decker, 1995, p. 88):

■ Future orientation; ability to minimize past failures
■ Ability to cope with life's problems and disappointments
■ Ability to help and accept help from others
■ Ability to see and value the uniqueness of all individuals
■ Ability to feel all aspects of emotion but not allow the feelings to affect behavior negatively or affect interactions with people who are not responsible for the situation

Because a person's subconscious mind acts positively or negatively on the information it receives, nurses can change their self-concepts by controlling what goes into the subconscious mind. Nurses who perceive themselves as successful will use their energy and creativity to explore ways to become even more successful. Positive thoughts help them to succeed.

To develop a positive self-concept, Strader and Decker (1995, 88–89) suggest the following steps:

■ Accept your present self but have a better self in mind.
■ Set goals that are high but attainable.
■ Develop expertise in some area to increase your value to yourself and to your employing agency. This may involve continuing education or obtaining certification in a specialized area of practice.

Managing Role Stress and Role Strain

Prevention of burnout in professional nursing can be approached by stress reduction. There are a number of approaches that can be applied, but common threads among them are personal goal setting, problem identification, and problem-solving strategies. Personal goals should include both long-term and short-term goals. Being goal-directed reduces the erratic activity that frequently keeps the person busy and working hard without accomplishing much and leading to frustration. These goals can be applied to personal life choices as well as professional career development. An important step in implementing a plan to pursue goals is identification of the problems that produce stress. Correctly identifying a problem allows the development of a plan that will appropriately and positively provide a solution. Problem solving is applied to the development of solutions that will result in stress reduction.

Table 2–4 Summary of Interventions for Professional Survival

Personal Self-Care	Professional Self-Care
Boundary Work	**Managing Negative Patient Behavior**
1. Self-awareness: pay attention to your own thoughts, feelings, and the effect of your behavior on others.	1. Recall that all behavior is the best adaptation that the person can make at the time.
2. Self-reflection: examine your own reactions to specific patients and what created that reaction.	2. Recall that behavior can be changed.
3. Accept feedback: develop a support system that will provide honest feedback you can trust.	3. Attempt to understand what needs and feelings are creating the behavior.
	4. Start all interactions with respect and empathy.
	5. Learn how to set limits on negative behaviors.
Goal Setting	**Conflict Resolution**
1. Let go of perfectionism.	1. Learn how to respond rather than react.
2. Formulate realistic outcome measures.	2. Seek win-win solutions.
3. Seek opportunities to exercise excellence.	3. Base peer relationships on integrity.
Stress Management	**Taking Professional Inventory**
1. Sustain a healthy diet.	1. What is working?
2. Maintain an exercise routine.	2. What is frustrating or unsatisfying?
3. Engage in positive self-talk.	3. What milestones have been attained?
4. Use affirmations.	4. What losses have been accrued?
5. Practice mindfulness.	5. In what areas are you feeling most competent?
6. Maintain adequate sleep and rest.	6. Do you have personal and professional balance?
7. Avoid toxins.	7. Are you feeling financially and physically secure?
8. Use humor.	**Sustaining Values and Vision**
9. Sustain a spiritual practice.	1. Speak the truth.
	2. Sustain an awareness of those behaviors that sap your energy and those that enhance your energy.
	3. Clarify personal and professional values.
	4. Compare your values with the mission statement of your agency/facility.
	Influencing Healthcare Policy
	1. Remain informed regarding public health policy changes.
	2. Join a professional organization.
	3. Support positive nursing standards at work and in the community.

Source: Used by permission of B. Cherry and S. R. Jacob, *Contemporary Nursing: Issues, Trends, and Management,* St. Louis: Mosby, 1999.

Time-management skills can be a valuable tool in stress reduction and may result in improvement in the nurse's personal life as well as in the practice setting. Assuming multiple roles creates heavy demands on time and multitasking tends to fragment attention and concentration. Delegation is one tool the nurse can use in time management. Overcoming procrastination is another time-management strategy. Simply starting a task is one of the best ways to overcome procrastination. Once begun, a task is usually completed. Prioritization may be needed when the number or scope of tasks seems insurmountable.

Taking care of one's self is important in stress management. Nurses must care for themselves before they can care for others effectively. Decompression is an important component, and the nurse can reduce tension by taking time for those things that meet personal needs and are pleasurable and restorative. Nursing support groups are also helpful. Using these techniques prevents stress and keeps problems from becoming overwhelming.

A summary of interventions for survival in the nursing profession is shown in Table 2–4. These include measures to set personal and professional boundaries and manage stress. The table is divided into activities for personal self-care and activities for professional self-care.

Consider . . .

- your own strategies for dealing with role stress. Which strategies have been effective? Which have not?

- how your practice setting supports nurses dealing with role stress. What resources are needed for the institution to provide a work environment that minimizes role stress and strain?

- three personal and three professional goals that you have. Develop a plan for achieving these goals and consider how the personal and professional goals might enhance one another.

Research Box

Wildman, S., Weale, A., Rodney, C., and Pritchard, J. 1999. The impact of higher education for post-registration nurses on their subsequent clinical practice: An exploration of students' views. *Journal of Advanced Nursing* 29(1): 246–253.

This study reports the results of a survey sent to nurses in the UK who completed postregistration education. The questionnaire was sent to 169 nurses who had successfully completed the course. A response rate of 66.8% resulted in a sample size of 113. These nurses reported themselves to be more questioning, to be more able to apply research findings, and to have a wider knowledge for practice following completion of the course. The author concludes that continuing professional education for nurses has a positive impact on clinical practice.

SUMMARY

Nurses must understand the roles they and others play and societal expectations associated with those roles. Any role consists of three elements: the ideal role, the perceived role, and the performed role. Role performance is influenced by such factors as health status, values, and situational pressures. Five determinants form boundaries for nursing roles: conceptual frameworks, the nursing process, standards of practice, nurse practice acts, and a code of ethics.

Socialization is a lifelong process by which people become functioning participants of a society or a group. It is a reciprocal learning process that is brought about by interaction with other people and establishes boundaries of behavior. Socialization to professional nursing practice is the process whereby the values and norms of the nursing profession are internalized into the nurse's own behavior and self-concept.

The nurse acquires the knowledge, skills, and attitudes characteristic of the profession.

Socialization for professional nursing requires the development of critical values, including a strong commitment to the service that nursing provides to the public, a belief in the dignity and worth of each person, a commitment to education, and autonomy.

Socialization into professional nursing has been challenging because of the different educational routes available. Controversy exists as to the appropriate level of entry into professional nursing, although professional organizations have stated that it is at the baccalaureate level.

Various models of the socialization process have been developed. Such models may serve as guidelines to establish the phase and extent of an individual's socialization.

Nurses are prone to role stress and strain for a variety of reasons unique to their role in the health care and social systems. Common problems are role conflict, role ambiguity, role overload, and role incongruity. Strategies to handle role stress differ from strategies to manage role strain. Nurses can positively influence their self-concepts and role images to improve work satisfaction and provide quality care.

SELECTED REFERENCES

American Nurses Association (ANA). 1998. *Standards of clinical nursing practice*. Kansas City, Mo.: ANA.

Benner, P. 1984. *From novice to expert: Excellence and power in clinical nursing practice*. Menlo Park, Calif.: Addison-Wesley Nursing.

Benner, P., and Wrubel, J. 1989. *The primary of caring: Stress and coping in health and illness*. Menlo Park, Calif.: Addison-Wesley Nursing.

Callinicos, A. 1999. *Social theory: A historical introduction*. New York: New York University Press.

Catalano, J. T. 2000. *Nursing now! Today's issues, tomorrow's trends*, 2d ed. Philadelphia: F.A. Davis.

Cherry, B., and Jacob, S. R. 1999. *Contemporary nursing: Issues, trends and management*. St. Louis: Mosby.

Dalton, G. W., Thompson, P. H., and Price, R. L. 1977, Summer. The four stages of professional careers—A new look at performance by professionals. *Organizational Dynamics*, 19–42.

Davis, F. 1966, September. Professional socialization as subjective experiences: The process of doctrinal conversion among student nurses. Paper. Evian, France: *Sixth World Congress of Sociology*.

DeYoung, L. 1985. *Dynamics of nursing*, 5th ed. St. Louis: Mosby.

Donaldson, S. K., and Crowley, D. M. 1978. The discipline of nursing. *Nursing Outlook*: 113–120.

Ellis, J. R., and Hartley, C. L. 2001. *Nursing in today's world: Challenges, issues, and trends*, 7th ed. Philadelphia: Lippincott.

Greenwood, E. 1957. Attributes of a profession. *Social Work* **2**(3): 45–55.

Hardy, M. E., and Conway, M. E. 1988. *Role theory: Perspectives for healthy professionals*, 2nd ed. Norwalk, Conn.: Appleton and Lange.

Hardy, M. E., and Hardy, W. L. 1988. Role stress and strain. In *Role theory: Perspectives for health professionals*, 2nd ed., pp. 159–239, edited by M. E. Hardy and M. E. Conway. Norwalk, Conn.: Appleton and Lange.

Hinshaw, A. S. 1977, November. *Socialization and resocialization of nurses for professional nursing practice*. National League for Nursing Pub. No. 15-1659. New York: National League for Nursing.

Hinshaw, A. S. 1986. Socialization and resocialization of nurses for professional nursing practice. In *Contemporary leadership behavior: Selected readings*, 2nd ed., edited by E. C. Hein and Nicholson, M. J. Boston: Little, Brown.

Kelman, H. 1961. Process of opinion changes. *Public Opinion Quarterly* **25**(1): 57.

Kramer, M. 1974. *Reality shock: Why nurses leave nursing*. St. Louis: Mosby.

Leddy, S., and Pepper, J. M. 1998. *Conceptual bases of professional nursing*, 4th ed. Philadelphia: Lippincott.

Lemert, C. C. 1997. *Social things: An introduction to the sociological life*. Lanham, Md.: Rowman and Littlefield.

Lindberg, J. B., Hunter, M. L., and Druszewski, A. Z. 1998. *Introduction to nursing: Concepts, issues, and opportunities*. Philadelphia: Lippincott-Raven.

Musolf, G. R. 1998. *Structure and agency in everyday life: An introduction to social psychology*. Dix Hills, N.Y.: General Hall.

Nunnery, R. K. 1997. *Advancing your career: Concepts of professional nursing*. Philadelphia: F.A. Davis.

Parsons, T. 1977. *Action theory and the human condition*. New York: Free Press.

Phaneuf, M. C., and Lang, M. 1985. *Issues in professional nursing practice 7: Standards of nursing practice*. Washington, D.C.: ANA.

Rafferty, A. M. 1996. *The politics of nursing knowledge*. New York: Routledge.

Redman, B. K. 1997. *The process of patient education*, 8th ed. St. Louis: Mosby.

Shead, H. 1991, June. Role conflict in student nurses: Towards a positive approach for the 1990s. *Journal of Advanced Nursing* **16,** 736–740.

Simpson, I. H. 1967, Winter. Patterns of socialization into professions: The case of student nurses. *Sociological Inquiry* **37**: 47–54.

Simpson, I. H. 1979. *From student to nurse: A longitudinal study of socialization*. New York: Cambridge University Press.

Strader, M. K., and Decker, P. J. 1995. *Role transition to patient care management.* Norwalk, Conn.: Appleton and Lange.

Strasen, L. L. 1992. *The image of professional nursing: Strategies for action.* Philadelphia: Lippincott.

Tappen, R. 2001. *Nursing leadership and management: Concepts and practice,* 4th ed. Philadelphia: F. A. Davis.

Watson, I. 1981, Summer. Socialization of the nursing student in a professional nursing education program. *Nursing Papers* **13:** 19–24.

Watson, J. (1979). *Nursing—The philosophy and science of caring.* Boston: Little, Brown.

Watt, E. 1997. An exploration of the way in which the concept of patient advacacy is perceived by registered nurses working in an acute care hospital. *International Journal of Nursing Practice* **3**(2):119–127.

Weedman, J. 1998. Burglar's tools: The use of collaborative technology in professional socialization. Paper presented at meeting of American Society for Information Science, May 17–20, 1998, Orlando, Fla.

CHAPTER 3

Historical Foundations of Professional Nursing

Objectives

■ Discuss the historical development of nursing from ancient times to the present.

■ Discuss the role of religion in the development of nursing.

■ Describe the contributions of selected nurses to nursing and society.

■ Analyze the contributions of selected nurses and the nursing profession to society from a historical perspective.

■ Discuss the development of professional nursing organizations and their role in advocating for nurses and health care.

N U R S E   C O N N E C T

Additional online resources for this chapter can be found on the companion web site at www.prenhall.com/blais.

One of the irrefutable laws of nature is dynamism, or change. Individual and group elements of society respond and adapt to historical events that may alter the behaviors, values, laws, beliefs, and even the daily living habits of society. Influencing events may be related to natural disasters, such as floods, earthquakes, famine, or epidemic disease, or they may be invented by people, such as the discovery of fire, the wheel, the printing press, the microscope, and penicillin. War, political upheaval, religious intolerance, and economic instability are systemic events that can alter individuals' lives and group progress.

As a subgroup of society, nursing must also respond and adapt to the influences of society. Nursing has been a continuous thread linking the past with the present—from the tribal groups of early societies to modern societies linked by jet-powered transportation and instant telecommunications. Just as human history has shown tremendous progress over the centuries, so has nursing evolved from the art of comforting, caring for, and nurturing the sick to a synthesis of this art with the science and technology of contemporary thinking.

CHALLENGES AND OPPORTUNITIES

Studying the history of nursing can lead to an appreciation of the development of the discipline and profession that challenges nurses to honor the leaders and carry forward the best of the values and traditions. The perspective provided by knowing the roots of nursing can contribute to professional identity. Although nursing is facing a time of change and challenge, the depth and breadth of nursing's historical foundations provide a broad base of experience to draw on as the profession evolves. One challenge is to continue the leadership within the profession in furthering the traditional values by understanding where nursing has been and how it got there as well as where it needs to go in the future. It is important to convey to new nurses a knowledge and value of the past. In a profession that can be intensely involved in immediate decision making, knowing the past may seem to be of low priority.

Knowing the past and understanding the roles of early nursing leaders provides an opportunity to use the experience and lessons learned to create the future. The mistakes and successes of the past provide examples and can help guide decisions of today. Appreciation of what has been contributed by the pioneers of nursing and the social influences of the past provides the opportunity to celebrate the accomplishments, take pride in what has been done, and carry the best of the past into the future.

NURSING IN PRIMITIVE SOCIETIES

It is impossible to describe nursing practice or the role of the nurse prior to recorded history. It is also difficult to differentiate between the role of the physician and that of the nurse or even to determine if there were two distinctly different roles. It is likely that any differentiation that existed was based on male-female role proscriptions, such as medicine man or herb woman. It may be postulated that individuals provided care or cure based on experience and oral transmission of available knowledge about health and illness. Traditional female roles of wife, mother, daughter, and sister always included the care and nurturing of other family members. The term *nurse* derives from the care mothers gave to their helpless infant children. Donahue (1996, p. 2) suggests that the very survival of the human race is evidence of the existence of nursing throughout history and is "inextricably intertwined with the development of nursing."

NURSING IN ANCIENT CIVILIZATIONS

In the early recordings of ancient civilizations, there is little information about those who cared for the sick. It is known that midwives provided care for the mother and infant during birthing and that wet nurses often suckled and cared for infant children of wealthy families. Often these roles were filled by female slaves. This fact contributes to the lack of recorded information about nursing, because slaves had no status and as such their work was not worthy of documentation. The slave-nurse depended on the master, healer, or priest for instruction or direction in the care of her charge. Often the care provided for the sick was related to physical maintenance and comfort.

During this time, beliefs about the cause of disease were imbedded in superstition and magic, so treatment often required magical cures. The priest or witch doctor enjoyed great status in ancient societies. But as these societies evolved, practical theories of medical care emerged as nonmagical causes of disease were observed. The earliest recording of healing practices is a 4000-year-old clay tablet attributed to the Sumerian civilization. It contains healing prescriptions but, unfortunately, neglects to describe the illnesses for which they were prescribed.

The earliest documentation of law governing the practice of medicine is the Code of Hammurabi, attributed to the Babylonians and dating to 1900 B.C. The code recorded regulations related to sanitation and public health, the practice of surgery, the differentiation between the practice of human and veterinary medicine, a table of fees for operations, and penalties for violators of the code. There is no specific record of nursing in the Babylonian civilization; however, there are references to tasks and practices traditionally provided by nurses. Medical illustrations from that period often include a nurselike figure providing patient support or comfort.

Important historic findings related to the Egyptian culture include the Ebers papyrus and the practice of mummification. The Ebers papyrus, which dates to approximately 1550 B.C., is believed to be the oldest medical text in the world. It describes many diseases known today and identifies specific symptomatology. It also lists more than 700 substances that were used as drugs and describes their preparation and medicinal use.

Mummification, or embalming, derived from the belief in life after death. The development of effective solutions to preserve the body from decay and the subsequent ability for modern-day anthropologists to examine the mummified body indicate a high level of knowledge of human anatomy, physiology, and pathophysiology.

The ancient Hebrew culture contributed the Mosaic Health Code to the history of health care. This code is considered the first sanitary legislation and contains the first record of public health requirements. The code, which covered every aspect of individual, family, and community health, differentiated between *clean* and *unclean*. Principles of personal health related to rest, sleep, and cleanliness were also provided. There were rules for women related to menstruation and childbearing. Dietary laws were a significant part of the Mosaic Code and provided for the "kosher" slaughter of animals as well as preparation and preservation of animal and plant foods.

The use of quarantine as a prevention against the transmission of communicable diseases, such as leprosy and diphtheria, is recorded in the Bible. Nurses are mentioned occasionally in the Old Testament as women who provided care for infants, children, the sick, and the dying and as midwives who assisted during pregnancy and at delivery.

In ancient African cultures, the nurturing functions of the nurse included roles as midwives, herbalists, wet nurses, and caregivers for children and the elderly (Dolan, Fitzpatrick, and Herrmann, 1983, p. 19). In ancient India, early hospitals were staffed by male nurses who were required to meet four qualifications: (1) "knowledge of the manner in which drugs should be prepared for administration, (2) cleverness, (3) devotedness to the patient, and (4) purity of mind and body" (Donahue 1996, 47). Indian women served as

midwives and nursed ill family members. There is no mention of the nurse role in ancient China; however, the contribution of ancient China to health care knowledge includes the effects of some 365 herbal remedies in the Pen Tsao (ca. 2700 B.C.), the use of acupuncture as a treatment method, and the publication of the Nei Ching (Canon of Medicine), which detailed the four steps of examination: look, listen, ask, and feel.

In the histories of ancient Greece and Rome, care of the sick and injured was advanced in mythology and reality. The Greek mythic God Asklepios was the chief healer; his wife, Epigone, was the soother, Hygeia, the daughter of Asklepios, was the goddess of health and was revered by some as the embodiment of the nurse. Temples built to honor Asklepios became centers of healing, and the priests of Asklepios provided healing through natural and supernatural remedies (Donahue, 1996, p. 54). The ancient Greek physician Hippocrates is honored today as the father of medicine. He believed that disease had a natural cause, in contrast to the magical and mystical causes pronounced by the priest healers of the temples.

After they conquered Greece in 200 B.C., the Romans borrowed gods from the Greeks, including Aesculapius (Asklepios) and Hygeia. Greek physician-slaves brought medical practices to the Roman empire. The Romans' contribution to health care was in public sanitation, the draining of marshes, and the building of aqueducts, public and private baths, drainage systems, and central heating.

THE ROLE OF RELIGION IN THE DEVELOPMENT OF NURSING

Many of the world's religions encourage benevolence, but it was the Christian value of "love thy neighbor as thyself" that impacted significantly on the development of Western nursing. The principle of caring was established with Christ's parable of the Good Samaritan providing care for a tired and injured stranger. Converts to Christianity during the third and fourth centuries included several wealthy women of the Roman Empire. See the box on page 32.

Women were not the sole providers of nursing services; in the third century in Rome there was an organization of men called the Parabolani brotherhood. This group of men provided care to the sick and dying during the great plague in Alexandria. During the Crusades, knighthood orders, such as the Knights Hospitallers of St. John of Jerusalem, the Teutonic Knights, and the Knights of Lazarus, often comprised brothers in arms who provided nursing care to their sick and in-

Dedicated Women of the Roman Empire

- Marcella converted her palace into a monastery and encouraged other Roman matrons to join her in caring for the sick poor. She is considered by some to be the first nurse educator, because she taught her followers how to care for the sick. She was also literate in Latin, Greek, and Hebrew and encouraged the education of women.

- Fabiola, a follower of Marcella, also contributed her great wealth to the care of the poor and sick. She is credited with establishing the first public hospital in Rome in A.D. 390. She is said to have personally nursed patients whose wounds and sores were ugly and repugnant. She was considered the patron saint of nursing.

- Paula was a wealthy and learned friend of Fabiola. Upon the death of her husband, she converted to Christianity. She, too, studied with Marcella. In A.D. 385 she moved with her daughter to Palestine, where she built hospitals for the sick and hospices for the pilgrims who followed the road to Bethlehem. She also provided direct care to the sick.

jured comrades. These orders were responsible for building great hospitals, the organization and management of which set a standard for the administration of hospitals throughout Europe at that time.

As the Christian church grew, more hospitals were built, as were specialized institutions providing care for orphans, widows, the elderly, the poor, and the sick. It is unfortunate that the religious beliefs of the church were in conflict with scientific thought and education during this period. The church encouraged care and comfort of the sick and poor but did not allow for the advancement of knowledge in preventing illness or curing disease. This attitude pervaded the period known as the Dark Ages, which endured for approximately 500 years.

During the Middle Ages (A.D. 500–1500), male and female religious, military, and secular orders with the primary purpose of caring for the sick were formed. Conspicuous among them were the Knights Hospitalers of St. John; The Alexian Brotherhood (organized in 1431); and the Augustinian sisters, which was the first purely nursing order.

In 1633, the Sisters of Charity were founded by St Vincent de Paul in France. It was the first of many such orders organized under various Roman Catholic Church auspices and largely devoted to caring for the sick.

The deaconess groups, which had their origins in the Roman Empire of the third and fourth centuries under Marcella, Fabiola, and Paula, were suppressed during the Middle Ages by the Western churches. However, these groups of nursing providers reoccurred occasionally throughout the centuries, most notably in 1836 when Theodor Fliedner reinstituted the Order of Deaconesses and opened a small hospital and training school in Kaiserswerth, Germany. Florence Nightingale received her "training" in nursing at the Kaiserswerth School.

THE DEVELOPMENT OF MODERN NURSING

In the eighteenth and nineteenth centuries, the world underwent a renaissance. The discoveries of Copernicus, Galileo, Newton, Kepler, Briggs, and Descartes precipitated an intellectual revolution. Vesalius, Harvey, Hooke, and van Leeuwenhoek contributed to the scientific revolution in medicine. With the discovery and exploration of new continents, an economic revolution evolved, after which nations became more interdependent through trade and mercantilism. The Industrial Revolution displaced workers from cottage craftspeople to factory laborers. With these changes came stressors to health. New illnesses, transmitted in the holds of ships by sailors and stowaway rodents, jumped national boundaries and continents. The closeness of factory work, the long hours, and the unhealthy working conditions led to the rapid transmission of communicable diseases such as cholera and plague. Lack of prenatal care, inadequate nutrition, and poor delivery techniques resulted in a high rate of maternal and infant mortality. Orphaned children died in workhouses of neglect or cruelty. These conditions have been effectively portrayed in the writings of Dickens, including *Oliver Twist* and *David Copperfield*.

A "proper" woman's role in life was to maintain a gracious and elegant home for her family. A common woman worked as a servant in a private home or was dependent on her husband's wages. The provision of care for the sick in hospitals or private homes fell to the uncommon women, often prisoners or prostitutes who had little or no training in nursing and even less enthusiasm for the job. Because of this, nursing had little acceptance and no prestige. The only acceptable nursing role was within a religious order, wherein services were provided to the hospital for little or no cost.

The development of the Deaconess Institute at Kaiserswerth, Germany changed all this. Associated with a religious organization, the Order of Deaconesses ignited recognition of the need for the services of women in the care of the sick, the poor, children, and female prisoners. The training school for nurses at Kaiserswerth included care of the sick in hospitals, instruction in visiting nursing, instruction in religious doctrine and ethics, and pharmacy. The deaconess movement eventually spread to four continents, including North America, North Africa, Asia, and Australia.

Florence Nightingale, the most famous Kaiserswerth pupil, was born to a wealthy and intellectual family. Her education included the mastery of several ancient and modern languages, literature, philosophy, history, science, mathematics, religion, art, and music. It was expected that she would follow the usual path of a wealthy and intelligent woman of the day: marry, bear children, and maintain an elegant home. She was determined, however, to become a nurse in order to diminish the suffering of the helpless. As a well-traveled young woman of the day, in 1847 she arranged to visit Kaiserswerth, where she received 3 months' training in nursing. In 1853 she studied in Paris with the Sisters of Charity, after which she returned to England to assume the position of superintendent of a charity hospital for ill governesses.

During the Crimean War, there was public outcry about the inadequacy of care for the soldiers. The death rate, estimated at 43%, was attributed to wounds, infection, cholera, inadequate nutrition, lack of drugs, and lack of care. Florence Nightingale was asked by Sir Sidney Herbert of the War Department to recruit a contingent of female nurses to provide care to the sick and injured in the Crimea. In spite of opposition from the Army medical officers, she and her nurses transformed the environment by setting up diet kitchens, a laundry, recreation centers, and reading rooms and organizing classes. She trained the orderlies to scrub the wards and empty wastes. In the course of 6 months, the mortality rate decreased to 2% (Donahue, 1996, p. 204).

When she returned to England, Nightingale was given an honorarium of £4500 by a grateful English public. She later used this money to develop the Nightingale Training School for Nurses, which opened in 1860. The school served as a model for other training schools. Its graduates traveled to other countries to manage hospitals and institute nurse-training programs. The efforts of Florence Nightingale and her nurses changed the status of nursing to a respectable occupation for women.

THE DEVELOPMENT OF NURSING IN THE AMERICAS

Between the American Revolution and the Civil War nursing in America probably paralleled nursing in Europe. Early public hospitals developed in the colonies included The Philadelphia Almshouse (1731) and Bellevue Hospital in New York (1658). These early "hospitals" provided care for the sick, indigent, insane, infirm, prisoners, and orphans. Caregivers or attendants were described as paupers or prisoners, who were often drunk.

In 1639 the Augustinian Sisters migrated to Canada and eventually established the first hospital, the Hotel Dieu, in Quebec City. In 1809 in the United States, Mother Elizabeth Seton established the first American order of the Sisters of Charity of St. Joseph's in Maryland. Eventually, other orders or branches of orders in the Roman Catholic Church evolved under the name of Sisters of Charity throughout the eastern United States and Canada. These religious orders developed programs of nursing education and provided nursing service. Following the westward expansion of the United States, Roman Catholic religious orders established hospitals in New Orleans, Chicago, and San Francisco. Religious sisterhoods of Protestant churches, including the Episcopal Sisterhood of the Holy Communion and the English Lutheran Church, also established hospitals and provided nursing care.

Much of nursing's development is related to the need to provide care to sick and injured soldiers during times of war. This fact is true in the development of nursing in the United States. During the Civil War, Dorothea Dix was appointed superintendent of the first nurse corps of the United States Army. She recruited only women who were over 30 and plain-looking. She was able to recruit 2000 women to care for the armed forces. These nurses dressed wounds, gave medicines, and attended to diets. In addition to war wounds, the soldiers suffered from dysentery and smallpox, and many nurses died as a result of disease contracted in the line of duty.

As with Nightingale in the Crimea, the nurses in the Civil War met with much opposition from the male physicians. Hospital ships were used to transport the wounded to hospitals, and nurses provided care along with medical orderlies. Many assertive women, who are known not only for their ability to nurse but also for their influence in other arenas, provided nursing service during the Civil War. Some of the most influential were Louisa May Alcott, who eventually became an important literary figure; Harriet Tubman, who as a nurse and abolitionist provided care and comfort to her fellow African Americans on the Underground Railroad; and Sojourner Truth, another African American nurse who provided care for the wounded soldiers of the Union Army and was active in the early roots of the women's movement.

During World War I approximately 23,000 nurses were assigned to military service. After the war, many of these nurses continued to provide care with relief programs in Europe and Asia. The need for trained nurses placed a strain on the supply of nurses, resulting in a fear that the admission and graduation standards of nurse training would be lowered. Rather than sacrifice the quality of nurses, a committee composed of M. Adelaide Nutting, Annie Goodrich, and Lillian Wald met to develop an alternative training program combining university and hospital training. The first such program was the "Vassar Training Camp," under the direction of Isabel Stewart. In 1918, in response to the need for trained nurses, the Secretary of War authorized the Army School of Nursing, with Annie Goodrich as its first dean.

World War II had a tremendous impact on nursing. Nurses served at the war front in field hospitals, on hospital ships, and in air ambulances. Again the need for nurses impacted on nursing education, resulting in the development of the United State Cadet Nurse Corps, a training program for nurses funded by federal funds under the Bolton Act of 1943. This was a forerunner of federal funding programs aiding nursing education. Provisions of this act forbade discrimination on the basis of race and marital status, required minimum educational standards, and forced nursing schools to review and revise their curricula (Kelly and Joel, 1999, p. 59).

As nursing developed its practice and training schools proliferated, nurse leaders considered the need to establish minimum standards for educational programs and for safe practice. In 1903, North Carolina, New Jersey, New York, and Virginia enacted voluntary licensure laws. These laws did not require licensure but regulated the use of the title Registered Nurse (RN). In 1915 the American Nurses Association drafted a model nurse practice act. By 1923, all 48 states had passed laws to regulate nursing licensure or registration. Licensure was still voluntary or permissive. It was not until 1935 that the first mandatory licensure act was passed in New York, but it did not go into effect until 1949. Now, licensure is mandatory throughout the United States and Canada. In 1971

Research Box

Fairman, J., and Kagan, S. 1999. Creating critical care: The case of the hospital of the University of Pennsylvania 1950–1965. *Advances in Nursing Science* **22(1): 63–77.**

This study uses social history to study the development of critical-care nursing using oral history interviews, archival material, and secondary sources. This critical-care unit was the third of its kind in 1955, preceded by North Carolina Memorial Hospital in 1953 and Chestnut Hill Hospital in Philadelphia in 1954.

Architectural changes were implemented at hospitals to create semiprivate and private rooms in response to social trends that placed high value on privacy. Because of their reliance financially on income from patients, hospitals depended on the loyalty of the local community to support the facilities. Patients also wanted to be sure they received adequate care and so they wanted private-duty nurses when they were ill. These three factors were major influences in the development of critical-care units.

An acute nursing shortage greatly reduced the availability of private-duty nurses. As more severely ill people required more complicated care, the demand for nurses further increased. By the 1950s, the hospital was having difficulty caring for the growing complexity of its patient population in semiprivate rooms. Having a special room for desperately ill patients that was well-staffed with nurses was proposed as a solution. Critical care was a response to the dangers posed by traditional staffing and was thought to be an economical strategy.

The study concludes that social factors, such as workforce and economic issues, architectural changes, and a more complex hospital population, rather than new technology led to the development of critical care. Many of the workforce issues parallel contemporary nurse workforce issues.

Idaho became the first state to recognize advanced nursing practice in its Nurse Practice Act, and in 1986 North Dakota became the first state to require the baccalaureate degree for licensure as a registered nurse (Ellis and Hartley, 2001).

Social change has continued to influence change within the profession. At the same time nurses change society through their education and practice. In 1992, Eddie Bernice Johnson was the first nurse elected to the United States House of Representatives. Today many nurses have been elected to local, state, and national office. These nurses effect change in the social systems in which nurses work and live. Nurses are involved in professional and civic organizations to effect change in society.

HISTORICAL LEADERS IN NURSING

Throughout the history of nursing, individuals have come forward to influence the profession and society. Many of the names are familiar. The people discussed are not the only leaders in nursing but are presented to provide a perspective of nurses as women and men, founders, risk takers, and social reformers.

The Founders

It is usually difficult to identify who was the first nurse in a specific country. Often the first person to provide nursing care was an unnamed slave, convict, pilgrim, rebel, mother, daughter, wife, or other unknown. Nurses as founders have established schools of nursing, hospitals, and organizations to promote the good health of the public. The accompanying box describes some of nursing's founders.

Nurses as Founders

- Jeanne Mance (1606–1673), founder of the Hotel Dieu hospital in Montreal, Quebec, Canada, is credited with being the first lay nurse not only in Canada, but also in North America.

- Florence Nightingale (1830–1910) is considered the founder of modern nursing. Her achievements in improving standards for the care of war casualties in the Crimea earned her the title "Lady of the Lamp." She was the first nurse to exert political pressure on government to improve health conditions. Through her contributions to nursing education, she is also recognized as nursing's first scientist/theorist for her work *Notes on Nursing: What It Is, and What It Is Not.*

- Mary Seacole (1805–1881) learned about nursing from her mother in Jamaica, British West Indies. When she learned about the war in the Crimea, she offered to go to the Crimea to tend the soldiers. Her request was denied, so she traveled at her own expense to the Crimea, where she opened a lodging house in which she cared for wounded and sick officers.

- Clara Barton (1821–1912) nursed in federal hospitals during the Civil War. Following the war she went to Europe, where she learned about the International Red Cross. She served with the Red Cross during the Franco-Prussian War. She returned to the United States, where she was instrumental in founding the American Red Cross in 1882.

- Lucy Osborne was a Nightingale-trained nurse who arrived in Australia in 1868 as superintendent of nurses, along with five head nurses, to provide nursing care to patients at the Sydney Hospital. She is credited with founding the Sydney training school, the first training school for nurses in Australia using the Nightingale model.

- Linda (Melinda) Richards (1841–1930) is considered the first trained nurse in the United States. She received her nursing certificate October 1, 1873, from the New England Hospital for Women and Children. She went to England in 1877 to study nursing with Florence Nightingale. She then went to Japan, where she organized the first nurse-training school.

- Mary Mahoney (1845–1926) is considered America's first African American professional nurse, receiving her nursing certificate from the New England Hospital for Women and Children in 1879.

- Cecilia Makiwane became South Africa's first Black African professional nurse in 1908. She was a pioneer for nurses in Africa.

- Lillian Wald (1858–1940) is considered the founder of public health nursing. She and Mary Brewster were the first to offer trained nursing services to the poor in the New York slums. Their home among the poor on the upper floor of a tenement, called the Henry Street Settlement and the Visiting Nurse Service, provided nursing services, social services, and organized educational and cultural activities.

- Mary Breckinridge (1881–1965) established the Frontier Nursing Service in 1925 to provide health care to the people of rural America. Within this organization, Breckinridge started one of the first midwifery training schools in the United States.

Research Box

Mackintosh, C. 1997. A historical study of men in nursing. *Journal of Advanced Nursing* 26(2): 232–236. This study uses primary archival sources, oral history, and secondary sources to outline a brief history of men as nurses in the United Kingdom. Men have had a place in nursing for as long as records have been available. Their place is detailed in records of the monastic movement in 1095, when St. Antonines was founded to nurse sufferers of erysipelas and the mentally ill. The Knight Hospitallers of St. John of Jersulem was founded in 1200 and records male nurses, as does the Knights of Lazarus, founded in 1490 to care for lepers. However, once the monasteries went through dissolution in the 1600s, records of organized nursing disappear.

Workhouses with attached infirmaries appeared in the mid-nineteenth century using inmates to nurse each other. Men worked in a strictly sex-segregated setting; however, they were referred to as attendants or keepers rather than nurses.

Nursing at this point in history was a low-status occupation, and nurses had dubious reputations. Reformers were influenced by the religious sisterhoods, so the occupation was placed in a female sphere that was furthered by Nightingale. The assumption was that this new nursing was more natural for females. Male nurses continued to fill roles outside the reformed sphere in private sectors. In the early 1900s the Royal Army Medical Corp was another avenue for employment.

In the mid-1920s, a chronic shortage of nurses allowed male nurses into the workforce. The Society of Registered Male Nurses was established in 1937; in 1949 formal legislative discrimination was ended, and 108 schools of nursing opened their doors to male students. The expansion of males in nursing has been dramatic since that time.

Stereotypes and assumptions regarding male nurses, their characteristics, employment, and role must be viewed within the historical perspective. Male nurses are a product of many years of biased and discriminatory employment practices. This is a by-product of moral squeamishness of earlier times. The contributions men have made to nursing history should be more positively recognized.

The Men

Although nursing is often thought of as a woman's profession, men have been influential in nursing's history. Often male caregivers were not called nurses; however, their activities of caring for and nurturing the sick and injured reflect the values and activities of nursing. For example, knighthood orders of the Middle Ages combined religion, chivalry, militarism, and charity. Their original purpose was to carry the wounded from the battlefield to the hospitals and to provide care. During the period of the Crusades, the organization and management of their battlefield hospitals became the standard for the development of hospitals throughout Europe. Some specific men who have been identified with their nursing roles are described in the box on page 37.

The Risk Takers

Many nurses have taken personal risks to uphold the values of nursing. Caring for those who are ill exposes nurses to the obvious risks of contagious illnesses or work-related injuries. Some nurses have risked loss of status, danger to family and friends, and even death. Some of these risk takers are described in the box on page 37.

The Social Reformers

Nurses have assumed roles in social reform throughout recorded history. Many of their efforts have been to improve the plight of the poor, the sick, the abandoned, or the hopeless. Often the focus has been on the particular difficulties experienced by women and children who did not have the support of male family members. It must be remembered that it has only been during the twentieth century that women and minorities achieved the right to vote or to own property in many of the Western nations. The box on page 38 describes the work of some these social reformers.

Consider . . .

- how the history of nursing has affected your own nursing practice.
- who the nursing leaders in your community or your area of practice are. What have they done to enhance the profession or the society in which we live?
- issues in health care today that ask nurses to become risk takers to uphold the values of nursing. What risks are you willing to take to uphold the values of nursing?

Men in Nursing

- John Ciudad (1495–1550) founded the order of the Brothers of St. John of God or the Brothers of Mercy in 1538. He opened a hospital in Granada and asked a group of friends to assist in providing nursing care to the mentally ill, homeless vagrants, crippled, derelicts, and abandoned children. Men of this order also visited the sick in their homes.
- St Camillus de Lellis (1550–1614) founded the Nursing Order of Ministers of the Sick. Men of this order cared for the dying, people stricken with the plague, and alcoholics. St. Camillus opened a hospital for alcoholics in Germany.

- James Derham was an African American man who worked as a nurse in New Orleans in 1783. He was able to save enough money to buy his freedom from slavery. He went on to become the first African American physician in the United States.
- Walt Whitman (1819–1892), poet and writer, served as a volunteer hospital nurse in Washington, D.C. during the Civil War. He recorded his experiences in a collection of poems called *Drumtaps* and in his diary, *Specimen Days and Collect.*

THE DEVELOPMENT OF PROFESSIONAL NURSING ORGANIZATIONS

As nursing has developed, an increasing number of nursing organizations have been formed. These organizations function at the local, regional, national, and international levels. When nurses participate in the activities of nursing organizations, they enhance their own professional growth and help all nurses collectively as they influence policies affecting nursing, nursing practice, and the health of the community. Nursing organizations can be divided into three types: organizations that represent all nurses (e.g., the American Nurses Association and the National League for Nursing), organizations that meet the needs of nurses within specific nursing specialties (e.g., the American Association for Critical Care Nurses, the Emergency Nurses Association, the Association of Operating Room Nurses), and organizations that represent special interests. Some of these organizations are discussed on the following pages.

Nurses as Risk Takers

- Clara Maass (1876–1901) volunteered to go to Havana, Cuba, where experiments on yellow fever were being conducted. She provided nursing care for victims of yellow fever through the spring of 1901. She allowed herself to be bitten by a mosquito to prove a theory that yellow fever was caused by mosquitoes. She experienced a mild attack of the fever in June but offered to be bitten again. She died following the second bite in August 1901, demonstrating that mosquitoes were indeed the cause of yellow fever.
- Edith Cavell (1865–1915) was an English nurse during World War I who had founded a training school for nurses in Belgium. During the war, her hospital cared for both Allied and German soldiers.

She also assisted Allied soldiers who were prisoners of the Germans in escaping. She was charged by the Germans with harboring British and French soldiers and aiding them in escape. She was shot on October 12, 1915.
- Sharon Lane, an Army nurse during the Vietnam conflict, was the only nurse to die as a result of enemy fire. She died on June 8, 1969, of wounds received while on duty.
- Barbara Fassbinder was an advocate for mandatory HIV testing of health care workers. She was infected with HIV in 1986 while caring for a patient with AIDS. She is recognized as the first health care provider to acquire AIDS on the job. She died in 1994 of AIDS.

Nurses as Social Reformers

- Sojourner Truth (1767–1881) was an early feminist and abolitionist who identified the similarity between the problems of African Americans and women. She was significant in helping African American women overcome the oppression caused by their race and sex.

- Dorothea Lynde Dix (1802–1887) was an early crusader for humane care for the mentally ill in the United States. She also advocated for humane care for criminals in prison after finding that many of them suffered from mental illness. Prior to her efforts, it was not uncommon to find mentally ill people imprisoned in jails along with criminals. Through her efforts, standards of care for the mentally ill were improved, and more than 30 psychiatric hospitals were established in the United States.

- Harriet Tubman (1820–1913) was called the "Moses of her people." She made numerous trips between the South and the North to assist slaves in their quest for freedom. She was an abolitionist who became active with the Underground Railroad. She provided nursing care to the sick and suffering slaves and former slaves.

- Lavinia Dock (1858–1956) was a feminist, prolific writer, political activist, and suffragette. She actively participated in protest movements for women's rights that resulted in the passage of the Nineteenth Amendment to the U.S. Constitution in 1920, which granted women the right to vote. She also campaigned for legislation to allow nurses rather than physicians to control the nursing profession. In 1893, she founded, with the assistance of Mary Adelaide Nutting and Isabel Hampton Robb, the American Society of Superintendents of Training Schools for Nurses of the United States and Canada, a forerunner of the National League for Nursing.

- Margaret Sanger (1879–1966) worked as a public health nurse in New York City. In 1912, she was called to care for a woman who had attempted to abort herself and who later died. It was illegal at the time to provide information about contraception and family planning. However, Sanger learned everything she could about contraception and family planning and published information about it in a journal. She was arrested, convicted, and sentenced to 30 days in a workhouse. She continued to provide information on family planning and lobbied to change the laws. She founded the National Committee on Federal Legislation for Birth Control, the forerunner of the Planned Parenthood Federation.

American Nurses Association

The American Nurses Association (ANA) is the national professional organization representing all registered nurses in the United States. It was founded in 1896 as the Nurses Associated Alumnae of the United States and Canada. In 1911 the name was changed to the American Nurses Association. It was a charter member of the International Council of Nurses in 1899, along with nursing organizations in Great Britain and Germany.

In 1982 the ANA became a federation of state nurses' associations. Nurses participate in the ANA by joining their state nurses' associations. The official journal of the ANA is the *American Journal of Nursing*, and *American Nurse* is the official newspaper.

The purposes of the ANA are to foster high standards of nursing practice, to promote the economic and general welfare of nurses in the workplace, to project a positive and realistic view of nursing, and to lobby Congress and regulatory agencies on health care issues affecting nurses and the public (ANA, 2001). Affiliate groups of the ANA are the American Nurses Credentialing Center (ANCC), which conducts the certification process at the nurse generalist and the advanced practice levels in many nursing specialities; the United American Nurses (UAN), which acts as the agent for those nurses who are organized for collective bargaining; the American Nurses Foundation (ANF), which supports nursing research and scholarship; and the American Academy of Nursing (AAN), which recognizes nursing leaders.

National Student Nurses Association

The National Student Nurses Association (NSNA) was established in 1952 to represent nursing students in associate degree, diploma, baccalaureate, generic masters and generic doctoral programs preparing students for registered nurse licensure, and registered nurses in BSN-completion programs. The organization "promotes self-governance, advocates for students' rights and the rights of patients, and advocates for collective, responsible action on vital social and political issues" (NSNA, 2001). The official journal of the NSNA is *Imprint.*

National League for Nursing

The National League for Nursing (NLN) is an organization whose mission is "to advance quality nursing education that prepares the nursing workforce to meet the needs of diverse populations in an ever-changing health care environment" (NLN, 2001). The National League for Nursing began in 1893 as part of the American Society of Superintendents of Training Schools for Nurses. In 1912, the society was renamed the National League for Nursing Education (NLNE). In 1952 the NLNE, the National Organization for Public Health Nursing, and the Association for Collegiate Schools of Nursing combined to form the National League for Nursing (NLN, 2001).

The NLN also provides professional development for nursing faculty; provides support for research related to nursing education; and provides information, services, and products to support nursing education. The official publication of the NLN is *Nursing and Health Care Perspectives.* The National League for Nursing Accrediting Commission (NLNAC), an affiliate of the NLN, serves as a national accreditation body for schools of nursing at the vocational, associate degree, baccalaureate, and graduate levels.

American Association of Colleges of Nursing

The American Association of Colleges of Nursing (AACN) is the national voice for baccalaureate- and higher-degree nursing education programs in the United States. The purpose of the AACN is to "establish standards for bachelor's and graduate degree nursing programs, to assist deans and directors to implement those standards, to influence the nursing profession to improve health care, and to promote public support of baccalaureate and graduate education, research, and practice in nursing" (AACN, 2001). To fulfill its purpose, AACN serves as an accrediting organization for baccalaureate- and higher-degree nursing programs.

International Council of Nurses

The International Council of Nurses (ICN) was formed in 1899 as the world's first and widest inter-

national organization for health professionals. The goals of the ICN are to "ensure quality nursing care for all, sound health policies globally, the advancement of nursing knowledge, and the presence worldwide of a respected nursing profession and a competent and satisfied nursing workforce" (ICN, 2001). In 2001, ICN represented nurses in more than 120 countries. The official journal of the ICN is *International Nursing Review.*

Sigma Theta Tau International

Sigma Theta Tau is the international honor society for nursing. It was founded in 1922 at the University of Indiana in Indianapolis. The Greek letters stand for the Greek words storga, tharos, and tima, meaning "love," "courage," and "honor." The society is a member of the Association of College Honor Societies. The purpose of the society is the advancement of the status of nursing as a profession. The organization recognizes the value of scholarship and the importance of excellence in nursing practice (STTI, 2001). The official publication of Sigma Theta Tau is the *Journal of Nursing Scholarship.*

Specialty Nursing Organizations

There are several organizations that represent nurses of specific ethnic groups, including the National Black Nurses Association, the National Hispanic Nurses Association, the Philippine Nurses Association, and the Jamaican Nurses Association. These organizations represent the issues and concerns of these nurses and the populations they serve. These organizations often conduct activities to provide service to their own ethnic groups; for example, the National Black Nurses Association provides education and conducts research to understand the health problems that adversely affect African Americans.

Additionally, there are organizations that represent the special interests of nurses either from a practice perspective or a civic perspective. Examples of such organizations include the Association for Nurses in AIDS Care (ANAC).

Consider . . .

■ why many nurses choose not to be involved in nursing organizations.

■ how involvement in professional nursing organizations can assist nurses in managing the stresses of the changing and challenging health care system.

■ the nursing organizations you are involved in. What benefits do you obtain from membership in these organizations?

SUMMARY

Nursing has existed throughout the history of humankind. From primitive to contemporary societies, care of the sick has been influenced by many factors, such as superstition and magic, Greek and Roman mythology, religion, male-female role proscriptions, legislation, wars, and other societal events. Male-female role proscriptions traditionally attributed the care and nurturing functions to women. In the third century in Rome, however, the Parabolani Brotherhood provided care to the sick and dying during the great plague in Alexandria, and early hospitals in India were staffed largely by male nurses.

The first sanitary legislation, the Mosaic Health Code, was contributed by the ancient Hebrew culture. This code differentiated between clean and unclean. The Christian value of "love thy neighbor as thyself" and the parable of the Good Samaritan impacted the development of Western nursing.

During the Dark Ages, religious beliefs of the church encouraged comfort of the sick and poor, but little was done to prevent illness or cure disease. During the Middle Ages, male and female religious, military, and secular orders, with the primary purpose of caring for the sick, were established. Examples are the Knights Hospitalers of St. John, the Alexian Brotherhood, the Augustinian Sisters, and the Sisters of Charity, founded by St. Vincent de Paul in France.

In 1835, the Order of Deaconesses operated a small hospital and training school in Kaiserswerth, Germany, where Florence Nightingale trained. Nightingale went to the Crimean with several nurses to provide care to the ill and wounded soldiers. As a result of a grateful English public, Nightingale opened her training school for nurses in London.

The development of nursing in the Americas started with the Augustinian Sisters in Canada. Jeanne Mance founded the Hotel Dieu in Montreal in 1644, and Mother Elizabeth Seton established the first American order of the Sisters of Charity of St. Joseph in Maryland.

Nursing education, knowledge, and practice have developed as a result of societal events, including wars, civil strife, changes in women's roles, and so on. Nurses

have demonstrated leadership as founders, risk takers, and social reformers.

Nursing organizations have developed to meet the professional needs of nurses and the health care needs of the public. There are several types of nursing organizations: organizations that represent and influence all of nursing, organizations that represent the needs of nurses practicing in specialty areas, organizations that represent the needs of nurses of specific ethnic groups, and organizations that represent nurses' special interests.

Bookshelf

Dossey, B. M. 2000. *Florence Nightingale: Mystic, visionary, healer.* **Springhouse, Penn.: Springhouse.**
This biography of Florence Nightingale describes her life as a social activist and visionary whose ideas about public health, holistic health, and women's place in society were decades ahead of their time.

Gollaher, D. 1995. *Voice for the mad: The life of Dorothea Dix.* **New York: The Free Press.**
This biography of Dorothea Dix describes her life as a social activist for people with mental health problems and for the homeless.

Oates, S. B. 1994. *A woman of valor: Clara Barton and the Civil War.* **New York: The Free Press.**
Clara Barton's role in advocating care for soldiers during the American Civil War is described in this biography of her life. The outcome of her experience was the founding of the American Red Cross.

Schorr, T. M., and Zimmerman, A. 1988. *Making choices: Taking chances: Nurse leaders tell their stories.* **St. Louis: Mosby.**
This book includes autobiographies of more than 40 nursing leaders of the twentieth century. These very personal stories, written by the leaders themselves, are rich in knowledge, history, and inspiration.

REFERENCES

American Association of Colleges of Nursing (AACN). 2001. www.aacn.nche.edu

American Nurses Association (ANA). 2001. www.ana.org

Baly, M. E. 1986. *Florence Nightingale and the nursing legacy.* London: Croom Helm.

Burchill, E. 1992. *Australian nurses since Nightingale: 1860–1990.* Richmond, Victoria, Australia: Spectrum Publications.

Carnegie, M. E. 1995. *The path we tread: Blacks in nursing worldwide, 1854–1994,* 3d ed. New York: NLN Press.

Dolan, J. A., Fitzpatrick, M. L., and Herrmann, E. K. 1983. *Nursing in society: A historical perspective,* 15th ed. Philadelphia: W.B. Saunders.

Donahue, M. P. 1996. *Nursing: The finest art,* 2d ed. St. Louis: Mosby.

Dossey, B. M. 2000. *Florence Nightingale: Mystic, visionary, healer.* Springhouse, Penn.: Springhouse.

Ellis, J. R., and Hartley, C. L. 2001. *Nursing in today's world: Challenges, issues, and trends,* 7th ed. Philadelphia: Lippincott.

International Council of Nurses (ICN). 2001. www.icn.org

Kalisch, P. A., and Kalisch, B. J. 1995. *The Advance of American Nursing,* 3d ed. Philadelphia: Lippincott.

Kelly, L. Y., and Joel, L. A. 1999. *Dimensions of professional nursing,* 8th ed. New York: McGraw-Hill.

Kozier, B., Erb, G., and Blais, K. 1992. *Concepts and issues in nursing practice,* 2d ed. Redwood City, Calif.: Addison-Wesley.

National League for Nursing (NLN). 2001. www.nln.org

National League for Nursing Accrediting Commission. 2001. www.nlnac.org

National Student Nurses' Association (NSNA). 2001. www.nsna.org

Sigma Theta Tau International (STTI). 2001. www.stti.iupui.edu

CHAPTER 4

Ethical Foundation of Professional Nursing

Outline

Objectives

- Explain how nurses can help clients clarify their values to facilitate ethical decision making.
- Explain the uses and limitations of professional codes of ethics.
- Discuss how cognitive development, values, moral frameworks, and codes of ethics affect moral decisions.
- Discuss common bioethical issues currently facing health care professionals.
- Analyze ways in which nurses can enhance their ethical decision-making abilities.
- Identify the moral principles involved in ethical decision making.
- Describe the advocacy role of the nurse.

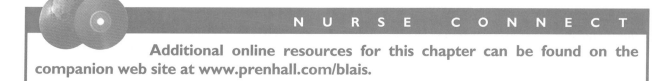

NURSE CONNECT

Additional online resources for this chapter can be found on the companion web site at www.prenhall.com/blais.

Professional nurses must attend to the ethical responsibilities and conflicts they may experience as a result of their unique relationships in professional practice. Advances in medical and reproductive technology, clients' rights, social and legal changes, and the allocation of scarce resources have contributed to an increase in ethical concerns. Standards of conduct for nurses are set forth in codes of ethics developed by international, national, and state or provincial nursing associations. Nurses need to be able to apply ethical principles in decision making and include values and beliefs of clients, of the profession, of the nurse, and of all other concerned parties. Nurses have a responsibility to protect the rights of clients by acting as client advocates. Advocacy derives from the ethical principles of beneficience (the duty to do good) and nonmaleficience (the duty to do no harm).

CHALLENGES AND OPPORTUNITIES

VALUES CONFLICTS Nursing has long advocated a nonjudgmental approach to care. However, nurses come into the profession with established values and beliefs, which may conflict with the values and beliefs of clients. Nurses sometimes feel compromised when they must provide care in such a situation. Sometimes beliefs are so strong that it is difficult not to judge the other person and act or react in a way that might compromise care. The nursing profession must be able to identify ways and means of assisting members of the profession so that values are not compromised by either party.

ETHICAL-LEGAL CONFLICTS *Ethical* and *legal* are not synonymous. There are times in professional practice when the legal requirement does not appear compatible with the ethical approach. Nurses may place themselves in legal jeopardy when they opt for what they see as the ethical, or "right" thing to do, in spite of what is inherent in the laws that apply. The same conflict may occur with institutional policy that may place the nurse in a similar position of risk. Advocacy for the profession is needed when such a conflict arises so that laws and/or policies may better serve the public.

VALUES

Values are freely chosen, enduring beliefs or attitudes about the worth of a person, object, idea, or action. Freedom, courage, family, and dignity are examples of values. Values frequently derive from a person's cultural, ethnic, and religious background; from societal traditions; and from the values held by peer group and family.

Values form a basis for behavior. Once a person becomes aware of his or her values, they become an internal control for behavior; thus, a person's real values are manifested in consistent patterns of behavior.

Values exist within a person in relationship to one another. A **value system** is the organization of a person's values along a continuum, that is, from most important to least important. Values form the basis of **purposive behavior,** which refers to actions that a person performs "on purpose," with the intention of reaching some goal or bringing about a certain result. Thus, purposive behavior is based on a person's decisions or choices, and these decisions or choices are based on the person's underlying values.

Values Transmission

Values are learned and are greatly influenced by a person's sociocultural environment. For example, if a parent consistently demonstrates honesty in dealing with others, the child will probably begin to value honesty. Acquiring values is a gradual process, usually occurring at an unconscious level. Because values are learned through observation and experience, they are heavily influenced by a person's sociocultural environment. For example, some cultures value the treatment of a folk healer over that of a physician. For additional information about cultural values relative to health and illness, see Chapter 21, "Nursing in a Culturally and Spiritually Diverse World."

Personal Values

Most people derive some values from the society or subgroup of society in which they live. A person may internalize some or all of these values and perceive them as *personal values.* People need societal values to feel accepted, and they need personal values to produce a sense of individuality. See the box on page 45 for examples of personal and societal values.

Professional Values

Professional values often reflect and expand on personal values. Nurses acquire professional values during socialization into nursing—from codes of ethics, nursing experiences, teachers, and peers. As members of a caring profession, nurses hold values that relate to both competence and compassion. Watson outlined four important values of nursing (1981, 20–21).

1. *Strong commitment to service.* Nursing is a helping, humanistic service. Because nurses are responsible for assessing and promoting health, they should value the caring aspect of nursing as well as their contribution to the health and well-being of people.

2. *Belief in the dignity and worth of each person.* This value means that the nurse acts in the best interest of the client regardless of nationality, race, creed, color, age, sex, politics, social class, or health status.

3. *Commitment to education.* This reflects a societal value of lifelong learning. In nursing, continuing education is needed to maintain and expand the nurse's

Examples of Societal and Personal Values

SOCIETAL VALUES	PERSONAL VALUES
• Human life	• Family unity
• Individual rights	• Worth of others
• Individual autonomy	• Independence
• Liberty	• Religion
• Democracy	• Honesty
• Equal opportunity	• Fairness
• Power	• Love
• Health	• Sense of humor
• Wealth	• Safety
• Youth	• Peace
• Vigor	• Beauty
• Intelligence	• Harmony
• Imagination	• Financial security
• Education	• Material things
• Technology	• Property of others
• Conformity	• Leisure time
• Friendship	• Work
• Courage	• Travel
• Compassion	• Physical activity
• Family	• Intellectual activity

level of competence and to increase the body of professional knowledge.

4. *Autonomy.* Nurses need to become more assertive in promoting nursing care and developing the ability to assume independent functions.

Nurses often need to behave in a *value-neutral* way, which means being nonjudgmental. This outlook permits nurses to establish effective relationships with clients who have values differing from theirs. Although nurses cannot and should not ignore or deny their own and the profession's values, they need to be able to accept a client's values and beliefs rather than assume their own are the "right ones." This acceptance and nonjudgmental approach requires nurses to be aware of their own values and how they influence behavior.

Consider . . .

■ what values you hold about life, health, illness, and death. How do your values influence the nursing care you provide?

■ whether a nurse who smokes can effectively help a client stop smoking or whether a nurse who is overweight can effectively help a client who needs to lose weight.

■ whether a nurse whose religious beliefs oppose the use of contraceptives can effectively teach a client about family planning.

■ how your values influence the career choices you make (e.g., your initial choice to become a nurse, your choice of practice setting, and your choice of specialty).

Values Clarification

Values clarification is a process by which people identify, examine, and develop their own individual values. A principle of values clarification is that no one set of values is right for everyone. When people are able to identify their values, they can retain or change them and thus act on the basis of freely chosen rather than unconscious values. Values clarification promotes personal growth by fostering awareness, empathy, and insight.

A widely used theory of values clarification was developed in 1966 by Raths, Harmin, and Simon (cited

Values Clarification

PROCESSES	DOMAINS	ACTIONS
Choosing	Cognitive	Reflection and consideration of alternatives result in freely choosing beliefs.
Prizing	Affective	Chosen beliefs are cherished.
Acting	Behavioral	Chosen beliefs are incorporated into behaviors that are affirmed to others and repeated consistently.

in Fowler and Levine-Ariff, 1987, p. 143). This "valuing process" includes cognitive, affective, and behavioral components, referred to as *choosing, prizing,* and *acting.* See the accompanying box.

Identifying Personal Values

Nurses need to know specifically what values they hold about life, health, illness, and death. Beginning as students, nurses should explore their own values and beliefs regarding such situations as the following:

- An individual's right to make decisions for self when conflicting with medical advice
- Abortion
- End-of-life issues
- Domestic violence
- Cloning
- Having a child to provide a bone marrow transplant

When considering these issues, the nurse should ask, Can I accept this or live with this? Why does this bother me? What would I do or want done in this situation? (Corey, Corey, and Callahan, 1984, pp. 57–94).

Because nurses are called upon to provide care to individuals who may have made decisions that conflict with the nurse's values, self-awareness is important. Nurses must be aware of their own values and attitudes in order to recognize when a situation might affect the care they are able to provide. Often, the awareness of the conflict of values allows nurses to hold their personal values in check and provide effective care. In those instances when nurses feel they cannot be effective due to their conflicting values, they need to be able to discuss the situation with colleagues who may be able to assist with providing care.

Helping Clients Identify Values

Nurses need to help clients identify values as they influence and relate to a particular health problem. Examples of behaviors that may indicate the need for values clarification are listed in the accompanying box.

The following process may help clients clarify their values.

Behaviors That May Indicate Unclear Values

BEHAVIOR	EXAMPLE
Ignoring a health professional's advice	A client with heart disease who values hard work ignores advice to exercise regularly.
Inconsistent communication or behavior	A pregnant woman says she wants a healthy baby but continues to drink alcohol and smoke tobacco.
Numerous admissions to a health agency for the same problem	A middle-aged, obese woman repeatedly seeks help for back pain but does not lose weight.
Confusion or uncertainty about which course of action to take	A woman wants to obtain a job to meet financial obligations but also wants to stay at home to care for an ailing husband.

Comparison of Moral Justice and Care Orientations

JUSTICE ORIENTATION	CARE ORIENTATION
Focuses on the moral vision of "not to treat others unfairly."	Focuses on the moral vision of "not to turn away from someone in need."
Requires understanding of what "fairness" means.	Requires understanding of what constitutes "care."
Draws attention to problems of inequality and oppression.	Draws attention to problems of detachment or abandonment.
Holds up an ideal of reciprocal rights and equal respect for individuals.	Holds up an ideal of attention and response to need.

1. *List alternatives.* Make sure that the client is aware of all alternative actions and has thought about the consequences of each. Ask, Are you considering other courses of action?

2. *Examine possible consequences of choices.* Ask, What do you think you will gain by doing that? What benefits do you foresee from doing that?

3. *Choose freely.* To determine whether the client chose freely, ask, Did you have any say in that decision? Did you have a choice?

4. *Feel good about the choice.* To determine how the client feels, ask, How do you feel about that decision (or action)? Because some clients may not feel satisfied with their decision, a more sensitive question may be, Some people feel good after a decision is made; others feel bad. How do you feel?

5. *Affirms the choice.* Ask, What will you say to others (family, friends) about this?

6. *Act on the choice.* To determine whether the client is prepared to act on the decision, ask, for example, Will it be difficult to tell your wife about this?

7. *Act with a pattern.* To determine whether the client consistently behaves in a pattern, ask, How many times have you done that before? or Would you act that way again?

When implementing these seven steps, the nurse assists the client to think each question through, never imposing personal values. When clarifying values, the nurse never offers an opinion (e.g., "It would be better to do it this way") or offers a judgment (e.g., "That's not the right thing to do"). The nurse offers an opinion only when the client asks the nurse for it, and then only with care.

MORALS

Morality (morals) is similar to ethics and many people use the two words interchangeably. Morality usually refers to an individual's personal standards of what is right and wrong in conduct, character, and attitude. Ethics usually refers to the moral standards of a particular group such as nurses. (See Table 4–1 for a comparison of morals and ethics.)

Sometimes the first clue to the moral nature of a situation is an aroused conscience, or an awareness of feelings such as guilt, hope, or shame. The tendency to respond to the situation with words such as *ought, should, right, wrong, good,* and *bad* is another indicator.

Table 4–1 Comparison of Morals and Ethics

Morals	Principles and rules of right conduct
	Private, personal
	Commitment to principles and values is usually defended in daily life
Ethics	Formal responding process used to determine right conduct
	Professionally and publicly stated
	Inquiry or study of principles and values
	Process of questioning, and perhaps changing, one's morals

Finally, moral issues are concerned with important social values and norms: they are not about trivial things.

Moral Development

Moral development is a complex process that is not fully understood. It is more than the imprinting of parents' rules and virtues or values upon children; rather, moral development is the process of learning what ought to be done and what ought not to be done. The terms *morality, moral behavior,* and *moral development* need to be distinguished. **Morality** refers to the requirements necessary for people to live together in society; **moral behavior** is the way a person perceives those requirements and responds to them; **moral development** is the pattern of change in moral behavior with age.

Kohlberg

The research of Lawrence Kohlberg has provided one of the most well-known approaches to moral development. He was directly affected by Jean Piaget's theory of cognitive development. Kohlberg's theory focuses on the structure of thought about moral issues rather than the specific content of moral values. It applies ways of thinking about issues that depend upon the specific issue and whether the person is very familiar with the topic. According to Kohlberg, moral development progresses through three levels and six stages. Levels and stages are not always linked to a specific developmental stage because some people progress to a higher level of moral development than others. The levels and stages range from egocentric actions to behaviors that show concern for society and rightness.

At Kohlberg's first level, called the *premoral* or *preconventional level,* children are responsive to cultural rules and labels of good and bad, right and wrong. However, children interpret these in terms of the physical consequences of their actions, that is, punishment or reward. At the second level, the *conventional level,* the individual is concerned about maintaining the expectations of the family, group, or nation and sees this as right. The emphasis at this level is conformity and loyalty to one's own expectations as well as society's. The third level is called the *postconventional, autonomous,* or *principled level.* At this level, people make an effort to define valid values and principles without regard to outside authority or to the expectations of others. For additional information about Kohlberg's levels, see Table 4–2.

With reference to Kohlberg's six stages, Munhall (1982, p. 14) writes that stage four, the "law-and-order"

orientation, is the dominant stage of most adults. It is recognized that there is a difference in action between nurses who act at the conventional level (level II) and those who act at the postconventional or principled level (level III): Refer to examples in Table 4–2.

Progression through the stages is determined by one's exposure to social complexity and the opportunity to question and discuss ethical decisions. Theoretically, formal operations (Piaget) are associated with stage 4; the ability to think abstractly is necessary to consider such things as social order. It is rare for an adult to reach stage 6. In his later writings, Kohlberg questioned the validity of including it as a stage.

There are questions about whether Kohlberg's stages, particularly 5 and 6, are universal across cultures. There is research supporting the sequence and achievement of these stages among various groups, such as South African blacks and whites, Chinese, Buddhists, British, and Hong Kong Chinese (Tudin, Straker, and Mendolsohn, 1994; Lei, 1994). Others question whether the universal ethical principle at stage 6 reflects Western ways of thinking (Miller, 1994; Heubner and Garrod, 1993).

Kohlberg developed this theory by conducting interviews using hypothetical dilemmas. Each dilemma described a character who finds himself or herself in a difficult situation and has to choose from conflicting values. The participant is asked how the character should resolve the problem in the right way. Analysis of the responses resulted in the formulation of Kohlberg's levels and stages (Colby and Kohlberg, 1987). Unfortunately, all the subjects in the study were male, which has led to serious criticism of the theory.

Gilligan

Carol Gilligan (1982) has been one of the major critics of Kohlberg's theory, particularly in its application to females. She contends that Kohlberg's stage sequence places the qualities most often stressed in the socialization of females in stage 3; these qualities are compassion, responsibility, and obligation. Men, who are taught to organize social relationships in a hierarchical order and subscribe to a morality of right, will be included in Kohlberg's higher stages of moral judgment.

After more than 10 years of research with women subjects, she found that women often considered the situations that Kohlberg used in his research to be irrelevant. Women scored consistently lower on his scale of moral development, in spite of the fact that they approached moral situations with considerable sophistication. Gilligan maintains that most frameworks do not include the concepts of caring and responsibility.

Table 4–2 Kohlberg's Stages of Moral Development

Level and Stage	Definition	Example
Level I Preconventional		
Stage 1: Punishment and obedience orientation	The activity is wrong if one is punished, and the activity is right if one is not punished.	A nurse follows a physician's order so as not to be fired.
Stage 2: Instrumental-relativist orientation	Action is taken to satisfy one's needs.	A client in hospital agrees to stay in bed if the nurse will buy the client a newspaper.
Level II Conventional		
Stage 3: Interpersonal concordance (good boy, nice girl)	Action is taken to please another and gain approval.	A nurse gives older clients in hospital sedatives at bedtime because the night nurse wants all clients to sleep at night.
Stage 4: Law and order orientation	Right behavior is obeying the law and following the rules.	A nurse does not permit a worried client to phone home because hospital rules stipulate no phone calls after 9:00 P.M.
Level III Postconventional		
Stage 5: Social contract, legalistic orientation	Standard of behavior is based on adhering to laws that protect the welfare and rights of others. Personal values and opinions are recognized, and violating the rights of others is avoided.	A nurse arranges for an East Indian client to have privacy for prayer each evening.
Stage 6: Universal-ethical principles	Universal moral principles are internalized. Person respects other humans and believes that relationships are based on mutual trust.	A nurse becomes an advocate for a hospitalized client by reporting to the nursing supervisor a conversation in which a physician threatened to withhold assistance unless the client agreed to surgery.

Source: Adapted from *Moral Development: A Guide to Piaget and Kohlberg* by Ronald Duska and Mariaellen Whelan. Copyright © 1975 by The Missionary Society of St. Paul the Apostle in the State of New York. Used by permission of Paulist Press. *www.paulistpress.com*

In contrast to Kohlberg's theory of moral development, which emphasizes fairness, rights, and autonomy in a *justice framework*, Gilligan focuses on a *care perspective*, which is organized around the notions of responsibility, compassion (care), and relationships. Gilligan contends that for women, moral maturity is less a matter of abstract, impersonal justice and more an ethic of caring relationships.

The ethic of *justice*, or fairness, is based on the idea of equality: that everyone should receive the same treatment. This is the development path usually followed by men. It is widely accepted by the theorists in

the field. By contrast, the ethic of *care* is based on a premise of nonviolence: that no one should be harmed or abandoned. This is the path typically followed by women. It is an approach that has been given very little attention in the literature. Distinctions between a justice orientation and a caring orientation are shown in the box on page 47.

Gilligan feels that a blend of justice and care perspectives is necessary for a person to reach maturity. The blending of these two perspectives could give rise to a new view of human development and a better understanding of human relations. To Gilligan, two intersecting dimensions characterize human relationships: equality and attachment. All relationships can be described as unequal or equal and as attached or detached. Most people have been vulnerable both to oppression and to abandonment. Thus, two moral visions—one of justice and one of care—recur in human experience.

Gilligan describes three stages in the process of developing an "ethic of care" (1982, 74). Each stage ends with a transitional period. A *transitional period* is a time when the individual recognizes a conflict or discomfort with some present behavior and considers new approaches.

- *Stage 1. Caring for oneself.* In this first stage of development, the person is concerned only with caring for the self. The individual feels isolated, alone, and unconnected to others. There is no concern or conflict with the needs of others because the self is the most important. The focus of this stage is survival. The end of this stage occurs when the individual begins to view this approach as selfish. At this time, the person also begins to see a need for relationships and connections with other people.
- *Stage 2. Caring for others.* During this stage, the individual recognizes the selfishness of earlier behavior and begins to understand the need for caring relationships with others. Caring relationships bring with them responsibility. The definition of *responsibility* includes self-sacrifice, where "good" is considered to be "caring for others." The individual now approaches relationships with a focus of not hurting others. This approach causes the individual to be more responsive and submissive to others' needs, excluding any thoughts of meeting one's own. A transition occurs when the individual recognizes that this approach can cause difficulties with relationships because of the lack of balance between caring for oneself and caring for others.
- *Stage 3. Caring for oneself and others.* During this last stage, a person sees that there is a need for a balance between caring for others and caring for the self. One's concept of responsibility is now defined as including both responsibility for the self and for other people. In this final stage, care still remains the focus on which decisions are made. However, the person now recognizes the interconnections between the self and others and thus realizes that it is important to take care of one's own needs, because if those needs are not met, other people may also suffer.

Consider . . .

- situations that may arise in health care where the cultural practices of a family conflict with the values of the dominant culture. For instance, child discipline practices that are accepted as appropriate by some may be interpreted as severe or abusive by others. How might the nurse respond to the delimma of mandatory reporting to a child protection agency at each stage or level of Kohlberg's and Gilligan's theories?

Moral Frameworks

Four general moral frameworks are teleology, deontology, intuitionism, and the ethic of caring. **Teleology** looks to the consequences of an action in judging whether that action is right or wrong. **Utilitarianism,** one specific teleologic theory, is summarized in the ideas "the greatest good for the greatest number" and "the end justifies the means."

Deontology proposes that the morality of a decision is not determined by its consequences. It emphasizes duty, rationality, and obedience to rules. For instance, a nurse might believe it is necessary to tell the truth no matter who is hurt. There are many deontologic theories; each justifies the rules of acceptable behavior differently. For example, some state that the rules are known by divine revelation; others refer to a natural law or social contract; still others propose both of these as sources.

The difference between teleology and deontology can be seen when each approach is applied to the issue of abortion. A person taking a teleologic approach might consider that saving the mother's life (the end, or consequence) justifies the abortion (the means, or act). A person taking a deontologic approach might consider any termination of life as a violation of the rule "Do not kill" and, therefore, would not abort the fetus, regardless of the consequences to the mother. It is important to note that the approach, or framework, guides making the moral decision; it does not determine the outcome (e.g., the person taking a teleologic approach might have considered that saving the life of the fetus justified the death of the mother).

A third framework is **intuitionism,** summarized as the notion that people inherently know what is right or wrong; determining what is right is not a matter of rational thought or learning. For example, a nurse inherently knows it is wrong to strike a client; the nurse does not need to be taught this or to reason it out.

Benner and Wrubel (1989) proposed **caring** as the central goal of nursing as well as a basis for nursing ethics. Unlike the preceding theories which are based on the concept of fairness (justice), an ethic of caring is based on relationships. Caring theories stress courage, generosity, commitment, and responsibility. Caring is a force for protecting and enhancing client dignity. Caring is of central importance in the client-nurse relationship. For example, guided by this ethic, nurses use touch and truth-telling to affirm clients as persons rather than objects and to assist them to make choices and find meaning in their illness experiences.

Moral Principles

Moral principles are statements about broad, general philosophic concepts such as autonomy and justice. They provide the foundation for **moral rules,** which are specific prescriptions for actions. For example, "People should not lie" (rule) is based on the moral principle of respect of autonomy for people. Principles are useful in ethical discussions because even people who do not agree on which action to take may be able to agree on the principles that apply. That agreement can serve as the basis for an acceptable solution. For example, most people would agree that nurses are obligated to respect their clients (a principle), even if they disagree about whether a nurse should deceive a client about the client's prognosis (action).

Autonomy refers to the right to make one's own decisions. Respect for autonomy means that nurses recognize the individual's uniqueness, the right to be what that person is, and the right to choose personal goals. People have "inward autonomy" if they have the faculty and ability to make choices. People have "outward autonomy" if their choices are not limited or imposed by others.

Nurses who follow the principle of autonomy respect a client's right to make decisions even when those choices seem not to be in the client's best interest. Respect for people also means treating others with consideration. In a health care setting, this principle is violated when a nurse disregards clients' subjective accounts of their symptoms (e.g., pain). Finally, respect for autonomy means that people should not be treated as "a means to an end"; this principle comes into play, for example, in the requirement that clients give informed consent before tests and procedures are carried out.

Nonmaleficence means the duty to do no harm. This principle is the basis of most codes of nursing ethics. Although this would seem to be a simple principle to follow in nursing practice, in reality it is complex. Harm can mean deliberate harm, risk of harm, and unintentional harm. In nursing, intentional harm is always unacceptable. However, the risk of harm is not always clear. A client may be at risk of harm during a nursing intervention that is intended to be helpful. For example, a client may react adversely to a medication. Sometimes, the degree to which a risk is morally permissible can be in dispute.

Beneficence means "doing good." Nurses are ob-ligated to do good, that is, to implement actions that benefit clients and their support persons. However, in an increasingly technologic health care system, doing good can also pose a risk of doing harm. For example, a nurse may advise a client about an intensive exercise program to improve general health but should not do so if the client is at risk of heart attack.

Justice is often referred to as fairness. Nurses frequently face decisions in which a sense of justice should prevail. For example, a nurse is alone on a hospital unit, and one client arrives to be admitted at the same time another client requires a medication for pain. Instead of running from one client to the other, the nurse weighs the situation and then acts based on the principle of justice.

Fidelity means to be faithful to agreements and responsibilities one has undertaken. Nurses have responsibilities to clients, employers, government, society, the profession, and to themselves. Circumstances often affect which responsibilities take precedence at a particular time.

Veracity refers to telling the truth. Most children are taught always to tell the truth, but for adults, the choice is often less clear. Does a nurse tell the truth when it is known that doing so will cause harm? Does a nurse tell a lie when it is known that the lie will relieve anxiety and fear? Bok (1992) concludes that lying to sick and dying people is rarely justified. The loss of trust in the nurse and the anxiety caused by not knowing the truth, for example, usually outweigh any benefits derived from lying.

ETHICS

The term **ethics** derives from the Greek *ethos*, meaning custom or character. It has several meanings in common usage. First, it refers to a method of inquiry that assists people to understand the morality of human behavior; that is, ethics is the study of morality. When used in this sense, ethics is an activity; it is a way of looking at or investigating certain issues about human behavior. Second, ethics refers to the practices, beliefs, and standards of behavior of a certain group (e.g., physicians' ethics, nursing ethics). These standards are described in the group's code of professional conduct. **Bioethics** is ethics as applied to life (i.e., to life and death decision making). Because of technologic advances, bioethics is receiving increased prominence in literature and discussions. Nursing ethics refers to ethical issues involved in nursing practice.

Nurses are accountable for their ethical conduct. In 1998, the American Nurses Association (ANA) re-

ANA Standards of Professional Performance

STANDARD V: ETHICS
The nurse's decisions and actions on behalf of patients are determined in an ethical manner.

MEASUREMENT CRITERIA
1. The nurse's practice is guided by the *Code for Nurses.*
2. The nurse maintains patient confidentiality within legal and regulatory parameters.
3. The nurse acts as a patient advocate and assists patients in developing skills so they can advocate for themselves.
4. The nurse delivers care in a nonjudgmental and nondiscriminatory manner that is sensitive to patient diversity.
5. The nurse delivers care in a manner that preserves patient autonomy, dignity, and rights.
6. The nurse seeks available resources in formulating ethical decisions.

Source: Standards of Clinical Nursing Practice, 2d ed. American Nurses Association, Washington, D.C., 1998.

vised *Standards of Clinical Nursing Practice.* Professional Performance Standard V relates to ethics; see the accompanying box.

Nurses need to understand their own values related to moral matters and to use ethical reasoning to determine and explain their moral positions. Sometimes it is not enough for nurses to be aware of an ethical issue; they also need moral principles and reasoning skills to explain their position. Otherwise they may give emotional responses, which often are not helpful.

Nursing Codes of Ethics

A **code of ethics** is a formal statement of a group's ideals and values. It is a set of ethical principles that is shared by members of the group, reflects their moral judgments over time, and serves as a standard for their professional actions. Codes of ethics are usually higher than legal standards, and they can never be less than the legal standards of the profession.

International, national, state, and provincial nursing associations have established codes of ethics. The International Council of Nurses (ICN) developed and adopted their first code of ethics in 1953. The ICN Code was revised in 1965 and again in 1973. The ANA first adopted a code of ethics in 1950; it was revised in 1968, 1976, and 1985 and is simply referred to as the *Code for Nurses.* In 1980, the Canadian Nurses Association (CNA) adopted a code of ethics; it was revised in 1991 and 1996. Increasingly, professional nursing associations are taking an active part in improving and enforcing standards. Nurses are responsible for being familiar with the code that governs their practice.

Nursing codes of ethics have the following purposes:

1. To inform the public about the minimum standards of the profession and to help them understand professional nursing conduct
2. To provide a sign of the profession's commitment to the public it serves
3. To outline the major ethical considerations of the profession
4. To provide general guidelines for professional behavior
5. To guide the profession in self-regulation
6. To remind nurses of the special responsibility they assume when caring for clients

Because the wording in a code of ethics is intentionally vague, such codes can serve as general guides. They do not give direction for actions to take in specific cases. For example, the first item in the ANA *Code for Nurses* refers to respect for human dignity and states that in caring for clients, nurses should be "unrestricted by considerations of the nature of health problems." Does that mean that it is wrong for a pregnant nurse to refuse to care for a client with active herpes? Or that it is wrong to refuse to care for a client who uses rude language? When making ethical decisions, nurses should consider their code of ethics together with a more unified ethical theory, ethical principles, and the relevant data about each situation.

Consider . . .

■ a situation in which your personal code of ethics might conflict with the client's. What would guide your practice?

■ how you might support a colleague whose personal code of ethics conflicts with the ANA *Code for Nurses.* How could you help to resolve the conflict?

Types of Ethical Problems

Nurses encounter two broad types of problems: decision-focused problems and action-focused problems. Each requires a different approach (Wilkinson, 1993, p. 4).

In **decision-focused problems,** the difficulty lies in deciding what to do. The question is, What *should* I do? For example:

> Because Leon is committed to the sanctity of life, he wishes his client to have artificial nutrition and hydration. As a nurse, Leon also believes in relieving suffering, so when he sees that the tube-feedings are prolonging the client's pain and even contributing to her discomfort, he wishes to have the feedings discontinued. He is not comfortable with either choice.

In this case, two principles clearly apply, so no matter what the nurse does, an important value must be sacrificed. This is the typical **ethical dilemma** that people commonly refer to as "being between a rock and a hard place." The nature of a dilemma dictates that there are no easy solutions. However, because the difficulty is personal and internal, nurses can address decision-focused problems by learning to make better decisions by, for example, reviewing their own personal value systems, taking advantage of staff development offerings, and attending ethics rounds.

In **action-focused problems,** the difficulty lies not in making the decision, but in implementing it. In these situations, nurses usually feel secure in their judgment about what is right but act on their judgment only at personal risk. The central question is, What *can* I do? or What risks am I willing to take to do what is right? **Moral distress,** one type of action-focused problem, occurs when the nurse knows the right course of action but cannot carry it out because of institutional policies or other constraints (Jameton, 1984, p. 6). This results in feelings of anger, guilt, and loss of integrity on the part of the nurse and can impact client care. For example:

> A resident physician has told the nurses to order complete blood count (CBC) and urinalysis on all clients and to get the results before calling him to the emergency room

to examine the clients. The nurses believe this is unethical because it is wasteful and poses unnecessary discomfort and possible risks for clients. However, they do not have the authority or the access to decision-making channels needed to change the situation. So they order the tests, but they feel guilty and upset because they believe what they are doing is wrong.

Unlike decision-focused problems, action-focused problems cannot be resolved by improving one's decision-making skills. Even after a nurse decides what is *right* to do, the issue becomes what the nurse actually can do given the conditions of practice. Research indicates that nurses' actions are influenced by such constraints as verbal threats, fear of losing their jobs or their nursing licenses, fear of physicians, fear of the law or lawsuits, and lack of support from both peers and administrators (Wilkinson, 1987/88, p. 21). Action-focused problems require knowledge, experience, communication, and the ability to make integrity-preserving compromises. To deal successfully with these problems, nurses must shift their attention away from "making the right decision" and focus on the factors that are preventing the "right action" (Wilkinson, 1993, p. 5).

Conflicts Within Nursing

Ethical conflicts also arise from nurses' unresolved questions about the nature and scope of their practice. High-technology and specialty roles (intensive care nurses, advanced practice nurses) have expanded the scope of nursing practice, often causing nursing and medical activities to overlap. This creates value conflicts for nurses. For example:

■ Although nurses value health promotion and wellness, many still work in hospitals, and many are involved in high-tech treatment of illness.
■ Although the profession values a humanistic, caring approach and emphasizes nurse-client relationships, many nurses spend much of their time attending to the client's machines.

Conflicting Loyalties and Obligations

Because of their unique position in the health care system, nurses experience conflicting loyalties and obligations to clients, families, physicians, employing institutions, and licensing bodies. The client's needs may conflict with institutional policies, physician preferences, needs of the client's family, or even laws of the state. According to the nursing code of ethics, the nurse's first allegiance is to the client. However, it is not always easy to determine which action best serves the client's needs. For instance, a nurse may believe that the client's interests require telling the client a truth that others have been withholding. But this might damage the client-physician relationship, in the long run causing harm to the client rather than the intended good.

Making Ethical Decisions

Responsible ethical reasoning is rational thinking. It is also systematic and based on ethical principles and civil law. It should *not* be based on emotions, intuition, fixed policies, or precedent. (A *precedent* is an earlier similar occurrence. For example, "We have always done it this way" is a statement reflecting a decision based on precedent.)

Catalano (1997) has developed an ethical decision-making algorithm for the nurse. See Figure 4–1. It involves five steps, beginning with the identification of a potential ethical delimma and resulting in either a resolution or a decision to take no action. Many components enter into the decision-making process. These include the following:

- Facts of the specific situation
- Ethical theories and principles
- Nursing codes of ethics
- The client's rights
- Personal values
- Factors that contribute to or hinder one's ability to make or enact a choice, such as cultural values, societal expectations, degree of commitment, lack of time, lack of experience, ignorance or fear of the law, and conflicting loyalties

Ethical decision making that entails a person's choices, values, and actions begins in desire: people are inspired by a desire to pursue the good as they each see it. However, to know that what they are pursuing truly is good, people must rely on reason. Ethical choices, values, and actions then become a *reasoned* desire (Husted and Husted, 1995, pp. 178–183).

Nurses are responsible for deciding on their own actions and for supporting clients who are making ethical decisions or coping with the results of decisions that other people have made. A good decision is one that is in the client's best interest and at the same time preserves the integrity of all involved. Nurses have multiple obligations to balance in moral situations.

An important first step in ethical decision making is to ensure that the problem has ethical or moral content. Not all nursing problems have moral con-

Figure 4–1

Ethical Decision-Making Algorithm.

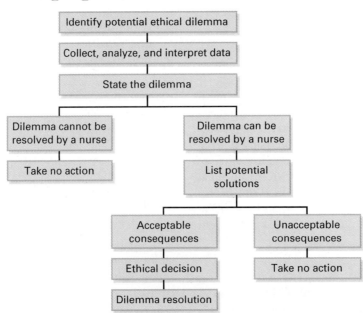

Source: Nursing Now! Today's Issues, Tomorrow's Trends, 2nd ed. by J. T. Catalano. 2000. Philadelphia: F A Davis.

tent. The following criteria may be used to determine whether a moral situation exists (Fry, 1989b, p. 491):

- There is a need to choose between alternative actions that conflict with human needs or the welfare of others.
- The choice to be made is guided by universal moral principles or theories, which can be used to provide some kind of justification for the action.
- The choice is guided by a process of weighing reasons.
- The decision must be freely and consciously chosen.
- The choice is affected by personal feelings and by the particular context of the situation.

In some cases, the most important question is *who* should make the decision. When the decision maker is the client, the nurse functions in a supportive role. Clients need knowledge about the probability and nature of consequences attending various courses of action. Nurses share their special knowledge and expertise with clients to enable them to make informed decisions.

The following questions may help the nurse determine who owns a problem:

- For whom is the decision being made?
- Who should be involved in making the decision, and why?
- What criteria (social, economic, psychologic, physiologic, or legal) should be used in deciding who makes the decision?
- What degree of consent is needed by the subject?

The accompanying box shows an example using a bioethical decision-making model proposed by Cassels and Redman (1989, 465–466).

Because they have ethical obligations to their clients, to the agency that employs them, and to the physician, nurses must weigh competing factors when making ethical decisions. In many health care settings, nurses do not always have the autonomy to act on their moral or ethical choices.

Integrity-preserving moral compromise is the settling of differences in which the conflicting values of all parties are respected and concessions are made. The compromises preserve each person's integrity because no one is forced to give up self-interests, principles, or moral integrity. All parties are encouraged to discuss personal values, their assessment of the situation, and the perceived "best decision" for the client (Fry, 1989a, p. 152). For example, a nurse with a profound moral conviction against abortion might agree to care for an abortion client if there were no other way for the client to receive adequate care (Fry, 1989a,

p. 152). The outcome of integrity-preserving moral compromise is for the parties involved to reach a decision that respects the values held by the decision makers; the outcome does not necessarily fall in line with what any one person thinks ought to be done. Each participant needs to recognize reasonable differences of opinion, see things from others' points of view, and reach an agreement that is mutual and peaceful for all concerned.

According to Winslow and Winslow (1991, 309, 315–320), an integrity-preserving moral compromise is one in which the following elements are present:

1. *Some basic moral language must be shared.* Currently, moral and ethical issues are expressed in the language of client care, client rights, autonomy, and client advocacy. One task of institutional ethics committees is to provide a setting in which a mutual moral language can be built.

2. *A context of mutual respect must exist.* All parties must listen with respect to those with whom they differ. Coercive measures are not used. Without mutual respect, compromise becomes capitulation or persuasion. Everyone's views must be considered.

3. *The moral perplexity of the situation must be honestly acknowledged.* Each person should retain a sense of humility, remembering that there are elements of uncertainty and that he or she could be wrong.

4. *Legitimate limits to compromise must be admitted.* There are times when one cannot compromise. Compromise is more likely when there is factual uncertainty, ambiguity, and an extremely complex situation. The more certain a person is of the facts and the more clearly convinced he or she is about the morality of a course of action, the less room there is for compromise. The limits of compromise are reached when a person is so certain about a particular course of action that to compromise on that point would be to compromise the sense of self as a moral agent.

Specific Ethical Issues

The changing scope of nursing practice has led to an increasing incidence of conflicts between clients' needs and expectations and nurses' professional values. Some of these conflicts center on end-of-life issues, abortion, organ transplantation, and the allocation of health care resources. With the development of sophisticated technology that impacts the course and outcome of illness, nurses and clients face more complex ethical decisions. Because today's public is better

Clinical Application Bioethical Decision-Making Model

SITUATION

Mrs. LaVesque, a 67-year-old woman, is hospitalized with multiple fractures and lacerations caused by an automobile crash. Her husband, who was killed in the crash, was taken to the same hospital. Mrs. LaVesque, who had been driving the automobile, constantly questions Kate Murillo, her primary nurse, about her husband. The surgeon, Dr. Mario Gonzales, has told the nurse not to tell Mrs. LaVesque about the death of her husband; however, he does not give the nurse any reason for these instructions. Ms. Murillo expresses concern to the charge nurse, who says the surgeon's orders must be followed. Ms. Murillo is not comfortable with this and wonders what she should do.

NURSING ACTIONS	CONSIDERATIONS
1. Identify the moral aspects. See the criteria provided on page 55 to determine whether a moral situation exists.	In this situation, the ethical dilemma is either to tell the truth or to withhold it. There is conflict between the values of honesty and loyalty: The primary nurse wants to be honest with Mrs. LaVesque without being disloyal to the surgeon and the charge nurse. Her choice will probably be affected by her concern for Mrs. LaVesque and perhaps by the surgeon's incomplete communication with her.
2. Gather relevant facts related to the issue.	Data should include information about the client's health problems. Determine who is involved, the nature of their involvement, and their motives for acting. In this case, the people involved are the client (who is concerned about her husband), the husband (who is deceased), the surgeon, the charge nurse, and the primary nurse. Motives are not known. Perhaps the nurse wishes to protect her therapeutic relationship with Mrs. LaVesque; possibly the physician believes he is protecting Mrs. LaVesque from psychologic trauma and consequent physical deterioration.
3. Determine ownership of the decision.	In this case, the decision is being made for Mrs. LaVesque. The surgeon obviously believes that he should be the one to decide, and the charge nurse agrees. It would be helpful if caregivers agreed on criteria for deciding who the decision maker should be.
4. Clarify and apply personal values.	We can infer from this situation that Mrs. LaVesque values her husband's welfare, that the charge nurse values policy and procedure, and that Ms. Murillo seems to value a client's right to have information. Ms. Murillo needs to clarify her own and the surgeon's values, as well as confirm the values of Mrs. LaVesque and the charge nurse.
5. Identify ethical theories and principles.	For example, failing to tell Mrs. LaVesque the truth can negate her autonomy. The nurse would uphold the principle of honesty by telling Mrs. LaVesque. The principles of beneficence and nonmaleficence are also involved because of the possible effects of the alternative actions on Mrs. LaVesque's physical and psychologic well-being.

Clinical Application Bioethical Decision-Making Model (cont.)

6. Identify applicable laws or agency policies.

Because Dr. Gonzales simply "gave instructions" rather than an actual order, agency policies might not require Ms. Murillo to do as he says. She should clarify this with the charge nurse. She should also be familiar with the nurse practice act in her state or province.

7. Use competent interdisciplinary resources.

In this case, Ms. Murillo might consult literature to find out whether clients are harmed by receiving bad news when they are injured. She might also consult with the chaplain.

8. Develop alternative actions and project their outcomes on the client and family. Possibly because of the limited time available for ethical deliberations in the clinical setting, nurses tend to identify two opposing, either-or alternatives (e.g., to tell or not to tell) instead of generating multiple options (DeWolf 1989, 80). This creates a dilemma even when none exists.

Two alternative actions, with possible outcomes, follow:
1. Follow the charge nurse's advice and do as the surgeon says. Possible outcomes: (a) Mrs. LaVesque might become increasingly anxious and angry when she finds out that information has been withheld from her; or (b) by waiting until Mrs. LaVesque is stronger to give her the bad news, the health care team avoids harming Mrs. LaVesque's health.
2. Discuss the situation further with the charge nurse and surgeon, pointing out Mrs. LaVesque's right to autonomy and information. Possible outcomes: (a) The surgeon acknowledges Mrs. LaVesque's right to be informed, or (b) he states that Mrs. LaVesque's health is at risk and insists that she not be informed until a later time.

Regardless of whether the action is congruent with Ms. Murillo's personal value system, Mrs. LaVesque's best interests take precedence.

9. Apply nursing codes of ethics to help guide actions. Codes of nursing usually support autonomy and nursing advocacy.

If Ms. Murillo believes strongly that Mrs. LaVesque should hear the truth, then as a client advocate, she should choose to confer again with the charge nurse and surgeon.

10. For each alternative action, identify the risk and seriousness of consequences for the nurse.

If Ms. Murillo tells Mrs. LaVesque the truth without the agreement of the charge nurse and surgeon, she risks the surgeon's anger and a reprimand from the charge nurse. If Ms. Murillo follows the charge nurse's advice, she will receive approval from the charge nurse and surgeon; however, she risks being seen as unassertive, and she violates her personal value of truthfulness. If Ms. Murillo requests a conference, she may gain respect for her assertiveness and professionalism, but she risks the surgeon's annoyance at having his instructions questioned.

11. Participate actively in resolving the issue.

The appropriate degree of nursing input varies with the situation. Sometimes nurses participate in choosing what will be done; sometimes they merely support a client who is making the decision. In this situation, if an action cannot be agreed upon, Ms. Murillo must decide whether this issue is important enough to merit the personal risks involved.

Clinical Application Bioethical Decision-Making Model (cont.)

12. Implement the action.

13. Evaluate the action taken.

Ms. Murillo can begin by asking, "Did I do the right thing?" Involve the client, family, and other health members in the evaluation, if possible. Ms. Murillo can ask herself whether she would make the same decisions again if the situation were repeated. If she is not satisfied, she can review other alternatives and work through the process again.

Source: Model adapted from Preparing students to be moral agents in clinical nursing practice by J. Cassells and B. Redman, *Nursing Clinics of North America* **24** (2):463–473, June 1989.

informed about medical advances and issues, it is important that nurses become comfortable in dealing with clients, families, and peers facing ethical decisions. Nurses are ethically obligated to maintain a nonjudgmental attitude, be honest, and protect the client's right to privacy and confidentiality.

ABORTION Abortion is a highly publicized issue about which many people, including nurses, feel very strongly. Debate continues, pitting the principle of the sanctity of life against the principle of autonomy and the woman's right to control her own body. This is an especially volatile issue because no public consensus has yet been reached.

Most state and provincial laws have provisions known as *conscience clauses* that permit individual physicians and nurses, as well as institutions, to refuse to assist with an abortion if doing so violates their religious or moral principles. However, nurses have no right to impose their values on a client, and nursing codes of ethics support clients' rights to information and counseling regarding abortion. For example, the CNA's *Code of Ethics for Nursing* (1996) states, "Based upon respect for clients and regard for their right to control their own care, nursing care reflects respect for the right of choice held by clients."

END-OF-LIFE ISSUES Advances in health care technology have made it possible to sustain life much longer than previously possible. Some people want everything possible done to maintain life, and others do not. Competent adults have a legal right to refuse or have withdrawn any medical treatment. Often family members of the dying patient cannot make end-of-life decisions or have conflicting desires about the care that should be provided. Advance directives and living wills allow patients to indicate their desires about end-of-life care. A durable power of attorney can designate a decision maker in the event that the patient is unable to make the choice. Information about advance directives are mandated for individuals admitted to health care facilities. Nurses are often called upon to present information and provide explanations.

Active and passive euthanasia are also end-of-life issues. Active euthanasia involves the administration of a lethal agent to end life and alleviate suffering; this approach can result in criminal charges of murder. Passive euthanasia involves the withdrawal of extraordinary means of life support, such as removing ventilator support and withholding resuscitation (DNR orders). The concept of death with dignity and the concerns about quality of life have brought about right-to-die legislative actions. These statutes absolve health care personnel from possible liability when they support a client's wishes not to prolong life. However, these statutes are complex and varied. Nurses are advised to familiarize themselves with the statutes in their particular state or province.

Withdrawing or withholding food and fluids and terminating or withholding treatment present difficult decisions. It is generally accepted that providing food and fluids is part of nursing practice and, therefore, a moral duty. A nurse is morally obligated, however, to withhold food and fluids when it is more harmful to administer them than to withhold them (ANA, 1988a, p. 2). In addition, "It is morally as well as legally permissible for nurses to honor the refusal of food and fluids by competent patients in their care" (ANA, 1988a, p. 3). The *Code for Nurses* supports this statement through the nurse's role as a client advocate and through the moral principle of autonomy.

Clients may specify that they wish to have life-sustaining measures withdrawn, they may have advance directives on this matter, or they may specify a surrogate decision maker. When these decisions are made, the nurse, as the primary caregiver, must ensure that sensitive care and comfort measures are given as the client's illness progresses. A decision to withdraw treatment is not a decision to withdraw care.

ORGAN DONATION Organs for transplantation may come from living donors or from donors who have just died. Ethical issues related to organ transplantation include the allocation of organs, the selling of body parts, the involvement of children as potential donors and recipients, and cloning for the manufacture of organs. Ethical decision making related to these issues is complex. In some situations, religious beliefs may be a source of conflict; for example, the mutilation of the body even for the benefit of another person may be forbidden.

Many people are choosing to become donors by giving consent under the Uniform Anatomical Gift Act. Making these decisions in advance can be helpful. When there is a death due to injury and organs are healthy enough to be harvested, it often falls upon the nurse and other members of the health care team to approach the grieving family about the possibility of organ donation. Many nurses feel uncomfortable about discussing this topic with the family. Some nurses have strong feelings about organ donation that make it difficult to remain neutral when a family faces that decision.

ALLOCATION OF HEALTH RESOURCES Allocation of health care goods and services, including such things as organ transplants, the services of medical specialists, and care involving expensive technology, has become an especially urgent issue as medical costs continue to rise and more stringent cost-containment measures are implemented. For example, decisions about the number of office visits and the length of hospital stay are increasingly being influenced not by medical considerations but by administrative policies of health care facilities and funding entities, such as insurance companies, HMOs, and Medicare. Coverage of some expensive and/or experimental treatments are being denied.

Critics dispute that health care is a scarce resource in North America; instead, they contend that access to health care is limited for segments of the population. Increasing people's access to health care is costly, however, and makes decisions about providing and financing health care difficult. An ethical argument arises as to whether health care is a right or a privilege.

Research Box

Hughes, K. K., and Dvorak, E. M. 1997. The use of decision analysis to examine ethical decision making by critical care nurses. *Heart and Lung* **26(3): 238–248.**

This study was done to examine the extent to which critical care nurses make ethical decisions that coincide with those recommended by a decision analytic model. The nurses completed two instruments, the ethical decision analytic model and a background inventory. The results showed a marked consensus among nurses when they used informal decision making. However, there was little consistency between the nurses' decisions using informal methods and the decisions recommended by the model. Results were unrelated to educational background or years of clinical experience. The authors suggest that more research is needed to clarify the type of decision analysis that is appropriate to a critical care setting.

Catlin, A. J. 1999. Physicians' neonatal resuscitation of extremely low-birth-weight preterm infants. *Image: Journal of Nursing Scholarship* **31(3): 269–275.**

The purpose of the study was to examine the perceptions of physicians who make decisions in the delivery room to resuscitate extremely low-birth-weight (ELBW) infants. Such decisions present ethical dilemmas due to the high incidence of morbidity and mortality. Naturalistic inquiry used interview for data collection. Ninety-six percent of the physicians made the decision to resuscitate and offered the following as factors affecting the decision: (1) training to save lives, (2) inability to determine gestational age, (3) the requests of parents to do everything, and (4) the need to move from the chaotic delivery room environment to the more controlled environment of the NICU. Physicians reported being burdened by these decisions, their inability to predict survival, and conflicts with colleagues over viability. Statistical probability of survival, legal constraints, and cost of care did not appear to affect greatly the decision. The physicians asked that society and national policy makers set parameters for resuscitation. The American Academy of Pediatrics' Neonatal Resuscitation Protocol needs revision to delineate the ethical criteria for resuscitation.

Consider . . .

- whether there should be a level of "essential" care that is provided for all individuals and a higher level that must be financed privately.
- whether preventive care services should receive the same financing as illness services.
- how you would help a client who is contemplating an abortion but has moral distress about doing so. She tells you her boyfriend is strongly opposed to an abortion. She, however, feels she is too young to be a mother but feels guilty about having an abortion.
- your views about organ donation from someone under the age of 18 years.

STRATEGIES TO ENHANCE ETHICAL DECISION MAKING

Rodney and Starzomski (1993, p. 24) and Davis and Aroskar (1991, p. 65) describe several strategies to help nurses overcome possible organizational and social constraints that may hinder the ethical practice of nursing and create moral distress for nurses. These strategies encompass areas of education, administration, practice, and research.

Become aware of one's own values and the ethical aspects of nursing situations. Much of this chapter has been devoted to discussions of nursing values and ethical situations. Most nursing programs include information about these topics at the undergraduate and graduate levels. Continuing education, in the form of inservice programs or other activities, also helps practicing professionals learn more about ethics.

Be familiar with nursing codes of ethics. The content and intent of codes center on supporting nursing practice based on ethical principles.

Understand the values of other health care professionals. An understanding of the values that other health care professionals hold enables nurses to appreciate and respect values, opinions, and responsibilities similar to and different from their own. For example, nurses may find it helpful to know that the American Medical Association considers it morally permissible to refrain from exercising or to discontinue extraordinary efforts to prolong life. In this context, the choice of action is decided on the basis of doing good and avoiding harm.

Some educational institutions now include interdisciplinary ethics education at both undergraduate and graduate levels to enhance the understanding of beliefs, responsibilities, and values among various members of the health care team. For example, nurses and medical students together take classes on bioethics, professional ethics, and business ethics. The goal of this type of interdisciplinary education is to bring about better team communication in the practice setting.

Participate on ethics committees. Because nurses have more contact with the client and family than other members of the health care team, they know the client better and have access to special kinds of information not available to other health care professionals. Nurses offer unique perspectives that can greatly improve the quality of the ethical decisions made in health care settings. One important way for nurses to provide input is to serve on institutional ethics committees. Standards established by the Joint Commission on Accreditation of Healthcare Organizations (JCAHO) support this involvement.

Ethics committees typically review cases, write guidelines and policies, and provide education and counseling. They ensure that relevant facts are brought out; provide a forum in which diverse views, such as views on resource allocation, can be expressed; reduce stress for caregivers; and can reduce legal risks. These factors tend to produce better decisions than would otherwise be made (Hosford, 1986, p. 15).

Institutional policies and guidelines about such issues as informed consent, the withdrawal or withholding of life-sustaining treatment, and do-not-

---

Examples of Nurses' Obligations in Ethical Decisions

- Maximizing the client's well-being
- Balancing the client's need for autonomy with family members' responsibilities for the client's well-being
- Supporting each family member and enhancing the family support system

- Carrying out hospital policies
- Protecting other clients' well-being
- Protecting the nurse's own standards of care

resuscitate (DNR) orders provide direction for all health care practitioners to resolve ethical conflicts. To encourage the most effective functioning, ethics committees need to include representatives of all parties involved—consumers, hospital administrators, nurses, physicians, attorneys, hospital chaplains, social workers, and bioethicists.

Participate in or establish a nursing ethics group. A nursing ethics group can address the specific ethical issues of nursing practice and explore ethical choices nurses consider on a daily basis. Nurses are most commonly involved in issues of client's refusal of treatment, informed consent, discontinuation of life-saving treatment, withholding of information from clients, confidentiality, client competence, and allocation of resources.

Nursing ethics committees can also provide an opportunity for nurse-to-nurse collaboration, facilitating effective cooperation among nurses and increasing nurses' power or capacity to produce change and to implement the care they believe to be most beneficial to their clients. For nurses to act freely as moral agents within any institution, collaboration among and support of peers are essential. Discussions with peers during difficult ethical situations helps to reduce nurses' moral distress.

Participate in or establish educational ethics rounds. Ethics rounds using hypothetical or real cases can be used to explore ethical principles and discuss ethical dilemmas. Ethics rounds incorporate the traditional teaching approach for clinical rounds, but the focus is on the ethical dimensions of client care rather than the client's clinical diagnosis and treatment. Discussions may be held at the bedside, where health care professionals can speak directly to the client. Consent from the client must first be obtained.

Ethics rounds help all those involved to articulate their own views, encourage discussion of value conflicts, and help individuals apply decision-making skills. There are various formats. The clients and issues to be discussed may be presented by staff nurses, advanced nursing students, clinical nurse specialists, or ethics consultants, among others. Rounds serve as examples for future situations the nurse may confront. Each health care facility establishes the format and procedure of ethics rounds to fit its particular situation.

Help to establish an ethical research base. Research is needed to establish effective ways to develop ethical health policies and to evaluate the effectiveness of specific strategies in enhancing the moral agency of health care professionals.

ADVOCACY

An **advocate** is one who pleads the cause of another, and a **client advocate** is an advocate for clients' rights. The origin of the word *advocate* derives from the Latin *advocatus,* meaning "one summoned to give evidence." The focus of the client advocacy role is to respect client decisions and enhance client autonomy. Values basic to client advocacy are shown in the box on page 62.

Levels and Types of Advocacy

Kohnke (1982) identifies three levels of advocacy: (1) advocacy for self, (2) advocacy for the client, and (3) advocacy for the community of which the nurse is a part. Kohnke postulates that one cannot be an advocate for others if one is unable to advocate for oneself. The nurse needs self-knowledge as well as professional knowledge about nursing and health care or needs to know where to obtain such knowledge to assist clients in their decision making. Nurses as knowledgeable professionals have an obligation and a right to share their unique knowledge with the community when needed (Kohnke, 1982, pp. 8–11). Today's health care crises of AIDS, homelessness, teenage pregnancy, child and spouse abuse, drug and alcohol abuse, and increasing health care costs all demand the nurse to fulfill the role of advocate in the community.

Gates (1995, 32) states that advocacy encompasses a range of approaches including legal, self, collective (class), and citizen advocacy. Citizen advocacy may be likened to client advocacy. See Table 4–3.

The Advocate's Role

The primary goal of the client advocate is to protect the rights of clients. The role of client advocate has three major components (Nelson 1988, p. 126): protector of the client's self-determination, mediator, and actor.

As a *protector,* the nurse assists the client to make informed decisions. As a *mediator,* the nurse acts as an intermediary between the client and other people in the environment. As an *actor,* the nurse directly intervenes on the client's behalf.

According to Kohnke (1982, p. 5) the actions of an advocate are to *inform* and *support.* An advocate informs clients about their rights in a situation, and provides them with the information they need to make an informed decision. The first step in informing is to make sure the client agrees to receiving the information. In addition, an advocate must (1) either have the necessary information or know how to get it, (2) want the client to have the information, (3) present informa-

Table 4–3 Types of Advocacy

Type	Description	Example
Legal advocacy	Related to various tribunals and other court case work.	Limited to the work of attorneys or other court-appointed agents.
Self-advocacy	Individual people or groups speaking or acting on behalf of other people on issues that are of mutual interest. Individuals are encouraged to speak for themselves in order to encourage an element of self-empowerment.	Individual clients or family members telling the physician their own requirements related to treatment. Nurses behaving assertively in describing their own needs to administrators.
Collective or class advocacy	Refers to relatively large organizations that pursue the interests of a category of people. Such organizations usually have a national resource that provides full-time officers, as well as volunteers who are able to act as advocates.	American Association for Retired Persons (AARP), National Association for the Advancement of Colored People (NAACP). Professional organizations: American Nurses Association (ANA), Canadian Nurses Association (CNA).
Citizen or client advocacy	Concerned primarily with empowering people through an individual relationship. One person represents, as if they were his or her own, the interests of another person who has needs that are unmet and are likely to remain unmet without special intervention.	Nurse, social worker, court appointed temporary guardian.

tion in a way that is meaningful to the client, and (4) deal with the fact that there may be those who do not wish the client to be informed.

An advocate supports clients in their decisions. Support can involve action or nonaction. An advocate must know how to provide support in an objective manner, being careful not to convey approval or dis-approval of the client's choices. Advocacy involves accepting and respecting the client's right to decide, even if the nurse believes the decision is wrong. As advocates, nurses do not make decisions for clients; clients must make their own decisions freely. For example: After being fully informed about the chemotherapy treatment, the alternative treatments, and the

Nursing Values Basic to Client Advocacy

- The client is a holistic, autonomous being who has the right to make choices and decisions.
- Clients have the right to expect a nurse-client relationship that is based on shared respect, trust, collaboration in solving problems related to health and health care needs, and consideration of their thoughts and feelings.
- Clients are responsible for their health.

- Nurses are responsible for helping clients use their strengths to achieve the highest level of health possible.
- It is the nurse's responsibility to ensure the client has access to health care services that meet health needs.
- The nurse and client are equally able and responsible for the outcomes of care.

possible consequences of the available choices, Mr. Rae decides against further chemotherapy for his cancer. The client advocate supports Mr. Rae in his decision. Underlying client advocacy are the beliefs that individuals have the following rights (Donahue, 1985, p. 1037):

- The right to select values they deem necessary to sustain their lives
- The right to decide which course of action will best achieve the chosen values
- The right to dispose of values in a way they choose without coercion by others

According to Leddy and Pepper (1998), the role of the advocate involves influencing others. Nurses implement the advocacy role in two supportive ways: acting on behalf of the client, and giving the client full or at least mutual responsibility in decision making. An example of acting on behalf of a client is asking a physician to review with the client the reasons for and the expected duration of combined chemotherapy and radiation therapy because the client says he always forgets to ask the physician. An example of mutual responsibility for decision making is nurse-client collaboration in planning an exercise schedule.

There are many occasions when the nurse may speak up for clients. Examples include issues of resuscitation status, inadequate pain control, lack of information, or the client's desire to refuse a treatment. It is often stated that nurses are in a unique position to be client advocates because they spend more time with clients and their families than any other health care professionals. However, a number of challenges face nurses who wish to act as client advocates. To be a client advocate involves the following:

- Being assertive
- Recognizing that the rights and values of their clients and families must take precedence when they conflict with those of health care providers
- Ensuring that clients and families are adequately informed to make decisions about their own health and health care
- Being aware that potential conflicts may arise over issues that require consultation, confrontation, or negotiation between the nurses and administrative personnel or between the nurse and physician
- Working with unfamiliar community agencies or lay practitioners

Advocacy may also require political action—communicating a client's health care needs to government and other officials who have the authority to do something about these needs.

Zusman (1982, 49) offers guidelines characteristic of responsible advocacy. These are shown in the accompanying box. Although Zusman says nurses should "think twice about being a patient advocate," Leddy and Pepper (1998) comment that "the choice of the nurse is not really between being or not being an advocate; rather it is between assuming the advocate role by using a collaborative process or operating as an adversary to those with whom conflict occurs." Collaboration is the obvious choice.

Professional/Public Advocacy

Advocacy is needed for the nursing profession as well as for the public. Gains that nursing makes in developing and improving health policy at the institutional and government levels help both the public and the nursing profession to achieve better health care. Pro-

Bookshelf

Bohjalian, C. 1997. *Midwives.* **New York: Harmony Books.** This book is a novel about a lay midwife accused of killing a patient during a difficult delivery. The story centers around her ethical dilemmas.

Caplan, A. L. 1997. *Am I my brother's keeper? The ethical frontiers of biomedicine.* **Bloomington, Ind.: Indiana University Press.** This book discusses the need for compassion in relation to the needs of others. It suggests that an excessive reliance on defense of rights and adversarial roles means that a moral framework is overlooked.

Hall, M. A. 1997. *Making medical spending decisions: The law, ethics, and economics of rationing mechanisms.* **New York: Oxford University Press.** Difficult questions about allocation of resources and care are analyzed.

Irving, J. 1999. *The cider house rules.* **Ballantine Books.** This is a fictional story of Dr. Wilbur Larch, an obstetrician and founder of an orphanage in rural Maine. Dr. Larch, who is also an ether addict and abortionist, raises an orphan, Homer Wells.

Kidder, R. M. 1996. *How good people make tough choices: Resolving the dilemmas of ethical living.* **New York: Simon and Schuster.** A good book for beginners in ethical analysis, it uses a practical approach.

Reed, D., and Moore, K. 1988. *Deadly medicine.* **New York: St. Martins Press.** This book describes why heart patients died in a disastrous clinical trial of a drug.

fessional advocacy involves the following broad concerns (Leddy and Pepper, 1998):

- Shaping policies aimed at removing financial barriers to health care
- Improving the quality of nursing care available
- Improving nurses' economic rewards
- Expanding nurses' independent roles within the delivery system
- Developing new roles outside the hospital

Nurses who function responsibly as advocates for themselves, their clients, and the community in which they reside are in a position to effect change. To act as an advocate, the nurse needs an objective understanding of the ethical issues in nursing and health care. The nurse also needs knowledge of the laws and regulations that affect nursing practice and the health of society.

Consider . . .

- risks the nurse takes when assuming an advocacy role. What benefits might the nurse realize when acting as an advocate?
- factors that would make the nurse an appropriate or inappropriate advocate for a client. In what situations might you feel personally compromised as the client's advocate?
- what client advocacy needs may be required as a result of changes in technology.
- what societal situations require professional nursing advocacy.

SUMMARY

Values give direction and meaning to life and guide a person's behavior. They are freely chosen, prized and cherished, affirmed to others, and consistently incorporated into one's behavior. Most people derive some values from the society or subgroup of society in which they live. A person may internalize some or all of these values and perceive them as *personal values*. *Professional values* often reflect and expand on personal values. They are acquired during socialization into nursing—from codes of ethics, nursing experiences, teachers, and peers.

Values clarification is a process in which people identify, examine, and develop their own values. Nurses need to help clients clarify their values as they influence and relate to a particular health problem or to end-of-life issues.

Morality refers to what is right and wrong in conduct, character, or attitude—that is, the requirements necessary for people to live together in society. *Moral behavior* is the way a person perceives those requirements and responds to them. *Moral development* is the pattern of change in moral behavior that occurs with age. According to Kohlberg, moral development progresses through three levels: the premoral or preconventional level; the conventional level; and the postconventional, autonomous, or principled level. Each level has two stages. Gilligan describes three stages in the process of developing an "ethic of care": caring for oneself, caring for others, and caring for self and others.

There are four general moral frameworks: teleology, deontology, intuitionism, and caring. Moral principles, such as autonomy, beneficence, nonmaleficence, justice, fidelity, and veracity, are broad, general philosophical concepts. Moral rules, by contrast, are specific prescriptions for actions. Moral issues are those that arouse conscience, are concerned with important values and norms, and evoke words such as *good, bad, right, wrong, should,* and *ought*.

Nursing codes of ethics are formal statements of the profession's ideals and values that serve as a standard for professional actions and inform the public of its commitment.

Ethical problems are created as a result of changes in society, advances in technology, conflicts within the nursing role itself, and nurses' conflicting loyalties and obligations to clients, families, employees, physicians, and other nurses. Decision-focused problems are those in which it is difficult to arrive at a decision; they can be relieved by improving one's decision-making skills. Action-focused problems arise when nurses believe they know the right action but cannot act on their judgment without great personal risk; improved decision-making skills will not relieve the effects of these problems. Nurses's ethical decisions are influenced by their role perceptions, moral theories and principles, nursing codes of ethics, level of cognitive development, and personal and professional values. The goal of ethical reasoning, in the context of nursing, is to reach a mutual, peaceful agreement that is in the best interests of the client; reaching the agreement may require compromise. Integrity-preserving moral compromise requires shared moral language, a context of mutual respect, and acknowledgment of a situation's moral complexity.

In all situations, nurses are ethically obligated to maintain a nonjudgmental attitude, be honest, and protect the client's right of privacy and confidentiality. To enhance their ethical decision making, nurses can gain a better understanding of their own values and those of other health care professionals; participate on ethics committees, nursing ethics groups, and educational rounds; and help establish an ethical research base. Ethics committees are multidisciplinary bodies that review cases, write guidelines and policies, and provide education and counseling.

The focus of client advocacy is to respect client decisions and enhance client autonomy. Its goal is to protect the rights of clients. Various levels and types of client advocacy include advocacy for self, advocacy for the client, and advocacy for the community of which the nurse is a part. Advocacy is also needed for the profession, which benefits not only nursing but also the public. Its goal is to achieve better health care. A number of challenges face nurses who assume the role of client advocacy.

SELECTED REFERENCES

American Nurses Association (ANA). 1985a. *Code for nurses with interpretive statements.* Kansas City, Mo.: ANA.

American Nurses Association. 1985b. *Ethical dilemmas confronting nurses.* Kansas City, Mo.: ANA.

American Nurses Association. 1988a. *Ethics in nursing: Position statements and guidelines.* Kansas City, Mo.: ANA.

American Nurses Association. 1988b. *Nursing and the human immunodeficiency virus: A guide for nursing's response to AIDS.* Kansas City, Mo.: ANA.

American Nurses Association. 1998. *Standards of clinical nursing practice,* 2d ed. Washington, D.C.: ANA.

Bandman, E. L., and Bandman, B. 1995. *Nursing ethics through the life span,* 3d ed. Norwalk, Conn.: Appleton and Lange.

Benner, P., and Wrubel, J. 1989. *The primacy of caring.* Redwood City, Calif.: Addison-Wesley Nursing.

Berkowitz, M. W., and Oser, F. (eds.). 1985. *Moral education: Theory and application.* Hillsdale, N.J.: Lawrence Earlbaum.

Bishop, A., and Scudder, J. 1987, April. Nursing ethics in an age of controversy. *Advances in Nursing Science* 9(3): 34–43.

Bok, S. 1992. *Moral choice in public and private life.* New York: Pantheon Books. As cited in J. R. Ellis and C. L. Hartley, 1992, *Nursing in today's world,* 4th ed. Philadelphia: Lippincott.

Brown, C. 1999. Ethics, policy, and practice: Interview with Emily Friedman. *Image: Journal of Nursing Scholarship* **31**(3): 259–262.

Canadian Nurses' Association (CNA). 1996. *Code of ethics for nursing.* CRNA. Ottawa: CNA.

Cassells, J., and Redman, B. 1989, June. Preparing students to be moral agents in clinical nursing practice. *Nursing Clinics of North America,* **24:** 463–473.

Catalano, J. 1997. Ethical decision making in the critical care patient. *Critical Care Nursing Clinics of North America* **9**(1): 45–52.

Catlin, A. J. 1999. Physician's neonatal resuscitation of extremely low-birth-weight preterm infants. *Image: Journal of Nursing Scholarship,* **31**(3): 269–275.

Colby, A., and Kohlberg, L. 1987. *The measurement of moral judgment: Theoretical foundations and research validation (Vol. 1).* New York: Cambridge University Press.

Corey, G., Corey, M., and Callahan, P. 1984. *Issues and ethics in the helping professions,* 2d ed. Monterey, Calif.: Brooks/Cole.

Curtin, L. L. 1993, Nov. Ethics and economic pressures: A case in point . . . ethics in management. *Nursing Management* **24:** 17–18, 20.

Curtin, L. L. 1994a, Jan. Ethical concerns of nutritional life support. *Nursing Management* **25:** 14–16.

Curtin, L. L. 1994b, Feb. DNR in the OR: Ethical concerns and hospital policies. *Nursing Management* **25:** 29–31.

Czerwinski, B. 1990, June. An autopsy of an ethical dilemma. *Journal of Nursing Administration* **20:** 25–29.

Davis, A., and Aroskar, M. 1991. *Ethical dilemmas and nursing practice,* 3rd ed. Norwalk, Conn.: Appleton and Lange.

Dierckx de Casterle, B., Roelens, A. and Gastmans, C. 1998. An adjusted version of Kohlberg's moral theory: Discussion of its validity for research in nursing ethics. *Journal of Advanced Nursing* **27**(4): 829–835.

Donahue, M. P. 1985 The viewpoints. Euthanasia: An ethical uncertainty, in McClosky, J. C. and Grace, H. K. *Current issues in nursing,* 2nd ed. Boston: Blackwell Scientific Publications.

Duska, R., and Whelan, M. 1975. *Moral development: A guide to Piaget and Kohlberg.* New York: Paulist Press.

Edwards, B. S. 1994, Jan. Ethical issues: When the family can't let go. *American Journal of Nursing* **94:** 52–56.

Eliason, M. J. 1993, Sept./Oct. Ethics and transcultural nursing care. *Nursing Outlook* **41:** 225–228.

Ericksen, J., Rodney, P., and Starzomski, R. 1995, Sept. When is it right to die? *Canadian Nurse* **91:** 29–33.

Erien, J. A. 1994, Feb. Ethical dilemmas in the high-risk nursery: Wilderness experiences. *Journal of Pediatric Nursing* **9:** 21–26.

Fowler, M. D. M., and Levine-Ariff, J. 1987. *Ethics at the bedside*. Philadelphia: Lippincott.

Fry, S. 1989a, May/June. The ethics of compromise. *Nursing Outlook* **37:** 152.

Fry, S. 1989b, June. Teaching ethics in nursing curricula. *Nursing Clinics of North America* **24:** 485–497.

Fry, S. 1989c, July. Toward a theory of nursing. *Advanced Nursing Science* **11:** 9–22.

Gadow, S. 1990. Existential advocacy: Philosophical foundations of nursing. In T. Pence and J. Cantrall (eds.), *Ethics in nursing: An anthology* (pp. 41–51). Pub. no. 20-2294. New York: National League for Nursing.

Gates, B. 1995, Jan 25. Advocacy: Whose best interest? *Nursing Times* **91**(4): 31–32.

Gearhart, S., and Young, S. 1990, April. Intuition, ethical decision making, and the nurse manager. *Health Care Supervisor* **8:** 45–52.

Gibson, C. H. 1993, Dec. Underpinnings of ethical reasoning in nursing. *Journal of Advanced Nursing* **18:** 2003–2007.

Gilligan, C. 1982. *In a different voice*. Cambridge, Mass.: Harvard University Press.

Gilligan, C., and Attanucci, J. 1988, July. Two moral orientations: Gender differences and similarities. *Merrill-Palmer Quarterly* **34**(3): 223–237.

Haddad, A. M. 1993, Fall. Problematic ethical experiences: Stories from nursing practice. *Bioethics Forum* **9:** 5–10.

Haddad, A. 1994, Jan. Acute care decisions: Ethics in action . . . terminally ill patient's pain . . . increased doses of morphine might directly cause the patient's death. *RN* **57:** 20, 22–23.

Hamric, A. B. 1999. Ethics: The nurse as moral agent in modern health care. *Nursing Outlook* **47**(3): 106.

Hawkey, M., and Steel, A. 1994, Sept. 14. Moral decisions. *Nursing Times* **90:** 58–59.

Heubner, A. M., and Garrod, A. C. 1993. Moral reasoning among Tibetian monks: A study of Buddhist adolescents and young adults in Nepal. *Journal of Cross Cultural Psychology* **24**(2): 167–185.

Hosford, B. 1986. *Bioethics committees*. Rockville, Md.: Aspen Publishers.

Hughes, K., and Dvorak, E. 1997. The use of decision analysis to examine ethical decision making by critical care nurses. *Heart and Lung* **26**(3): 238–248.

Husted, G. L., and Husted, J. H. 1995. *Ethical decision-making in nursing*, 2d ed. St. Louis: Mosby-Year Book.

International Council of Nurses. 1973. *ICN code for nurses: Ethical concepts applied to nursing*. Geneva: Imprimeries Populaires.

Jameton, A. 1984. *Nursing practice: The ethical issues*. Upper Saddle River, N.J.: Prentice Hall.

Joint Commission on Accreditation of Healthcare Organizations. 1992. *Accreditation manual for hospitals*. Oakbrook Terrace, Ill.: JCAHO.

Kohnke, M. F. 1982. *Advocacy: Risk and reality*. St. Louis: Mosby.

Leddy, S., and Pepper, J. M. 1998. *Conceptual bases of professional nursing*, 4th ed. Philadelphia: Lippincott.

Lei, T. 1994. Being and becoming moral in a Chinese culture: Unique or universal? *Cross-Cultural Research: The Journal of Comparative Social Science* **28**(1): 59–91.

Mallick, M., and McHale, J. 1995, Jan. 25. Support for advocacy. *Nursing Times* **91**(4): 28–30.

Milholland, D. K. 1994, Feb. Privacy and confidentiality of patient information: Challenges for nursing. *Journal of Nursing Administration* **24:**19–24.

Miller, J. 1994. Cultural diversity in the morality of caring: Individually oriented versus duty-based interpersonal moral codes, *Cross-Cultural Research: The Journal of Comparative Social Science* **28**(1): 3–39.

Milton, C. L. 1999. Ethical issues. Ethical codes and principles: The link to nursing theory. *Nursing Science Quarterly* **12**(4): 290–291.

Miya, P. A. 1994, Jan. Ethical dilemmas: On camera . . . A little white lie. *American Journal of Nursing* **94:** 16.

Moore, S., and Fowler, G. A. 1993, Oct. Twelve nurses tell their ethical stories. *Nursing Management* **24:** 63, 66.

Munhall, P. L. 1982, June. Moral development. A prerequisite. *Journal of Nursing Education* **21:** 11–15.

Nelson, M. L. 1988, May/June. Advocacy in nursing: How has it evolved and what are its implications for practice? *Nursing Outlook* **36**(3): 136–141.

Parker, R. S. 1990, Sept. Nurses stories: The search for a relational ethic of care. *Advances in Nursing Science* **13:** 31–40.

Pearson, C. 1994, April. Facing ethical dilemmas in the neonatal intensive care unit. *Journal of Pediatric Nursing* **9:** 131–132.

Raths, L., M. Harmin, and Simon, S. 1966. Values clarification. In M. D. M. Fowler and J. Levine-Ariff. 1987. *Ethics at the Bedside*. Philadelphia: Lippincott.

Raths, L., Harmin, M., and Simon, S. 1978. *Values and teaching,* 2d ed. Columbus, Ohio: Merrill.

Rich, S. 1995, Jan. 25. Meeting the challenges: Advocacy/ethics. *Nursing Times* **91**(4): 34–35.

Rodney, P., and Starzomski, R. 1993, Oct. Constraints on the moral agency of nurses. *Canadian Nurse* **89:** 23–26.

Rubin, S. B. 1998. *When doctors say no: The battleground of medical futility.* Bloomington, Ind.: Indiana University Press.

Salladay, S. A. 1994a, Aug. H.I.V. Status: Co-worker confidentiality. *Nursing94* **24:** 30.

Salladay, S. A. 1994b, Aug. Organ donation: Family affair. *Nursing94* **24:** 28–29.

Salladay, S. A. 1994c, Sept. Patient self-determination: Assessing competence. *Nursing94* **24:** 22.

Salladay, S. A. 1994d, Nov. Terminal illness: Withholding the truth. *Nursing94* **24:** 30.

Salladay, S. A., and McDonnell, M. M. 1992, Feb. Facing ethical conflicts. *Nursing92* **22:** 44–47.

Savage, T. 1999. Pediatric ethics, issues, and commentary. Ethics, the outpatient pediatric nurse and managed care. *Pediatric Nursing* **25**(2): 197–209.

Steel, A., and Hawkey, M. 1994, Sept. 14. Moral dimensions. *Nursing Times* **90:** 58–59.

Steele, S. M., and Harmon, V. M. 1983. *Values clarification in nursing,* 2d ed. Norwalk, Conn.: Appleton-Century-Crofts.

Stephens, P. 1999. Development of standards for differentiated competencies of the nursing workforce at time of entry/advanced beginner. *Journal of Nursing Education* **38**(7): 298–300.

Sundin-Huard, D., and Fahy, K. 1999. Moral distress, advocacy and burnout: Theorizing the relationships. *International Journal of Nursing Practice* **5**(1): 8–13.

Thompson, J. E., and Thompson, H. O. 1985. *Bioethical decision-making for nurses.* Norwalk, Conn.: Appleton-Century-Crofts.

Thompson, J., and Thompson, H. 1990, June. Moral development. *Neonatal Network* **8:** 77–78.

Tudin, P., Straker, G., and Mendolsohn, M. 1994. Social and political complexity and moral development. *South African Journal of Psychology* **24**(3): 163–168.

Tschudin, V. 1994. *Deciding ethically: A practical approach to nursing challenges.* London: Ballière Tindall.

Uustal, D. 1990, Sept. Enhancing your ethical reasoning. *Critical Care Nursing Clinics of North America* **2:** 437–442.

van Hooft, S. 1990, Feb. Moral education for nursing decisions. *Journal of Advanced Nursing* **15:** 210–215.

Van Weel, H. 1995, Sept. Euthanasia: Mercy, morals and medicine. *Canadian Nurse* **91:** 35–40.

Vergara, M., and Lynn-McHale, D. J. 1995, Nov. Ethical issues. Withdrawing life support: Who decides? *American Journal of Nursing* **95:** 47–49.

Watson, J. 1985. *Nursing: Human science and human care.* Norwalk, Conn.: Appleton-Century-Crofts.

Wilkinson, J. 1993, Jan. All ethics problems are not created equal. *The Kansas Nurse* **68**(1): 4–6.

Winslow, B. J., and Winslow, G. R. 1991, June. Integrity and compromise in nursing ethics. *The Journal of Medicine and Philosophy* **16:** 307–323.

Wurzback, M. E. 1999. The moral metaphors of nursing. *Journal of Advanced Nursing* **30**(1): 94–99.

Zusman, J. 1982, Nov./Dec. Want some good advice? Think twice about being a patient advocate. *Nursing Life* **6:** 49.

Legal Foundations of Professional Nursing

Objectives

- Identify primary sources of law and types of legal actions.

- Describe how nurse practice acts direct nursing.

- Discuss essential legal aspects of malpractice, informed consent, incident reports, DNR orders, euthanasia, and death-related issues.

- Examine the nurse's role in identifying and assisting the chemically impaired nurse.

- Examine the problem of sexual harassment in nursing.

- Consider how the collective bargaining process is used to improve nursing practice.

N U R S E   C O N N E C T

Additional online resources for this chapter can be found on the companion web site at www.prenhall.com/blais.

Knowledge of legal rights and responsibilities related to nursing practice is essential to the nurse.

■ Laws prohibit extremes of behavior so that individuals can live without fear for their person and their property (Hall, 1990, p. 35).

■ In the past, nurses were not considered responsible for their actions. In fact, the hospital, physician, or clinic assumed responsibility for a nurse's actions. However, as nursing practice has become more autonomous, nurses have held increasing responsibility for their actions.

■ Understanding one's own rights and responsibilities as well as those of others is essential for competent and safe nursing practice.

■ In 1938, New York State passed the first nurse practice act. BY 1952, all states had nurse practice acts. Nurse practice acts control the practice of nursing through licensing. They legally define the practice of nursing, thereby describing the scope of nursing and protecting the public. They also set the requirements for licensure, including educational requirements, and they describe the legal titles and abbreviations that a nurse may use.

Standards of practice, codes of ethics, and established laws act as guides for nursing practice. In the nineteenth century, life was fairly simple, and questions were uncomplicated. Medical advances were few. The roles of physicians and nurses were to support patients through times of illness, helping them toward recovery or keeping them comfortable until death (Tappen, Weiss, and Whitehead, 2001). The nurse acted as a caregiver and physician-helper.

CHALLENGES AND OPPORTUNITIES

The latter part of the twentieth century introduced life-saving technology. The creation of critical care units, new surgical techniques for organ transplants and the development of medications to prevent rejection, and the ability to keep individuals alive on life support presented challenges for nurses. These advances led to the development of advance directives, such as living wills, and the creation of health care surrogates. In many situations, nurses needed to act as client advocates.

Scientific development and new technological advances in the 21st century will create situations and questions that may be resolved only in courts of law. Genetic engineering and the identification of disease-carrying genes present problems regarding confidentiality and possible discrimination. As client advocates, nurses find themselves on the frontline in many of these situations. Analysis, discussion, and debate among nurses, other health care providers, and attorneys will take place to develop an understanding and agreement on public policy and laws regarding these scientific advances.

Changes in the health care system have provided new opportunities for nursing. The roles of the advanced practice nurse (APN) and clinical specialist have taken on new dimensions. APNs act as primary care providers in areas such as emergency care, critical care, and community health. Many work as first surgical assistants. With these expanded roles come added responsibilities and legal issues.

Nurses will need to understand the legalities involved with these new technologies to practice safely and effectively. Dock (1907, 896) emphasized, "it is essential that nurses as trained workers exercise social awareness." Scientific achievements have opened up new ground for nursing exploration. Nurses can find career opportunities as forensic nurses, legal nurse consultants, and nurse-attorneys.

THE JUDICIAL SYSTEM

The judicial systems in both the United States and Canada have their origins in the English common law system. Three primary sources of law are constitutions, statutes, and decisions of court (common law).

Constitutions

The constitution of a country constitutes the supreme laws of the country. The Constitution of the United States, for example, establishes the general organization of the federal government, grants certain powers to them, and places limits on what federal and state governments may do. Constitutions create legal rights and responsibilities and are the foundation for a system of justice.

Legislation (Statutes)

Laws enacted by any legislative body are called statutory laws. When federal and state laws (or, in Canada, provincial laws) conflict, federal law supersedes. Likewise, state or provincial laws supersede local laws.

The regulation of nursing is a function of state or provincial law. State or provincial legislatures pass statutes that define and regulate nursing; these statutes are known as nurse practice acts. These acts, however, must be consistent with constitutional and federal provisions. The Patient Self-Determination Act of 1991 enables clients to participate in decisions about their care, including the right to refuse treatment, even if such treatment is necessary to preserve life. This act requires that hospitals and other health care organizations receiving payment through Medicare and Medicaid do the following:

■ Tell clients that they have the right to declare their personal wishes regarding treatment decisions, including the right to refuse medical treatment.
■ Inform the client regarding the hospital's policy on how advance directives are honored.
■ Provide a written statement on the client's chart indicating whether the client has an advance directive. A copy of the advance directive should be included on the client's chart.
■ Provide staff and community education on advance directives.

Nurse practice acts, Good Samaritan laws, and laws regarding spouse or child abuse are other examples of statutes that affect nurses.

Common Law

The body of principles that evolves from court decisions is referred to as common law, or *decisional law.* Common law is continually being adapted and expanded. To arrive at a ruling in a particular case, a court applies the same rules and principles applied in previous, similar cases; this practice is known as following precedent. Courts may depart from precedent when slight differences are noted between cases or when it is thought that a particular common law rule no longer applies to the needs of society.

See Table 5–1 for types of laws that affect nurses.

Types of Legal Actions

There are two kinds of legal actions: civil, or private, actions and criminal actions. Civil actions deal with issues between individuals; for example, a man may file a suit against a person who he believes cheated him. Criminal actions deal with disputes between an individual and the society as a whole; for example, if a man shoots a person, society brings him to trial.

SAFEGUARDING THE PUBLIC

The first laws applicable to nursing in the United States were passed in the 1890s. These were "permissive" laws because they placed no restrictions on nursing practice, stating that the registered nurse (RN) title could be used by individuals who were registered and paid the required fee. By 1923 all states had nurse registration laws.

In 1981 the ANA described nursing practice as in-

Table 5–1 Types of Laws Affecting Nurses

Category	Examples
Constitutional	Due process
	Equal protection
Statutory (legislative)	Nurse practice acts
	Good Samaritan acts
	Child and adult abuse laws
	Living wills
	Sexual harassment laws
	Americans with Disabilities Act
Criminal (public)	Homicide, manslaughter
	Theft
	Arson
	Active euthanasia
	Sexual assault
	Illegal possession of controlled drugs
Contracts (private/civil)	Nurse and client
	Nurse and employer
	Nurse and insurance
	Client and agency
Torts (private/civil)	Negligence
	Libel and slander
	Invasion of privacy
	Assault and battery
	False imprisonment
	Abandonment

cluding but not limited to "administration, teaching, counseling, supervision, delegation, and evaluation of practice and execution of the medical regimen, including the administration of medications and treatments prescribed by any person authorized by state law to prescribe" (ANA, 1981, p. 6).

In 1990, the ANA published *A Guideline for Suggested State Legislation* to help state nurses' associations revise their nurse practice acts. This guide suggests that a nurse practice act contain the following:

■ A distinct differentiation between professional and technical nursing practice
■ Authority for boards of nursing to regulate advanced nursing practice, including the authority to write prescriptions

- Clarification of nurses' responsibilities for supervising and delegating other personnel
- Authority of nursing boards to oversee unlicensed assistive personnel

Nurse practice acts are administered by state boards of nursing by authority of the governor of the state. The boards are appointed by the governor and usually consist of RNs, licensed practical nurses (LPNs), and consumers of nursing. State boards may be independent agencies of the state government or part of a bureau or department, such as the department of licensure and regulation.

State nursing practice acts permit professional nurses to delegate, but they do not permit delegating by licensed vocational/practical nurses. An important aspect of the delegating process is the ethical responsibility of delegatees to refuse any responsibilities for activities that they do not have the expertise to carry out safely and competently. This applies even if hospital policies, physicians, and other nurses request these activities be carried out.

Credentialing is the process of determining and maintaining competence in nursing practice. The credentialing process is one way in which the nursing profession maintains standards of practice and accountability for the educational preparation of its members. Credentialing includes licensure, registration, certification, and accreditation.

Licensure

Licenses are legal permits a government agency grants to individuals to engage in the practice of a profession and to use a particular title. A particular jurisdiction or area is covered by the license.

There are two types of licensure: mandatory and permissive. Under *mandatory licensure,* anyone who practices nursing *must* be licensed. Under *permissive licensure,* the title RN is reserved for licensed or, in Canada, registered practitioners, but the practice of nursing is not prohibited to others who are not licensed or registered. In the United States, nursing licensure is mandatory in all states. In Canada, most provinces and territories have mandatory registration.

In each state there is a mechanism by which licenses (or registration in Canada) can be revoked for just cause, for example, incompetent nursing practice, professional misconduct, or conviction of crime, such as using illegal drugs or selling drugs illegally. In each situation, all the facts are generally reviewed by a committee at a hearing. Nurses are entitled to be represented by legal counsel at such a hearing. If the nurse's license is revoked as a result of the hearing, either the nurse can appeal the decision to a court of law, or, in some states, an agency is designated to review the decision before any court action is initiated.

For advanced nursing practice, many states require a different license or have an additional clause that pertains to actions that may be performed only by nurses with advanced education. For example, an additional license may be required to practice as a nurse midwife, nurse anesthesiologist, or nurse practitioner. The advanced practice nurse also requires a license to be able to prescribe medication or order treatment from physical therapists or other health professionals. There is some controversy about the requirement for additional licensure for advanced practice. The ANA's position is that it is the function of the professional association, not the law, to establish the scope of practice for advanced nursing practice and that the state boards of nursing can regulate advanced nursing practice within each state (ANA, 1993b).

Registration

Registration is the listing of an individual's name and other information on the official roster of a governmental or nongovernmental agency. Nurses who are registered are permitted to use the title "Registered Nurse."

In the United States, all registered nurses are licensed by the board of nursing of the state; in Canada, they are licensed or registered by the provincial nursing association or college of nursing. The requirements for licensure vary by state and province. In the United States, all nursing candidates write the National Council Licensure Examinations (NCLEX) for registered nursing or practical nursing.

Canada has a national comprehensive registered nurse examination, offered in both French and English. Nurses from other countries are granted registration by endorsement after successfully completing these examinations. Both licensure and registration must be renewed on an annual basis (in some states, every two years) to remain valid.

Certification

Certification is the voluntary practice of validating that an individual nurse has met minimum standards of nursing competence in specialty or advanced practice areas, such as maternal-child health, pediatrics, mental health, gerontology, and school nursing. Certification programs are conducted by the ANA and by specialty nursing organizations. In Canada, the Canadian Nurses

Association (CNA) certifies nurses in a number of specialized fields of nursing.

Accreditation

Accreditation is a process by which a voluntary organization, such as the National League for Nursing Accrediting Commission (NLNAC) or the American Association of Colleges of Nursing (AACN), or governmental agency, such as the state board of nursing, appraises and grants accredited status to institutions and/or programs or services that meet predetermined standards and measurement criteria. Minimum standards for basic nursing education programs are established in each state of the United States and in each province in Canada. State accreditation or provincial approval is granted to schools of nursing meeting the minimum criteria.

According to the National League for Nursing Accrediting Commission (1999, 1–2) accreditation provides "assurance that schools and programs meet or exceed agreed upon standards and criteria. . . . Achievement of accreditation indicates to the general public and to the educational community that a nursing program has clear and appropriate educational objectives and is providing the conditions under which its objectives can be fulfilled." The NLNAC provides accreditation for schools of nursing from practical or vocational nursing through master's level nursing education. The American Association of Colleges of Nursing accredits nursing programs at the baccalaureate and master's levels.

Standards of Care

Another way the nursing profession attempts to ensure that its practitioners are competent and safe to practice is through the establishment of standards of practice. These standards are often used to evaluate the quality of care nurses provide. In addition to this basic set of standards, which are applicable in any practice setting, the ANA has developed standards of nursing practice for specific areas such as maternal-child, medical-surgical, geriatric, psychiatric, and community health nursing.

Standards have also been developed for Medicare and Medicaid clients. In addition, the Joint Commission for Accreditation of Healthcare Organizations (JCAHO) has developed accreditation standards that help ensure specific levels of care. In addition, individual health care agencies have developed standard care plans intended to reflect a standard of care. Specific nursing measures that promote safe nursing practice are shown in the accompanying box.

POTENTIAL LIABILITY AREAS

Malpractice

Malpractice refers to the negligent acts of persons engaged in professions or occupations in which highly technical or professional skills are employed. The elements of proof for nursing malpractice are (1) a duty of the nurse to the client to provide care and follow an acceptable standard, (2) a breach of the duty on the part of the nurse, (3) an injury to the client, and (4) a causal relationship between the breach of the duty and the client's subsequent injury. A nurse could be liable for malpractice if the nurse injured a client while performing a procedure differently from the way other nurses would have done it.

Malpractice suits may result from untoward patient outcomes or injury related to patient falls, operating room errors, medication errors, or other negligent acts on the part of the health care provider. "According to

Nursing Measures That Protect Nurses and Clients

- Know your job description.
- Follow the policies and procedures of the agency in which you are employed.
- Always identify clients before implementing nursing activities.
- Report all incidents or accidents involving clients.
- Maintain your clinical competence.
- Know your own strengths and weaknesses.

- Question any order a client questions.
- Question any order if a client's condition has changed since it was written.
- Question and record verbal orders to avoid miscommunication.
- Question standing orders if you are inexperienced in the particular area.

the Institute of Medicine (IOM), 44,000 to 98,000 deaths occur from medical errors each year" (Kohn, 2000). This report suggested a mandatory medical-error-reporting system, including a national patient safety center. The reporting system and safety center would work together to decrease system errors. To create this system, *error* must be defined. The IOM defines error "as the failure of a planned action to be completed as intended or the use of a wrong plan to achieve an aim" (Kohn, 2000). In court, error is not necessarily equated with legal liability. Therefore, an error in judgment may not necessarily have the elements necessary to constitute professional negligence.

Nurses are responsible for their own actions, whether they are independent practitioners or employees of a health agency. The descriptions of malpractice do not mention good intentions; it is not pertinent that the nurse did not intend to be negligent. If a nurse administers an incorrect medication, even in good faith, the fact that the nurse failed to read the label correctly indicates malpractice if all the conditions of negligence are met.

Another significant aspect of malpractice is that it encompasses both omissions and commissions; that is, a nurse can be negligent by forgetting to give a medication as well as by giving the wrong medication.

To avoid charges of malpractice, nurses need to recognize nursing situations in which negligent actions are most likely to occur and to take measures to prevent them. The most common situations are medication errors, burning a client, client falls, and failure to assess and take appropriate action.

Medication errors account for a large number of deaths each year (Kohn, 2000). Many individuals receive either the wrong medication or the right medication but the wrong dosage. Some patients never receive their ordered medication.

Because of the increase in the number of malpractice lawsuits against health professionals, nurses are advised in many areas to carry their own liability insurance. Most hospitals have liability insurance that covers all employees, including all nurses. However, some smaller facilities, such as "walk-in" clinics, may not. Thus the nurse should always check with the employer at the time of hiring to see what coverage the facility provides. A physician or a hospital can be sued because of the negligent conduct of a nurse, and the nurse can also be sued and held liable for negligence or malpractice. Because hospitals have been known to countersue nurses when they have been found negligent and the hospital was required to pay, nurses are advised to provide their own insurance coverage and not rely on hospital-provided insurance.

Liability insurance coverage usually defrays all costs of defending a nurse, including the costs of retaining an attorney. The insurance also covers all costs incurred by the nurse up to the face value of the policy, including a settlement made out of court. In return, the insurance company may have the right to make the decisions about the claim and the settlement.

In the United States, insurance can be obtained through the ANA or private insurance companies; in Canada, it can usually be obtained through provincial nurses' associations. Nursing students in the United States can also obtain insurance through the National Student Nurses Association. In some states, hospitals do not allow nursing students to provide nursing care without liability insurance.

Documentation

The old adage, not documented, not done holds true in nursing. According to the law, if something is not documented, then the responsible party did not do whatever needed to be done. If the nurse did not carry out or complete an activity or documented it incorrectly, he or she is open to a charge of negligence or malpractice. Nursing documentation needs to be legally credible, that is, it must give an accurate accounting of the care the client received. Tappen, Weiss, and Whitehead (2001) assert that documentation is credible when it is the following:

- Contemporaneous—care is documented at the time it is provided.
- Accurate—a factual account is given of what the nurse did and how the client responded.
- Truthful—documentation includes an honest account of what was actually done or observed.
- Appropriate—only what one would be comfortable discussing in a public setting is documented.

The client's medical record is a legal document and can be produced in court as evidence. Often, the record is used to remind a witness of events surrounding a lawsuit, because several months or years usually elapse before the suit goes to trial. The effectiveness of a witness's testimony can depend on the accuracy of such records. Therefore, nurses need to keep accurate and complete records of nursing care provided to clients. Failure to keep proper records can constitute negligence and be the basis for tort liability. Insufficient or inaccurate assessments and documentation can hinder proper diagnosis and treatment and result in injury to the client. The box on page 75 provides guidelines for appropriate documentation.

Guidelines for Documentation

MEDICATIONS

- Always chart the time, route, dose, and response.
- Always chart prn medications and the client response.
- Always chart when a medication was not given, the reason, and the nursing intervention.
- Chart all medication refusals and report them to the appropriate person.

PHYSICIANS

- Document each time a call to a physician is made, even if he or she is not reached. Include the exact time of the call. If the physician is reached, document the details of the message and the physician's response.
- Read verbal orders back to the physician and clarify the client's name on the chart to confirm the client's identity.
- Chart verbal orders only if you have heard them, not those told to you by another nurse or unit personnel.

FORMAL ISSUES IN CHARTING

- Before writing, check to be sure you have the correct client record.
- Check to make sure each page has the client's name and date stamped in the appropriate area.
- If you forget to make an entry, chart "late entry" and place the date and time at the entry.
- Correct all charting mistakes according to the policy and procedures of your institution.
- Chart in an organized fashion following the nursing process.
- Write legibly and concisely avoiding subjective statements.
- Write specific and accurate descriptions.
- When charting a symptom or situation, chart the interventions taken and the client response.
- Document your own observations, not those that were told to you.
- Chart frequently to demonstrate ongoing care, and chart routine activities.
- Chart client and family teaching and the response.

Source: Tappen, R. M., S. A. Weiss, and D. K. Whitehead. *Essentials of Nursing Leadership and Management,* 2d ed. Philadelphia, Pa: F.A. Davis, 2001.

Delegation

The American Nurses Association Code for Nurses (1985a, 10) states, "the nurse exercises informed judgment and uses individual competence and qualifications as criteria in seeking consultation, accepting responsibilities, and delegating nursing activities to others." The nurse is accountable for the care given to his or her clients even if that care has been delegated to a subordinate. In 1990 the National Council of State Boards of Nursing (NCSBN) defined delegation as the

Components of the Delegation Decision-Making Grid

- Level of client acuity
- Level of unlicensed assistive personnel (UAP) capability
- Level of licensed nurse capability
- Possibility for injury

- Number of times the skill has been performed by the UAP
- Level of decision making needed for the activity
- Client's ability for self-care

Source: Adapted from the National Council of Sate Boards of Nursing Delegation Decision-Making Grid. National Council of State Boards of Nursing, Inc., 1997. http//www.ncsbn.com

Research Box

M. K. Anthony, Standing, T., and Hertz, J. E. Factors Influencing Outcomes after Delegation to Unlicensed Assistive Personnel, *Journal of Nursing Administration* **30(10); 474–481, 2000.**

The purpose of the study was to examine factors related to the outcomes of delegated nursing activities. There were four research questions:

1. How do characteristics of the practice setting influence outcomes of delegated nursing activities?

2. How do the educational and experiential backgrounds of licensed nurses and UAPs influence the outcomes of delegated nursing activities?

3. How do factors related to supervision influence outcomes of delegated nursing activities?

4. Is there a pattern among critical factors related to practice, education, supervision, and the outcome of delegated nursing activities?

A cross-sectional sample of 516 licensed nurses (both RNs and LPNs) working in long-term care, home health care, and acute care settings across the United States were sent questionnaires; 148 were returned. The respondents were asked to write about two events of which they had personal knowledge that involved delegation to and supervision of UAPs. One event resulted in a positive outcome and the other had a potential or actual negative outcome. Several questions asking for specific information about the events were included. A chi-square analysis showed no significant differences between patient conditions and positive or negative outcomes. There was no significant difference between positive and negative outcomes and the nurse's educational preparation. The manner in which the UAP was supervised was significantly different between positive and negative events; no direct observation was associated with more negative outcomes. Routine observations resulted in more positive outcomes. The greater the length of time the UAP had worked in the area was also associated with greater frequency of positive outcomes. In the delegation process, outcomes were affected by the experience of the UAP and the supervisory behaviors of the nurse.

"transferring to a competent individual the authority to perform a selected nursing task in a selected situation" (p. 2). This definition was reaffirmed in 1995. To delegate tasks safely, nurses must delegate appropriately and supervise adequately (Barter and Furmidge, 1994).

In 1997, the NCSBN developed a Delegation Decision-Making Grid to help nurses delegate appropriately. The grid provides a scoring instrument for seven categories the nurse should consider when making delegation decisions. The categories for the grid are listed in the box on page 75. The scoring of the components helps the nurse evaluate situations, client needs, and health care personnel available to meet client needs. A low score on the grid states that the activity may be safely delegated to personnel other than the registered nurse, whereas a high score indicates that delegation may not be advisable.

Nurses who delegate tasks to unlicensed assistive personnel should evaluate the activities being considered for delegation (Herrick et al., 1994). The American Association of Critical Care Nurses (AACN) (1990) recommends consideration of five factors affecting the decision to delegate: (1) potential for harm, (2) complexity of task, (3) problem solving and necessary innovation, (4) unpredictability of outcome, and (5) level of interaction with the client required.

It is the responsibility of the nurse to be well acquainted with the state nurse practice acts and regulations issued by the state board of nursing regarding unlicensed assistive personnel. State laws and regulations supersede any publications or opinions set forth by professional organizations.

Informed Consent

Informed consent is an agreement by a client to accept a course of treatment or a procedure after complete information, including the risks of treatment and facts relating to it, has been provided by the physician. Informed consent, then, is an exchange between a client and a physician. Usually, the client signs a form provided by the agency. The form is a record of the informed consent, not the informed consent itself.

Obtaining informed consent for specific medical and surgical treatments is the responsibility of a physician. Although this responsibility is delegated to nurses in some agencies and there are no laws that prohibit the nurses from being part of the information-giving process, the practice nevertheless is highly undesirable (Aiken and Catalano, 1994, p. 104). Often, the nurse's responsibility is to witness the giving of informed consent. This involves the following:

- Witnessing the exchange between the client and the physician
- Establishing that the client really did understand, that is, was really informed
- Witnessing the client's signature

If a nurse witnesses only the client's signature and not the exchange between the client and the physician, the nurse should write "witnessing signature only" on the form. If the nurse finds that the client really does not understand the physician's explanation, then the physician must be notified.

There are three major elements of informed consent:

1. The consent must be given voluntarily.
2. The consent must be given by an individual with the capacity and competence to understand.
3. The client must be given enough information to be the ultimate decision maker.

To give informed consent voluntarily, the client must not feel coerced. Sometimes fear of disapproval by a health professional can be the motivation for giving consent; such consent is not voluntarily given.

To give informed consent, the client must receive sufficient information to make a decision; otherwise, the client's right to decide has been usurped. Information needs to include benefits, risks, and alternative procedures. It is also important that the client understand. Technical words and language barriers can inhibit understanding. If a client cannot read, the consent form must be read to the client before it is signed. If the client does not speak the same language as the health professional who is providing the information, an interpreter must be acquired.

If given sufficient information, the client can make decisions regarding health. To do so, the client must be competent and an adult. A competent adult is a person over 18 years of age who is conscious and oriented. A person under 18 years who is considered "an emancipated minor" (i.e., self-supporting or married) can also give consent. A client who is confused, disoriented, or sedated is not considered functionally competent at that time.

There are three groups of people who cannot provide consent. The first is *minors*. In most areas, a parent or guardian must give consent before minors can obtain treatment. The same is true for adults who are not mentally competent to make decisions for themselves and have a legal guardian. In some states, however, minors are allowed to give consent for such procedures as blood donations, treatment for drug dependence and sexually transmitted disease, and procedures for obstetric care. The second group is *persons who are unconscious or injured* in such a way that they are unable to give consent. In these situations, consent is usually obtained from the closest adult relative if existing statutes permit. In a life-threatening emergency, if consent cannot be obtained from the client or a relative, then the law generally agrees that consent is assumed. This is referred to as implied consent. The third group is *mentally ill persons* who have been judged to be incompetent. State and provincial mental health acts or similar statutes generally provide definitions of mental illness and specify the rights of the mentally ill under the law as well as the rights of the staff caring for such clients.

Incidents and Risk Managment

An incident report is an agency record of an incident or unusual occurrence that is required by JCAHO. Incident reports are used to make all the facts about an unusual occurrence available to agency personnel, to contribute to statistical data about incidents, and to help health personnel prevent future incidents. All incidents are usually reported on incident forms and are

Information to Include in an Incident Report

- Identify the client by name, initials, and hospital or identification number.
- Give the date, time, and place of the incident.
- Describe the facts of the incident. Avoid any conclusions or blame. Describe the incident as you saw it even if your impressions differ from those of others.

- Identify all witnesses to the incident.
- Identify any equipment by number and any medication by name and number.
- Document any circumstance surrounding the incident, for example, that another client was experiencing cardiac arrest.

usually filed with the agency's risk-management department. The box on page 77 lists information to be included in an incident report. The report should be completed as soon as possible, always within 24 hours of the incident, and filed according to agency policy. Because incident reports are not part of the client's medical record, the facts of the incident should also be noted in the medical record. Incident reports are used not only to report incidents related to direct client care, but also to report occupational injuries of employees, such as needle-stick or back injuries, and injuries to visitors to the agency, such as falls.

Incident reports are reviewed by the risk-management department. The purpose of risk management is to "identify risks, control occurrences, prevent damage, and control legal liability" (Huber, 2000, p. 628). The risk-management department decides whether to investigate the incident further. The nurse may be required to answer such questions as what the nurse believes precipitated the incident, how it could have been prevented, and whether any equipment should be adjusted. Nurses who believe they may be dismissed or that a suit may be brought against them should obtain legal advice. Even if the risk-management department clears the nurse of responsibility, the client or the client's family may file suit. The plaintiff, however, bears the burden of proving that the incident occurred because reasonable care was not taken. Even if the accepted standard of care was not met, the plaintiff must prove that the incident was the direct result of failure to meet the acceptable standards of care and that the incident caused physical, emotional, or financial injury.

When an incident occurs, the nurse should first assess the client and intervene to prevent injury. If the client is injured, nurses must take steps to protect the client, themselves, and their employer. Most agencies have policies regarding incidents. It is important to follow these policies and not to assume someone is negligent. Although negligence may be involved, incidents can and do happen even when every precaution has been taken to prevent them.

Wills

A **will** is a declaration by a person about how the person's property is to be disposed of after death. In order for a will to be valid the following conditions must be met:

- The person making the will must be of sound mind, that is, able to understand and retain mentally the general nature and extent of the person's property, the relationship of the beneficiaries and of relatives to whom none of the estate will be left, and the disposition being made of the property. A person, therefore, who is

seriously ill and unable to carry out usual roles may be still able to direct preparation of a will.
- The person must not be unduly influenced by anyone else. Sometimes a client may be persuaded by someone who is close at that particular time to make that person a beneficiary. Clients sometimes are persuaded to leave their estates to persons looking after them rather than to their relatives. Frequently, the relatives contest the will in such situations and take the matter to court, claiming undue influence.

Nurses may be requested from time to time to witness a will, although most agencies have policies that nurses not do so. In most states and provinces, a will must be signed in the presence of two witnesses. In some situations, a mark can suffice if the person making the will cannot write a signature. When witnessing a will, the nurse (1) attests that the client signed a document that is stated to be the client's last will and (2) attests that the client appears to be mentally sound and appreciates the significance of their actions (Bernzweig, 1996).

If a nurse witnesses a will, the nurse should note on the client's chart the fact that a will was made and the nurse's perception of the physical and mental condition of the client. This record provides the nurse with accurate information if the nurse is called as a witness later. The record may also be helpful if the will is contested. If a nurse does not wish to act as a witness—for example, if in the nurse's opinion undue influence has been brought on the client—then it is the nurse's right to refuse to act in this capacity.

Do-Not-Resuscitate Orders

Physicians may order "no code" or **do-not-resuscitate (DNR)** for clients who are in a stage of terminal, irreversible illness or expected death. DNR orders require that no effort be made to resuscitate the client in the event of a respiratory or cardiac arrest. The ANA believes that "the appropriate use of DNR orders can prevent suffering for many clients who choose not to extend their lives after experiencing cardiac arrest" (ANA, 1992a, p. 2). The ANA makes the following recommendations related to DNR orders:

- The competent client's values and choices should always be given highest priority, even when these wishes conflict with those of the family or health care providers.
- When the client is incompetent, an advance directive or the surrogate decision makers acting for the client should make health care treatment decisions.
- A DNR decision should always be the subject of explicit discussion between the client, family, any designated surrogate decision maker acting on the client's behalf, and the health care team.

- DNR orders must be clearly documented, reviewed, and updated periodically to reflect changes in the client's condition. Such documentation is required to meet standards of the Joint Commission on Accreditation of Healthcare Organizations (JCAHO, 1996).

- A DNR order is separate from other aspects of a client's care and does not imply that other types of care should be withdrawn, for example, nursing care to ensure comfort or medical treatment for chronic but non-life-threatening illnesses.

- If it is contrary to a nurse's personal beliefs to carry out a DNR order, the nurse should consult the nurse-manager for a change in assignment.

The ANA also recommends that each health care organization put into place mechanisms to resolve conflicts between clients, their families, and health care professionals, or between different health care professionals. Institutional ethics committees usually deal with such conflicts. It is important that nurses be represented on these institutional ethics committees, so that nursing perspectives can be heard and nurses can be involved in developing DNR policies.

Advance Medical Directives

An **advance medical directive** is a statement the client makes prior to receiving health care, specifying the client's wishes regarding health care decisions. There are three types of advance medical directives, the **living will,** the **health care proxy** or **surrogate,** and the **durable power of attorney for health care.** The living will states what medical treatment the client chooses to omit or refuse in the event that the client is unable to make those decisions and is terminally ill. For example, the client can indicate a wish not to be kept alive by artificial means such as cardiopulmonary resuscitation (CPR), respiratory ventilation, or tube feeding. With a health care proxy, the client appoints a proxy, usually a relative or trusted friend, to make medical decisions on the client's behalf in the event that the client is unable to do so. The health care proxy is not limited to terminal situations but can apply to any illness or injury in which the client is incapacitated. A durable power of attorney is a notarized statement appointing someone else to manage health care treatment decisions when the client is unable to do so.

The specific requirements of advance medical directives are directed by individual state legislation. In most states, advance directives must be witnessed by two people but do not require review by an attorney. Some states do not permit relatives, heirs, or physicians to witness advance directives.

The ANA (1991) supports the client's right to self-determination and believes that nurses must play a primary role in implementation of the law. The nurse is often the facilitator of discussions between clients and their families about health care and end-of-life decisions. The ANA recommends that the following questions be part of the nursing admission assessment regarding advance directives:

- Does the client have basic information about advance care directives, including living wills and durable power of attorney?
- Does the client wish to initiate an advance care directive?
- If the client has prepared an advance care directive, did the client bring it to the health care agency?
- Has the client discussed end-of-life-choices with the family and/or designated surrogate, physician, or other health care team worker?

Nurses should learn the law regarding client self-determination for the state in which they practice, as well as the policy and procedures for implementation in the institution where they work.

Euthanasia

Euthanasia is the act of painlessly putting to death persons suffering from incurable or distressing disease. It is commonly referred to as "mercy killing." Regardless of compassion and good intentions or moral convictions, euthanasia is *legally wrong* in both Canada and the United States and can lead to criminal charges of homicide or to a civil lawsuit for withholding treatment or providing an unacceptable standard of care. Because advanced technology has enabled the medical profession to sustain life almost indefinitely, people are increasingly considering the meaning of quality of life. For some people, the withholding of artificial life-support measures or even the withdrawal of life support is a desired and acceptable practice for clients who are terminally ill or who are incurably disabled and believed unable to live their lives with some happiness and meaning.

Voluntary euthanasia refers to situations in which the dying individual desires some control over the time and manner of death. All forms of euthanasia are illegal except in states where right-to-die statutes and living wills exist. Currently, the legality of assisted suicide in the United States is being tested in the court of law. Right-to-die statutes legally recognize the client's right to refuse treatment.

In 1994, Oregon approved the first physician-assisted suicide law in the United States. This law permits physicians to prescribe lethal doses of medications.

The Oregon Death with Dignity Act was challenged in court and was not finally enacted until November 1997 (Kirk, 1998). Since the enactment of Oregon's law, several other states have proposed similar laws. Right-to-die statutes legally acknowledge a client's right to refuse treatment.

Death and Related Issues

Legal issues surrounding death include issuing the death certificate, labeling of the deceased, autopsy, organ donation, and inquest. By law, a death certificate must be made out when a person dies. It is usually signed by the attending physician and filed with a local health or other government office. The family is usually given a copy to use for legal matters, such as insurance claims.

Nurses have a duty to handle the deceased with dignity and label the corpse appropriately. Mishandling can cause emotional distress to survivors. Mislabeling can create legal problems if the body is inappropriately identified and prepared incorrectly for burial or a funeral. Usually, the deceased's wrist identification tag is left on, and another tag is tied to the client's ankles, in case one of the tags becomes detached. Tags tied to the ankles are preferred, because any tissue damage they cause will be concealed by bed linen or clothing. A third tag is attached to the shroud. All identification tags should include the client's name, hospital number, and physician's name.

An **autopsy,** or **postmortem examination,** is an examination of the body after death. It is performed only in certain cases. The law describes under what circumstances an autopsy must be performed, for example, when death is sudden or occurs within 48 hours of admission to a hospital. The organs and tissues of the body are examined to establish the exact cause of death, to learn more about a disease, and to assist in the accumulation of statistical data.

It is the responsibility of the physician or, in some instances, of a designated person in the hospital to obtain consent for autopsy. Consent must be given by the decedent (before death) or by the next of kin. Laws in many states and provinces prioritize the family members who can provide consent as follows: surviving spouse, adult children, parents, siblings. After autopsy, hospitals cannot retain any tissues or organs without the permission of the person who consented to the autopsy.

Organ Donation

Under the Uniform Anatomical Gift Act in the United States or the Human Tissue Act in Canada, any person 18 years or older and of sound mind may make a gift of all or any part of the body for the following purposes: for medical or dental education, research, advancement of medical or dental science, therapy, or transplantation. The donation can be made by a provision in a will or by signing a cardlike form in the presence of two witnesses. This card is usually carried at all times by the person who signed it. In most states and provinces, the gift can be revoked, either by destroying the card or by revoking the gift orally in the presence of two witnesses. Nurses may serve as witnesses for persons consenting to donate organs. In some states health care workers are required to ask survivors for consent to donate the deceased's organs.

Inquest

An **inquest** is a legal inquiry into the cause or manner of a death. When a death is the result of a motor-vehicle crash, for example, an inquest is held into the circumstances of the crash to determine any blame. The inquest is conducted under the jurisdiction of a coroner or medical examiner. A *coroner* is a public official, not necessarily a physician, appointed or elected to inquire into the causes of death, when appropriate. A *medical examiner* is a physician who usually has advanced education in pathology or forensic medicine. Agency policy dictates who is responsible for reporting deaths to the coroner or medical examiner.

THE IMPAIRED NURSE

An impaired nurse is one whose practice has deteriorated because of substance abuse, specifically the use of alcohol and/or drugs. Chemical dependence in health care workers has become a problem because of the high levels of stress involved in many health care settings and the easy access to addictive drugs. In addition to substance abuse, mental illnesses such as depression or secondary posttraumatic stress disorder may also affect the nurse's ability to deliver safe, competent care (Tappen, Weiss, and Whitehead, 2001).

Impaired nurses adversely affect client care, staff retention, and morale (Damrosch and Scholler-Jacquish, 1993). There are three victims of the nurse who is impaired: the client, whose care may be compromised by the nurse whose judgment and skills are impaired, the colleagues, who must pick up after the impaired worker, and the impaired nurse, whose illness may go undetected and untreated for years. The primary concern is for the protection of clients, but it is also critically important that the nurse's problem be identified quickly so that appropriate treatment can be instituted. In 1981 the ANA appointed a task force on

Behavioral Indicators of Chemical Abuse

- Increasing isolation from colleagues, friends, and family
- Frequent reports or illness, minor accidents, and emergencies
- Complaints about poor work performance
- Inability to meet schedules and deadlines
- Tendency to avoid new and challenging assignments
- Mood swings, irritability, and depression
- Request for night shifts

- Social avoidance of staff
- Illogical and sloppy charting
- Excessive errors
- Increasing carelessness about personal appearance
- Medication "errors" that require many changes in charting
- Arriving on duty early or staying late for no reason
- Volunteering to administer client medications, especially pain medications

addiction and psychological disturbance to develop guidelines for identifying, treating, and assisting nurses impaired by alcohol or drug abuse or psychologic disturbance. The accompanying box lists behaviors that may be seen in the impaired nurse.

Several programs have been developed to assist impaired nurses to recovery. In many states, impaired nurses who enter an intervention program for treatment do not have their nursing license revoked, but their practice is closely supervised within the limitations placed by the intervention program.

SEXUAL HARASSMENT

Sexual harassment is a violation of the individual's rights and a form of discrimination. The Equal Employment Opportunity Commission (EEOC) defines sexual harassment as "unwelcome sexual advances, requests for sexual favors, and other verbal or physical conduct of a sexual nature" occurring in the following circumstances (EEOC, 1980, sections 3950.10–3950.11):

- When submission to such conduct is considered, either explicitly or implicitly, a condition of an individual's employment
- When submission to or rejection of such conduct is used as the basis for employment decisions affecting the individual
- When such conduct interferes with an individual's work performance or creates an "intimidating, hostile, or offensive working environment"

In 1993, the Supreme Court determined that a plaintiff is not required to prove any psychological injury to establish a harassment claim. A proven hostile or abusive environment was sufficient for a claim.

In health care, both clients and health care professionals may experience sexual harassment. Because sexual harassment is generally related to a power imbalance, female nurses are more likely to experience sexual harassment from male physicians or administrators. Nurses may report having been "sexually propositioned," "suggestively touched," or "sexually insulted" by physicians during their career. Such behavior is considered sexual harrassment and can negatively affect client care. For example, to avoid uncomfortable situations, the nurse may refuse to care for the clients of a particular offensive physician or work on a unit with an offensive administrator, or the nurse may avoid calling a physician to report changes in client status or to suggest changes to improve client care.

The victim of the harasser may be male or female. The victim does not have to be of the opposite sex. Moreover, the victim does not have to be the person harassed; anyone who is affected by the offensive conduct may be considered a victim (ANA, 1992b, p. 2). Nurses must be familiar with the sexual harassment policy and procedures in their employing agency. Many organizations provide educational programs to provide information about sexual harassment, including what incidents are considered sexual harassment and how to prevent them. They also review sexual harassment policies and procedures, including grievance procedures, determine to whom incidents should be reported, and provide the process for resolution. See the box on page 82 for strategies to deter sexual harassment.

Strategies to Deter Sexual Harrassment

- Confront the harasser, repeatedly if necessary, and clearly ask that the behavior stop.
- Report the harassment to authorities, using the "chain of command" and whatever formal complaint channels are available.

- Document the harassment, recording in detail the "who," "what," "where," and "when" of the situation and how you responded. Include witnesses if any.
- Seek support from others, such as friends, colleagues, relatives or an organized support group.

Source: Reprinted with permission from *Sexual Harrassment: It's Against the Law,* © 1992 American Nurses Association, Washington, D.C.

NURSES AS WITNESSES

A nurse may be called to testify in a legal action for a variety of reasons. The nurse may be a defendant in a malpractice or negligence action or may have been a health professional that provided care to the plaintiff. It is advisable that any nurse who is asked to testify in such a situation seek the advice of an attorney before providing testimony. In most cases, the attorney for the institution will provide support and counsel during the legal case. If the nurse is the defendant, however, it is advisable for the nurse to retain an attorney to protect the nurse's own interests.

A nurse may also be asked to provide testimony as an expert witness. An **expert witness** is one who has special training, experience, or skill in a relevant area and who is allowed by the court to offer an opinion on some issue within the nurse's area of expertise (Bernzweig, 1996). Such a witness is usually called to help a judge or jury understand evidence pertaining to the extent of damage and the standard of care.

When called into court as a witness, the nurse has a duty to assist justice as far as possible. The nurse should always respond directly and truthfully to the questions asked. The nurse is not expected to volunteer additional information, nor is the nurse expected to remember completely all the details of a situation that may have occurred months or even years prior to the legal action. The nurse may ask to refer to the client record or to personal notes related to the incident. If the nurse does not remember the details of the incident, it is advisable to say so rather than to report an inaccurate recollection. In any case, it is the nurse's professional responsibility to provide accurate testimony, both during the pretrial discovery phase and the trial phase of a legal action.

Consider . . .

■ being called as a witness in a malpractice case. The incident occurred more than three years ago. The case is against the health care institution and a nurse whom you know was overtly negligent. This negligence resulted in harm to the client in question. On several previous occasions you observed the nurse violating standards of care. You reported these incidents to the administration. At the time of the incident in question, you kept personal anecdotal notes because you were concerned about a possible lawsuit in the future. You are still an employee of the health care institution involved. You are asked if you have ever witnessed other incidents of negligence performed by this nurse and, if so, what you did. What is your responsibility to your employer, the nurse being sued, the client in question, and the institution's clients? What do you do? To whom is your obligation?

COLLECTIVE BARGAINING

Collective bargaining is the formalized decision-making process between representatives of management and representatives of labor to negotiate wages and conditions of employment, including work hours, working environment, and fringe benefits of employment (e.g., vacation time, sick leave, and personal leave). Through a written agreement, both employer and employees legally commit themselves to observe the terms and conditions of employment. Collective bargaining is a controversial issue among nurses. Some nurses consider collective bargaining to be unprofessional and contrary to the altruistic nature of nursing. Others argue that collective bargaining is necessary to obtain control of nursing practice and economic security.

The collective bargaining process involves the recognition of a certified bargaining agent for the employees. This agent can be a union, a trade association, or a professional organization. The agent represents the employees in negotiating a contract with management.

In the 1930s, the National Labor Relations Act (NLRA) established the regulation of collective bargaining. In nursing, the NLRA provides guidelines for the resolution of conflicts between nurse employees and their employers. Nurses who are supervisors are not covered by the NLRA. There is still debate regarding whether all nurses who oversee the nursing care provided by other nurses, such as team leaders, are supervisors as defined by the NLRA (Brent, 1997).

In 1999 the American Nurses Association established the United American Nurses as the labor union for registered nurses in the United States. As a subsidiary of the American Nurses Association, the UAN is the largest labor union for registered nurses in the country (UAN, 2000). Examples of resolutions approved at the 2000 National Labor Assembly included "Documenting the Relationship Between Working Conditions Related to Patient Safety and Working Conditions Related to Nurses' Safety," "Emergency Action to Prevent Musculoskeletal Disorders," and "Preventing Violence in the Healthcare Workplace."

When collective bargaining breaks down because an agreement cannot be reached, the employees usually call a strike. A **strike** is an organized work stoppage by a group of employees to express a grievance, enforce a demand for changes in conditions of employment, or solve a dispute with management.

Because nursing practice is a service to people (often ill people), striking presents a moral dilemma to many nurses. Actions taken by nurses can affect the safety of people. When faced with a strike, each nurse must make an individual decision to cross or not to cross a picket line. Nursing students may also be faced with decisions about crossing picket lines in the event of a strike at a clinical agency used for learning experiences. The ANA supports striking as a means of achieving economic and general welfare.

Collective bargaining is more than the negotiating of salary terms and hours of work; it is a continuous process in which day-to-day working problems and relationships can be handled in an orderly and democratic manner. Day-to-day difficulties or grievances are handled through the grievance procedure, a formal plan established in the contract that outlines the channels for handling and settling grievances through progressively higher levels of administration. A grievance is any dispute, difference, controversy, or disagreement arising out of the terms and conditions of employment. Grievances fall into four main categories, outlined in Table 5–2.

Consider . . . .

■ what would happen if your workplace downsized and closed several units. The administration is requesting nurses to take leave days without pay when the census drops. At the same time, administration is asking nurses to work 4 to 6 hours overtime to cover units

Table 5–2 Categories and Examples of Grievances

Category	Examples
Contract violations	Shift or weekend work is assigned inequitably. A nurse is dismissed without cause.
Violations of federal and state law	A female nurse is paid less than a male nurse for the same work. Appropriate payment is not given for overtime work. Minority group nurses are not promoted.
Management responsibilities	Appropriate locker room facilities are not provided. Safe client care is jeopardized by inadequate staffing.
Violation of agency rules	Performance evaluations are conducted only at termination of employment, but the contract requires annual evaluations. A vacation period is assigned without the nurse's agreement, as required in personnel policies.

Source: The Grievance Procedure, American Nurses Association, Kansas City, Mo.: ANA, 1985, pp. 2–4. Used by permission.

when staffing is inadequate. Nurses are also being floated to areas where they have no expertise. The nurses want to organize for collective bargaining. What is your position? What can be gained by organizing? Are there disadvantages to organizing in a union?

- health care settings where nurses choose not to organize for collective bargaining. What are the characteristics of these employment settings?
- health care settings where nurses choose to organize for collective bargaining. What are the characteristics of these employment settings?

Bookshelf

Cook, Robin. 1990. *Harmful intent.* **New York: J. P. Putnam**

The ethical principle do no harm guides medical and nursing practice. In this fictional novel, a mother dies during delivery and the baby is born with brain damage. The anesthesiologist is blamed and charged with malpractice. He believes that he did nothing wrong. The author blends legal and medical issues together in this medical mystery.

Cook, Robin. 1995. *Acceptable risk.* **New York: J. P. Putnam**

The use of personality-altering drugs raises complex moral and legal issues, particularly pertaining to research and informed consent. The enormous profits available from marketing these drugs acts as a strong motivator for both the pharmaceutical companies and the researchers. In this novel, the author describes how far an individual and the medical community will go regarding testing and marketing.

Levy, H. 1999. *Chain of custody.* **New York: Random House**

When a highly respected deputy district attorney is found murdered, her physician husband becomes suspect. Forensic evidence connects him to the crime scene. The author pursues the legal issues regarding forensic evidence discovered at crime scenes and how such evidence is used to confirm the guilt or innocence of an individual.

SUMMARY

Accountability is an essential concept of professional nursing practice under the law. Nurses need to understand laws that regulate and affect practice to ensure that their actions are consistent with current legal principles and to protect themselves from liability. Nurse practice acts legally define and describe the scope of nursing practice that the law seeks to regulate. Competence in nursing practice is determined and maintained by various credentialing methods, such as licensure, registration, certification, and accreditation, which protect the public's welfare and safety. Standards of practice published by national and state or provincial nursing associations and agency policies, procedures, and job descriptions further delineate the scope of a nurse's practice.

Negligence or malpractice of nurses can be established when (1) the nurse (defendant) owed a duty to the client, (2) the nurse failed to carry out that duty, (3) the client (plaintiff) was injured, and (4) the client's injury was caused by the nurse's failure to carry out that duty. When a client is injured or involved in an unusual incident, the nurse's first responsibility is to take steps to protect the client and then to notify appropriate agency personnel.

The nurse is responsible for ensuring that informed consent from clients (or from the closest relative in emergencies or from parents or guardians when the client is a minor) are in the medical record before treatment regimens and procedures begin. Informed consent implies that (1) the consent was given voluntarily; (2) the client was of age and had the capacity and competence to understand; and (3) the client was given enough information on which to make an informed decision.

Nurses must be knowledgeable about their responsibilities in regard to legal issues surrounding death: ensuring completion of the death certificate, labeling of the deceased, autopsy, organ donation, and inquest. Physicians may order no-code or do-not-resuscitate (DNR) for clients who are in a stage of terminal, irreversible illness or expected death. Nurses need to know their responsibility to clients who have a DNR order.

Nurses need to be aware of their responsibility when identifying a colleague who is impaired. Nurses also need to know the legal protections available for them when confronted with sexual harassment. Nurses may be called as witnesses for a variety of reasons. When called as a witness, a nurse has a duty to assist justice. Nurses also must be knowledgeable about collective bargaining as a means of ensuring just compensation, including wages and benefits and a safe and positive work environment.

SELECTED REFERENCES

Aiken, T. D., and Catalano, J. T. 1994. *Legal, ethical, and political issues in nursing.* Philadelphia: F. A. Davis.

American Association of Critical Care Nurses. 1990. *Delegation of nursing and non-nursing activities in critical care: A framework for decision-making.* Irvine, Calif.: AACN.

American Nurses Association. 1981. The Nursing Practice Act: Suggested state legislation. Kansas City, Mo.: ANA.

American Nurses Association. 1985a. *The code for nurses.* Kansas City, Mo.: ANA.

American Nurses Association. 1985b. *The grievance procedure.* Kansas City, Mo.: ANA.

American Nurses Association. 1990. *A guideline for suggested state legislation.* Kansas City, Mo.: ANA.

American Nurses Association. 1991. Position statement on nursing and the Patient Self-Determination Act. Washington, D.C.: ANA.

American Nurses Association. 1992a. Position statement on nursing care and do-not-resuscitate decisions. Washington, D.C.: ANA.

American Nurses Association. 1992b. Report to the Constituent Assembly on Sexual Harassment in the Workplace. Washington, D.C.: ANA.

American Nurses Association. 1993a. *Sexual harassment: It's against the law.* Washington, D.C.: ANA.

American Nurses Association. 1993b. Regulation of advanced nursing practice. In *Summary of Proceedings, 1993, House of Delegates.* Washington, D.C.: ANA.

American Nurses Association. 1995. *Registered professional nurses and unlicensed assistive personnel.* Washington, D.C.: ANA.

Barter, M., and Furmidge, M. L. 1994. Unlicensed assistive personnel: Issues relating to delegation and supervision. *Journal of Nursing Administration* **24:** 36–43.

Bernzweig, E. P. 1996. *The nurse's liability for malpractice: A programmed course,* 6th ed. St. Louis: Mosby.

Brent, N. J. 1997. *Nurses and the law.* Philadelphia: Saunders.

Damsrosch, S., and Scholler-Jaquish, A. 1993. Nurses' experiences with impaired coworkers. *Applied Nursing Research* **6** (4): 154–160.

Diaz, A. L., and McMillin, F. D. 1991, Feb. A definition and description of nurse abuse. *Western Journal of Nursing Research* **13:** 97–109.

Dock, L. L. 1900. What we may expect from the law. *American Journal of Nursing* **1**(1): 8–12.

Dock, L. L. 1907. Some urgent social claims. *American Journal of Nursing* **7**(11): 895–911.

Equal Employment Opportunity Commission. 1980. Sex discrimination guideline. In *EEOC Rules and Regulations.* Chicago: Commerce Clearing House.

Hall, J. K. 1990, Oct. Understanding the fine line between law and ethics. *Nursing* **90** (20): 34–39.

Herrick, K., Hansten, R., O'Neill, L., Hayes, P., and Washburn, M. 1994. My license is on the line: The art of delegation. *Nursing Management* **25**(2), 48–50.

Huber, D. 2000. *Leadership and nursing care management,* 2nd edition. Philadelphia: Saunders.

Joint Commission on the Accreditation of Healthcare Organizations. 1996. *1997 accreditation manual for hospitals.* Oak Bluffs Terrace, Ill.: JCAHO.

Kirk, K. 1998. How Oregon's Death with Dignity Act affects practice. *American Journal of Nursing* **98** (8): 54–55.

Kohn, L. T. 2000. *To err is human: Building a safer health system.* Washington, D.C.: National Academy Press.

Lee, N. G. 2000. Proving nursing negligence. *American Journal of Nursing* **7** (11), 55–56.

National Council of State Boards of Nursing. 1995. *Delegation Concepts and Decision Making Process.* National Council Position Paper. NCSBN. http://ncsbn.org/files/publications/positions/delegati.asp

National Council of State Boards of Nursing. 1997. *Delegation Decision-Making Grid.* NCSBN. http://www.ncsbn.org

National League for Nursing Accrediting Commission. 1999. *1999 accreditation manual.* New York: NLNAC.

Nguyen, B. Q. 2000. If you are replaced by a younger nurse. *American Journal of Nursing* **100** (3), 82.

Sheehy, S. B. 2000. Law and the emergency room nurse: Infections in pregnant women. *Journal of Emergency Nursing.* **26:** 155–157.

Tappen, R. M., Weiss, S. A., and Whitehead, D. K. 2001. *Essentials of nursing leadership and management,* 2d ed. Philadelphia: F. A. Davis.

United American Nurses. 2001. http.//www.ana.org/uan.

CHAPTER 6

Theoretical Foundations of Professional Nursing

Objectives

■ Describe the nature of knowledge development.

■ Differentiate between the terms *concept, conceptual framework, conceptual model, theory, construct, proposition,* and *hypothesis.*

■ Analyze the development of theory in nursing.

■ Compare the theoretical approach of selected nurse theorists.

■ Identify the relationship between nursing process and nursing theory.

N U R S E   C O N N E C T

Additional online resources for this chapter can be found on the companion web site at www.prenhall.com/blais.

Knowledge development in nursing has proliferated since the 1960s. To be meaningful, this knowledge must be organized and information must be linked in a way that can be understood and used to continue to generate new knowledge. Theory and conceptual frameworks allow that organization and linking of data in the building of a body of knowledge for nursing. This chapter presents the development of theoretical foundations for professional nursing practice.

CHALLENGES AND OPPORTUNITIES

GAP BETWEEN THEORY AND PRACTICE Traditionally there has been a gap between academia and practice in nursing, which has resulted in nursing theory being developed and articulated by academicians and proposed to guide practice for those nurses in clinical practice. The collegial contact and communication between nurse educators and nurses in practice has been limited, with the result that nursing theory has been viewed by the practicing nurse as ethereal and unrelated to the "real world" of nursing. Nursing must bridge the gap to achieve theory-based practice. Nursing theories must be seen as supporting and guiding practice and must be communicated in ways that are compelling to nurses who must apply them.

ONE THEORY OR MANY The development of nursing theory has resulted in multiple diverse approaches with a language all its own. Theories have been drawn from a number of other disciplines and have been developed at varying levels of abstraction. This has the advantage of allowing nurses to match their own thinking and reasoning styles with the theory that is the "best fit." But is this diverse approach one that best serves the profession? Should nursing continue on its current course of numerous theories from which to choose or should nursing theorists now begin to converge on one theoretical approach?

WORLD VIEWS AND KNOWLEDGE DEVELOPMENT

Einstein is credited with saying that there is nothing so practical as a good theory. Theory is defined as a system of ideas proposed to explain something. Theory helps provide knowledge to improve practice by describing, explaining, predicting, and controlling phenomena. It guides practice, education, and research and provides professional autonomy as knowledge is systematically developed, producing practices that are more likely to be successful. The study of theory helps nurses develop analytical skills and critical thinking ability. Each nurse

Purposes of Nursing Theories and Conceptual Frameworks

Provide direction and guidance for (1) structuring professional nursing practice, education, and research; and (2) differentiating the focus of nursing from other professions.

IN PRACTICE

- Assist nurses to describe, explain, and predict everyday experiences.
- Serve to guide assessment, intervention, and evaluation of nursing care.
- Provide a rationale for collecting reliable and valid data about the health status of clients, which are essential for effective decision making and implementation.
- Help to establish criteria to measure the quality of nursing care.
- Help build a common nursing terminology to use in communicating with other health professionals. Ideas are developed and words defined.

- Enhance autonomy (independence and self-governance) of nursing through defining its own independent functions.

IN EDUCATION

- Provide a general focus for curriculum design.
- Guide curricular decision making.

IN RESEARCH

- Offer a framework for generating knowledge and new ideas.
- Assist in discovering knowledge gaps in the specific field of study.
- Offer a systematic approach to identify questions for study; select variables, interpret findings, and validate nursing interventions.

uses concepts and theories daily, which may or may not be articulated or perceived as such, to guide nursing action. Each time a decision is made based upon ideas that explain the situation or event, theory is used, even though it may not be formalized as such. Nursing theory has not been formally integrated at an everyday level. The gap between nurse theorists and practicing nurses can be attributed, at least in part, to the development of nursing theories in the 1960s by nurses who were pursuing graduate degrees in nursing and related fields. Few other nurses knew or cared about such matters; it was not part of nursing education at that time. Until the 1950s nursing practice was based upon principles and traditions passed on through an apprenticeship form of education and common sense that came from years of experience. Florence Nightingale, in the mid-1800s, proposed that nursing knowledge was based upon knowledge of persons and their environment and was different and distinct from medical knowledge. It was nearly a century later that nursing theory began to emerge and be valued by the profession.

Different theories represent different worldviews, which are different ways of conceiving of knowledge. Theories are not discovered; individuals who think and see the world in different ways create them. These worldviews provide contrasting paradigms (structure for organizing theory) and provide different traditions and approaches to science and knowledge development.

One paradigm is derived from the positivist approach that comes from the nineteenth century Age of Enlightenment and represents what many people regard as hard science. It deals with natural law and assumes that there is a body of facts and principles to be discovered and understood that is independent of the context. This approach is linear and attempts to look at cause and effect using experimental research methods. The theories generated by quantitative methods are normative, and they suggest propositions to explain relationships. They start with a generalization and bring it to a more specific level. Hypotheses are deduced from the theory to be tested in research, but some suggest that this is inappropriate for investigating and understanding complex and subtle nursing phenomena (Booth, Kenrick, and Woods, 1997).

The second paradigm began as a countermovement to positivism and sees science as necessarily embedded in time because truth is dynamic. That is, reality is not a fixed entity but, instead, is relative. Truth is found in one's experiences, and research uses naturalistic settings and observational methods to describe phenomena. This approach is sometimes referred to as constructivist. These theories are inductively constructed and give insights in social contexts and personal meanings; they start with a specific observation or relationship and make generalizations from it.

Theories differ in their scope and have been categorized as philosophies, grand theories, or middle-range theories. These theories can all be used to explain more specific situations. Table 6–1 lists theorists whose work can fall into these categories.

Table 6–1 Nursing Theorists and Their Theoretical Scope

Philosophies	Grand Theory	Middle-Range Theory
Florence Nightingale	Dorothea Orem	Hildegard Peplau
Ernestine Wiedenbach	Myra Levine	Ida Orlando
Virginia Henderson	Martha Rogers	Joyce Travelbee
Faye Abdellah	Dorothy Johnson	Kathryn Barnard
Lydia Hall	Callista Roy	Madeleine Leininger
Jean Watson	Betty Neuman	Rosemarie Parse
Patricia Benner	Imogene King	Margaret Newman
		Joyce Fitzpatrick
		Nola Pender

Based upon A. M. Tomey and M. R. Alligood, *Nursing Theorists and Their Work*, 4th ed. St. Louis: Mosby Yearbook, Inc., 1998.

Middle-Range Theory of Unpleasant Symptoms

The theory of unpleasant symptoms has three major components: the symptoms that the individual is experiencing, the influencing factors of the symptom experience, and the consequences of the symptom experience. Multiple symptoms can occur together as a result of a single event, such as surgery, and this is likely to result in an experience that is multiplicative rather than additive. Three categories of variables are identified as influencing the occurrence, intensity, timing, distress level, and quality of the symptoms; these variables are physiologic factors, psychologic factors, and situational factors. The factors can interact with each other.

This middle-range theory was developed from deductive and inductive research on the concepts of dyspnea and fatigue. Subsequent research looked at the resulting model as it applied to other symptoms and found consistent results.

The clinical applicability of this theory goes beyond a symptom-specific approach and looks at the way symptoms interact. It allows individualized interventions. It has been applied in an emergency department to develop a symptom assessment scale.

Source: E. R. Lenz, L. C. Pugh, R. A. Milligan, A. Gift, and F. Suppe, The Middle-Range Theory of Unpleasant Symptoms: An Update. *Advances in Nursing Science* **19**(3): 14–27, 1997.

A *philosophy* looks at the nature of things and aims to provide the meaning of nursing phenomena. Philosophies represent the early works leading to nursing theory. A *grand theory* is broad and complex and tends to be very general; grand theories are abstract but may provide insights useful for practice. They are conceptual and have concepts, definitions, and propositions. *Middle-range theory* has a narrower focus and is derived from earlier works, such as philosophies and grand theories, or from works in other disciplines. Middle-range theories may be refined through a series of studies, each providing increased focus. The accompanying boxes describe two such middle-range theories.

The Middle-Range Theory of Experiencing Transitions

Changes in health and illness create transitions, and clients in transition tend to be more vulnerable to risks that may affect their health. Examples of transitions are illness experiences, developmental and lifespan transitions, and social and cultural transitions. This theory was developed by reviewing inductively and deductively studies of the experiences of the following: pregnancy and childbirth, menopause, diagnostic events, migration, and family care giving. A theoretical framework emerged, consisting of types and patterns of transitions, properties of transition experiences, transition conditions (facilitators and inhibitors), process indicators, outcome indicators, and nursing therapeutics.

Transitions are complex and multidimensional. Several properties have been identified: awareness, engagement, change and difference, time span, and critical points and events. Several conditions affect transitions; these are personal, community, and societal. Personal conditions include meanings attributed to the event, cultural beliefs and attitudes, socioeconomic status, and preparation for the transition and knowledge about what to expect.

Patterns of response are feeling connected, interacting, location and being situated, developing confidence and coping. Outcome indicators are mastery and fluid integrative identities. Understanding the process allows nursing therapeutics congruent with the unique experience of the client to promote a healthy transition.

Source: A. I. Meleis, L. M. Sawyer, E. Im, D. K. Hilfinger-Messias, and K. Schumacher, Experiencing Transitions: An Emerging Middle-Range Theory, *Advances in Nursing Science* **23**(1): 12–28, 2000.

DEFINING TERMS

Before specific theories and conceptual frameworks can be understood, the terms *concept, conceptual framework, conceptual model,* and *theory* must be clarified. **Concepts,** the building blocks of theory, are abstract ideas or mental images of phenomena. Concepts are words that bring forth mental pictures of the properties and meanings of objects, events, or things. Concepts may be (1) readily observable, or *concrete,* ideas such as thermometer, rash, and lesion; (2) indirectly observable, or *inferential,* ideas such as pain and temperature; or (3) nonobservable, or *abstract,* ideas such as equilibrium, adaptation, stress, and powerlessness.

Four concepts have been identified as the *metaparadigm* of nursing—the most global philosophical or conceptual framework of a profession. The term originates from two Greek words: *meta,* meaning "with"; and *paradigm,* meaning "pattern." The four concepts are as follows:

1. *Person or client,* the recipient of nursing care (includes individuals, families, groups, and communities)
2. *Environment,* the internal and external surroundings that affect the client, including people in the physical environment, such as families, friends, and significant others
3. *Health,* the degree of wellness or well-being that the client experiences
4. *Nursing,* the attributes, characteristics, and actions of the nurse providing care on behalf of or in conjunction with the client

Each nurse theorist's definitions of these four concepts vary in accordance with philosophy, scientific orientation, experience, and view of nursing held by the theorist. At the time the metaparadigm was conceived, it assisted nurse scholars and students of nursing to analyze, compare, and contrast theories within a nursing framework. Not all theorists embrace the four concepts as distinct concepts. The theories representing more holistic and phenomenological approaches do not necessarily separate person from environment or health.

THEORY DEVELOPMENT IN NURSING

The terms *theory* and *conceptual framework* are often used interchangeably in nursing literature. Strictly speaking, they differ in their levels of abstraction; conceptual framework is more abstract than theory. A **conceptual framework,** viewed simply, is a group of related concepts. It provides an overall view or orientation to focus thoughts. A conceptual framework can be thought of as an umbrella under which many concepts can exist. A **conceptual model,** a term also used interchangeably with *conceptual framework,* is a graphic illustration or diagram of a conceptual framework. A **theory** is a supposition or system of ideas that is proposed to explain a given phenomenon. For example, Newton proposed his theory of gravity to explain why objects always fall from a tree to the ground. A *theory* goes one step beyond a *conceptual framework;* a theory relates concepts by using definitions that state significant relationships between concepts.

Theories generally include three elements:

1. A set of well-defined constructs or concepts. A **construct** is a concept that has been invented to suit a special purpose. It is measurable and can be observed in relation to other constructs. For example, *id, ego,* and *superego* are constructs Sigmund Freud developed to explain the concept of personality. To use a nursing example, the constructs in Imogene King's (1981) theory of goal attainment include perception, communication, interaction, transaction, self, role, growth and development, stress, time, and space.
2. A set of **propositions,** statements that specify the relationships among the constructs. For example, one of the eight propositions King developed to describe the relationship among the concepts in her theory of goal attainment is that "if perceptual accuracy is present in nurse-client interactions, transactions (goal attainment) will occur" (King, 1981).
3. **Hypotheses,** conjectures that test the relationships between the constructs and propositions. Because theory is abstract, it cannot be applied to practice. Instead, hypotheses derived from the theory are tested. For example, a testable hypothesis derived from King's goal-attainment theory is that "perceptual accuracy in nurse-client interactions increases mutual goal setting" (King, 1981).

Knowledge development may use a deductive or inductive approach. These two approaches represent theory testing or theory generation. Theory testing compares observed outcomes with the relationship predicted by the hypothesis that was drawn from the theory and linked the concepts. Theory generation comes from descriptive data that results in new concepts that may be related to other concepts. Generally speaking, theory testing uses a deductive approach and applies quantitative research methods. Theory generation uses an inductive approach and is a result of qualitative research. Chapter 10 discusses the role of the nurse as a research consumer.

Not all knowledge comes about as a result of research. Ways of knowing have been identified and described that include but are not limited to empirical methods. Kneller (1971) described five kinds of knowledge:

Revealed knowledge—that disclosed by God

Intuitive knowledge—that coming from a process of discovery nurtured by experience with the world

Rational knowledge—that using principles of formal logic

Empirical knowledge—information tested by observation or experiment

Authoritative knowledge—that vouched for by authorities in the field

Carper (1978) organized ways of knowing according to the following framework: empirical, esthetic, personal, and ethical. Empirical knowing represents the science of nursing that emphasizes generation of theory that is systematic and controllable by factual evidence. Esthetic knowing represents the art of nursing and emphasizes expressiveness, creativity, perceptions, subjectivity, and empathy. Personal knowledge focuses on interpersonal processes and the therapeutic use of self. Ethical knowing represents a pattern of knowing related to what ought to be done and focuses on matters of obligation.

Efforts to develop theory in nursing have resulted in discussion and debate about what is unique to nursing. Do nurses need basic scientific knowledge that they apply in practice, or is there a distinct body of knowledge for the discipline? Historically, nursing practice has been linked to the use of medical knowledge and has embraced the scientific bases of social and behavioral sciences as well as education. Some have suggested that theories in nursing are borrowed and shared theories. Other disciplines have provided the foundation of theory more unique to nursing. Nurse theorists have borrowed from others and applied these theories to nursing. Other theories are shared with other disciplines. For instance, Maslow's hierarchy of needs and Erikson's psychosocial development are applied to nursing without modification to the theories.

This has resulted in a diversity of theories. An overview of some selected nursing theories representing a range of scope and worldviews is included in this chapter. For further examination of particular theories, the student is referred to one of the many books available on nursing theory.

OVERVIEW OF SELECTED NURSING THEORIES

Nursing theories have been developed by nurses who were, in most instances, involved in their own graduate education at a time when there were few doctoral programs in nursing. Therefore, they were studying in related fields and, consequently, their developing theories were influenced by and borrowed from disciplines such as anthropology and sociology and applied to nursing. This can be seen in the description of the selected theories discussed here.

Nightingale's Environmental Theory

Florence Nightingale, often considered the first nurse theorist, defined nursing more than 100 years ago as utilizing the environment of the patient to assist him in his recovery (Nightingale, 1860). She linked health with five environmental factors: (1) pure or fresh air, (2) pure water, (3) efficient drainage, (4) cleanliness, and (5) light, especially direct sunlight. Deficiencies in these five factors produced lack of health or illness.

These factors are especially significant when one considers that sanitation conditions in hospitals of the mid-1800s were extremely poor and that women working in the hospitals were often unreliable, uneducated, and incompetent to care for the ill.

In addition to the preceding factors, Nightingale also stressed the importance of keeping the client warm, maintaining a noise-free environment, and attending to the client's diet in terms of assessing intake, timeliness of the food, and its effect on the person.

Nightingale set the stage for further work in the development of nursing theories. Her general concepts about ventilation, cleanliness, quiet, warmth, and diet remain integral parts of nursing and health care today.

Peplau's Interpersonal Relations Model

Hildegard Peplau, a psychiatric nurse, introduced her interpersonal concepts in 1952 (Peplau, 1952) and based them on available theories at the time: psychoanalytic theory, principles of social learning, and concepts of human motivation and personality development. *Psychodynamic nursing* is defined as understanding one's own behavior to help others identify felt difficulties and applying principles of human relations to problems arising during the experience.

Peplau views nursing as a maturing force that is realized as the personality develops through educational, therapeutic, and interpersonal processes. Nurses enter into a personal relationship with an individual when a felt need is present. This nurse-client relationship evolves in four phases:

1. *Orientation.* During this phase, the client seeks help, and the nurse assists the client to understand the problem and the extent of the need for help.
2. *Identification.* During this phase, the client assumes a posture of dependence, interdependence, or independence in relation to the nurse (relatedness). The nurse's focus is to assure the person that the nurse understands the interpersonal meaning of the client's situation.
3. *Exploitation.* In this phase, the client derives full value from what the nurse offers through the relationship. The client uses available services on the basis of self-interest and needs. Power shifts from the nurse to the client.
4. *Resolution.* In this final phase, old needs and goals are put aside and new ones adopted. Once older needs are resolved, newer and more mature ones emerge.

During the nurse-client relationship, nurses assume many roles: stranger, teacher, resource person, surrogate, leader, and counselor. Today, Peplau's model continues to be used by clinicians when working with individuals who have psychological problems.

Henderson's Definition of Nursing

Virginia Henderson is well known for her *Textbook on the Principles and Practices of Nursing*, co-authored with Canadian nurse Bertha Harmer (Harmer and Henderson, 1955); her subsequent publications, including *The Nature of Nursing* (1966); and numerous scholarly papers. She was motivated to develop her ideas because she was dissatisfied with the emphasis that nursing education programs placed on technical competence and mastery of nursing procedures; her experiences in psychiatric, pediatric, and community health nursing were other major influences.

In 1955, Henderson formulated a definition of the unique function of nursing. This definition was a major stepping-stone in the emergence of nursing as a discipline separate from medicine. She wrote, "The unique function of the nurse is to assist the individual, sick or well, in the performance of those activities contributing to health or its recovery (or to peaceful death) that he would perform unaided if he had the necessary strength, will, or knowledge, and to do this in such a way

as to help him gain independence as rapidly as possible" (Henderson, 1966, p. 3). Like Nightingale, Henderson described nursing in relation to the client and the client's environment. Unlike Nightingale, Henderson saw the nurse as concerned with both well and ill individuals, acknowledged that nurses interact with clients even when recovery may not be feasible, and mentioned the teaching and advocacy roles of the nurse.

Basic to her definition are various assumptions about the individual: namely, that the individual (1) needs to maintain physiologic and emotional balance, (2) requires assistance to achieve health and independence or a peaceful death, and (3) needs the necessary strength, will, or knowledge to achieve or maintain health. These needs give direction to the nurse's role.

Henderson conceptualized the nurse's role as assisting sick or well individuals in a supplementary or complementary way. The nurse needs to be a partner with the client, a helper to the client, and, when necessary, a substitute for the client. The nurse's focus is to help individuals and families (which she viewed as a unit) to gain independence in meeting 14 fundamental needs (Henderson, 1966):

1. Breathing normally
2. Eating and drinking adequately
3. Eliminating body wastes
4. Moving and maintaining a desirable position
5. Sleeping and resting
6. Selecting suitable clothes
7. Maintaining body temperature within normal range by adjusting clothing and modifying the environment
8. Keeping the body clean and well-groomed to protect the integument
9. Avoiding dangers in the environment and avoiding injuring others
10. Communicating with others in expressing emotions, needs, fears, or opinions
11. Worshipping according to one's faith
12. Working in such a way that one feels a sense of accomplishment
13. Playing or participating in various forms of recreation
14. Learning, discovering, or satisfying the curiosity that leads to normal development and health, and using available health facilities

Henderson published many works and continues to be cited in current nursing literature. Her emphasis on the importance of nursing's independence from and interdependence with other health care disciplines is well recognized.

Consider . . .

- the relationship between Henderson's 14 fundamental needs and Maslow's hierarchy of needs. How might one have built upon the other?

Rogers' Science of Unitary Human Beings

Martha Rogers first presented her theory of unitary human beings in 1970. It contains complex conceptualizations related to multiple scientific disciplines. Her theory was influenced by Einstein's theory of relativity, which introduced the four coordinates of space-time; Burr and Northrop's electrodynamics theory of life, which revealed the pattern and organization of the electrodynamics field; Von Bertalanffy's general systems theory; and many other disciplines, such as anthropology, psychology, sociology, astronomy, religion, philosophy, history, biology, and literature.

Rogers views the person as an irreducible whole, the whole being greater than the sum of its parts. *Whole* is differentiated from *holistic,* the latter often being used to mean only the sum of all the parts. She states that humans are dynamic energy fields in continuous exchange with environmental fields, both of which are infinite. Both human and environmental fields are characterized by pattern, a universe of open systems, and pandimensionality. According to Rogers, *unitary man*

- Is an irreducible energy field identified by pattern;
- Manifests characteristics different from the sum of the parts;
- Interacts continuously and creatively with the environment;
- Behaves as a totality;
- As a sentient being, participates creatively in change.

Key concepts Rogers uses to describe the individual and the environment are energy fields, openness, pattern and organization, and pandimensionality. *Energy fields* are the fundamental level of humans and the environment (all that is outside a given human field). Energy fields are dynamic, constantly exchanging energy from one to the other. The concept of *openness* holds that the energy fields of humans and the environment are open systems, that is, infinite, integral with one another, and in continuous process. *Pattern* refers to the unique identifying behaviors, qualities, and characteristics of the energy fields that change continuously and innovatively. Pandimensionality expresses the idea of unitary whole; it provides for an infinite domain without limits.

To Rogers, the life process in humans is homeodynamic, involving continuous and creative change. She provides three principles of homeodynamics to offer a way of perceiving how unitary human beings develop: integrality (formerly complementarity), resonancy, and helicy. According to the principle of *integrality,* the human and environmental fields interact mutually and simultaneously. *Resonancy* means the wave pattern in the fields change continuously and from lower- to higher-frequency patterns. *Helicy* is spiral development, that is, continuous and nonrepeating.

When Rogers' theory is applied in practice, nurses (1) focus on the person's wholeness, (2) seek to promote symphonic interaction between the two energy fields (human and environment) to strengthen the coherence and integrity of the person, (3) coordinate the human field with the rhythmicities of the environmental field, and (4) direct and redirect patterns of interaction between the two energy fields to promote maximum health potential.

Some find Rogers' concepts difficult to understand, but a specific example can help clarify them. Nurses' use of therapeutic touch is based on the concept of human energy fields. The human energy field is identified by pattern. The qualities of the field vary from person to person and are affected by pain and illness. Although the field is infinite, realistically it is most clearly "felt" within several feet of the body. The nurse trained in therapeutic touch can assess and feel the energy field and manipulate it to help a person manage pain.

Orem's General Theory of Nursing

Dorothea Orem's theory, first published in 1971, has been widely accepted by the nursing community and has resulted from the work of the Nursing Development Conference Group. This general theory of nursing is referred to as the *self-care deficit theory of nursing,* and it consists of the articulation of the theories of self-care, self-care deficit, and nursing systems. It provides a way of looking at and investigating what nurses do and what they should do in social groups.

SELF-CARE Self-care theory postulates that self-care and the self-care of dependents are learned behaviors that individuals initiate and perform on their own behalf to maintain life, health, and well-being. Self-care theory is based upon four concepts: self-care, self-care agency, self-care requisites, and therapeutic self-care demand. *Self-care* refers to those activities an individual performs independently throughout life to promote and maintain personal well-being. *Self-care agency* is the individual's ability to perform self-care activities. It consists of two agents: a *self-care agent* (an individual who performs self-care independently) and a *dependent-care agent* (a person other than the individual who provides the care). Adults care for themselves, whereas infants, the aged, the ill, and the disabled require assistance with self-care activities.

Self-care requisites, also called *self-care needs,* are measures or actions taken to regulate functioning and development. There are three categories of self-care requisites:

1. *Universal requisites* are common to all people. They include maintaining intake and elimination of air, water, and food; balancing rest, solitude, and social interaction; preventing hazards to life and well-being; and promoting normal human functioning.
2. *Developmental requisites* result from maturation and are related to stage of development or are associated with conditions or events, such as adjusting to a change in body image or to the loss of a spouse.
3. *Health deviation requisites* result from illness, injury, or disease or its treatment. They include actions such as seeking health care assistance, carrying out prescribed therapies, and learning to live with the effects of illness or treatment.

Therapeutic self-care demand refers to all self-care activities required to meet the requisites for certain conditions and circumstances, such as an illness.

SELF-CARE DEFICIT Self-care deficit theory asserts that people benefit from nursing because they have health-related limitations in providing self-care. These limitations may result from illness, injury, or from the effects of medical tests or treatments. Two variables affect these deficits: self-care agency (ability) and the therapeutic self-care demands (the measures of care required to meet the existing requisites). *Self-care deficit* results when the self-care agency is not adequate to meet the known self-care demand. Orem's self-care deficit theory explains not only when nursing is needed but also how people can be assisted through five methods of helping: acting or doing for, guiding, teaching, supporting, and providing an environment that promotes the individual's abilities to meet current and future demands.

NURSING SYSTEMS Nursing systems theory postulates that nursing systems form when nurses prescribe, design, and provide nursing that regulates the individual's self-care capabilities and meets therapeutic self-care requirements. Orem identifies three types of nursing systems:

1. *Wholly compensatory* systems are required for individuals who are unable to control and monitor their environment and process information.
2. *Partly compensatory* systems are designed for individuals who are unable to perform some (but not all) self-care activities.
3. *Supportive-educative (developmental)* systems are designed for persons who need to learn to perform self-care measures and need assistance to do so.

Development of the theory continues with contributions from researchers, scholars, nursing faculty, nursing students, and practicing nurses.

King's Goal-Attainment Theory

Imogene King's theory of goal attainment is based on systems theory, the behavioral sciences, and deductive and inductive reasoning. She first published *Toward a Theory of Nursing: General Concepts of Human Behavior* in 1971. Initially, King formulated her theory as a conceptual framework for nursing when, as an associate professor of nursing at Loyola University in Chicago, she developed a master's degree program in nursing. King refined her concepts in her 1981 publication, *A Theory for Nursing: Systems, Concepts, Process.*

King's theory consists of three dynamic interacting systems: (1) personal systems (individuals), (2) interpersonal systems (groups), and (3) social systems (society). Key concepts are identified for each system as follows:

1. Personal-system concepts: perception, self, body image, growth and development, space and time
2. Interpersonal-system concepts: interaction, communication, transaction, role, stress, and coping
3. Social-system concepts: organization, authority, power, status, and decision making

The client and nurse are personal systems or subsystems within interpersonal and social systems. To identify problems and to establish goals, the nurse and client perceive one another, act and react, interact, and transact. *Transactions* are defined as purposeful interactions that lead to goal attainment. Transactions have the following characteristics:

- They are basic to goal attainment and include social exchange, bargaining and negotiating, and sharing a frame of reference toward mutual goal setting.
- They require perceptual accuracy in nurse-client interactions and congruence between role performance and role expectation for nurse and client.

■ They lead to goal attainment, satisfaction, effective care, and enhanced growth and development.

King postulates seven hypotheses in goal-attainment theory:

1. Perceptual congruence in nurse-client interactions increases mutual goal setting.
2. Communication increases mutual goal setting between nurses and clients and leads to satisfactions.
3. Satisfaction in nurses and clients increase goal attainment.
4. Goal attainment decreases stress and anxiety in nursing situations.
5. Goal attainment increases client learning and coping ability in nursing situations.
6. Role conflict experienced by clients, nurses, or both decreases transactions in nurse-client interactions.
7. Congruence in role expectations and role performance increases transactions in nurse-client interactions.

King's theory highlights the importance of the participation of all individuals in decision making and deals with the choices, alternatives, and outcomes of nursing care. The theory offers insight into nurses' interactions with individuals and groups within the environment.

Neuman's Systems Model

Betty Neuman, a community health nurse and clinical psychologist, began developing her model while lecturing in community health nursing at the University of California at Los Angeles. The model is based on Gestalt theory, Selye's stress theory, and general systems theory. Neuman's model was first published in 1972 in *Nursing Research* in an article coauthored by R.J. Young, "A Model for Teaching Total Person Approach to Patient Problems." Refinements were published as the Neuman Systems Model in 1974, 1982, 1989, and 1995.

Neuman's systems model is based on the individual's relationship to stress, the reaction to it, and reconstitution factors that are dynamic in nature. *Reconstitution* is the state of adaptation to stressors.

Neuman views the client as an open system consisting of a basic structure or central core of energy resources (physiologic, psychologic, sociocultural, developmental, and spiritual) surrounded by two concentric boundaries or rings referred to as *lines of resistance* (Figure 6–1). The lines of resistance represent internal factors that help the client defend against a stressor; one

example is an increase in the body's leukocyte count to combat an infection. Outside the lines of resistance are two lines of defense. The inner, or *normal, line of defense,* depicted as a solid line, represents the person's state of equilibrium or the state of adaptation developed and maintained over time and considered normal for that person. The *flexible line of defense,* depicted as a broken line, is dynamic and can be rapidly altered over a short period of time. It is a protective buffer that prevents stressors from penetrating the normal line of defense. Certain variables (e.g., sleep deprivation) can create rapid changes in the flexible line of defense.

Neuman describes a *stressor* as any environmental force that alters the system's stability. Stressors are categorized as *intrapersonal stressors,* those that occur within the individual (e.g., an infection); *interpersonal stressors,* those that occur between individuals (e.g., unrealistic role expectations); and *extrapersonal stressors,* those that occur outside the person (e.g., financial concerns). The individual's reaction to stressors depends on the strength of the lines of defense. When the lines of defense fail, the resulting reaction depends on the strength of the lines of resistance. As part of the reaction, a person's system can adapt to a stressor, an effect known as *reconstitution.*

Nursing interventions focus on retaining or maintaining system stability. These interventions are carried out on three preventive levels.

1. *Primary prevention* identifies risk factors, attempts to eliminate the stressor, and focuses on protecting the normal line of defense and strengthening the flexible line of defense. A reaction has not yet occurred, but the degree of risk is known.
2. *Secondary prevention* relates to interventions or active treatment initiated after symptoms have occurred. The focus is to strengthen internal lines of resistance, reduce the reaction, and increase resistance factors.
3. *Tertiary prevention* refers to intervention following that in the secondary stage. It focuses on readaptation and stability and protects reconstitution or return to wellness following treatment. The nurse emphasizes educating the client in strengthening resistance to stressors and ways to help prevent recurrence of reaction or regression.

Betty Neuman's model of nursing has been widely accepted by the nursing community, nationally and internationally. It is applicable to a variety of nursing practice settings involving individuals, families, groups, and communities.

Figure 6–1

Neuman's Client System

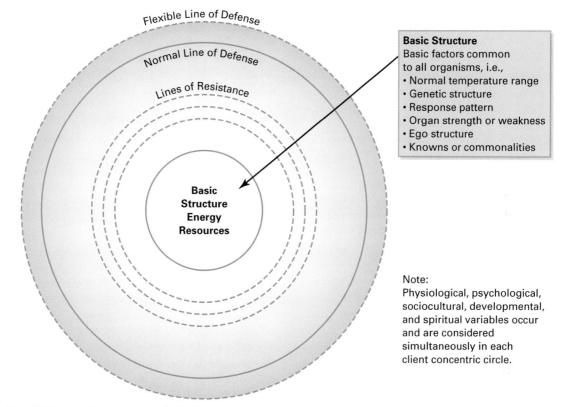

Flexible Line of Defense

Normal Line of Defense

Lines of Resistance

Basic
Structure
Energy
Resources

Basic Structure
Basic factors common
to all organisms, i.e.,
• Normal temperature range
• Genetic structure
• Response pattern
• Organ strength or weakness
• Ego structure
• Knowns or commonalities

Note:
Physiological, psychological,
sociocultural, developmental,
and spiritual variables occur
and are considered
simultaneously in each
client concentric circle.

Source: From *The Newman Systems Model* (3rd ed.) by B. Neuman, 1995, Norwalk CT: Appleton & Lange, p. 26. Used with permission.

Roy's Adaptation Model

Sister Callista Roy's adaptation model, widely used by nurse educators, researchers, and practitioners, was introduced in *Nursing Outlook* as "Adaptation: A Conceptual Framework in Nursing" (Roy, 1970). The model was published in book form in 1976 and 1984 as *Introduction to Nursing: An Adaptation Model* (Roy, 1976, 1984) and in 1991 and 1999 as *The Roy Adaptation Model* (Roy and Andrews, 1991, 1997). Roy, a nurse and sociologist, based her theory on Harry Helson's work in psychophysics and on her observations of the great resilience of children and their ability to adapt to major physical and psychologic changes.

Roy focuses on the individual as a biopsychosocial adaptive system that employs a feedback cycle of input, throughput, and output. Both the individual and the environment are sources of stimuli that require modification to promote adaptation, an ongoing purposive response. Adaptive responses contribute to health, which she defines as the process of being and becoming integrated; ineffective or maladaptive responses do

not contribute to health. Each person's adaptation level is unique and constantly changing.

As an open system, an individual receives *input* or stimuli from both the self and the environment. Roy identifies three classes of stimuli:

1. *Focal stimuli:* the internal or external stimuli most immediately confronting the person and contributing to behavior

2. *Contextual stimuli:* all other internal or external stimuli present

3. *Residual stimuli:* beliefs, attitudes, or traits having an indeterminate effect on the person's behavior but whose effects are not validated.

Throughput makes use of a person's (1) *processes,* which are control mechanisms that a person uses as an adaptive system, and (2) *effectors,* which refer to the physiologic function, self-concept, and role function involved in adaptation. *Output* of the system refers to the individual's behaviors, which can be either adaptive responses promoting the system's integrity or ineffective responses, such as not following a prescribed therapy. These outputs or responses provide feedback for the system.

Roy's adaptive systems consist of two interrelated subsystems. The *primary subsystem* is a functional or internal control process that consists of the regulator and the cognator. The *regulator* processes input automatically through neural-chemical-endocrine channels. The *cognator* processes input through cognitive pathways, such as perception, information processing, learning, judgment, and emotion. Roy views the regulator and cognator as methods of coping.

The *secondary subsystem* is an effector system that manifests cognator and regulator activity. It consists of four adaptive modes:

1. The *physiologic mode* involves the body's basic physiological needs and ways of adapting in regard to fluid and electrolytes, activity and rest, circulation and oxygen, nutrition and elimination, protection, the senses, and neurologic and endocrine function.
2. The *self-concept mode* includes two components: the *physical* self, which involves sensation and body image, and the *personal* self, which involves self-ideal, self-consistency, and the moral-ethical self.
3. The *role-function mode* is determined by the need for social integrity and refers to the performance of duties based on given positions within society.
4. The *interdependence mode* involves one's relations with significant others and support systems that provide help, affection, and attention.

Roy's work has been shaped by the current influences in nursing of holism and spiritualism. She has proposed some changes to guide nursing through the 21st century. Adaptation has been redefined as "the process and outcome whereby the thinking and feeling person uses conscious awareness and choice to create human and environmental integration." (Roy, 1997, p. 44). Two sets of assumptions of the Roy model, scientific and philosophic, have been examined for applicability in the new century. These are listed in the accompanying boxes on this page and page 99.

Parse's Human Becoming Theory

Rosemarie Rizzo Parse has broad experience in nursing theory, research, administration, and practice. Her theory has been used to guide practice in many countries, including Canada, Finland, Sweden, and the United States. As founder and president of Discovery International, Inc., she promoted excellence in nursing science and provided health guidance services to individuals, families, and groups in Pittsburgh. Parse first published her theory in *Man-Living-Health: A Theory of Nursing* (Parse, 1981) and has since retitled it as human becoming theory, substituting human for man and becoming for health. The retitled theory was published in *The Human Becoming School of Thought. A Perspective for Nurses and Other Health Professionals* (Parse 1998). Major influences on her work include existential philosophers such as Martin Heidegger, Jean-Paul Sartre, and Maurice Merleau-Ponty. Parse draws upon the concepts and theoretical assumptions of Martha Rogers' Science of Unitary Human Beings. She has blended integrality, resonancy, helicy, complementarity, energy field, openness, pattern, and pandimensionality (Rogers) with the following beliefs from existential-phenomenologic theory:

Roy's Adaptation Model: Scientific Assumptions for the 21st Century

Systems of matter and energy progress to higher levels of complex self-organization.

Consciousness and meaning are constitutive of person and environment integration.

Awareness of self and environment is rooted in thinking and feeling.

Human decisions are accountable for the integration of creative processes.

Thinking and feeling mediate human action.

System relationships include acceptance, protection, and fostering interdependence.

Persons and the earth have common patterns and integral relations.

Person and environment transformations are created in human consciousness.

Integration of human and environment meanings results in adaptation.

From C. Roy, Future of the Roy Model: Challenge to Redefine Adaptation, *Nursing Science Quarterly* **10**(1): 42–48, 1997.

Roy's Adaptation Model: Philosophical Assumptions for the 21st Century

Persons have mutual relationships with the world and with a God figure.

Human meaning is rooted in an omega point convergence of the universe.

God is intimately revealed in the diversity of creation and is the common destiny of creation.

Persons use human creative abilities of awareness, enlightenment, and faith.

Persons are accountable for the processes of deriving, sustaining and transforming the universe.

From C. Roy, Future of the Roy Model: Challenge to Redefine Adaptation, *Nursing Science Quarterly* **10**(1): 42–48, 1997.

human subjectivity, intentionality, coconstitution, coexistence, and situational freedom. *Human subjectivity* means that people grow in a dialectic (reasoning) relationship with the world that gives meaning to what emerges in the process of becoming. *Intentionality* is involvement with the world through a fundamental nature of knowing, being present, and being open. *Coconstitution* refers to the idea that the meaning that emerges in any situation is related to the particular components or constituents of that situation. *Coexistence* means that people as emerging beings are in the world with others. *Situational freedom* refers to the idea that people participate in choosing the situations in which they find themselves, as well as their attitudes toward the situation. Humans are, therefore, always choosing.

Parse's theory claims that nursing must focus on quality of life from the perspective of the patient or client. The means by which the nurse achieves this is what Parse calls "true presence." The person is in a process of continuous becoming, and Parse offers three principles that characterize human becoming.

Principle 1. Human becoming is freely choosing personal *meaning* in situations in the intersubjective process of relating value priorities.

Principle 2. Human becoming is cocreating *rhythmic patterns* or relating in open process with the universe.

Principle 3. Human becoming is *cotranscending* multidimensionally with emerging possibles.

These three principles focus on meaning, rhythmicity, and cotranscendence.

■ *Meaning* arises from a person's interrelationship with the world and refers to happenings to which the person attaches varying degrees of significance.

Imaging—structuring the meaning of an experience

Valuing—confirming cherished beliefs

Languaging—expressing valued images

■ *Rhythmicity* is the movement toward greater diversity.

Revealing-concealing—simultaneously disclosing some aspects of self and hiding others

Enabling-limiting—the result of making choices; in choosing, one is both enabled in some things and limited in others

Connecting-separating—a simultaneous process; connecting with some phenomena results in separating from others

■ *Cotranscendence* is the process of reaching out beyond the self.

Powering—moving toward all future possibilities

Originating—distinguishing self from others

Transforming—an ongoing process of change; moving toward greater diversity by transcending the present

Parse's theory enables nurses to understand how individuals choose and bear responsibility for patterns of personal health. According to Parse, the client is the authority figure and decision-maker. The nurse's role is helping individuals and families choose the possibilities, specifically illuminating meaning (uncovering what was and what will be), synchronizing rhythms (leading through discussion to recognize harmony), and mobilizing transcendence (dreaming of possibilities and planning to reach them). Edwards (2000), in a critical review of Parse's work, explains the three principles in this way. In interpreting situations, persons also create them. This is the cocreation of reality. In leading a human life, a person's relationships inevitably have a rhythmical pattern that exhibits the three kinds of paradoxes: revealing-concealing, enabling-limiting, and connecting-separating. In cotranscending, one considers possible courses of action and, after considering them, may undertake one of them.

The Caring Theorists

A current thrust in nursing theory development is based on the concept of caring. This movement grew out of humanism and was given considerable impetus by the work of Mayeroff (1971) that made the link between generic caring and the uniqueness of caring in nursing. In 1998, the American Association of Colleges of Nursing (AACN, 1998) published *The Essentials of Baccalaureate Education for Professional Nursing Practice,* a document prepared to guide education for practice in the 21st century. It defines caring as a concept central to the practice of professional nursing and identifies it as a core value encompassing altruism, autonomy, human dignity, integrity, and social justice.

Caring as a central concept in nursing has its own substantive area of nursing science and has been a focus of scholarly inquiry. Jean Watson (1979, 1985, 1988) may be the best known and most widely recognized caring theorist. Madeleine Leininger (1978, 1980, 1984) was also a forerunner in the caring movement, although her work may be better known for its transcultural focus. Roach (1992) and Boykin and Schoenhofer (1993) further developed the concepts of caring. Each of these theorists identifies caring as the essence of nursing and a central and unifying feature. Table 6–2 shows a comparison of four caring theories.

Critics of caring theory question whether practitioners can use these theories with a limited understanding of the philosophies that underpin and contribute to the language used in describing them. The

Table 6–2 Comparison of Caring Theories

	Leininger	Watson	Roach	Boykin and Schoenhofer
Origin of Theory	Anthropology	Human science and metaphysics	Philosophy and theology	Philosophy and human science
Description of Caring	Actions and activities directed toward assisting, supporting, or enabling another individual or group with evident or anticipated needs to ameliorate or improve a human condition or lifeway, or to face death	A value and an attitude that has to become a will, an intention, or a commitment, that manifests itself in concrete acts	Caring is the human mode of being	Caring is the intentional and authentic presence of the nurse with another who is recognized as a person living caring and growing in caring
Key Concepts	Caring; culture; culture care universality and diversity	Transpersonal caring and the ten carative factors	The five Cs of caring: compassion, competence, conscience, confidence, commitment	Personhood and the nursing situation
Goal/outcome	To improve and provide care that is culturally acceptable and is beneficial and useful to the client and family	To protect, enhance, and preserve humanity by helping a person find meaning in illness, suffering, pain, and existence	Roach does not clearly state a goal or outcome	Enhancement of personhood

Based on T. V. McCance, H. P. McKenna, and J. R. P. Boore, Caring: Theoretical Perspectives of Relevance to Nursing, *Journal of Advanced Nursing* 30(6): 1388–1395, 1999.

existential-phenomenological-spiritual forces may be poorly understood by nurses from mainstream nursing curricula. This raises the issue of the gap between academia and practice and the educational preparation needed to make them relevant and useful to practice.

The caring movement has produced an organization dedicated to the dissemination of research and scholarly activity in caring; The International Association for Human Caring began in 1978, and Madeleine Leininger convened the first conference. It continues to meet on an annual basis at a different location each year.

Leininger and Watson's theories are the best known of the caring theories and have had the most exposure in nursing literature and critical review. They are the least abstract and have been the basis of research and clinical applications. Both of these theories will be briefly described.

Consider . . .

■ whether caring is the essence of nursing. If so, should it be studied and have its own body of knowledge? How does this knowledge apply in situations where fast responses and highly technologic care are critical to outcomes?

Watson's Human Caring Theory

Jean Watson was educated in psychiatric and mental health nursing and received her doctorate in educa-tional psychology and counseling. Her theory of the science of caring was first published in *Nursing: The Philosophy and Science of Caring* (Watson, 1979). She refined her ideas in *Nursing: Human Science and Human Care* (Watson, 1985, 1988).

Watson believes the practice of caring is central to nursing; it is the unifying focus for practice. Two major assumptions underlie human care values in nursing: (1) care and love constitute the primal and universal psychic energy, and (2) care and love are requisite for our survival and the nourishment of humanity. Watson's major assumptions about caring are shown in the accompanying box.

Nursing interventions related to human care are referred to as *carative factors*. Watson outlines the following ten factors:

1. Forming a *humanistic-altruistic system of values*. This factor relates to satisfaction through giving and extending the sense of self. Although the values are learned early in life, they can be greatly influenced by educators.

2. Instilling *faith and hope*. Feelings of faith and hope promote wellness by helping the client to adopt health-seeking behaviors. By developing an effective nurse-client relationship, the nurse facilitates feelings of optimism, hope, and trust.

3. Cultivating *sensitivity to one's self and others*. Nurses who are able to recognize and express their feel-

Watson's Assumptions of Caring

- Human caring in nursing is not just an emotion, concern, attitude, or benevolent desire. *Caring* connotes a personal response.

- Caring is an intersubjective human process and is the moral ideal of nursing.

- Caring can be effectively demonstrated only interpersonally.

- Effective caring promotes health and individual or family growth.

- Caring promotes health more than does curing.

- Caring responses accept a person not only as they are now but also for what the person may become.

- A caring environment offers the development of potential while allowing the person to choose the best action for the self at a given point in time.

- Caring occasions involve action and choice by nurse and client. If the caring occasion is transpersonal, the limits of openness expand, as do human capacities.

- The most abstract characteristic of a caring person is that the person is somehow responsive to another person as a unique individual, perceives the other's feelings, and sets one person apart from another.

- Human caring involves values, a will and commitment to care, knowledge, caring actions, and consequences.

- The ideal and value of caring is a starting point, a stance, and an attitude that has to become a will, an intention, a commitment, and a conscious judgment that manifests itself in concrete acts.

ings are better able to allow others to express theirs.

4. Developing a *helping-trusting (human care) relationship.* This kind of relationship involves effective communication, empathy, and nonpossessive warmth. It promotes and accepts the expression of positive and negative feelings.

5. Expressing *positive and negative feelings.* Sharing feelings of sorrow, love, and pain is a risk-taking experience. The nurse must be prepared for negative feelings.

6. Using a *creative problem-solving, caring process.* Caring linked to the nursing process contributes to a creative problem-solving approach to nursing care.

7. Promoting *transpersonal teaching-learning.* This factor separates caring from curing and shifts responsibility for wellness to the client.

8. Providing a *supportive, protective, or corrective mental, physical, sociocultural, and spiritual environment.* Because the client can experience change in any aspect of the internal and external environments, the nurse must assess and facilitate the client's abilities to cope with mental, emotional, and physical changes.

9. Assisting with *gratification of human needs.* Caring is conveyed by recognizing and attending to the physical, emotional, social, and spiritual needs of the client.

10. Being sensitive to the *existential-phenomenologic-spiritual force.* Phenomenology describes data relative to the immediate situation that help people understand the concept or event in question. The *phenomenal field* is the individual's frame of reference; this field can be known only to the person. A phenomenal field involves many levels of consciousness, such as awareness, perceptions of self, body sensations, thoughts, values, feelings, intuitive insights, beliefs, and hopes. When nurse and client come together, two phenomenal fields come together. Both are in a process of being, becoming, and developing transpersonal understanding. Existential psychology is a science of human existence that employs the method of phenomenologic analysis. Persons possess three spheres of being: mind, body, and soul. Allowing for expression of these forces leads to a better understanding of self and others.

Leininger's Culture Care Diversity and Universality Theory

Madeleine Leininger, a well-known nurse anthropologist, has written extensively on transcultural nursing concepts and is a proponent of the science of human caring. She first published her cultural care diversity and universality theory in 1985 in the journal *Nursing and Health Care,* explained it further in 1988 and then in 1991, in her book *Culture Care Diversity and Universality: A Theory of Nursing* (Leininger, 1984, 1988, 1991). In this book she produced the sunrise model to depict her theory. (See also Chapter 21, "Nursing in a Culturally and Spiritually Diverse World.")

Leininger postulates that caring and culture are inextricably linked. Educated in cultural and social anthropology, Leininger observed a marked number of differences between Western and non-Western cultures in caring and health practices. She defines *transcultrual nursing* as a major area of nursing that focuses on comparative study and analysis of different cultures and subcultures in the world, with respect to their caring behavior, nursing care, health values, beliefs, and patterns. The goal of transcultural nursing is to develop a scientific and humanistic body of knowledge in order to provide culture-specific and culture-universal nursing practices. She believes culture is the broadest and the most holistic way to conceptualize, understand, and be effective with people.

Leininger states that *care* is the essence of nursing and the dominant, distinctive, and unifying feature of nursing. She says that there can be no cure without caring, but that there may be caring without curing. She emphasizes that human caring, although a universal phenomenon, varies among cultures in its expressions, processes, and patterns; it is largely culturally derived. These differences in caring values and behaviors lead to differences in the expectations of those seeking care. For example, cultures that perceive illness primarily as a personal and internal body experience—caused by physical, genetic, and intra-body stresses—tend to use more medications and

---

Leininger's Descriptions of Care and Caring

- Caring includes assistive, supportive, and facilitative acts toward or for another individual or group with evident or anticipated needs.
- Caring serves to ameliorate or to improve human conditions or life ways. It emphasizes healthful, enabling activities of individuals and groups that are based on culturally defined, ascribed, or sanctioned helping modes.
- Caring is essential to human development, growth, and survival.

- Caring behaviors include comfort, compassion, concern, coping behavior, empathy, enabling, facilitating, interest, involvement, health consultative acts, health instruction acts, health maintenance acts, helping behaviors, love, nurturance, presence, protective behaviors, restorative behaviors, sharing, stimulating behaviors, stress alleviation, succor, support, surveillance, tenderness, touching, and trust.

---

physical techniques than cultures that view illness as an extrapersonal experience.

Leininger identifies many caring constructs (see the box on page 103). Leininger believes that the goal of health care personnel should be to work toward an understanding of care and the values, health beliefs, and lifestyles of different cultures, which will form the basis for providing culture-specific care.

Consider . . .

- how Leininger's description of caring compares and contrasts to Watson's description of caring. When applied to clinical practice would each lead to differing or similar nursing interventions?

ONE MODEL VERSUS SEVERAL MODELS

Many nurses believe that having a single, universal model for nursing would offer the following advantages:

- Further the development of nursing as a profession.
- Give all nurses a common framework, enhancing communication and research.
- Promote understanding about the nurse's role in nontraditional nursing settings, such as independent nurse practitioner practices, self-help clinics, and health maintenance organizations (HMOs), correcting the common misconception that nurses provide care only for sick persons.

In contrast, advocates of several different conceptual models point out the following:

- Most disciplines have several conceptual models, which allow members to explore phenomena in different ways and from different viewpoints.
- Several models increase an understanding of the nature of nursing and its scope.
- Several models foster development of the full scope and potential of the discipline.

It is possible that in the 21st century more models for nursing will be developed and that existing ones will be refined in accordance with societal needs and with their tested usefulness. More research on existing theory may result in the development of middle-range theories that have the potential to direct practice in more specific situations. This direction would help narrow the gap between theory and practice.

RELATIONSHIP OF THEORIES TO THE NURSING PROCESS AND RESEARCH

Conceptual models for nursing are abstractions that are operationalized or made real by the use of the nursing process.

1. *Assessing.* The specific data collected about a client's health needs relate directly to the theorist's view of the client. For example, if the client is seen as having 14 fundamental needs, the nurse collects data about these 14 needs.
2. *Diagnosing.* In this step, the nurse analyzes assessment data to identify actual, potential, and possible nursing diagnoses. The nurse outlines or writes the client's actual or potential health problems as a nursing diagnostic statement in accordance with the nursing model used.

Research Box

Watson, R., Deary, I. J., and Lea, A. 1999. A longitudinal study into the perceptions of caring and nursing among student nurses. *Journal of Advanced Nursing* 29(5): 1228–1237.
The relationship between nursing and caring was investigated with a sample of student nurses to determine whether changes in perceptions of nursing and caring take place and how perceptions of nursing and caring are related. Questionnaires were used to collect data at the time of entry into nursing school and again 12 months later. Items that changed significantly over the time of the study suggest that nurses lose some idealism about nursing and caring. However, the relationship between the two increased indicating that nursing and caring became more synonymous to the students.

Campbell, J. C., and Soeken, K. L. 1999. Women's responses to battering: A test of the model. *Research in Nursing and Health* 22: 49–58.
A study of battered women was done to test a model based on Orem's theory. The effects of physical and nonphysical abuse and self-care agency were investigated in relation to physical and emotional health outcomes. Tools to measure index of spouse abuse were used to screen the sample. Self-care agency tools measured self-esteem, power, and capability for self-care operations. Functional health and mental health were measured. Structural equation modeling supported the model that both battering and self-care agency have direct effects on health. In addition, age and education have indirect effects on health through self-care agency.

Nuamah, I. F., Cooley, M. E., Fawcett, J., and McCorkle, R. 1999. Testing a theory for health-related quality of life in cancer patients: A structural equation approach. *Research in Nursing and Health* 22: 231–242.
This study tested a Roy adaptation model–based theory of health-related quality of life in patients with newly diagnosed cancer. The four biopsychosocial response modes were tested by the Symptom Distress Scale, Depression Scale, Enforced Social Dependency Scale, and availability of a caregiver. The results revealed that severity of illness and adjuvant cancer treatment had the strongest association with the biopsychosocial responses and should be considered the focal environmental stimuli. The remaining environmental stimuli should be considered contextual. The proposition that initial biopsychosocial responses predict later response was supported.

3. *Planning*. Planning also relates directly to the conceptual nursing model. The nurse establishes goals for resolution of client problems, nursing interventions aimed at achieving those goals, and outcome criteria by which the nurse can evaluate whether or not the goals are met. These goals, interventions, and criteria are established in accordance with the modes of intervention outlined in the conceptual model.

4. *Implementing*. Implementing the planned interventions draws on scientific knowledge from many sources. The nursing model instructs the nurse what to do and directly influences what nursing interventions are planned, but it does not tell the nurse how to do it.

5. *Evaluating*. Evaluating is a continuous nursing function. How is the client adjusting and reacting? What does the client see as needs? How does the client see these needs changing? Has the client achieved the desired consequences? The answers to these questions help the nurse evaluate the effectiveness of the total nursing process and the nursing model.

Table 6–3 outlines how two selected nurse theorists have addressed the nursing process.

The conceptual models for nursing drive nursing research and provide a way to organize finding of research in a meaningful way. Variables selected for study are selected according to the suggested relationships drawn from theories; research then validates theory and confirms the presence of the proposed relationships. Research can also be theory generating by describing concepts and suggesting relationships between and among variables that have not previously been proposed. For more discussion of the relationship between research and theory, the student is directed to Chapter 10, "The Nurse as Research Consumer."

Table 6–3 Selected Nursing Theories and the Nursing Process

Theory	Nursing Process	Application
Orem's general theory of nursing	Assessing	Involves collecting data about the client's capacities (knowledge, skills, and motivation) to perform universal, developmental, and health-deviation self-care requisites; determines self-care deficits.
	Diagnosing	Stated in terms of the client's limitations to maintain self-care (a deficit in self-care agency).
	Planning	Involves considering and designing, with the client's participation, an appropriate nursing system (wholly compensatory, partially compensatory, and/or supportive-educative) that will help the client achieve an optimal level of self-care (i.e., enhance the client's self-care agency).
	Implementing	Assisting the client by acting for or doing for, guiding, supporting, providing a developmental environment, and teaching.
	Evaluating	Determining the client's level of achievement in resolving self-care deficits and in performing self-care.
Roy's adaptation model	Assessing	Involves two levels: *First-level assessment* includes collecting data about output behaviors related to the four adaptive modes (physiologic, self-concept, role function, and interdependence modes); *second-level assessment* includes collecting data about internal and external stimuli (focal, contextual, or residual) that are influencing the identified behaviors.
	Diagnosing	Focuses on adaptation problems and uses one of three alternative methods: 1. Stating behaviors within one mode with their most relevant influencing stimuli. 2. Clustering behavioral information and labeling it according to indicators of positive adaptation and a typology of common adaptation problems related to each mode. Roy provides a typology of indicators of positive adaptation and a typology of commonly recurring adaptation problems according to each of the four modes. 3. Labeling a behavioral pattern when more than one mode is being affected by the same stimuli.
	Planning	Setting goals in terms of behaviors the client is to achieve and planning nursing interventions to promote the effectiveness of the client's coping mechanisms and adaptive behaviors.
	Implementing	Altering and manipulating the focal, contextual, and residual stimuli by increasing, decreasing, or maintaining them.
	Evaluating	Determining the client's output behaviors with those identified in the goals.

SUMMARY

Nursing is deeply involved in identifying its own unique knowledge base, the body of knowledge needed for practice. Knowledge development in nursing comes from science generated by varying worldviews. Theories and conceptual frameworks help to unify the knowledge into a science of nursing. They offer ways of conceptualizing a discipline in clear, explicit terms that can be easily communicated. Because opinions about the nature and structure of nursing vary, theories continue to be developed. Some theories are broad in scope and others are limited. They vary in level of abstraction, conceptualization, and ability to describe, explain, or predict.

A major distinction between a theory and a conceptual framework or model is the level of abstraction with the conceptual framework being more abstract than the theory. A conceptual model is a system of related concepts or a conceptual diagram. Its major purpose is to give clear and explicit direction to the three areas of nursing: practice, education, and research. A theory generates knowledge in a field. Theories can be categorized as philosophy, grand theory, and middle-range theory based upon the scope and structure.

Theory development in nursing had its origins with Florence Nightingale, but it was about a century later when theory development accelerated. The 1960s produced a flurry of activity as nurses pursued graduate education in nursing and related fields. Much of the early theory was inspired by related science in other fields. A current focus in nursing theory development is caring, which has been identified by the AACN as a core value for the profession. It is identified by some as the essence of nursing, a view that is growing in popularity.

Challenges in the 21st century include making theory-based practice a reality. Direct application of theory to clinical situations will depend upon the ability to develop models that are operationalized with the nursing process. A question for the future is whether there should be one grand theory for nursing or the continued use of multiple theories and models. To be considered professionals, nurses must be able to com-

municate about the science of nursing. Theory can offer a way of communicating to others what is unique about nursing and direct practice in a meaningful way. Theory can be either generated by or tested by research.

> ## Bookshelf
>
> ***Nightingale Songs.*** **www.fau.edu/divisions/collegeof nursing**
> Esthetic expressions of caring written by students in nursing.
> **O'Brien, J., and Kollock, P. 1997.** *The production of reality: Essays and readings on social interaction.* **Thousand Oaks, Calif.: Pine Forge Press.**
> A collection of essays written by well-known authors. These essays focus on perceptions of reality from a variety of perspectives in an entertaining way.
> **Parse, R. R. 1999.** *Hope: An international human becoming perspective.* **Sudbury, Mass.: Jones and Bartlett Publishers, Inc.**
> Phenomenolgic findings regarding the experience of hope.

REFERENCES

American Association of Colleges of Nursing. 1998. *The essentials of baccalaureate education for professional nursing practice.* Washington, D.C.: AACN.

Booth, K., Kenrick, M., and Woods, S. 1997. Nursing knowledge, theory, and method revisited. *Journal of Advanced Nursing* **26**(4): 804–811.

Boykin, A., and Schoenhofer, S. 1993. *Nursing as caring: A model for transforming practice.* New York: National League for Nursing Press, Pub. No. 15-2549.

Campbell, J. C., and Soeken, K. L. 1999. Women's responses to battering: A test of the model. *Research in Nursing and Health* **22**: 49–58.

Carboni, J. T. 1995, Spring. A Rogerian process of inquiry. *Nursing Science Quarterly* **7**(3): 128–133.

Carper, B. 1978. Fundamental patterns of knowing in nursing. *Advances in Nursing Science* **1**: 33–54.

Edwards, S. D. 2000. Critical review of R.R. Parse's *The Human Becoming School of Thought.* A perspective for nurses and other health professionals. *Journal of Advanced Nursing,* **31**(1): 190–196.

Gaut, D. A. 1995. *Historical review of the IAHC*

1978–1995. International Association for Human Caring. Royal Palm Beach, Fla.

Harmer, B., and Henderson, V. 1955. *Textbook of the principles and practice of nursing,* 5th ed. Riverside, N.J.: Macmillan.

Henderson, V. 1966. *The nature of nursing: A definition and its implications for practice, research, and education.* Riverside, N.J.: Macmillan.

Henderson, V. 1991. *The nature of nursing: Reflections after 25 years.* New York: National League for Nursing Press, Pub. No. 15-2346.

King, I. M. 1971. *Toward a theory for nursing: General concepts of human behavior.* New York: Wiley.

King, I. M. 1981. *A theory for nursing: Systems, concepts, process.* New York: Wiley.

Leininger, M. M. 1978. *Transcultural nursing: Concepts, theories, and practices.* New York: Wiley.

Leininger, M. M. 1980, Oct. Caring: A central focus of nursing and health care services. *Nursing and Health Care* **1**(3): 135–143.

Leininger, M. M. 1984. *Care: The essence of nursing and health.* Thorofare, N.J.: Charles B. Slack.

Leininger, M. M. 1985, April. Transcultural care diversity and universality: A theory of nursing. *Nursing and Health Care* **6**(4): 208–212.

Leininger, M. M. 1988, Nov. Leininger's theory of nursing: Cultural care, diversity and universality. *Nursing Science Quarterly* **1**(4): 152–160.

Leininger, M. M., ed. 1991. *Culture care diversity and universality: A theory of nursing.* New York: National League for Nursing Press, Pub. No. 15–2402.

Lenz, E. R., Pugh, L. C., Milligan, R. A., Gift, A., and Suppe, F. 1997. The middle-range theory of unpleasant symptoms: An update. *Advances in Nursing Science* **19**(3): 14–27.

Madrid, M., and Barrett, E. A. M., eds. 1994. *Rogers' scientific art of nursing practice.* New York: National League for Nursing Press, Pub. No. 15-2610.

McCance, T. V., McKenna, H. P., and Boore, J. R. P. 1999. Caring: Theoretical perspectives of relevance to nursing. *Journal of Advanced Nursing* **30**(6): 1388–1395.

Mayeroff, M. 1971. *On caring.* London: Harper Row.

Meleis, A. I., Sawyer, L. M., Im, E., Hilfinger-Messias, D. K., and Schumacher, K. 2000. Experiencing transitions: An emerging middle-range theory. *Advances in Nursing Science* **23**(1): 12–28.

Neuman, B. 1974. The Betty Neuman health-care systems model: A total person approach to patient problems. In *Conceptual models for nursing practice,* edited by J. P. Riehl and C. Roy. New York: Appleton-Century-Crofts.

Neuman, B. 1982. *The Neuman systems model: Applications to nursing education and practice.* New York: Appleton-Century-Crofts.

Neuman, B. 1989. *The Neuman systems model: Applications to nursing education and practice,* 2d ed. Norwalk, Conn.: Appleton and Lange.

Neuman, B. 1995. *The Neuman systems model,* 3d ed. Norwalk, Conn.: Appleton and Lange.

Neuman, B., and Young, R. J. 1972, June. A model for teaching total person approach to patient problems. *Nursing Research* **21**: 264–269.

Nicoll, L. H. 1997. *Perspectives on nursing theory,* 3d ed. Philadelphia: Lippincott.

Nightingale, F. 1860. *Notes on nursing.* Reprint, Philadelphia: Lippincott, 1957.

Nuamah, I. F., Cooley, M. E., Fawcett, J., and McCorkle, R. 1999. Testing a theory for health-related quality of life in cancer patients: A structural equation approach. *Research in Nursing and Health* **22**: 231–242.

Orem, D. E. 1971. *Nursing: Concepts of practice.* Hightstown, N.J.: McGraw-Hill.

Orem, D. E. 1980. *Nursing: Concepts of practice,* 2d ed. Hightstown, N.J.: McGraw-Hill.

Orem, D. E. 1985. *Nursing: Concepts of practice,* 3d ed. Hightstown, N.J.: McGraw-Hill.

Orem, D. E. 1991. *Nursing: Concepts of practice,* 4th ed. Hightstown, N.J.: McGraw-Hill.

Orem, D. E. 1995. *Nursing: Concepts of practice,* 5th ed. Hightstown, N.J.: McGraw-Hill.

Orem, D. E., and Vardiman, E. M. 1995, Winter. Oren's theory and positive mental health: Practical considerations. *Nursing Science Quarterly* **8**(4): 165–173.

Parse, R. R. 1981. *Man-living-health: Theory of nursing.* New York: Wiley.

Parse, R. R. 1987. *Nursing science: Major paradigms, theories, and critiques.* Philadelphia: W.B. Saunders.

Parse, R. R. 1989. *Man-living-health: A theory of nursing.* In *Conceptual models for nursing practice,* 3d ed., edited by J. Riehl-Sisca, pp. 253–257. Norwalk, Conn.: Appleton-Lange.

Parse, R. R., ed. 1995. *Illuminations: The human becoming theory in practice and research.* New York: National League for Nursing Press, Pub. No. 15-2670.

Parse, R. R. 1998. *The human becoming school of thought: A perspective for nurses and other health professionals.* Thousand Oaks, Calif.: Sage.

Peplau, H. E. 1952. *Interpersonal relations in nursing.* New York: Putnam.

Peplau, H. E. 1963, Oct/Nov. Interpersonal relations and the process of adaptations. *Nursing Science.* **1**(4): 272–279.

Peplau, H. E. 1980. The Peplau developmental model for nursing practice. In *Conceptual models for nursing practice,* 2d ed., edited by J. P. Riehl and C. Roy, pp. 53–75. New York: Appleton-Century-Crofts.

Roach, M. S. 1992. *The human act of caring: A blueprint for the health professions,* rev. ed. Ottawa, Canada: Canadian Hospital Association Press.

Rogers, M. E. 1970. *An introduction to the theoretical basis of nursing.* Philadelphia: F. A. Davis.

Rogers, M. E. 1989. Nursing: A science of unitary human beings. In *Conceptual models for nursing practice,* 3d ed., edited by J. Riehl-Sisca, pp. 181–188. Norwalk, CT: Appleton and Lange.

Rogers, M. E. 1994, Spring. The science of unitary human beings: Current perspectives. *Nursing Science Quarterly* **7**(1): 33–35.

Roy, C. 1970, March. Adaptation: A conceptual framework in nursing. *Nursing Outlook* **18:** 42–45.

Roy, C. 1976. *Introduction to nursing: An adaptation model.* Upper Saddle River, N.J.: Prentice Hall.

Roy, C. 1984. *Introduction to nursing: An adaptation model,* 2nd ed. Upper Saddle River, N.J.: Prentice Hall.

Roy, C., 1997. Future of the Roy model: Challenge to redefine adaptation. *Nursing Science Quarterly* **10**(1): 42–48.

Roy, C., and Andrews, H. A. 1991. *The Roy adaaptation model: The definitive statement.* Norwalk, Conn.: Appleton and Lange.

Roy, C., and Andrews, H. A. 1999. *The Roy adaptation model,* 2d ed. Stamford, Conn.: Appleton and Lange.

Sarter, B. 1988. *The stream of becoming: A study of Martha Rogers' theory.* New York: National League for Nursing Press, Pub. No. 15–2205.

Tomey, A. M., and Alligood, M. R. 1998. *Nursing theorists and their work,* 4th ed. St. Louis: Mosby Yearbook, Inc.

Watson, J. 1979. *Nursing: The philosophy and science of caring.* Boston: Little, Brown.

Watson, J. 1985. *Nursing: Human science and human care. A theory of nursing.* Norwalk, Conn.: Appleton-Century-Crofts.

Watson, J. 1988. *Nursing: Human science and human care. A theory of nursing.* New York: National League for Nursing Press, Pub. No. 15-2236.

Watson, R., Deary, I. J., and Lea, A. 1999. A longitudinal study into the perceptions of caring and nursing among student nurses. *Journal of Advanced Nursing* **29**(3): 1228–1237.

Wesley, R. L. 1995. *Nursing theories and models,* 2d ed. Springhouse, Pa.: Springhouse.

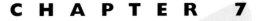
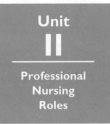

CHAPTER 7

Unit
II
Professional
Nursing
Roles

The Nurse as Health Promoter and Care Provider

Objectives

- Differentiate health preventive or protective care and health promotion.

- Discuss essential components of health promotion.

- Discuss the goals, focus areas, and leading health indicators of *Healthy People 2010*.

- Identify various types and sites of health-promotion programs.

- Compare three health promotion models: those of Pender, Kulbock, and Neuman.

- Discuss Prochaska and DiClemente's five-stage model of behavior change.

- Analyze the nurse's role in health promotion.

NURSE CONNECT

Additional online resources for this chapter can be found on the companion web site at www.prenhall.com/blais.

Health promotion is an important component of nursing practice. It is a way of thinking that revolves around a philosophy of wholeness, wellness, and well-being. In the past three decades, the public has become increasingly aware of and interested in health promotion. Many people are aware of the relationship between lifestyle and illness and are developing health-promoting habits, such as getting adequate exercise, rest, and relaxation; maintaining good nutrition; and controlling the use of tobacco, alcohol, and other drugs.

The vision of health promotion was expressed nationally in Canada in 1974 with the publication of the Lalonde Report, *A New Perspective on the Health of Canadians* (Lalonde, 1974), and in the United States in 1979 in the Surgeon General's report, *Healthy People* (U.S. Surgeon General, 1979). Both reports emphasized the role that individuals could play in modifying their lifestyles and personal behaviors to improve their health status. These reports also consider, to a lesser extent, environmental factors influencing health.

In 1980 the U.S. Public Health Service developed *Health Promotion/Disease Prevention: Objectives for the Nation* (U.S. Surgeon General, 1980). This report addressed more specifically the broad goals set forth in *Healthy People* by listing strategies to achieve each objective. These strategies included not only personal behavior changes but also the roles of institutions, legislation, and policy. In the mid-1980s, the Canadian government undertook a large restructuring of its approach to health care. This report, known as the Epp Report, emerged from a synthesis of the Lalonde Report and initiatives of the World Health Organization. The Epp Report focused on achieving health for all citizens by reducing inequities between low- and high-income groups, increasing prevention, and enhancing coping (Epp, 1986). See Figure 7–1.

In September 1990, *Healthy People 2000* was presented to the American public. This document encompassed 298 health-related objectives that provided a framework for a national health promotion, health protection, and preventive service strategy (U.S. Department of Health and Human Services, 1990). Individual nurses and 24 national nursing organizations were involved in the development of *Healthy People 2000* (Brown et al., 1992, p. 204).

Currently, *Healthy People 2010* builds on the initiatives developed over the previous two decades. It states national health objectives "designed to identify the most significant preventable threats to health and to establish national goals to reduce these threats" (web.health.gov/healthypeople). *Healthy People 2010* was developed through the Healthy People Consortium, an alliance consisting of 350 national organizations, including professional nursing and medical associations, and 250 state health, mental health, substance abuse, and environmental agencies. The public had opportunity to be involved in the development of *Healthy People 2010* through an interactive website. Thus, *Healthy People 2010* is a collaborative effort of private, professional, and governmental agencies, with consumer input to determine the future health of the people of the United States.

CHALLENGES AND OPPORTUNITIES

Health care and nursing have traditionally been more oriented toward curing and treating than preventing illness, injury, and disability. Shifting the focus toward maintaining and promoting health and wellness is a current challenge. Many forces in society, including cost containment and allocation of resources, have provided the impetus toward maintaining health rather than providing more resource-intensive care

Figure 7–1

A Framework for Health Promotion

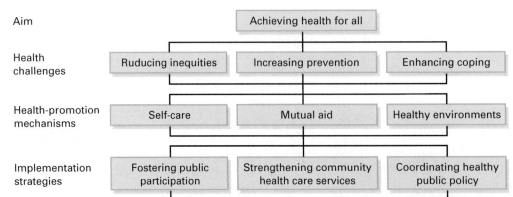

Source: *Achieving Health for All: A Framework for Health Promotion: Report of the Minister of National Health and Welfare,* by J. Epp, Ottawa, Canada: Government Printing Office, November 1986.

once health has been compromised. A number of nursing theories have been developed that focus on prevention and health promotion. The profession is challenged to use these theories and continue to develop its abilities to keep people healthy.

The role of health promoter provides the nurse with many opportunities to contribute to improved health. The nurse has an opportunity to educate individuals and groups in the community about prevention and maintaining health. Nurses practice in a variety of community settings, such as school-based clinics, primary care clinics, prenatal and well-baby clinics, and health departments, where they interact with healthy people and can provide guidance. However, the opportunities for health promotion can be found in more traditional health care settings as well. People with acute and chronic illnesses can learn ways of caring for themselves that will enhance health and increase well-being.

DEFINING HEALTH PROMOTION

Considerable differences appear in the literature regarding the use of the terms *health promotion, primary prevention, health protection,* and *illness prevention.* Leavell and Clark (1965, 21) define three levels of prevention: primary, secondary, and tertiary. There are five steps that describe these levels: **Primary prevention** focuses on (1) health promotion and (2) protection against specific health problems. **Secondary prevention** focuses on (1) early identification of health problems and (2) prompt intervention to alleviate health problems. **Tertiary prevention** focuses on restoration and rehabilitation to an optimal level of functioning.

In the model used by Leavell and Clark, primary prevention precedes any disease symptoms. The purpose of primary prevention is to encourage optimal health and to increase the person's resistance to illness. Examples of primary prevention include health education concerning the hazards of smoking and specific protection against a particular disease, such as the vaccine against poliomyelitis.

The second level, secondary prevention, presumes the presence of a disease or illness. Screening procedures, such as a blood sugar test for a client with diabetes mellitus, and the Denver Developmental Screening Tests to assess developmental delays, are facets of secondary prevention. Screening procedures facilitate early discovery and allow treatment to begin before the illness progresses. Disability limitation, another step in secondary prevention, is also more effective in the early stages of a disease.

Tertiary prevention relates to situations where a disability is already present. The goal of tertiary prevention is to restore individuals to their optimal level of functioning within the limitations imposed by their condition.

Pender (1996, p. 34) identifies the three levels of prevention (primary, secondary, and tertiary) as health protection. Health protection "is directed toward decreasing the probability of experiencing health problems by active protection against pathologic stressors or detection of health problems in the asymptomatic stage. Health protection focuses on efforts to move away from or avoid the negatively valenced states of illness and injury." In contrast, health promotion is "directed toward increasing the level of well-being and self actualization of a given individual or group. Health promotion focuses on efforts to approach or move toward a positively valenced state of high-level health and well-being." In this instance, health promotion is considered to be an approach behavior, whereas primary prevention is considered avoidance behavior. Health promotion is not disease oriented; that is, no specific problem is being avoided. By contrast, primary prevention activities are geared toward avoiding specific problems (p. 7).

Stachtchenko and Jenicek (1990, p. 53) support Pender's conceptual differences between the terms *health promotion* and *primary prevention* (or health protection). They describe health promotion as broad in scope, involving not only lifestyle changes but also the process of granting individuals and communities more control over determinants of health. Health prevention programs focus on risk reduction and are targeted toward specific populations.

Healthy People 2000 differentiated among health promotion, health protection, and preventive health services, outlining specific activities for each category:

- Health promotion: individual and community activities to promote healthful lifestyles. Examples of health-promotion activities include improving nutrition, preventing alcohol and drug misuse, restricting smoking, maintaining fitness, and exercising.
- Health protection: actions by government and industry to minimize environmental health threats. Health protection relates to activities such as maintaining occupational safety, controlling radiation and toxic agents, and preventing infectious diseases and accidents.
- Preventive health services: actions that health care providers take to prevent health problems. These services include control of high blood pressure, control of sexually transmitted diseases, immunization, family planning, and health care during pregnancy and infancy.

The difficulty in separating the terms *health promotion, disease prevention,* and *health protection* lies in the fact that an activity may be carried out for numerous reasons. For example, a 40-year-old male may begin a program of walking 3 miles each day. If the goal of his program is to "decrease the risk of heart disease," then the activity would be considered prevention. By contrast, if his walking regimen is instituted to "increase his overall health and feeling of well-being," then the activity would be considered health promotion behavior.

A chief scientist for nursing from WHO, Amelia Mangay Maglacas, uses the terms *positive health* and *positive health promotion* and presents them in a broader context. According to Maglacas, *positive* health for all does not mean the eradication of every disease or the healing of every body part. Rather, health should be considered in the context of its contribution to social and economic development, so that all people have the necessary social and economic support to lead satisfying lives (1988, p. 67). *Positive health promotion* is the process of enabling people to improve and to increase their control over their own health. The aim of positive health promotion is to improve health potential and maintain health balance. One attains this goal of positive health by caring for oneself and for others, by controlling life's circumstances with careful and conscientious decision making, and by ensuring that conditions in society allow people to attain health.

A summary of essential concepts of health promotion proposed by Schultz (1995, p. 32) is shown in the accompanying box. These points are incorporated into her definition of health promotion:

> Health promotion facilitates an individual or a community in a process of self-determining a present health status, in order to actively choose ways of altering personal or communal health habits for improvement, and to develop resources and skills to alter the environment so that health is being maintained or a self-determined higher level of health can be achieved.

Consider . . .

■ whether you agree with Pender's conceptual differences between the terms *health promotion* and *primary prevention.*

■ whether health promotion can be offered to all clients regardless of their age, health, and illness status.

HEALTHY PEOPLE 2010

Healthy People 2010 builds on prior *Healthy People* documents by identifying two overall goals:

1. Increase quality and years of healthy life.
2. Eliminate health disparities.

Increasing Quality and Years of Healthy Life

In 1995 Japan had the highest life expectancy in the world for nations with populations of more than 1 million: 82.9 years for women and 76.4 years for men; the United States ranked 19th for women (78.9) and 25th for men (72.5). (See Table 7–1.) Such data suggest the need for improvement in the United States as well as other nations. However, increasing the number of years is not sufficient if the quality of those years is not also improved. Quality of life is the general sense of well-being or satisfaction with one's life within one's environment. Quality of life embraces all aspects of life, including physical and mental health, recreation, culture, rights, values, beliefs, aspirations, and the conditions that support a life containing these elements (*Healthy People 2010*).

Concepts of Health Promotion

- Health promotion maintains and enhances health.
- Health promotion develops the resources and skills of the person or community.

- Health promotion alters personal or communal habits and the environment.
- Health promotion defines health as a continuum.
- Health promotion is self-directed.

Source: "What Is Health Promotion?" by A. Schultz, *Canadian Nurse* **91** (7), 31–34, 1995.

Table 7–1 Life Expectancy at Birth by Gender Ranked by Selected Countries

Female		Male	
Country	**Years of Life Expectancy**	**Country**	**Years of Life Expectancy**
Japan	82.9	Japan	76.4
France	82.6	Sweden	76.2
Switzerland	81.9	Israel	75.3
Sweden	81.6	Canada	75.2
Spain	81.5	Switzerland	75.1
Canada	81.2	Greece	75.1
Australia	80.9	Australia	75.0
Italy	80.8	Norway	74.9
Norway	80.7	Netherlands	74.6
Netherlands	80.4	Italy	74.4
Greece	80.3	England & Wales	74.3
Finland	80.3	France	74.2
Austria	80.1	Spain	74.2
Germany	79.8	Austria	73.5
Belgium	79.8	Singapore	73.4
England & Wales	79.6	Germany	73.3
Israel	79.3	New Zealand	73.3
Singapore	79.0	Northern Ireland	73.1
United States	78.9	Belgium	73.0
		Cuba	73.0
		Costa Rica	73.0
		Finland	72.8
		Denmark	72.8
		Ireland	72.5
		United States	72.5

Source: U.S. Department of Health and Human Services. *Healthy People 2010: A Systematic Approach to Health Improvement,* 2001, p. 3–4. www.health.gov/healthypeople.

Eliminating Health Disparities

The focus of this goal is to eliminate health disparities among segments of the population. The principle of *Healthy People 2010* is that every person in the United States, "regardless of age, gender, race or ethnicity, income, education, geographic location, disability, and sexual orientation, deserves equal access to comprehensive, culturally competent, community-based health care systems that are committed to serving the needs of the individual and promoting community health" (USDHHS 2001, 10).

In the United States, women currently live approximately six years longer than men. The infant death rate among Africans Americans is more than double that of whites. African Americans have higher death rates than whites related to heart disease (40% higher), cancer (30% higher), HIV/AIDS (700%), and homicide (600%). Hispanics living in the United States are more likely to die from diabetes than non-Hispanic whites. They have higher rates of hypertension and obesity than non-Hispanic whites. Native Americans and Alaska natives have higher infant-mortality rates, higher rates of diabetes, and higher death rates associated with unintentional injuries and suicide. People with higher levels of education and income have lower incidence of heart disease, diabetes, obesity, hypertension, and low birth weight. People with disabilities report more anxiety, pain, sleeplessness, and days of depression than do those who do not have disabilities. People in rural areas are more likely to have heart disease, cancer, and diabetes than those who live in urban areas. These disparities are inconsistent with the constitutional philosophy of the equality of all people. Efforts must be made to reduce these disparities.

To determine the nation's progress toward achieving the goals, 28 focus areas will be monitored via 467 objectives. (See the accompanying box.) The objectives focus on interventions designed to reduce or eliminate illness, disability, and premature death and to improve access to quality health care, strengthen public health services, and approve the availability and dissemination of health-related information. The focus areas relate to individual, group, and community efforts to achieve the overall goals.

Leading health indicators were developed reflecting the major public health concerns in the United States. (See the box on page 115.) They were chosen because they have the ability to motivate action, they can be measured by objective data to determine their progress, and they are relevant to broad public health issues. For each of the leading health indicators, spe-

---

Healthy People 2010 Focus Areas

- Access to quality health services
- Arthritis, osteoporosis, and chronic back conditions
- Cancer
- Chronic kidney disease
- Diabetes
- Disability and secondary conditions
- Educational and community-based programs
- Environmental health
- Family planning
- Food safety
- Health communication
- Heart disease and stroke
- HIV
- Immunization and infectious diseases

- Injury and violence prevention
- Maternal, infant, and child health
- Medical product safety
- Mental health and mental disorders
- Nutrition and overweight
- Occupational safety and health
- Oral health
- Physical activity and fitness
- Public health infrastructure
- Respiratory diseases
- Sexually transmitted diseases
- Substance abuse
- Tobacco use
- Vision and hearing

Source: U.S. Department of Health and Human Services. *Healthy People 2010: A Systematic Approach to Health Improvement,* 2001. web.health.gov/healthypeople.

Leading Health Indicators

- Physical activity
- Overweight and obesity
- Tobacco use
- Substance abuse
- Responsible sexual behavior

- Mental health
- Injury and violence
- Environmental quality
- Immunization
- Access to health care

Source: U.S. Department of Health and Human Services. *Healthy People 2010: Leading Health Indicators,* 2001. web.health.gov/healthy-people.

cific objectives will be used to track progress. For example, for the leading health indicator, physical activity, the objectives are to (1) "increase the proportion of adolescents who engage in vigorous physical activity that promotes cardiorespiratory fitness three or more days per week for 20 or more minutes per occasion" and (2) "increase the proportion of adults who engage regularly, preferably daily, in moderate physical activity for at least 30 min per day." (USDHHS, 2001, p. 3).

HEALTH-PROMOTION ACTIVITIES

Health-promotion organizations, wellness centers, and traditional health care centers all offer a different approach to client care. Table 7–2 demonstrates these differences. Health promotion activities can be carried out on a governmental level (e.g., a national program to improve knowledge of nutrition) or on a personal level (e.g., an individual exercise program).

Health-promotion programs on an individual level can be active or passive. With *passive* strategies, the client is a recipient of the health-promotion effort. Many health professionals participate in national programs to define and institute these passive strategies. Examples of passive government strategies are maintaining the cleanliness of water and promoting a healthy environment by enforcing sewage regulations to decrease the spread of disease. *Active* strategies depend on individu-

Table 7–2 Focus of Traditional Health Care Contrasted with Health Promotion and Wellness

	Traditional	Health Promotion	Wellness
Primary goal	Identify and correct problem	Disease prevention and risk reduction	Increased health
Dominant message	"Health care professionals will take care of you."	"You will live longer if you avoid illness."	"You are responsible, and your efforts to be well will be supported."
Change agent	Treatment	Information and behavior change	Positive experience and cultural influences
Target	The problem	Individuals, families, and communities	Clients within cultures
Duration of intervention	Ends when the problems clear up	Length of class or program	Ongoing

Source: Adapted from *A Primer of Health Promotion: Creating Healthy Organizational Cultures* by J. P. Opatz, Washington, D.C.: Oryn Publications, 1985, p. 101.

als' commitment to and involvement in adopting a program directed toward their health promotion. Active strategies are important in that they encourage individuals to take control of their lives and assume the responsibility for their health. Examples of active strategies that involve changes in lifestyle are (1) a diet-management program to improve nutrition, (2) a self-help program to reduce stress related to parenting, (3) an exercise program to improve muscle strength and endurance, or (4) a combination diet and exercise regimen for weight reduction or control. For optimal health and well-being, a combination of both active and passive strategies is suggested.

Types of Health-Promotion Programs

A variety of programs can be used for the promotion of health, including (1) information dissemination, (2) health appraisal and wellness assessment, (3) lifestyle and behavior change, and (4) environmental control programs.

Information dissemination is the most basic type of health promotion program. This method makes use of a variety of media to offer information to the public about the risk of particular lifestyle choices and personal behavior, as well as the benefits of changing that behavior and improving the quality of life. Billboards, posters, brochures, newspaper features, books, and health fairs all offer opportunities for the dissemination of health-promotion information. Alcohol and drug abuse, driving under the influence of alcohol, hypertension, sexually transmitted diseases (including HIV/AIDS), and the need for immunizations are some of the topics frequently discussed. Information dissemination is a useful strategy for raising the level of knowledge and awareness of individuals and groups about health habits.

Health risk appraisal/wellness assessment programs are used to apprise individuals of the risk factors that are inherent in their lives in order to motivate them to reduce specific risks and develop positive health habits. Wellness assessment programs are focused on more positive methods of enhancement, in contrast to the risk factor approach used in the health appraisal. A variety of tools are available to facilitate these assessments. Some of these tools are computer based and can therefore be offered to educational institutions and industries at a reasonable cost.

Lifestyle- and behavior-change programs require the participation of the individual and are geared toward enhancing the quality of life and extending the life span. Individuals generally consider lifestyle changes after they have been informed of the need to change their health behavior and become aware of the potential benefits of the process. Many programs are available to the public, both on a group and individual basis, some of which address stress management, nutrition awareness, weight control, smoking cessation, and exercise.

Environmental-control programs have been developed in response to the recent growth in the number of contaminants of human origin that have been introduced into our environment. The amount of contaminants that are already present in the air, food, and water will affect the health of our descendants for several generations. The most common concerns of community groups are toxic and nuclear wastes, nuclear power plants, air and water pollution, and herbicide and pesticide spraying.

Sites for Health-Promotion Activities

Health-promotion programs are found in many settings. Programs and activities may be offered to individuals and families in the home or in the community setting, at schools, in hospitals, at worksites, or at shopping malls. Some individuals may feel more comfortable having the nurse, diet counselor, or fitness expert come to their home for teaching and follow-up on individual needs. This type of program, however, is not cost-effective for most individuals. Many people prefer the group approach, find it more motivating, and enjoy the socializing and group support. Most programs offered in the community are group oriented.

Community programs are frequently offered by cities and towns. The type of program depends on the current concerns and the expertise of the sponsoring department or group. Program offerings may include health promotion, specific protection, and screening for early detection of disease. The local health department may offer a communitywide immunization program or blood pressure screening. The fire department may disseminate fire-prevention information; the police may offer bicycle safety programs for children, safe-driving campaigns for young adults or gun safety programs for all citizens.

Hospitals began the emphasis on health promotion and prevention by focusing on the health of their employees. Because of the stress involved in caring for the sick and the various shifts that nurses and other health care workers must work, the lifestyles and health habits of health care employees were given priority.

Programs offered by health care organizations initially began with the specific focus of prevention. Examples include infection control, fire prevention and fire drills, limiting exposure to X rays, and the prevention of back injuries. Gradually, issues related to the health and lifestyle of the employee were addressed with programs on topics such as smoking cessation, exercise and fitness, stress reduction, and time management. Increasingly, hospitals have offered a variety of these programs and others (e.g., women's health) to the community as well as to their employees. This community activity of the health care institution enhances the public image of the hospital, increases the health of the surrounding population, and generates some additional income.

School health-promotion programs may serve as a foundation for children of all ages to learn basic knowledge about personal hygiene and issues in the health sciences. Because school is the focus of a child's life for so many years, the school provides a cost-effective and convenient setting for health-focused programs. The school nurse may teach programs about basic nutrition, dental care, activity and play, drug and alcohol abuse, domestic violence, child abuse, and issues related to sexuality and pregnancy. Classroom teachers may include health-related topics in their lesson plans, for example, the way the normal heart functions or the need for clean air and water in the environment.

Worksite programs for health promotion have developed out of the need for businesses to control the rising cost of health care and employee absenteeism. Many industries feel that both employers and employees can benefit from healthy lifestyle behavior. The convenience of the worksite setting makes these programs particularly attractive to many adults who would otherwise not be aware of them or motivated to attend them. Health-promotion programs may be held in the company cafeteria so that employees can watch a film or have a discussion group during their lunch break. Worksite programs may include programs that address air-quality standards for the office, classroom, or plant; programs aimed at specific populations, such as accident prevention for the machine worker or back-saver programs for the individual involved in heavy lifting; programs to prevent repetitive stress injuries; programs to screen for high blood pressure; or health-enhancement programs, such as fitness information and relaxation techniques. Benefits to the worker may include an increased feeling of well-being, fitness, weight control, and decreased stress. Benefits to the employer may include an increase in employee motivation and productivity, an increase in employee morale, a decrease in absenteeism, and a lower rate of employee turnover, all of which may decrease business and health care costs.

Increasingly, health information is available on the Worldwide Web. Internet sites such as WebMD offer information on prevention, screening, and management of many illnesses. It is important that health professionals inform patients and consumers of the reliability of information on the Internet. Although there are many reliable sources of health information on the web, there are also websites that present opinions of the website developer, which may or may not be supported by scientific evidence. An example of health information disseminated on the Internet that must be viewed with caution are websites espousing various alternative medicine strategies.

Consider . . .

- the accessibility of preventive care services to people of all ages and economic status in your community.
- places where health information is made available to the public in your community.
- how you would improve your current worksite wellness program.
- the effectiveness of environmental control programs in your community.
- health-promotion activities you would like to see implemented in your community if there were no limits in such resources as time, expertise, and money.
- health-promotion activities you would plan for (a) elderly clients, (b) adolescents, and (c) school-age children in your community.
- health-promotion interventions that could be incorporated into a nursing care plan for a client with an existing health problem, such as chronic lung disease, diabetes mellitus, or cardiac disease.

HEALTH-PROMOTION MODELS

The health belief model (HBM) discussed in Chapter 17, "Nursing in an Evolving Health Care Delivery System," focuses on a person's susceptibility to disease. According to Pender (1996, p. 34), the HBM is considered appropriate for explaining health-protecting or preventive behaviors, but it is not considered an appropriate model for health-promoting behaviors. Three health-promotion models follow.

Pender's Health-Promotion Model

Nola Pender's health-promotion model (1996, pp. 51–75) focuses on *health-promoting* behaviors rather than health-protecting or preventive behaviors (Figure 7–2). Its organization is similar to that of the health belief model. Determinants of health-promoting behaviors are categorized into (1) cognitive-perceptual factors, (2) modifying factors, and (3) cues to action.

Figure 7–2

Health Promotion Model

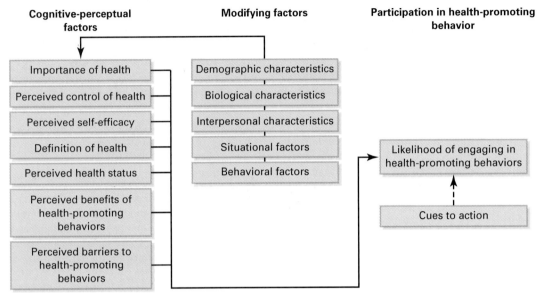

Source: Health Promotion in Nursing (3d ed.) by N. J. Pender, Norwalk, Conn.: Appleton and Lange, 1996, p. 52. Reprinted with permission.

Cognitive-Perceptual Factors

Cognitive-perceptual factors are considered to be the *primary motivational mechanisms* for acquiring and maintaining health-promoting behaviors. They include the following:

- *The importance of health.* Placing a high value on health results in information-seeking behavior, such as reading health-related pamphlets.
- *Perceived control.* People who perceive that they have control over their own health are more likely to use preventive services than people who feel powerless. Control over health can relate to such behaviors as not smoking and using seat belts in automobiles.
- *Perceived self-efficacy.* This concept refers to the conviction that a person can successfully carry out the behavior necessary to achieve a desired outcome, such as maintaining an exercise program to lose weight. Often people who have serious doubts about their capabilities decrease their efforts and give up, whereas those with a strong sense of efficacy exert greater effort to master problems or challenges.
- *Definition of health.* A person's definition of health may influence the extent to which the person engages in health-promoting behaviors.
- *Perceived health status.* Perceived health status may affect the frequency and intensity of health-promoting behaviors.
- *Perceived benefits of health-promoting behaviors.* Perceived benefits (e.g., physical fitness, psychologic well-being,

and stress reduction) affect the person's level of participation in health-promoting behaviors and may facilitate continued practice. Repetition of such behavior itself can strengthen and reinforce beliefs about benefits.
- *Perceived barriers.* A person's perceptions about available time, access to facilities, and difficulty performing the activity may act as barriers to health-promoting behaviors. These barriers may be imagined or real.

Modifying Factors

Factors that modify the cognitive-perceptual factors include the following:

- *Demographic factors,* such as age, sex, race, ethnicity, education, and income
- *Biologic characteristics,* such as percentage of body fat and total body weight, which are related to exercise adherence
- *Interpersonal influences,* such as expectations of significant others, family patterns of health care, and interactions with health professionals
- *Situational factors,* such as ease of access to health-promotion alternatives and availability of environmental options (e.g., vending machines and restaurant menus that provide healthful options)
- *Behavioral factors,* such as previous experience, knowledge, and skill in health-promoting actions

Research Box

Choudhry, U. K. 1998. Health promotion among immigrant women from India living in Canada. *Image: The Journal of Nursing Scholarship* 30(3): 269–274.

The purpose of this study was to describe the health-promoting practices of immigrant women from India and how cultural knowledge, norms, and values influence their behavior. Using ethnographic methods, 20 women between the ages of 40 and 70 were interviewed individually using open-ended questions. The women were all first-generation immigrants from India living in metropolitan Toronto, Canada.

The dominant themes that emerged were value of being healthy, lifestyle behaviors, relationships, spiritual well-being, traditional health practices, and barriers to health promotion. The women placed value on health and equated it with happiness. Health was discussed as part of the connectedness of body, mind, and spirit, and religious and spiritual belief was important. Barriers to health promotion identified were the cold climate that prevented regular walks, not having informative materials in their native language, and keeping up a fast pace.

Cues to Action

The likelihood that a person will take health-promoting action may depend on (a) cues of *internal origin,* such as personal awareness of the potential for growth or increased feelings of well-being; and (b) cues of *external origin,* such as conversations with others about their health behavior patterns and mass media information about personal and family health and environmental concerns.

Kulbok's Resource Model of Preventive Health Behavior

The resource model of preventive health behavior developed by Kulbok (1985, pp. 67–81) proposes that people act in ways that maximize their "stock in health." It hypothesizes that the greater a person's social and health resources, the more frequently the person will perform preventive behaviors.

Social resources refer to education level and family income. *Health resources* refer to general psychologic well-being; perceptions about health, health status,

and energy level; the capability to take care of one's own health; participation in social groups; and number and closeness of friends and relatives. *Preventive health behaviors* relate to physical activity, diet, sleeping, smoking, drinking alcoholic beverages, drinking caffeinated beverages, dental hygiene, use of seat belts, use of professional health services for prevention of disease, and behavior to control high blood pressure.

Neuman's Systems Model

In her health-promotion model, nurse theorist Betty Neuman (1995) includes levels of prevention (primary, secondary, and tertiary) and factors that strengthen a person's lines or barriers of defense. For additional information, see Chapter 6, "Theoretical Foundations of Professional Nursing," and the book *The Neuman Systems Model.*

Consider . . .

- determinants of health-promoting behaviors cited in Pender's and Kulbok's models that may influence your own health behavior.
- what barriers can deter positive health-promoting behaviors in adolescents and older adults.
- how demographic factors such as age, sex, race, ethnicity, education, and income may influence health-promoting behaviors.

STAGES OF HEALTH BEHAVIOR CHANGE

Health behavior change is a cyclic phenomenon in which people progress through several stages. In the first stage, the person does not think seriously about changing a behavior; by the time the person reaches the final stage, he or she is successfully maintaining the change in behavior. Several behavior change models have been proposed. The stage model proposed by Prochaska and DiClemente (1982, 1992) is discussed here. The stages are (1) precontemplation, (2) contemplation, (3) preparation, (4) action, and (5) maintenance. If the person does not succeed in changing behavior, relapse occurs.

In the *precontemplation stage,* the person does not think about changing behavior, nor is the person interested in information about the behavior. The negative aspects of making the change outweigh the benefits. Some people may believe the behavior is not under their control and may become defensive when confronted with information.

During the *contemplative stage,* the person seriously considers changing a specific behavior, actively gathers information, and verbalizes plans to change the behavior in the near future. Belief in the value of the change and self-confidence in the ability to change both increase in this phase. It is common for a person to feel some ambivalence when weighing the losses against the rewards of changing the behavior. Some people may stay in the contemplative stage for months or years.

The *preparation stage* occurs when the person undertakes cognitive and behavioral activities that prepare the person for change. At this stage, the person believes that the advantages of changing the behavior outweigh the disadvantages and makes specific plans to accomplish the change. Some people in this stage change small aspects of the behavior, such as cutting out sugar in their coffee.

The *action stage* occurs when the person actively implements behavioral and cognitive strategies to interrupt previous behavior patterns and adopt new ones. To prevent recurrences of previous behavior, the action stage needs to continue for several weeks or months.

During the *maintenance stage,* the person integrates newly adopted behavior patterns into his or her lifestyle. This stage lasts until the person no longer experiences temptation to return to previous unhealthy behaviors.

These five stages are cyclical; people generally move through one stage before progressing to the next. However, at any point in time a person may regress to any previous stage. Sudden or gradual relapses to previous behavior patterns may occur during the action or maintenance stages, for example. Individuals who relapse may return to the stage of precontemplation, contemplation, or preparation before their next attempt to change. To identify whether the client is in the precontemplative or contemplative stages, ask whether the client is thinking about changing a behavior in the next 6 months or a year. Those in precontemplation will answer no; those in contemplation or preparation will answer yes. Table 7–3 relates nursing strategies appropriate for each stage of health behavior change.

Consider . . .

■ a client under your care who is considering a health behavior change. At what stage of Prochaska and DiClemente's model is the client? What barriers exist in the client's experience that might interfere with the client's goal? What activities or interventions might you suggest or do to help the client successfully make the health behavior change?

■ your own experience in changing an unhealthy behavior (e.g., quitting smoking, losing weight,

maintaining proper nutrition, reducing stress). How did you progress through the stages of the Prochaska and DiClemente model? What barriers to health behavior change did you experience? How did you overcome the barriers and effect a successful health behavior change?

■ what barriers exist in your community that interfere with individual and family health behavior changes. What supports exist in your community to assist individuals and families in making health behavior changes? How might you promote and support health behavior changes in your community?

THE NURSE'S ROLE IN HEALTH PROMOTION

Individuals and communities who seek to increase their responsibility for personal health and self-care require health education. The trend toward health promotion has created the opportunity for nurses to strengthen the profession's influence on health promotion, disseminate information that promotes an educated public, and assist individuals and communities to change long-standing health behaviors. Health-promotion activities involve collaborative relationships with both clients and physicians. The role of the nurse is to work *with* people, not *for* them—that is, to act as a facilitator of the process of assessing, evaluating, and understanding health. The nurse may act as advocate, consultant, teacher, or coordinator of services. For examples of the nurse's role in health promotion, see the box on page 122.

In these roles, the nurse may work with individuals of all age groups and diverse family units or concentrate on a specific population, such as new parents, school-age children, or older adults. In any case, the nursing process is a basic tool for the nurse in a health-promotion role. Although the process is the same, the nurse emphasizes teaching the client (who can be either an individual or a family unit) self-care responsibility. Adult clients decide the goals, determine the health-promotion plans, and take the responsibility for the success of the plans.

Consider . . .

■ types of health-promotion activities you have previously been involved in.

■ any difficulties you have previously encountered in initiating or maintaining clients' health-promoting behaviors.

■ what personal responsibility means in relation to health and how that affects the nurse's role in health promotion.

Table 7–3 Examples of Nursing Strategies for Each Stage of Health Behavior Change

Stage	Nursing Strategies
Precontemplation	• Raise the client's awareness of healthy behaviors, such as exercising, altering the diet, quitting smoking, using sunscreen, and undergoing regular mammography screening. • Provide personalized information about the benefits of specific health behaviors; for example, relate the client's cough to smoking or excessive fat intake to heart disease. • Explore the client's beliefs and feelings related to the health behavior. • Identify previous successful changes (e.g., previous weight loss) to increase the client's self-confidence, and offer positive feedback.
Contemplation	• Continue to provide the interventions cited in the previous stage. In addition, provide adequate and accurate information about available alternatives to encourage clients to make appropriate choices and actively participate in decision making. • Encourage the client to express ambivalent feelings. Include spouses, if appropriate (e.g., for dietary alterations). • Help the client further clarify values in relation to the health behavior, and encourage the client to consider how it would feel, for example, to be at an appropriate weight or to be an ex-smoker. • Help the client identify social pressures that encourage positive health behaviors, such as exercise facilities or bans on smoking at work.
Preparation	• Assist the client to make specific plans to implement the change; for example, discuss self-help groups and other available support persons or groups. • Help the client identify stimuli that trigger unhealthy behavior and consider ways to remove or minimize these stimuli (e.g., altering the environment or removing oneself from a troublesome area). • Teach the client to substitute activities to counteract the unhealthy behavior, such as relaxation exercises, internal dialogues, or thought stopping (suddenly saying "stop" loudly). • Plan appropriate rewards (e.g., a movie, dining out) for clients to give themselves for having achieved their goals.
Action	• Review plans and instructions discussed in the preparation phase. • Help the client set realistic goals. • Encourage positive self-talk that supports the behavior change. • Provide positive feedback, support, and encouragement for partial or complete achievement of goals.
Maintenance	• Encourage continuing use of support networks and open discussion of problems related to maintaining healthy behavior. • Identify and encourage strategies that support healthy behavior.

Sources: "Toward a More Integrative Model of Change" by J. Prochaska and C. DiClemente, *Psychotherapy: Theory, Research, and Practice* **19:** 276–288, 1982; "Stages of Change in the Modification of Problem Behaviors" by J. Prochaska and C. DiClemente, *Progress in Behavior Modification* **28:** 183–218, 1992; "A Stage-Based Approach to Helping People Change Health Behaviors" by V. S. Conn, *Clinical Nurse Specialist* **8**(4): 187–193, 1994.

SUMMARY

The goal of health promotion is to raise the level of health of an individual, family, or community. Health-promotion activities are directed toward developing client resources that maintain or enhance well-being. Health-protection activities are geared toward pre-venting specific diseases, such as obtaining immunizations to prevent measles.

Healthy People 2010 is focused on improving the health of individuals, families, communities, and the nation. The goals of *Healthy People 2010* are (1) to in-

The Nurse's Role in Health Promotion

- Model health lifestyle behaviors and attitudes.
- Facilitate client involvement in the assessment, implementation, and evaluation of health goals.
- Teach clients self-care strategies to enhance fitness, improve nutrition, manage stress, and enhance relationships.
- Assist individuals, families, and communities to increase their levels of health.
- Educate clients to be effective health care consumers.

- Assist clients, families, and communities to develop and choose health-promoting options.
- Guide clients' development in effective problem solving and decision making.
- Reinforce clients' personal and family health-promoting behaviors.
- Advocate in the community for changes that promote a healthy environment.

crease the quality and years of healthy life and (2) to eliminate health disparities.

Health-promotion strategies may be active or passive. With active strategies, the client participates in making lifestyle changes. With passive strategies, the client is the recipient of a health-promotion effort, such as maintaining an appropriate water supply. A variety of programs can be used for health promotion, including (1) information dissemination, (2) health appraisal and wellness assessment, (3) lifestyle and behavior change, and (4) environmental control programs. These programs are found in many settings—in the home, schools, community centers, hospitals, worksites, and shopping malls.

Three health-promotion models are described. Pender's health-promotion model categorizes determinants of health-promoting behaviors as cognitive-perceptual factors, modifying factors, and variables affecting the likelihood of action. Cognitive-perceptual factors, the primary motivational factors, include the person's perception of the importance of health, perceived control, perceived self-efficacy, definition of health, perceived health status, perceived benefits of health-promoting behaviors, and perceived barriers. These factors may be modified by demographic factors, biological characteristics, interpersonal influences, situational factors, and behavioral factors. Cues to action may be of either internal origin or external origin.

Kulbok's resource model of preventive health behavior hypothesizes that the greater the person's social and health resources, the more frequently the person will perform preventive behaviors. Neuman's systems model includes dimensions of health promotion designed to strengthen a person's lines of defense and addresses primary, secondary, and tertiary levels of prevention.

Prochaska and DiClemente propose a five-stage model for health behavior change. The stages are (1) precontemplation, (2) contemplation, (3) prepara-

Bookshelf

Edelman, C. L., and Mandle, C. L. 1998. *Health promotion throughout the lifespan,* 4th ed. St. Louis: Mosby. This reference text is a must for nurses who work in settings that promote health. Units include "Foundations of Health Promotion," "Assessment for Health Promotion," "Interventions for Health Promotion," "Application of Health Promotion," and "Challenges as We Enter the New Millennium." Health-promotion activities for people from the prenatal period through older adults are presented from a developmental perspective.

Murray, R. B., and Zentner, J. P. 2001. *Health promotion strategies through the life span,* 7th ed. Upper Saddle River, N.J.: Prentice Hall.

This text provides a comprehensive guide to health promotion and disease- and injury-prevention interventions for all age groups. The authors use a holistic approach to the health care of individuals and families. The text offers guidelines for nursing assessment with suggested interventions and health-promotion strategies for each developmental stage from birth to death.

tion, (4) action, and (5) maintenance. If the person is not successful in changing behavior, relapse may occur during the action or maintenance stages. However, at any point in these stages, people may move to any previous stage. An understanding of these stages enables the nurse to provide appropriate nursing interventions.

The nurse's role in health promotion is to act as a facilitator of the process of assessing, evaluating, and understanding health.

SELECTED REFERENCES

Brown, K. C., Mattson, A. H., Newman, K. D., and Sirles, A. T. 1992, Winter. A community health nursing curriculum and Healthy People 2000. *Clinical Nurse Specialist* **6**(4): 203–208.

Choudhry, U. K. 1998. Health promotion among immigrant women from India living in Canada. *Image: The Journal of Nursing Scholarship* **30**(3): 269–274.

Conn, V. S. 1994. A stage-based approach to helping people change health behaviors. *Clinical Nurse Specialist* **8**: 187–193.

Epp, J. 1986, November. *Achieving health for all: A framework for health promotion. Report of the Minister of National Health and Welfare.* Ottawa, Canada: Government Printing Office.

Kulbok, P. P. 1985, June. Social resources, health resources, and preventive behaviors: Patterns and predictions. *Public Health Nursing* **2**: 67–81.

Lalonde, M. 1974. *A new perspective on the health of Canadians.* Ottawa: Government of Canada.

Leavell, H. R., and Clark, E. G. 1965. *Preventive medicine for the doctor in the community,* 3d ed. New York: McGraw-Hill.

Lewis, F. M. 1982, March/April. Experienced personal control and quality of life in late-stage cancer patients. *Nursing Research* **31**: 113–118.

Maglacas, A. M. 1988, March/April. Health for all: Nursing's role. *Nursing Outlook* **36**: 266–271.

Neuman, B. 1995. *The Neuman systems model,* 3d ed. Norwalk, Conn.: Appleton and Lange.

Opatz, J. P. 1985. *A primer of health promotion: Creating healthy organizational cultures.* Washington, D.C.: Oryn Publications, p. 101.

Pender, N. J. 1996. *Health promotion in nursing practice,* 3d ed. Stamford, Conn.: Appleton-Lange.

Prochaska, J., and DiClemente, C. 1982. Toward a more integrative model of change. *Psychotherapy: Theory, Research, and Practice* **19**: 276–288.

Prochaska, J., and DiClemente, C. 1992. Stages of change in the modification of problem behaviors. *Progress in Behavior Modification* **28**: 183–218.

Salsbury, P. J. 1993, Sept./Oct. Assuming responsibility for one's health: An analysis of a key assumption in nursing's agenda for health care reform. *Nursing Outlook* **41**: 212–216.

Schultz, A. 1995, Aug. What is health promotion? *Canadian Nurse* **91**: 31–34.

Smillie, C. 1992, July/Aug. Preparing health professionals for a collaborative health promotion role. *Canadian Journal of Public Health* **93**: 279–282.

Stachtchenko, S., and Jenicek, M. 1990, Jan.–Feb. Conceptual differences between prevention and health promotion: Research implications for community health programs. *Canadian Journal of Public Health* **81**: 53–59.

Travis, J. W., and Ryan, R. S. 1988. *The wellness workbook.* Berkeley, Calif.: Ten Speed Press.

United States Department of Health and Human Services. 1990, Sept. *Healthy people 2000: National health promotion and disease prevention objectives.* DHHS Pub. No. (PHS) 91-50212. Washington, D.C.: Government Printing Office.

United States Department of Health and Human Services. 2001. *Healthy people 2010.* Washington, D.C.: USDHHS. web.health.gov/healthypeople.

United States Department of Health and Human Services. 2001. *Healthy people 2010: A systematic approach to health improvement.* Washington, D.C.: USDHHS. web.health.gov/healthypeople.

United States Department of Health and Human Services. 2001. *Healthy people 2010: Leading health indicators.* Washington, D.C.: USDHHS. web.health.gov/healthypeople.

U.S. Surgeon General. 1979. *Healthy people: The Surgeon General's report on health promotion and disease prevention.* DHHS Pub. No. 79-55071. Washington, D.C.: Government Printing Office.

U.S. Surgeon General. 1980. *Health promotion/disease prevention: Objectives for the nation.* Washington, D.C.: Department of Health and Human Services.

World Health Organization. 1984. *Report of the working group on the concept and principles of health promotion.* Copenhagen: WHO.

World Health Organization. 1986. *Framework for health promotion training.* Copenhagen: WHO.

The Nurse as Learner and Teacher

Objectives

- Discuss selected learning theories.
- Explain the three domains of learning.
- Describe the various teaching roles of the nurse.
- Identify guidelines for effective teaching and learning.
- Develop a teaching plan.
- Identify strategies for teaching learners of different cultures.

N U R S E   C O N N E C T

Additional online resources for this chapter can be found on the companion web site at www.prenhall.com/blais.

Nurses have both learning and teaching responsibilities. They must continue to learn so that they can maintain their knowledge and skills amid the many changes in health care. They teach clients and their families, other health care professionals, and nursing assistants to whom they delegate care, and they share their expertise with other nurses and health professionals. Some teach their profession to others.

Teaching and learning is not limited to classroom experiences and can occur in all settings for practice.

Learning is a complex process, and there are many theories about how learning occurs. These learning theories are generally based on assumptions about people, the nature of knowledge, and how people learn. The eclectic approach presumes that no one theory is more correct than another. More information is becoming available regarding people's learning styles.

There are also beliefs about how teaching can be most effective. These are commonly referred to as principles of teaching. Both learning and teaching are active and interactive processes. Currently, there is increasing focus on outcome-based teaching and evidence-based learning.

CHALLENGES AND OPPORTUNITIES

The challenges associated with teaching and learning in the current health care system are many. Federal and state regulations impact the content to be taught and the documentation required. Health care clients vary in age, ethnic diversity, socioeconomic status, primary language, and previous knowledge and experience. Today's resources are numerous and readily available through the Worldwide Web (www). Information is constantly changing as new research becomes available. Providing clients with accurate, current information is a challenge for nurses. Teaching is a major role of nurses, and it is often performed without adequate preparation. Effective teaching is a challenge.

Nurses today must also keep up to date with theory and practice. Nursing education programs prepare the new practitioner with effective beginning nursing skills. Changes occur quickly and often in nursing and health care; consequently nurses must continue learning to keep current. Many states require nurses to complete continuing education programs designed to increase knowledge and skill. Often employers provide programs at the work site for updating nurses' knowledge and skills. Sometimes nurses need to travel to specialized centers to gain advanced specialized skills.

The importance of the learning and teaching roles of nurses creates new opportunities for nurses as teachers of clients and their families, subordinates in the health care system, and peers and colleagues. Nurses can also influence the health of communities by participating in community health education programs. Nurses not only teach clients directly but also participate in the development of health education literature and Internet-based health information.

NURSES AS LEARNERS

There are several ways in which the nurse may learn, including continued formal academic education, institution-based human resource development (HRD) programs, encouraged or legislatively mandated continuing education, or episodic individual-selected educational pursuits.

Continued formal academic education includes postbaccalaureate study at the master's or doctoral degree levels. Education at the graduate level requires critical thinking and knowledge of the research process. Graduate study may be in nursing or in other disciplines that potentiate the nurses' practice. For example, nurses in administration may choose to pursue master's degrees in nursing administration, health care administration, or business administration. There are many factors the nurse must consider in choosing a graduate program. Chapter 22, "Advanced Nursing Education and Practice," provides guidelines for preparing for graduate study and selecting and applying to a graduate program.

Institution-based human resource development programs are administered by the employer. Swansburg (1995, p. 2) defines human resource development as "the process by which corporate management stimulates the motivation of employees to perform productively. HRD provides the stimuli that motivate nursing personnel to provide nursing care services to clients at quality and quantity standards that keep the health care entity reputable and financially solvent, the nurses satisfied with their professional accomplishments and quality of work life, and the clients treated successfully." Human resource development programs are designed to upgrade the knowledge and skills of employees. For example, an employer might offer programs to orient new staff members, to inform nurses about a new institutional policy, to familiarize nurses with a new piece of equipment or a new technique, to prepare nurses for certification at specialty or advanced levels of practice, or to implement a nurse theorist's conceptual framework as the guideline for nursing practice within the institution. Some human resource development programs also offer nurses tuition benefits to enroll in work-related courses or to attend professional conferences. It is important for the nurse to remember that the primary intended benefit of human resource development programs is for the institution; however, nurses who take advantage of institution-based programs can also benefit their own professional practice.

The term *continuing education* refers to formalized experiences designed to expand the knowledge or skills of nurses. Continuing education programs tend to be more specific and shorter than formal advanced academic degree study. Continuing education is the responsibility of each practicing nurse. Constant updating and growth are essential for the nurse to keep abreast of scientific and technologic change and changes within the nursing profession. Continuing education can be part of an employer's human resource development program or may be offered by professional organizations or continuing education departments of colleges or universities. Continuing education may also be obtained through self-study programs offered through professional journals or through home study programs provided by private, public, and professional educational organizations.

Some states require nurses to obtain a certain number of continuing education (CE) credits to renew their professional licenses. In these states, required CE contact hours vary from 15 to 30 hours for every two-year licensure period. Depending on the state, all, some, or none of these hours may be acquired through home study. Some states require specific content instruction as part of the legislated continuing education requirement, for example, current study in violence or AIDS. Nurses who hold licensure in several states must meet the continuing education requirements for each state.

Some professional organizations require continuing education to meet certification and recertification requirements for specialty practice. For example, to be certified as a pediatric nurse by the American Nurses Association, the nurse must have completed 30 contact hours of continuing education applicable to pediatric nursing within the previous 3 years (American Nurses Credentialing Center [ANCC], 2001). This continuing education requirement is in addition to other requirements.

Episodic learning activities are determined by the individual nurse. Episodic learning activities are those activities that are distinct and separate from formal or planned education. Subscribing to and reading professional journals and newsletters or commercial newspapers are examples of nurses' episodic educational activities. The learning the nurse gains through these activities can be just as important as formal educational pursuits. Through reading about the contemporary understanding of health care in professional or commercial literature, the nurse gains an awareness of how nurses can influence the health care system. Nurses can also gain knowledge of personal benefit, such as liability and malpractice issues, advanced practice and licensure issues, and portable pension plans.

Consider . . .

■ the various learning activities you have participated in during the last year. How many were episodic activities? How many were part of the human resource development program of your employer? How many were done to meet continuing education requirements for relicensure or recertification? How many were done for personal satisfaction?

■ your personal goals related to professional learning activities. Are your learning activities directed toward becoming certified? To achieving an academic degree? For personal satisfaction?

THE LEARNING PROCESS

People, including clients, have a variety of learning needs. A learning need is evidenced by a desire or requirement to change behavior or "a gap between the information an individual knows and the information necessary to perform a function or care for self" (Gessner, 1989, p. 593). **Learning** is a change in human disposition or capability that persists over a period of time and that cannot be solely accounted for by growth. Learning is represented by a change in behavior. See the accompanying box for attributes of learning.

Attributes of Learning

Learning is:

• An experience that occurs inside the learner.

• The discovery of the personal meaning and relevance of ideas.

• A consequence of experience.

• A collaborative and cooperative process.

• An evolutionary process.

• A process that is both intellectual and emotional.

An important aspect of learning is the individual's desire to learn and to act on the learning. This desire is best illustrated when the person recognizes and accepts the need to learn, willingly expends the energy required to learn, and then follows through with the appropriate behaviors that reflect the learning. For example, a person diagnosed as having diabetes willingly learns about the special diet needed and then plans and follows the learned diet.

Andragogy is "the art and science of helping adults learn" (Knowles, 1980, p. 43) in contrast to **pedagogy,** the discipline concerned with helping children learn. Nurses can use the following andragogic concepts about learners as a guide for client teaching (Knowles, 1984):

- As people mature, they move from dependence to independence.
- An adult's previous experiences can be used as a resource for learning.
- An adult's readiness to learn is often related to a developmental task or social role.
- An adult is more oriented to learning when the material is immediately useful, not useful sometime in the future.

Theories of Learning

Theories about how and why people learn can be traced back to the seventeenth century. Psychologists first focused on the mental phenomena. Today, there is more focus on the behaviors or activities of learning. There are a number of theories and numerous psychologists associated with theories of learning. Five contemporary theoretical constructs are behaviorism, cognitivism, humanism, constructivism, and multiple intelligence.

Behaviorism

Behaviorism was originally advanced by Edward Thorndike, who believed that transfer of knowledge could occur if the new situation closely resembled the old situation. To Thorndike, the term *understanding* was used in the context of building connections. One of his major contributions applicable to teaching is that learning should be based on the learner's behavior. He is known for his "laws of learning." In addition to Thorndike, major behaviorist theorists include Pavlov, Skinner, and Bandura.

Behaviorists believe that the environment influences behavior and how a person controls it; moreover, they maintain that it is the essential factor determining human action. In the behaviorist school of thought, an act is called a response when it can be traced to the effects of a stimulus.

SKINNER'S OPERANT CONDITIONING THEORY Skinner postulates two types of **conditioning** (behavioral responses to a stimulus) that cause the response or behavior. The first type of conditioning, termed *classical conditioning,* is illustrated by Pavlov's well-known experiments with dogs. Pavlov (1849–1936) conditioned dogs to salivate in response to the sound of a tuning fork, a sound they heard when they received food. Classical conditioning is a procedure in which conditioned responses are established by the association of a new stimulus that is known to cause an unconditioned response. The resulting response is the conditioned response to the *new* (unrelated) stimulus.

The second type of conditioning is what Skinner refers to as *operant conditioning,* a process by which the frequency of a response can be increased or decreased depending on when, how, and to what extent it is reinforced. Skinner believes that humans, like animals, will always repeat actions that bring pleasure. He considers the consequences of an action, what he terms **reinforcement,** to be all-important. Positive consequences foster repetition of the action; negative consequences or the absence of consequences can cause the action to cease.

Extinction is the process in which a conditioned behavior is "unlearned" because the reinforcement has been removed. Greater effort, however, is required to extinguish a behavior than to condition it. The procedure involves removing the *unconditional stimulus* or the reward from the training situation. When the conditioning procedure is again instigated following complete extinction, it does not take the subject as long to show the conditioned response as it did in the original conditioning.

Studies of conditioning produced a number of laws of learning that were thought to be universal; that is, they were thought to apply to all ages, all cultures, and all types of behavior—motor, cognitive, emotional, and social. Examples follow:

- The more quickly reinforcement follows a response, the more effective the reinforcement.
- A response made in the presence of one stimulus generalizes to similar stimuli.
- Behavior that is reinforced only part of the time takes longer to extinguish than behavior that is reinforced continuously.

BANDURA'S MODELING THEORY Social learning theorists such as Bandura agree with Skinner that the environment exerts a great deal of control over overt behavior; however, they believe that the entire learning process involves three highly interdependent factors:

1. Characteristics of the person
2. The person's behavior
3. The environment

These factors influence and control each other through a process that Bandura calls *reciprocal determinism.* The major contribution of Bandura's reciprocal determinism is the concept that the child's behavior affects or "creates" that child's environment. This differs from Skinner's belief that the environment, viewed as a set of stimuli, controls behavior.

Bandura claims that most learning comes from observational learning and instruction rather than from overt trial-and-error behavior. **Observational learning** is the acquisition of new skills or the alteration of old behaviors simply by watching other children and adults. It is especially important for acquiring behavior in situations where mistakes are life-threatening or costly, e.g., driving a car or performing brain surgery.

Bandura's research focuses on **imitation,** the process by which individuals copy or reproduce what they have observed, and **modeling,** the process by which a person learns by observing the behavior of others. Imitation is regarded as one of the most powerful socialization forces. Various imitative behaviors are reinforced by a process of operant conditioning. For example, a boy may be praised for being "just like his father." The child may even self-reinforce the imitations by repeating an adult's words of praise. According to Bandura, models influence others mainly by providing information rather than by eliciting matching behavior, so that learning can occur without even once performing the model's behavior.

In recent years, Bandura's theory has become more cognitive, and he now calls his theory a "social cognitive theory." Learning is defined as "knowledge acquisition through cognitive processing information" (1971, p. xii). For example, television's effects on children depend on both cognitive and imitative processes. Whether the child can comprehend the story affects the child's perceptions of the model and the tendency to imitate the model.

Cognitivism

Cognitivism depicts learning as a complex cognitive activity. Major cognitive theorists include Piaget, Lewin, Gagne, Bloom, and Bruner. Cognitivists view learning as the development of understandings and apprecia-

tion that help the individual function in a larger context. Learning is based on a change of perception, which itself is influenced by the senses and both internal and external variables. In other words, learning is largely a mental, intellectual, or thinking process. The learner structures and processes information based on his or her perceptions of the information. The learner's perceptions are influenced by their personal characteristics and their experiences. Cognitivists also emphasize the importance of social, emotional, and physical contexts in which learning occurs, such as the teacher-learner relationship and environment. Developmental readiness and individual readiness (expressed as motivation) are other key factors associated with cognitive approaches.

PIAGET'S PHASES OF COGNITIVE DEVELOPMENT According to Piaget, cognitive development is an orderly sequential process in which a variety of new experiences (stimuli) must exist before intellectual abilities can develop. Piaget's cognitive developmental process is divided into four major phases: sensorimotor, preoperational, concrete operations, and formal operations. A person develops through each of these phases, and each phase has unique characteristics.

The *sensorimotor* phase lasts from birth to 2 years of age. It includes reflexive actions, perceptions of events centered on the body, objects as an extension of self, mental acknowledgment of the external environment, and discovery of new goals and ways to attain these goals. The preoperational phase occurs from 2 to 7 years of age and includes an egocentric approach to accommodate the demands of the environment. Everything is significant and relates to "me." The child is able to think of one idea at a time, can use words to express thoughts, and includes others in the environment. The *concrete operations* phase (7 to 11 years old) involves a beginning understanding of relationships such as size, right and left, different viewpoints, and the ability to solve concrete problems. In the *formal operations* phase, occurring at 11 to 15 years of age, the person is able to use rational thinking and reasoning that is deductive and futuristic.

In each phase, the person uses three primary abilities: assimilation, accommodation, and adaptation. *Assimilation* is the process through which humans encounter and react to new situations by using the mechanisms they already possess. In this way, people acquire new knowledge and skills as well as insights into the world around them. *Accommodation* is the process of change whereby cognitive processes mature sufficiently to allow the person to solve problems that were unsolvable before. This adjustment is possible chiefly because new knowledge has been assimilated. *Adaptation,* or coping behavior, is the ability to handle the demands made by the environment.

Consider . . .

- how a nurse can employ Piaget's theory of cognitive development when developing teaching strategies for learners of different ages and developmental stages, e.g., a toddler (egocentric and literal) or teenager (rational thinking).

LEWIN'S FIELD THEORY Lewin's field theory involves theories of motivation and perception, which were considered precursors of the more recent cognitive theories. Lewin believed that learning involved four different types of changes: change in cognitive structure, change in motivation, change in one's sense of belonging to the group, and gain in voluntary muscle control. His well-known theory of change has three basic stages: unfreezing, moving, and refreezing. These stages are discussed in Chapter 14, "Change Process."

GAGNE'S INFORMATION PROCESSING THEORY Gagne postulates eight levels of intellectual skills: (1) signal; (2) stimulus-response; (3) chaining, which involves at least two stimulus-response connections; (4) verbal association, which involves assembling verbal chains from previous learning; (5) multiple discrimination involving differentiated responses to variable stimuli; (6) concept formation, which involves identifying and responding to a class of objects that serve as stimuli; (7) principle formation, which involves applying a principle that is made up of at least one chain of two or more concepts; and (8) problem solving, which involves processing at least two or more principles to produce a higher-level principle.

BLOOM'S DOMAINS OF LEARNING Bloom (1956) identified three domains, or areas of learning: cognitive, affective, and psychomotor. The *cognitive domain* includes six intellectual skills such as knowing, comprehending, and applying in order from simple to complex. The *affective domain* includes feelings, emotions, interests, attitudes, and appreciations. It involves five major categories. The *psychomotor domain* includes motor skills such as giving an injection. It includes seven categories from perception (lowest level) to origination (highest level). See Table 8–1. Nurses should include each of these three domains in client teaching plans. For example, teaching a client how to irrigate a colostomy is the psychomotor domain. An important part of such a teaching plan is to teach the client why a specific amount of fluid is used and when the irrigation should be carried out; this is the cognitive domain. Helping the client accept the colostomy and maintain self-esteem is in the affective domain.

Each of these domains has a developed hierarchical classification system; that is, the behaviors in each category are arranged from the simplest to the most complex.

Consider . . .

- how a nurse would teach a new diabetic client how to inject insulin using each of the domains of learning.
- how a nurse would teach a family member about organ donation in the cognitive domain and in the affective domain.

Humanism

Humanistic learning theory focuses on both cognitive and affective (feelings and attitudes) areas of the learner. It focuses on the whole person and therefore is pertinent to a holistic philosophy of care. Prominent members of this school of thought include Abraham Maslow and Carl Rogers. According to humanistic theory, learning is believed to be self-motivated, self-initiated, and self-evaluated. Each individual is viewed as a unique composite of biologic, psychologic, social, cultural, and spiritual factors. Learning focuses on self-development and achieving full potential; it is best when it is relevant to the learner. Autonomy and self-determination are important; the learner identifies the learning needs and takes the initiative to meet these needs. The learner is thus an active participant and takes responsibility for meeting individual learning needs.

Maslow's hierarchy of needs suggests a way of prioritizing nursing interventions so that physiologic needs are met first, followed by safety and security needs, love and belonging needs, esteem and self-esteem needs, and ultimately growth needs. Carl Rogers was particularly concerned with personalized approaches. He emphasized that independence, creativity, and self-reliance are all facilitated when self-criticism and self-evaluation are of primary importance; evaluation by others is of secondary importance.

Categorization

According to Jerome Bruner, perception, conceptualizing, learning, and decision making all depend on categorizing information. People interpret information in terms of the similarities and differences detected and arrange the information in related categories. For ex-

Table 8–1 Major Categories in Each Learning Domain

Category/Description	Client Learning Example
Cognitive Domain	
Knowledge Remembers previously learned material	A client lists the side effects of a medication 2 days following instruction.
Comprehension Understands the meaning of learned material	A client describes how the side effects of a medication can be recognized and what to do about them.
Application Applies newly learned material in new concrete situations	A client learns to take the medication after meals to minimize side effects.
Analysis Breaks learned material into component parts and separates important from unimportant material	A client describes which side effects are serious and when the physician is to be notified.
Synthesis Takes parts of learned material and puts them together to form new material	A client takes steps to prevent side effects of a medication.
Evaluation Judges the value of the learned material	A client describes how the knowledge of new material can help prevent accidents at work.
Affective Domain	
Receiving Willingness to attend to particular stimuli	A female client is willing to listen to a nurse's description of the preparation for breast surgery.
Responding Actively participates by listening and responding	The female client asks questions about the preparation for the scheduled surgery.
Valuing Attaches a value or worth to a particular object, phenomenon, or behavior	The female client refuses to look at the incision following her breast removal.
Organization Develops a value system by bringing together different values and resolving conflicts	The client accepts changes brought about by the breast surgery.
Characterization Acts according to a value system	After surgery, the client returns to a lifestyle consistent with her value system.
Psychomotor Domain	
Perception Uses the senses to obtain cues to guide motor activity	A male client immediately calls a nurse when he sees another client fall from his bed.
Set Refers to readiness to take immediate action: includes mental, physical, and emotional sets	The client becomes ready to act when he sees the client who fell from his bed preparing to get out of his chair.
Guided Response Performs an act under the guidance of a nurse	A client moves himself from his bed to a wheelchair with a nurse's guidance.
Mechanism Performs a learned activity with confidence and proficiency	The client moves himself between his bed and a wheelchair quickly and competently.
Complex Overt Response Performs a motor skill competently, accurately, and smoothly	The client moves between the bed and the wheelchair at the same time adjusting his intravenous line and his catheter.
Adaptation Performs skills and adapts them to special circumstances	The client stops transferring to the wheelchair and adjusts his intravenous line when it stops dripping.
Origination Creates new movement patterns to suit a particular problem	The client transfers from his bed to the wheelchair in a different way to avoid pull on the intravenous line.

Sources: Adapted from *Starting Objectives for Classroom Instruction,* 3d ed. by N. E. Gronlund, New York: Macmillan, 1985, pp. 34–40; and *Taxonomy of Educational Objectives. Vol. 1: Cognitive Domain,* ed. B. S. Bloom, New York: David McKay, 1956, pp. 18–24.

ample, there are hundreds of bones in the body. By categorizing them into major bone types (e.g., long bones, flat bones) or areas of the body (e.g., bones of the head, bones of the hand, vertebrae), it is easier to learn them. This theory of cognitive learning emphasizes the formation of a coding system. These systems serve to facilitate transfer, enhance retention, and increase problem-solving motivation. Bruner advocates discovery-oriented learning to help students discover relationships between categories. Bruner's work is sometimes considered among the theories of the constructivists.

Constructivism

Constructivism is a relatively recent term. It represents a collection of theories with a common thread of individuals actively constructing knowledge to solve realistic problems, often in collaboration with others. The ideas of constructivism emerged with John Dewey and continued with Bruner (learning as discovery). The constructivist described learning as a change in meaning constructed from experience. Knowledge becomes an individual interpretation of experience; learning is the construction of new interpretations. Gagne, Bruner, and Ausubel, as well as the social development theorist Vygotsky and social learning theorist Bandura, are associated with the constructionists. Their focus is more on the learning, not the teaching, with language as a process. Constructivists encourage learning inquiry and acknowledge the critical role of experience in learning. Constructivists encourage cooperative learning. Constructivist theory is applicable to learning with technology.

Multiple Intelligence

Early psychologists gauged intelligence by the use of the intelligence quotient, or IQ. They felt that intelligence at too low a level inhibited individuals from participating in intellectually demanding learning situations and that intelligence at a higher level indicated a genius. Those in between were considered to be normal. Many individuals were incorrectly labeled and as a result were never encouraged to reach higher potential. Intelligence was thought to be fixed and unchangeable by training. Recent research studies suggest that this is not so. Today, new theories have emerged disputing IQ as the only indicator of intelligence. Intelligence has a number of dimensions. Howard Gardner, head of the Project of Human Potential at Harvard, has presented a theory of multiple intelligence. This was based on observations of how brain damage

from a stroke might affect one area, such as language, while other areas of mental functioning remained intact. Gardner first cited seven intelligences; linguistic, musical/rhythmic (music), logical/mathematical, spatial (visual), body/kinesthetic/movement (body), personal, and symbols as intellectual strengths or ways of knowing (Gardner, 1983). He has since added naturalist as the eighth intelligence. Gardner offers a fresh perspective to learning.

Applying Learning Theories

The major attributes of *behaviorist* theories include the careful identification of what is to be taught and the immediate identification of and reward for correct responses. However, the theory is not easily applied to complex learning situations and is limiting in terms of the learner's role in the teaching process. Nurses applying behavioristic theory will do the following:

- Provide sufficient practice time and both immediate and repeat testing and redemonstration.
- Provide opportunities for learners to solve problems by trial and error.
- Select teaching strategies that avoid distracting information and evoke the desired response.
- Praise the learner for correct behavior and provide positive feedback at intervals throughout the learning experience.
- Provide role models of desired behavior.

The major attributes of *cognitive* theory are its recognition of developmental levels of learners, and acknowledgments of the learner's motivation and environment. However, some or many of the motivational and environmental factors may be beyond the teacher's control. Nurses applying cognitive theory will do the following:

- Assess a person's developmental and individual readiness to learn and adapt teaching strategies to the learner's developmental level.
- Provide a social, emotional, and physical environment conducive to learning.
- Encourage a positive teacher-learner relationship.
- Select multisensory teaching strategies since perception is influenced by the senses.
- Recognize that personal characteristics have an impact on how cues are perceived and develop appropriate teaching approaches to target different learning styles.
- Select behavioral objectives and strategies that encompass the cognitive, affective, and psychomotor domains of learning.

The major attributes of *humanism* are its focus on the feeling and attitudes of learners, the importance of the individual in identifying learning needs, in taking responsibility for them, and on the self-motivation of the learners to work toward self-reliance and independence. Nurses applying humanistic theory will do the following:

■ Encourage the learners to establish goals and promote self-directed learning.

■ Encourage active learning by serving as a facilitator, mentor, or resource for the learner.

■ Expose the learner to new relevant information and ask appropriate questions to encourage the learner to seek answers.

Cognitive Learning Processes

Learning involves three cognitive (mental) processes: acquiring information, processing the information, and using the information. These three processes can occur sequentially or simultaneously.

Acquiring Information

Acquiring information involves two processes: sensory reception and discrimination. Sensory reception is made possible by the neurosensory system. Stimuli in the environment signal the appropriate sense, such as sight, hearing, or smell, Impulses then travel by the nervous system to the brain. Sensory reception generally is continuous, but it is not always a conscious process.

The second aspect of acquiring information is discrimination. Discrimination is the ability to determine which stimuli are relevant in a particular situation. Stimuli can be objects, ideas, actions, or facts. They may be internal (i.e., inside the body) or external. Discrimination is the most difficult when there are multiple, complex stimuli.

Processing Information

Processing provides meaning to the information. Information is processed in three steps: association, generalization, and the formation of concepts. *Association* is the joining of two or many ideas. For example, a person may associate an object such as a needle with the word *needle* and/or with the experience of pain. *Generalization* is the perceiving of similarities among various stimuli, for example, the similarities between three different computers. *Concept formation* is the organization of stimuli that have some attributes in common. For example, a nurse who understands the concept of caring appreciates the characteristics associated with caring. The nurse can then help others to convey caring in the health care setting.

Using Information

Using information is the application of information in the cognitive, affective, and psychomotor areas. See "Bloom's Domains of Learning," earlier in this chapter. The ability to formulate and relate concepts is an essential critical thinking skill. In addition, relating concepts is essential for creative thinking and problem solving.

Factors Facilitating Learning

Learning is a complex phenomenon. It is an interactive process between the learner, the teacher, the environment, and many elements, including learning style and teaching style. Certain conditions or principles have been identified throughout years of research. Following are some of these to be considered by the nurse.

Motivation

Motivation to learn is the desire to learn. It greatly influences how quickly and how much a person learns. Motivation is generally greatest when a person recognizes a need and believes the need will be met through learning. It is not enough for the need to be identified and verbalized by the nurse; it must be experienced by the client. Often the nurse's task is to help the client personally work through the problem and identify the need. Sometimes clients or support persons need help identifying relevant situational elements before they can see a need. For instance, clients with heart disease may need to know the effects of smoking before they recognize the need to stop smoking. Or adolescents may need to know the consequences of an untreated sexually transmitted disease before they see the need for treatment.

Readiness

Readiness to learn is the behavior that reflects motivation at a specific time. Readiness reflects a client's willingness and ability to learn. The nurse's role is often to encourage the development of readiness.

Active Involvement

Active involvement in the process makes learning more meaningful. If the learner actively participates in planning and discussion, learning is faster and retention is better. Passive learning, such as listening to a lecture or watching a film, does not foster optimal learning.

Once learners have succeeded in accomplishing

a task or understanding a concept, they gain self-confidence in their ability to learn. This reduces their anxiety about failure and can motivate greater learning. Successful learners have increased confidence with which to accept failure. People learn best when they believe they are accepted and will not be judged. The person who expects to be judged as a "poor" or "good" client will not learn as well as the person who feels no such threat.

Feedback

Feedback is information relating a person's performance to a desired goal. It has to be meaningful to the learner. Feedback that accompanies practice of psychomotor skills helps the person to learn those skills. Support of desired behavior through praise, positively worded corrections, and suggestions of alternative methods are ways of providing positive feedback. Negative feedback such as ridicule, anger, or sarcasm can lead people to withdraw from learning. Such feedback, viewed as a type of punishment, may cause the client to avoid the teacher in order to avoid punishment.

Simple to Complex

Learning is facilitated by material that is logically organized and proceeds from the *simple to the complex.* Such organization enables the learner to comprehend new information, assimilate it with previous learning, and form new understandings. Of course, simple and complex are relative terms, depending on the level at which the person is learning. What is simple for one person may be complex for another.

Repetition

Repetition of key concepts and facts facilitates retention of newly learned material. Practice of psychomotor skills, particularly with feedback from the nurse, improves performance of those skills and facilitates their transfer to another setting. Also when a person appreciates the relevance of specific material, learning is facilitated.

Timing

People retain information and psychomotor skills best when the *time between learning and use is short;* the longer the time interval, the more is forgotten. For example, a woman who is taught to administer her own insulin but is not permitted to do so until discharge from hospital is unlikely to remember much of what she learned. However, if she is allowed to give her own injections while in hospital, her learning will be enhanced and reinforced.

Timing can also include opportunity, sometimes referred to as a *teachable moment.* When a nurse is caring for a patient's colostomy site, the patient may start asking questions about the procedure. Because the client has expressed interest in the procedure, the time, or opportunity, for learning is at that time. Learning occurs best when the learner is free from worry, fear, or pain. It would not be an appropriate time to teach clients about lifestyle changes following surgery when they are still fearful about the outcome of the surgery.

Environment

An *optimal learning environment* facilitates learning by reducing distraction and providing physical and psychologic comfort. It has adequate lighting that is free from glare, a comfortable room temperature, and good ventilation. Most students know what it is like to try to learn in a hot, stuffy room; the subsequent drowsiness interferes with concentration. Noise can also distract the student and interfere with listening and thinking. To facilitate learning in a hospital setting, nurses should choose a time when there are no visitors present and interruptions are unlikely. Privacy is essential for some learning. For example, when a client is learning to irrigate a colostomy, the presence of others can be embarrassing and thus interfere with learning. When a client is particularly anxious, having support persons present often gives the client confidence.

Consider . . .

- your own learning experiences. What are the circumstances of your most effective learning experiences? What were the circumstances of your least effective learning experiences? What does this tell you about your learning style?
- your experiences with teaching others. What were the circumstances of your most effective teaching experiences? What were the circumstances of your least effective teaching experiences? What is your teaching style?

Factors Inhibiting Learning

Many factors inhibit learning. Some of the most common are described next and in Table 8–2.

Emotions

A greatly elevated *anxiety* level can impede learning. Clients or families who are very worried may not hear spoken words or may retain only part of the commu-

Table 8–2 Barriers to Learning

Barrier	Explanation	Nursing Implications
Acute illness	Client requires all resources and energy to cope with illness.	Defer teaching until client is less ill.
Pain	Pain decreases ability to concentrate.	Deal with pain before teaching.
Age	Vision, hearing, and motor control can be impaired in the elderly.	Consider sensory and motor defects in teaching plan.
Prognosis	Client can be preoccupied with illness and unable to concentrate on new information.	Defer teaching to a better time.
Biorhythms	Mental and physical performances have a circadian rhythm.	Adapt time of teaching to suit client.
Emotion (e.g., anxiety, denial, depression, grief)	Emotions require energy and distract from learning.	Deal with emotions first and possible misinformation.
Language and ethnic background	Client may not be fluent in the nurse's language.	Obtain services of an interpreter or nurse with appropriate language skills.
Iatrogenic barriers	The nurse may set up barriers by appearing condescending or hurried, ignoring client cues, or appearing incompetent or unsure.	Establish a helping relationship and be sensitive to the client's needs. Plan and prepare for teaching ahead of time with current information appropriate for the learner.

nication. Extreme anxiety might be reduced by medications or by information that relieves uncertainty. By contrast, clients who appear disinterested and unconcerned may need to be cautioned about potential problems to enhance their motivation to learn.

Physiologic Events

Learning can be inhibited by *physiologic events* such as a critical illness, pain, or impaired hearing. Because the client cannot concentrate and apply energy to learning, the learning itself is impaired. The nurse should try to reduce the physiologic barriers to learning as much as possible before teaching. Providing analgesics and rest before teaching is often helpful.

Cultural Barriers

There are also *cultural barriers* to learning, such as language or values. Obviously, the client who does not understand the nurse's language will learn little. Western medicine may conflict with cultural healing beliefs and practices. Nurses must deal directly with this conflict to be effective; otherwise the client may be partially or totally nonadherent to recommended treatments. An-

other impediment to learning is *differing values* held by the client and the health team. For example, a client who comes from a culture that does not value slimness may have difficulty learning about a reducing diet.

Consider . . .

■ a new mother who believes a fat baby is a healthy baby. She has grown up with this value and is told this repeatedly by her mother (the baby's grandmother). Develop a plan for teaching infant nutrition to this mother.

NURSES AS TEACHERS

Nurses have many teaching roles. They may teach individual learners, such as patients who need instruction about treatments, or they may teach groups of learners, such as prospective parents enrolled in a Lamaze class. They also teach different types of learners. They teach patients or clients and their families or caregivers. They teach health professionals, including other nurses and physicians. They teach subordinates in various health care settings, including patient-care assistants, home health aides, and others. Nurses also teach in the community, providing instruction in disease and injury prevention and health promotion.

The primary teaching role of a nurse is in teaching patients and their families. Such instruction includes discharge teaching, about how to perform self-care, instruction about taking medications, including side effects, and how to perform prescribed treatments. Most teaching is done with patients directly. However, family members or caregivers also may be instructed in care of the patient. This is especially important for patients who have difficulty in performing self-care. For example, parents who need to give medication to their children must be instructed in the proper administration of that medication. A diabetic client who has visual impairment may need assistance in administering insulin or in assessing his or her feet and lower extremities for skin breakdown. The caregiver or family member must be included in the diabetic patient's instruction. When diet teaching is done, it is important to include the person who purchases and prepares the food.

Nurses also teach other nurses and health professionals. Experienced nurses often act as preceptors, teaching new nurses the policies and procedures of the nursing unit. Nurses teach continuing education programs for other nurses. Continuing education programs may include specialty nursing courses such as intensive-care nursing or perioperative nursing, or they may be classes updating nurses' knowledge regarding new research, medications, or procedures, such as new information about care of people with HIV/AIDS. Nurses teach nursing students either informally when students are on the nursing unit or formally in the classroom. Nurses also teach other health care team members, including physicians. Nurse-educators often provide classes in the work setting about new policies, and the learners may include all those who are affected by the policy, such as when a new documentation system is implemented.

Nurses teach subordinate or ancillary staff. Patient-care assistants, volunteers, dietary aides, housekeeping personnel, and unit secretaries participate in patient care at various levels. Nurses may be responsible for teaching these staff members about their responsibilities.

Nurses also participate in community education activities. Nurses may teach high school students about sexually transmitted diseases, teenage pregnancy, and alcohol and drug abuse. They may teach senior citizens about self-medication or other self-care activities. They may teach community classes on hypertension, risk factors for heart disease, or other illnesses. In order to prevent illness or injury, the public must be provided with information. Nurses are respected and knowledgeable and in a position to provide such information.

Consider . . .

- what teaching activities you are involved in (on the nursing unit, in your practice setting, in the community).
- what your feelings are about teaching others (patients, nursing students, others nurses, other health care providers).

THE ART OF TEACHING

Teaching is a system of activities intentionally designed to produce specific learning. It is a goal-directed activity that results in improved learning for the learner. Teaching is more than giving information; the art of teaching lies in providing the knowledge, skill, and desire within the learner to change some aspect of his or her life. Effective teaching requires knowledge of the subject matter, understanding of the learning process, judgment, and intuition.

The teaching/learning process involves dynamic interaction between teacher and learner. Each participant in the process communicates information, emotions, perceptions, and attitudes to the other.

The relationship between the teacher and the learner is essentially one of trust and respect. The learner trusts that the teacher has the knowledge and skill to teach, and the teacher respects the learner's ability to attain the recognized goals. Once a nurse starts to instruct a client and/or a coworker, it is important that the teaching process continue until the participants reach the learning goals, change the goals, or decide that the goals cannot be met.

Nurses have a responsibility to keep their clinical knowledge current. The American Nurses Association (ANA) lists four standards of clinical nursing practice that relate directly to learning and teaching. See the box on page 137.

Guidelines for Learning and Teaching

The following guidelines for effective learning/teaching may be helpful to nurses:

- Teaching activities should help a learner meet individual learning objectives. These objectives should be mutually determined by the client (learner) and the nurse (teacher). If certain activities do not assist the learner, these need to be reassessed; perhaps other activities can replace them. For example, explanation alone may not be sufficient to teach a client how to

American Nurses Association Standards of Clinical Nursing Practice Related to Teaching and Learning

- *Standard II. Performance Appraisal:* The nurse evaluates his/her own nursing practice in relation to professional practice standards and relevant statutes and regulations. This standard infers that the nurse should regularly engage in professional appraisal, evaluating strengths and areas for development. Also the nurse participates in peer reviews, seeks feedback from others, and takes action to achieve identified goals. Through such actions, the nurse can identify learning needs and devise a plan to meet them.

- *Standard III. Education:* The nurse acquires and maintains current knowledge and competency in nursing practice. This standard requires the nurse to participate in educational activities related to clinical knowledge and professional issues. Also, the

nurse seeks experience to maintain clinical skills and seeks knowledge and skills appropriate to the practice setting.

- *Standard IV. Collegiality:* The nurse interacts with and contributes to the professional development of peers and other health providers as colleagues. This standard suggests that nurses share information and skills with others and give constructive feedback to others regarding their performance. The nurse also contributes to an environment that is conducive to learning of nursing students.

- *Standard VII. Research:* The nurse uses research findings in practice. This standard suggests that the nurse participate in research according to individual educational level and practice environment and use research findings in practice.

Source: Adapted from American Nurses Association *Standards of Clinical Nursing Practice,* 2d ed. Washington, D.C., 1998.

handle a syringe. Actually handling the syringe may be more effective.

- Rapport between teacher and learner is essential. A relationship that is both accepting and constructive will best assist learning. The nurse should take time to establish rapport before teaching.
- The teacher who uses the client's previous learning in the present situation encourages the client and facilitates learning new skills. For example, a person who already knows how to cook can use this knowledge when learning to prepare food for a special diet.
- The nurse-teacher must be able to communicate clearly and concisely. The words the nurse uses need to have the same meaning to the learner as to the teacher. For example, a client who is taught not to put water on an area of skin may think a wet washcloth is permissible for washing the area. In effect, the nurse needs to explain that no water or moisture should touch the area.
- A knowledge of the learners and the factors that affect their learning should be established before planning the teaching.
- When a person is involved in planning, learning is often enhanced.
- Teaching that involves a number of the learners' senses often enhances learning. For example, when learning about changing a surgical dressing, the nurse can tell the client about the procedure (hearing), show how to change the dressing (sight), and

demonstrate how to manipulate the equipment (touch).

- The anticipated behavioral changes that indicate that learning has taken place must always be within the context of the client's lifestyle and resources. For example, it would probably not be reasonable to expect a woman to soak in a tub of hot water four times a day if she did not have a bathtub and had to heat water on a stove.

See the box on page 138 of the characteristics of effective teaching.

Assessing Learning Needs

The first step in teaching others is to assess their learning needs and the factors that may affect their learning. These factors include the learner's (1) age, (2) health beliefs and practices, (3) cultural factors, (4) economic factors, (5) learning styles, (6) readiness to learn, (7) motivation, and (8) reading level.

AGE Age provides information about the learner's developmental status that may indicate specific health teaching content and teaching approaches. Simple questions to school-age children and adolescents will elicit information about what they know. Observing children in play provides information about their motor and intellectual development as well as relation-

Characteristics of Effective Teaching

- Holds the learner's interest.
- Involves the learner in the learning process. Makes partners of the learner and the teacher.
- Fosters a positive self-concept in the learner; learner believes learning is possible and probable.
- Sets realistic goals.
- Is directed at helping the learner meet learner objectives.
- Supports the learner with positive reinforcement.
- Is accurate and current.

- Is appropriate for the learner's age, condition, and abilities.
- Is optimistic, positive, and nonthreatening.
- Uses several methods of teaching to accommodate a variety of learning styles; provides learning opportunities through hearing, seeing, and doing.
- Gathers information from reliable sources.
- Is cost-effective (cost of nurse's time spent teaching is less than the cost of treating health problems occurring when clients do not follow recommended treatments, fail to take medications correctly, or do not adapt lifestyle to changing health needs.

ships with other children. For the elderly person, conversation and questioning may reveal slow recall, limited psychomotor skills, diminished senses, or learning difficulties.

The age of learners also affects the duration of the instruction. Young children have a short attention span; therefore, instruction of children should be of shorter duration. Older adults may be uncomfortable sitting for long periods of time or may require more frequent bathroom breaks.

HEALTH BELIEFS AND PRACTICES A learner's health beliefs and practices are important to consider in any teaching plan. However, even if a nurse is convinced that a particular learner's health beliefs should be changed, doing so may not be possible because so many factors are involved in a person's health beliefs.

CULTURAL FACTORS Many cultural groups have their own beliefs and practices: a number of them related to diet, health, illness, and lifestyle. It is therefore important to know how the practices and values held by learners impinge on their learning needs.

Folk beliefs of certain groups may also affect learning. Although the learner may readily understand the health care information being taught, this learning may not be implemented in the home, where folk healing practices prevail.

ECONOMIC FACTORS Economic factors can also affect learning. For example, a learner who cannot afford to obtain a new sterile syringe for each injection of insulin may find it difficult to learn to administer the

insulin when the nurse teaches that a new syringe should be used each time.

LEARNING STYLE Considerable research has been done on people's learning styles. The best way to learn varies with the individual. Some people are visual learners and learn best by watching. Other people do not visualize an activity well; they learn best by actually manipulating equipment and discovering how it works. Other people can learn well from reading things presented in an orderly fashion. Still other people learn best in groups relating to other people. For some, stressing the thinking part of a skill and the logic of something will promote learning. For other people, stressing the feeling part or interpersonal aspect motivates and promotes learning. When material is presented in more than one learning domain, the chances for learning and retaining information are greatly increased.

The nurse seldom has the time or skills to assess each learner, identify the person's particular learning style, and then adapt teaching accordingly; what the nurse can do, however, is to ask learners how they have learned things best in the past or how they like to learn. Many people know what helps them learn, and the nurse can use this information in planning the teaching. Using a variety of teaching techniques and varying activities during teaching are good ways to match learners with learning styles. One technique will be most effective for some learners, whereas other techniques will be suited to learners with different learning styles.

READINESS TO LEARN People who are ready to learn often behave differently from those who are not.

A learner who is ready may search out information, for instance, by asking questions, reading books or articles, talking to others, and generally showing interest. Today people have access to information with computers and the Worldwide Web. The person who is not ready to learn is more likely to avoid the subject or situation. In addition, the unready learner may change the subject when it is brought up by the nurse.

In assessing readiness to learn, the nurse observes for the following:

- Physical readiness. Is the learner able to focus on things other than physical status, or are fatigue, pain, or disability using up all the learner's time and energy?
- Emotional readiness. Is the learner emotionally ready to learn? People who are extremely anxious, depressed, or grieving are not ready to learn.
- Cognitive readiness. Can the learner think clearly at this point? For example, a client who has an altered level of consciousness is not cognitively ready to learn.

Nurses can promote readiness to learn by providing physical and emotional support prior to and during learning activities.

MOTIVATION As discussed earlier, motivation relates to whether the learner wants to learn and is usually greatest when the learner is ready, the learning need is recognized, and the information being offered is meaningful to the learner. Nurses can increase a learner's motivation in several ways:

- By relating the content to something the learner values and helping the learner see the relevance of the content
- By making the learning situation pleasant and nonthreatening
- By encouraging self-direction and independence
- By demonstrating a positive attitude about the learner's ability to learn
- By offering continuing support and encouragement as the learner attempts to learn (i.e., positive reinforcement)
- By creating a learning situation where the learner is likely to succeed
- By rewarding the learner for his or her success

READING LEVEL The nurse should not assume that a learner's reading level is equal to the highest grade or level of formal education the learner has completed. An eighth-grade reading level or lower is recommended for health education material designed for the general client population (Estey, Musseau, and Keehn, 1991). The nurse can use the SMOG index to assess the reading levels of educational material and thereby determine its appropriateness for the population who will be reading it. See the box on page 140.

Planning Content and Teaching Strategies

Developing a teaching plan (see a sample teaching plan for wound care in the box on page 141) is accomplished in a series of steps. Involving the learner at this time promotes the formation of a meaningful plan and stimulates their motivation. The learner who helps formulate the teaching plan is more likely to achieve the desired outcomes.

Determining Teaching Priorities

Learning needs must be ranked according to priority. The client and the nurse should do this together, with the client's priorities always being considered. Once a client's priorities have been addressed, the client is generally more motivated to concentrate on other identified learning needs. For example, a man who wants to know all about coronary artery disease may not be ready to learn how to change his lifestyle until he meets his own need to learn more about the disease. Nurses can also use theoretical frameworks, such as Maslow's hierarchy of needs, to establish priorities.

Setting Learning Objectives or Outcomes

Outcome-based learning is prevalent in education today. Learning objectives can be considered the same as outcome criteria for other nursing diagnoses. They are written in the same way. Like client outcomes, learning objectives

- State the learner behavior or performance, not nurse behavior. For example, "Will choose her own diet as instructed" (client behavior), not "To teach the client about his diet" (nurse behavior).
- Reflect an observable, measurable activity. The performance may be visible (e.g., walking) or invisible (e.g., adding a column of figures). However, it is necessary to be able to deduce whether an unobservable activity has been mastered from some performance that represents the activity. Therefore, the performance of an objective might be written: "Writes the total for a column of figures in the indicated space" (observable), not "Adds a column of figures" (unobservable). Selected measurable verbs used for learning objectives are shown in the box on page 142. Avoid using words such as knows, understands, believes, and appreciates; they are neither observable nor measurable.

Determining Readability Level of Written Materials Using the SMOG Index

To determine the reading level of learning materials for clients, choose 30 sentences in the reading. Pick 10 from the beginning, 10 from the middle, and 10 from the end of the reading. Count all the words with 3 or more syllables; total these. Find the number in the list below, and read across to find the reading grade level.

NUMBER OF WORDS WITH 3 OR MORE SYLLABLES	READING GRADE LEVEL
0–2	4
3–6	5
7–12	6
13–20	7
21–30	8
31–42	9
43–56	10
57–72	11
73–90	12

To decrease the reading level of and simplify the client educational material,

- Use smaller words.
- Avoid words with several syllables.
- Write shorter sentences.
- Explain terms that must be used.
- Use easy, common words.

Sources: Adapted from "Patient Educational Materials: Are They Readable?" by S. T. Stephens, *Oncology Nursing Forum,* **19:** 84, January/February 1992; and "Self-Care Instructions: Do Patients Understand Educational Materials?" by M. Wong, *Focus on Critical Care* **19:**47–49, February 1992.

■ May add conditions or modifiers as required to clarify what, where, when, or how the behavior will be performed. Examples are "Walks to the end of the hall and back *without crutches*" (condition), "Irrigates his colostomy *independently* (condition) as taught," or "States *three* (condition) factors that affect blood sugar level."

■ Include criteria specifying the time by which learning should have occurred. For example, "The client will state three things that affect blood sugar level *by end of second diabetic class.*"

Choosing Content

The content, or what is to be taught, is determined by learning objectives. For instance, "Identify appropriate sites for insulin injection" means the nurse must include content about the body sites suitable for insulin injections. Nurses can select among many sources of information including books, nursing journals, and other nurses and physicians. Whatever sources the nurse chooses, content should be

■ Accurate
■ Current
■ Based on learning objectives
■ Adjusted for the learner's age, culture, language, and ability
■ Consistent with information the nurse is teaching
■ Selected with consideration for how much time and resources are available for teaching

Selecting Teaching Strategies

The method of teaching the nurse chooses should be suited to the individual, to the material to be learned, and to the teacher. For example, the person who cannot read needs material presented in other ways; a discussion is usually not the best strategy for teaching to give an injection; and a teacher using group discussion

Teaching Plan: Wound Care

Assessment of Learner: A 24-year-old male college student suffered a 2.5 in. (7-cm) laceration on the left lower anterior leg during a hockey game. The laceration was cleansed, sutured, and bandaged. The client was given an appointment to return to the health clinic in 10 days for suture removal. Client states that he lives in the college dormitory and is able to care for wound if given instructions. Client is able to read and understand English.

Nursing Diagnosis: **Knowledge deficit** related to care of sutured wound.

Long-Term Goal: Client's wound will heal completely without infection or other complication.

Intermediate Goal: At clinic appointment, client's wound will be healing without signs of infection, loss of function, or other complication.

Short-Term Goal: Client will respond to questions regarding wound care and perform return demonstration of wound cleansing and bandaging.

BEHAVIORAL OBJECTIVES	CONTENT OUTLINE	TEACHING METHODS
Upon completion of the instructional session, the client will		
1. Describe normal wound healing	I. Normal wound healing	Describe normal wound healing with the use of audiovisuals.
2. List signs and symptoms of wound infection	II. Infection Signs and symptoms include wound warm to touch, malalignment of wound edges, and purulent wound drainage. Signs of systemic infection include fever and malaise.	Discuss the mechanism of wound infection. Use audiovisuals to demonstrate infected wound appearance. Provide handout describing signs and symptoms of wound infection.
3. Correctly use equipment needed for wound care	III. Wound care equipment a. Cleansing solution as prescribed by physician (e.g., clear water, mild soap and water, antimicrobial solution, or hydrogen peroxide). b. Bandaging material: Telfa, gauze wrap, adhesive tape.	Demonstrate equipment needed for cleansing and bandaging wound. Provide handout listing equipment needed.
4. Demonstrate wound cleansing and bandaging	IV. Demonstration of wound cleansing and bandaging on the client's wound or a mannikin	Demonstrate wound cleansing and bandaging on the client's wound or a mannikin. Provide handout describing procedure for cleansing and bandaging wound.
5. Develop a plan for appropriate action if questions or complications arise	V. Resources available for client questions include health clinic, emergency department.	Discuss available resources. Provide handout listing available resources and follow-up treatment plan.
6. Identify date, time, and location of follow-up appointment for suture removal	VI. Follow-up treatment plan; where and when	Provide written instructions.

Evaluation: The client will
1. Respond to questions regarding self-care of wound
2. Return demonstration of wound cleansing and bandaging
3. State contact person and telephone number to obtain assistance
4. State date, time, and location of follow-up appointment

Selected Verbs for Learning Objectives

COGNITIVE DOMAIN	AFFECTIVE DOMAIN	PSYCHOMOTOR DOMAIN
compares	alters	adapts
contrasts	answers	arranges
defines	attends	assembles
describes	chooses	begins
draws	complies	calculates
differentiates	conforms	calibrates
explains	completes	changes
identifies	defends	constructs
labels	differentiates	creates
lists	discusses	demonstrates
matches	displays	dismantles
names	follows	manipulates
prepares	helps	measures
plans	initiates	moves
recites	joins	organizes
restates	justifies	proceeds
selects	modifies	rearranges
solves	participates	reacts
sorts	responds	shows
states	revises	starts
summarizes	shares	works
underlines	uses	
writes	verifies	

Source: Adapted from *Stating Objectives for Classroom Instruction,* 3d ed. by N. E. Gronlund, Toronto: Collier Macmillan, 1985, pp. 37–40.

for teaching should be a competent group leader. As stated earlier, some people are visually oriented and learn best through seeing; others learn best through hearing and having the skill explained. See Table 8–3 for selected teaching strategies.

Ordering Learning Experiences

To save nurses time in constructing their own teaching guides, some health agencies have developed teaching guides for teaching sessions that nurses commonly give. These guides standardize content and teaching methods and make it easier for the nurse to plan and implement client teaching. Whether the nurse is implementing a plan devised by another or developing an individualized teaching plan, some guidelines can help the nurse order the learning experience.

- Start with something the learner is concerned about; for example, before learning how to administer insulin to himself, an adolescent wants to know how he can adjust his lifestyle and still play football.
- Begin with what the learner knows, and proceed to the unknown. This gives the learner confidence. Sometimes you will not know the client's knowledge or skill base and will need to elicit this information, either by asking questions or by having the client fill out a form, such as a pretest.
- Address first any area that is causing the learner anxiety. A high level of anxiety can impair concentration in other areas. For example, a woman highly anxious about turning her husband in bed might not be able to learn about bathing him until she has successfully learned to turn him.
- Teach the basics first; then proceed to the variations or adjustments. It is very confusing to learners to have to consider possible adjustments and variations before they master the basic concepts. For example, when teaching a female client how to insert a retention catheter, it is best to teach the basic procedure before teaching any adjustments that

Table 8–3 Selected Teaching Strategies

Strategy	Major Type of Learning	Characteristics
Explanation or description (e.g., lecture)	Cognitive	Teacher controls content and pace. Learner is passive; therefore retains less information than when a participant. Feedback is determined by teacher. May be given to individual or group.
One-to-one discussion	Affective, cognitive	Encourages participation by learner. Permits reinforcement and repetition at learner's level. Permits introduction of sensitive subjects.
Answering questions	Cognitive	Teacher controls most of content and pace. Teacher must understand question and what it means to learner. Learner may need to overcome cultural perception that asking questions is impolite and may embarrass the teacher. Can be used with individuals and groups. Teacher sometimes needs to confirm whether question has been answered by asking learner, for example, "Does that answer your question?"
Demonstration	Psychomotor	Often used with explanation. Can be used with individuals, small or large groups. Does not permit use of equipment by learners; learner is passive.
Discovery	Cognitive, affective	Teacher guides problem-solving situation. Learner is active participant; therefore retention of information is high.
Group discussions	Affective, cognitive	Learner can obtain assistance from supportive group. Group members learn from one another. Teacher needs to keep the discussion focused and prevent monopolization by one or two learners.
Practice	Psychomotor	Allows repetition and immediate feedback. Permits "hands-on" experience.
Printed and audiovisual materials	Cognitive	Forms include books, pamphlets, films, programmed instruction, and computer learning. Learners can proceed at their own speed. Nurse can act as resource person, need not be present during learning. Potentially ineffective if reading level is too high. Teacher needs to select language that meets learner needs if English is a second language.
Role playing	Affective, cognitive	Permits expression of attitudes, values, and emotions. Can assist in development of communication skills. Involves active participation by learner. Teacher must create supportive, safe environment for learners to minimize anxiety.
Modeling	Affective, psychomotor	Nurse sets example by attitude, psychomotor skill.
Computer-assisted learning programs	All types of learning	Learner is active. Learner controls pace. Provides immediate reinforcement and review. Use with individuals or groups.

might be needed if the catheter stops draining after insertion.

■ Schedule time for review of content and questions the learner(s) may have to clarify information.

Implementing a Teaching Plan

The nurse needs to be flexible in implementing any teaching plan, because the plan may need revising. The learner may tire sooner than anticipated or be faced with too much information too quickly; the learner's needs may change; or external factors may intervene. For instance, the nurse and the learner, Mr. Brown, have planned to irrigate his colostomy at 10 A.M. but when the time comes, Mr. Brown wants additional information before actually doing it himself.

In this case, the nurse alters the teaching plan and discusses the desired information, provides written information, and defers teaching the psychomotor skill until the next day. It is also important for nurses to use teaching techniques that enhance learning and reduce or eliminate any barriers to learning such as pain or fatigue.

Guidelines for Teaching

When implementing a teaching plan, the nurse may find the following guidelines helpful.

1. The optimal time for each session depends largely on the learner. Some people, for example, learn best at the beginning of the day, when they are most rested; others prefer late afternoon, when no other activities are scheduled. Whenever possible, ask the prospective learner(s) for help in choosing the best time.

2. The pace of each teaching session also affects learning. Nurses should be sensitive to any signs that the pace is too fast or too slow. A learner who appears confused or does not comprehend material when questioned may be finding the pace too fast. When the learner appears bored and loses interest, the pace may be too slow, the learning period may be too long, or the learner may be tired.

3. An environment can detract from or assist learning; for example, noise or interruptions usually interfere with concentration, whereas a comfortable environment promotes learning.

4. Teaching aids can foster learning and help focus a learner's attention. To ensure the transfer of learning, the nurse should use the type of supplies or equipment the learner will eventually use. Before the teaching session, the nurse needs to assemble all equipment and visual aids and ensure that all audiovisual equipment is functioning properly.

5. Learning is more effective when the learners discover the content for themselves. Ways to increase learning include stimulating motivation and stimulating self-direction, for example, by providing specific, realistic, achievable objectives, giving feedback, and helping the learner derive satisfaction from learning. The nurse may also encourage self-directed independent learning by encouraging the client to explore sources of information required.

6. Repetition—for example, summarizing content, rephrasing (using other words), and approaching the material from another point of view—reinforces learning. For instance, after discussing the kinds of foods that can be included in a diet, the nurse describes the foods again, but in the context of the three meals eaten during one day.

7. It is helpful to employ "organizers" to introduce material to be learned. Advanced organizers provide a means of connecting unknown material to known material and generating logical relationships. For example: "You understand how urine flows down a catheter from the bladder. Now I will show you how to inject fluid so that it flows up the catheter into the bladder." The details that follow are then seen within its framework, and the details have added meaning.

8. Using a layperson's vocabulary enhances communication. Often nurses use terms and abbreviations that have meaning to other health professionals but make little sense to clients. Even words such as *urine* or *feces* may be unfamiliar to clients, and abbreviations such as RR (recovery room) or PAR (postanesthesia room) are often misunderstood.

9. Provide the learner with a handout that captures the key points of your instruction. Written material to which the learner can refer during and following the instruction provides security and reinforcement.

Evaluating Learning and Teaching
Evaluating Learning

Evaluating is both an ongoing and a final process in which the learner, the nurse, and, often, the support persons determine what has been learned. Learning is measured against the predetermined learning objectives selected in the planning phase of the teaching process. Thus, the objectives serve not only to direct the teaching plan but also to provide outcome criteria for evaluation. For example, the objective "Selects foods that are low in carbohydrates" can be evaluated by asking the learner to name such foods or to select low-carbohydrate foods from a list.

The best method for evaluating depends on the type of learning. In *cognitive learning*, the learner demonstrates acquisition of knowledge. Examples of the evaluation tools for cognitive learning include the following:

- Direct observation of behavior (e.g., observing the learner selecting the solution to a problem using the new knowledge).
- Written measurements (e.g., tests).
- Oral questioning (e.g., asking the learner to restate information or correct verbal responses to questions).
- Self-reports and self-monitoring. These can be useful during follow-up phone calls and home visits. Evaluating individual self-paced learning, as might occur with computer-assisted instruction, often incorporates self-monitoring.

The acquisition of *psychomotor skills* is best evaluated by observing how well the learner carries out a procedure such as changing a dressing or carrying out a urinary self-catheterization.

Affective learning is more difficult to evaluate. Whether attitudes or values have been learned may be inferred by listening to the learner's responses to questions, noting how the learner speaks about relevant subjects, and by observing the learner's behavior that expresses feelings and values. For example, have parents learned to value health sufficiently to have their children immunized? Do learners who state that they value health actually use condoms every time they have sex with a new partner?

Following evaluation, the nurse may find it necessary to modify or repeat the teaching plan if the objectives have not been met or have been met only partially. For the hospitalized client, follow-up teaching in the home or by phone may be needed.

Behavior change does not always take place immediately after learning. Often individuals accept change intellectually first and then change their behavior only periodically (for example, Mrs. Green, who knows that she must lose weight, diets and exercises off and on). If the new behavior is to replace the old behavior, it must emerge gradually; otherwise, the old behavior may prevail. The nurse can assist learners with behavior change by allowing for vacillation and by providing encouragement.

Evaluating Teaching

It is important for nurses to evaluate their own teaching. Evaluation should include a consideration of all factors—the timing, the teaching strategies, the amount of information, whether the teaching was helpful, and so on. The nurse may find, for example, that the learner was overwhelmed with too much information, was bored, or was motivated to learn more.

Both the learner and the nurse should evaluate the learning experience. The learner may tell the nurse what was helpful, interesting, and so on. Feedback questionnaires and videotapes of the learning sessions can also be helpful.

The nurse should not feel ineffective as a teacher if the learner forgets some of what is taught. Forgetting is normal and should be anticipated. Having the learner write down information, repeating it during teaching, giving handouts on the information and having the learner be active in the learning process all promote retention.

Special Teaching Strategies

There are a number of special teaching strategies that nurses can use: contracting, group teaching, computer-assisted instruction, multimedia presentations, discovery/problem solving, and behavior modification. Any strategy the nurse selects must be appropriate for the learner and the learning objectives.

Contracting

Contracting involves establishing a contract with a learner that specifies certain objectives and when they are to be met. The contract, drawn up and signed by the learner and the nurse, specifies not only the learning objectives but also the responsibilities of the learner and the nurse and the teaching plan. The agreement allows for freedom, mutual respect, and mutual responsibility.

Group Teaching

Group instruction is economical, and it provides members with an opportunity to share with and learn from others. A small group allows for discussion in which everyone can participate. A large group often necessitates a lecture technique or use of films, videos, slides, or role-playing by teachers.

It is important that all members involved in group instruction have a need in common (e.g., prenatal health or preoperative instruction). It is also important that sociocultural factors be considered in the formation of a group. Whereas middle-class Americans may value sharing experiences with others, people from a culture such as Japan may consider it inappropriate to reveal their thoughts and feelings.

Research Box

Macdonald, S. A. 1999, May. The cardiovascular health education program: Assessing the impact on rural and urban adolescents' health knowledge. *Applied Nursing Research* 12(2):86–90.
The purpose of the study was to determine the effectiveness of a cardiovascular health education program (CHEP) for grade 8 adolescents in Canada. The sample consisted of 146 adolescents. Knowledge scores for subjects of nutrition and exercise, cholesterol and plaque formation, and heart disease and smoking were obtained pretest and posttest. Findings indicated that the program had a positive impact on the cardiovascular health knowledge of the urban adolescents.

The implications are as follows: There appears to be a need for cardiovascular health education programs for adolescents in both urban and rural settings. School-based health education programs that are targeted to the adolescent population can be implemented by school and community health nurses. Nurses as health educators are needed to provide leadership to promote health programs in schools.

Computer-Assisted Instruction (CAI)

Computer-assisted instruction (CAI) has become popular. Initially, cognitive learning of facts was the primary use of computer educational methods. Now, however, computers can also be used to teach the following:

- Complex problem-solving skills
- Application of information
- Psychomotor skills

Programs can be used for

- Individual health care professionals or learners using one computer.
- Small groups of three to five learners gathered around one computer taking turns running the program and answering questions together.
- Large groups, with the computer display screen projected onto an overhead screen and a teacher or one learner using the keyboard.

Individuals using a computer are able to set the pace that meets their learning needs. Small groups are less able to do this, and large groups progress through the program at a pace that may be too slow for some learners and too fast for others. It is therefore helpful to group learners of similar needs and abilities together. Whether using the computer alone or in large groups, learners read and view informational material, answer questions, and receive immediate feedback. The correct answer is usually indicated by the use of colors, flashing signs, or written praise. When the learner selects an incorrect answer, the computer responds with an explanation of why that was not the best answer and encouragement to try again. Many programs ask learners whether they want to review material on which the question and answer were based. Some computer programs feature simulated situations that allow learners to manipulate objects on the screen to learn psychomotor skills. When used to teach such skills, CAI must be followed up with practice on actual equipment supervised by the teacher.

Some learners may have a negative attitude about computers that could act as a barrier to learning. The nurse helps these learners by explaining the steps to start and run the program, to turn the computer on and off, and where and when to insert the computer disk so that the learner can use the program when the nurse is not present. Most media catalogs, professional journals, and health care libraries contain information about computer programs available to the nurse for client education. The media specialist or librarian in a health care facility or college is an excellent resource to help the nurse locate appropriate computer programs. Computer educational material is also available for learners with different language needs, for learners with special visual needs, and for learners at different growth and development levels.

Multimedia Presentations

Multimedia presentations combine audio, film, video, and computers to stimulate many senses. This enhances learning and provides consistent instruction. Learners can stop the instruction and replay it as needed. Nurse-educators can use presentation software to create professional-looking lessons for clients. Storing the lessons on CD-ROM makes them transportable from one computer to another.

Discovery/Problem Solving

In using the discovery/problem-solving technique, the nurse presents some initial information and then asks the learners a question or presents a situation related to the information. The learner applies the new information to the situation and decides what to do. Learn-

Research Box

Suderman, E. M., Deatrich, J. V., Johnson, L. S., and Sawatzky-Dickson, D. M. 2000. Action research sets the stage to improve discharge preparation. *Pediatric Nursing* **26**(6):571–576.

The purpose of this study was to determine parents' perspectives of the discharge process of their children from a hospital. The researchers interviewed 14 urban families and 6 rural families. The children were admitted for respiratory problems. Lewin's change theory served as the theoretical framework underpinning this study. Four major themes were identified in the analysis of data. These included the parent as learner, the content taught, the timing of discharge, and the continued impact of hospitalization after discharge. Results indicated the importance of the nurse as discharge planner and educator.

The implications are as follows: Obtaining the parents' perspective about the discharge planning process provides valuable information for the nurse-educator, who needs to consider the diversity of the parents as learners, the extent and depth of their knowledge of the health issue, the care required following discharge, and information about styles and home situations.

ers can work alone or in groups. This technique is well suited to family learning. The teacher guides the learners through the thinking process necessary to reach the best solution to the question or the best action to take in the situation. This may also be referred to as anticipatory problem solving. For example, the nurse-educator might present information on diabetes and blood glucose management. Then, the nurse might ask the learners how they think their insulin and/or diet should be adjusted if their morning glucose was too low. In this way, clients learn what critical components they need to consider to reach the best solution to the problem.

Behavior Modification

Behavior modification is an outgrowth of behavioral learning theory. Its basic assumptions include (1) human behaviors are learned and can be selectively strengthened, weakened, eliminated, or replaced and (2) a person's behavior is under conscious control. Under this system, desirable behavior is regarded and un-

desirable behavior is ignored. The learner's response is the key to behavior change. For example, learners trying to quit smoking are not criticized when they smoke, but they are praised or rewarded when they go without a cigarette for a certain period of time. For some people a learning contract is combined with behavior modification and includes the following pertinent features.

- Positive reinforcement (e.g., praise) is used.
- The learner participates in the development of the learning plan.
- Undesirable behavior is ignored, not criticized.
- The expectation of the learner and the nurse is that the task will be mastered (i.e., the behavior will change).
- Success is maximized through positive reinforcement; failure and the threat of failure are minimized.

Consider . . .

- the teaching strategies you employ with clients in your clinical setting. Based on the strategies discussed on pages 145–147, which do you consider the most and least effective? Why?
- barriers that may influence the learning ability of older adults and children. What strategies would you employ to overcome these barriers? What teaching tools would you select for children?
- strategies you would use to teach a 15-year-old diabetic about insulin injections. Include strategies for the cognitive, affective, and psychomotor domains.
- teaching strategies that would be more effective with individual learners than groups of learners. Which would be more effective with groups?

Transcultural Client Teaching

The nurse and learners of different cultural and ethnic backgrounds have additional barriers to overcome in the teaching-learning process. These barriers include language and communication problems, differing concepts of time, conflicting cultural healing practices, beliefs that may positively or negatively influence compliance with health teaching, and unique high-risk or high-frequency health problems needing health-promotion instruction. See Chapter 7, "The Nurse as Health Promoter and Care Provider," and Chapter 21, "Nursing in a Culturally and Spiritually Diverse World," for detailed information. Nurses should consider the following guidelines when teaching learners from various ethnic backgrounds:

- *Obtain teaching materials, pamphlets, and instructions in languages used by clients in the health care setting.* Nurses who are unable to read the foreign language material for themselves can have the translator read the material to them. The nurse can then evaluate the quality of the information and update it with the translator's help as needed.

■ *Use visual aids, such as pictures, charts or diagrams, to communicate meaning.* Audiovisual material may be helpful if the English is spoken clearly and slowly. Even if understanding the verbal message is a problem for the learner, seeing a skill or procedure may be helpful. In some instances, a translator can be asked to clarify the video. Alternatively the video may be available in several languages, and the nurse can request the necessary version from the company.

■ *Use concrete rather than abstract words.* Use simple language (short sentences, short words), and present only one idea at a time.

■ *Allow time for questions.* This helps the learner mentally separate one idea or skill from another.

■ *Avoid the use of medical terminology or health care language,* such as "taking your vital signs" or "apical pulse." Rather, nurses should say they are going to take a blood pressure or listen to the client's heart.

Bookshelf

Deck, M. 1995. *Instant teaching tools for health care educators.* **St. Louis, Mo.: Mosby.**

Deck, M. L. 1998. *More teaching tools for health care educators.* **St. Louis, Mo.: Mosby.**

These books are useful resources for health care educators. The first provides how-to teaching strategies for a variety of learning situations. The second provides exercises and tricks for teaching allied health professionals.

Loring, K., Stewart, A., and Ritter, P., eds. 1996. *Outcome measures for health educators and other health care interventions.* **Thousand Oaks, Calif.: Sage Publications.**

This reference provides scales for measuring health behaviors, health status, self-efficacy, and health care utilization useful in planning for educational interventions. It also provides a report on the Stanford Patient Education Research Center's chronic disease self-measurement study.

Rankin, S. H., and Stallings, K. D. 2001. *Patient education: Principles and practice,* **4th ed. Philadelphia: Lippincott.**

This reference provides helpful approaches for creating client-education programs for clients of all ages, their families and caregivers, and groups of client learners in various practice settings. A special feature is the inclusion of material on teaching clients of diverse cultures.

■ *If understanding another's pronunciation is a problem, validate information in writing.* For example, during assessments, write down numbers, words, or phrases, and have the client read them to verify accuracy.

■ *Use humor very cautiously.* Meaning can change in the translation process.

■ *Do not use slang words or colloquialisms.* These may be interpreted literally.

■ *Do not assume that a learner who nods, uses eye contact or smiles is indicating an understanding of what is being taught.* These responses may simply be the learner's way of indicating respect. The learner may feel that asking the nurse questions or stating a lack of understanding is inappropriate because it might embarrass the nurse or cause the nurse to "lose face."

■ *Invite and encourage questions during teaching.* Let learners know they are urged to ask questions and be involved in making information more clear. When asking questions to evaluate learner understanding, avoid asking negative questions. These can be interpreted differently by people for whom English is a second language. "Do you understand how far you can bend your hip after surgery?" is better than the negative question "You don't understand how far you can bend your hip after surgery, do you?" With particularly difficult information or skills teaching, the nurse might say, "Most people have some trouble with this. May I help you go through this one more time?" In some cultures, expressing a need is not appropriate, and expressing confusion or asking to be shown something again is considered rude.

■ *When explaining procedures, or functioning related to personal areas of the body, it may be appropriate to have a nurse of the same sex do the teaching.* Because of modesty concerns in many cultures and beliefs about what is considered appropriate and inappropriate male-female interaction, it is wise to have a female nurse teach female learners about personal care, birth control, sexually transmitted diseases (STDs), and other potentially sensitive areas. If a translator is needed during explanation of procedures or teaching, the translator should also be female.

■ *Include the family in planning and teaching.* This promotes trust and mutual respect. Identify the authoritative family member and incorporate that person into the planning and teaching to promote adherence and support of health teaching. In some cultures, the male head of household is the critical family member to include in health teaching; in other cultures, it is the eldest female member.

DOCUMENTATION OF TEACHING

Documentation of the teaching process is essential when teaching clients in the clinical setting, because it provides a legal record that the teaching took place and communicates the teaching to other health professionals. If teaching is not documented, legally it did not occur. It is also important to document the response of the client and support persons. What did the client or support person say or do to indicate that learning occurred? The nurse records this in the client's chart as evidence of learning. The parts of the teaching process that should be documented in the client's chart include the following:

- Diagnosed learning needs
- Learning objectives
- Topics taught
- Client outcomes
- Need for additional teaching
- Resources provided

The written teaching plan that the nurse uses as a resource to guide future teaching sessions might also include these elements:

- Actual information and skills taught

- Teaching strategies used
- Time framework and content for each class

Consider . . .

- the learning needs of clients in your specific practice setting. Is the instruction given by different health care providers consistent in its content? What problems might occur if there is inconsistency in instruction? How might you go about correcting these inconsistencies?
- the specific health problems of your community (e.g., AIDS, teenage pregnancy, sexually transmitted disease, domestic violence). How might the nurse assist in solving community health problems through the teaching role?
- how the nurse might influence through education others' understanding of nurses' knowledge, skill, and roles. Do nurses speak in community education programs? In what way are nurses involved in the education of other health professionals? In what ways are nurses politically proactive regarding health care and nursing practice?

SUMMARY

Teaching clients, families, and other health professionals is a major nursing role. Learning is represented by a change in behavior.

Five main theories of learning are behaviorism, cognitivism, humanism, constructivism, and multiple intelligence. Behaviorism focuses on careful identification of what is to be taught and the immediate identification of a reward for correct responses. Cognitivism, which has a more holistic view of learning, emphasizes the importance of an integrated learning experience, one that develops understandings and appreciations that help the person function in a larger context. It also stresses the importance of social, emotional, and physical contexts in which learning occurs. The teacher-learner relationship is also an important factor in cognitive learning theory. Humanism focuses on the feelings and attitudes of the learner and stresses that individuals can become highly self-motivated learners. The learner identifies the learning needs and takes responsibility for meeting them. Constructivism is a collection of theories whereby the individual is actively involved in constructing knowledge. Learning is often collaborative. Multiple intelligence focuses on the many ways individuals are "smart."

Bloom has identified three learning domains: cognitive, affective, and psychomotor. The cognitive domain includes six intellectual skills: knowledge, comprehension, application, analysis, synthesis, and evaluation. The affective domain includes five categories: receiving,

responding, valuing, organization, and characterization. The psychomotor domain includes seven categories: perception, set, guided response, mechanism, complex overt response, adaptation, and origination.

A number of factors facilitate learning, including motivation, readiness, active involvement, success at learning, feedback, and moving from simple to complex. Factors such as extreme anxiety, certain physiologic processes, and cultural barriers impede learning.

Teaching is a system of activities intended to produce learning. Rapport between the teacher and the learner is essential for effective teaching. Teaching consists of five activities: assessing the learner, diagnosing learning needs, developing a teaching plan, implementing the plan, and evaluating learning outcomes and teaching effectiveness. Learning objectives guide the content of the teaching plan and are written in terms of client behavior. Teaching strategies should be suited to the client, the material to be learned, and the teacher. It should be adjusted to the client's developmental level and health status.

A teaching plan is a written plan consisting of learning objectives, content to teach, a time frame for teaching, and strategies to use in teaching the content. The plan must be revised when the client's needs change or the teaching strategies prove ineffective. Adaptations in teaching will facilitate learning for clients who are illiterate, elderly, or from non-Western cultural and ethnic backgrounds. Barriers to overcome transcultural teaching include language and communication problems, different concepts of time, and cultural beliefs and practices that conflict with those of Western medicine.

Evaluation of the teaching/learning process is both an ongoing and a final process. Documentation of client teaching is essential to communicate the teaching to other health professionals and to provide a record for legal purposes.

REFERENCES

American Nurses Association. 1998. *Standards of clinical nursing practice,* 2d ed. Washington, D.C.: ANA.

American Nurses Credentialing Center. 2001. ANCC Board Certification. http://www.ana.org/ancc/certify/cert/catalogs/2000/bcc/spec.htm.

Bandura, A. 1971. Analysis of modeling processes. In *Psychological modeling,* edited by A. Bandura. Chicago: Aldine.

Bloom, B. S. (ed.). 1956. *Taxonomy of educational objectives.* Book 1, *Cognitive domain.* New York: Longman.

Brooks, J. G., and Brooks, M. G. 1993. *In search of understanding: The case for constructivist classrooms.* Alexandria, Va.: Association for Supervision and Curriculum Development.

Driscoll, M. 2000. *Psychology of learning for instruction,* 2d ed. New York: Allyn and Bacon.

Estey, A., Musseau, A., and Keehn, L. 1991, Oct. Comprehensive levels of patients reading health information. *Patient Education and Counseling* **18:** 165–169.

Gagne, R. M. 1974. *Essentials of learning of instruction.* Hinsdale, Ill.: Dryden Press.

Gardner, H. 1983. *Frames of mind: The theory of multiple intelligences.* New York: Basic Books.

Gerty, C. 1997. *Learning with Bruner.* New York: Review of Books.

Gessner, B. A. 1989, Sept. Adult education: The cornerstone of patient teaching. *Nursing Clinics of North America* **24:** 589-595.

Gredler, M. E. 2001. *Learning and instruction: Theory into practice,* 4th ed. Columbus, Ohio: Merrill.

Gronlund, N. E. 1985. *Stating objectives for classroom instruction,* 3rd ed. New York: Macmillan.

Knowles, M. S. 1980. *The modern practice of adult education: From pedagogy to andragogy.* Chicago: Follet.

Knowles, M. S. 1984. *Andragogy in action.* San Francisco: Jossey-Bass.

Lewin, K. 1951. *Field theory in social science.* New York: Harper and Row.

MacDonald, S. A. 1999, May. The cardiovascular health education program: Assessing the impact on rural and urban adolescents' health knowledge. *Applied Nursing Research* **12**(2): 86–90.

Maslow, A. H. 1970. *Motivation and personality.* New York: Harper and Row.

North American Nursing Diagnosis Association. 1992. *NANDA nursing diagnoses: Definitions and classification 1994–1995.* Philadelphia: NANDA.

Pavlov, I. P. 1927. *Conditioned reflexes* (trans. G. V. Anrep). London: Oxford U. Press.

Piaget, J. 1966. *Origins of intelligence in children.* New York: Norton.

Rogers, C. R. 1961. *On becoming a person.* Boston: Houghton-Mifflin.

Rogers, C. R. 1969. *Freedom to learn.* Columbus, Ohio: Merrill.

Schoenly, L. 1994, Sept./Oct. Teaching in the affective domain. *Journal of Continuing Education in Nursing* **25:** 209–212.

Skinner, B. F. 1953. *Science and human behavior.* New York: Macmillan.

Stephens, S. T. 1992. Patient educational materials: Are they readable? *Oncology Nursing Forum* **19**(1): 84.

Suderman, E. M., Deatrich, J. V., Johnson, L. S., and Sawatzky-Dickson, D. M. 2000. Action research sets the stage to improve discharge preparation. *Pediatric Nursing* **26**(6): 571–576.

Swansburg, R. C. 1995. *Nursing staff development: A component of human resource development.* Boston: Jones and Bartlett.

Thorndike, E. L. 1913. *The psychology of learning.* New York: Teachers College.

Wong, M. 1992. Self-care instructions: Do patients understand educational materials? *Focus on Critical Care* **19**(2): 47–49.

The Nurse as Leader and Manager

Objectives

- Differentiate leadership from management.

- Compare and contrast the following leadership styles: charismatic, authoritarian, democratic, laissez-faire, situational, transactional, and transformational.

- Describe the management concepts of authority, accountability, planning, organizing, leading, controlling, and power.

- Compare and contrast the following nursing delivery models: case method, functional method, team nursing, primary nursing, case management, managed care, differentiated practice, and shared governance.

- Discuss the impact of downsizing and restructuring on the role of the professional nurse.

N U R S E   C O N N E C T

Additional online resources for this chapter can be found on the companion web site at www.prenhall.com/blais.

Today's professional nurses assume leadership and management responsibilities regardless of the activity in which they are involved. Although leadership and management roles are different, they are frequently intertwined. Leadership is defined as "the process of influencing others" (Tappen, 2001, p. 5). Management involves not only leadership but also "coordination and integration of resources through planning, organizing, coordinating, directing, and controlling to accomplish specific institutional goals and objectives (Huber 2000). Leaders focus on people, whereas managers focus on systems and structures. See Table 9–1 for a comparison of leader and manger roles.

The ability to advocate for the client is linked to the nurse's leadership ability. The nurse may be a leader or manager in the care of the individual client, the client's family, groups of clients, or the community. Regardless of the setting, the nurse must demonstrate leadership and management skills in interacting with nursing colleagues, nursing students, physicians, and other health professionals.

CHALLENGES AND OPPORTUNITIES

Leadership challenges for nurses in the current U.S. health care system are the need to provide care for high numbers of uninsured or underinsured individuals, limited access to health care services, especially for the poor, and limited resources for providing care. Nurse-managers and -administrators are faced with the need to recruit and retain high-quality nurses during a time of rapidly changing nursing roles and cycles of nursing shortages.

These challenges provide opportunities to develop innovative approaches to nursing care delivery and to redefine the roles of professional nurses. These innovations and changes provide opportunities to develop new recruitment and retention strategies that increase nursing satisfaction and commitment to the profession.

NURSING LEADERSHIP

Nurses may assume leadership roles in their work setting, their profession, and their community, whether or not they have designated positions of leadership. As leaders in the workplace, they may advocate for improvements in the quality of patient care. As leaders in the profession, nurses may advocate not only for improvements in client care, but also for improvements in the working environment of nurses and other health professionals. Because of their special knowledge and skill, nurses may also assume leadership roles in the community, advocating for changes that pro-

Table 9–1 Comparison of Leader and Manager Roles

Leaders	Managers
• Do not have delegated authority; power derives from other means, such as personal influence	• Have an assigned position in the formal organization
• Have a wider variety of roles	• Have a legitimate source of power because of the delegated authority that is part of their position
• May not be a part of the formal organization	• Are expected to carry out specific functions, duties, and responsibilities
• Focus on group process, information gathering, feedback, and empowering others	• Emphasize control, decision making, decision analysis, and results
• Emphasize interpersonal relationships	• Manipulate personnel, the environment, money, time, and other resources to achieve organizational goals
• Direct willing followers	• Have a greater formal responsibility and accountability
• Have goals that may or may not reflect those of the organization	• Direct willing and unwilling subordinates

Source: B. L. Marquis and C. J. Huston. *Leadership Roles and Management Function in Nursing,* 3d ed. Philadelphia: Lippincott, 2000.

mote physical, psychologic, and social well-being in the society as a whole.

On a wider scope, nurses must apply leadership skills as they apply nursing knowledge to personal concerns. Nurses can demonstrate these leadership skills in their involvement in such organizations as Mothers Against Drunk Drivers (MADD), the American Cancer Society, and the American Heart Association. Nurses demonstrate leadership activities as they advocate for the homeless, older adults, persons living with AIDS, victims of violence, and environmental protection programs. In recent years, professional nurses have demonstrated a wide range of leadership and management skills to politicians and legislators in all parts of the country in their efforts to advocate and plan for a system of affordable health care for all residents of the United States through Nursing's Agenda for Health Care Reform (ANA, 1991a).

Leadership occurs when someone influences others to act. Whereas managers are assigned their roles, leaders achieve their roles. One may be designated the manager and demonstrate no leadership skills, while another person may have no formal management title yet demonstrate excellent leadership skills.

Leadership Characteristics

What are the characteristics of successful leadership? Hellriegel and Slocum (1993, pp. 469–479) emphasize the following core leadership skills:

- *Empowerment.* Leaders who empower others share influence and control with group members in deciding how to achieve the organization's goals. Through empowerment, the leader gives others a sense of achievement, belonging, and self-esteem. One way in which the nursing leader can empower the staff is to discuss with them ideas about providing client care.
- *Intuition.* By using intuition, a leader can build trust with others, scan a situation, anticipate the need for change, and quickly move to institute appropriate change. Intuition involves having a "feel" for the environment and the needs and desires of others. Effective nurse leaders heighten their sense of intuition in order to keep abreast of the needs of clients and staff.
- *Self-understanding.* Self-understanding includes an ability to recognize one's strengths and weaknesses. Building on one's strengths and correcting or working on weaknesses are essential for effective leadership.
- *Vision.* Leaders with a vision imagine a different and better situation and identify ways of achieving it. Visionary leadership does not mean constantly imagining new and original goals; a vision may be as simple as incorporating caring and efficiency in meeting the needs of employees and clients.

- *Values congruence.* Values congruence is the ability to understand and accept the mission and objectives of the organization and the values of employees and to reconcile them. In this era of health reform and cost containment, values congruence is an important leadership characteristic.

Does the fact that effective leaders share certain characteristics imply that they all act the same? Not necessarily. Besides having the preceding characteristics, most effective leaders demonstrate the following: (1) achievement and ambition, (2) the ability to learn from adversity, (3) high dedication to the job, (4) sound analytic and problem-solving skills, (5) a high level of people skills, and (6) a high level of innovation.

Leadership Style

Leadership styles are defined "as different combinations of task and relationship behaviors used to influence others to accomplish goals" (Huber, 2000, p. 51). Several leadership styles have been described: charismatic leadership; authoritarian, or directive, leadership; democratic, or participative, leadership; laissez-faire, or nondirectional, leadership; situational leadership; transactional leadership; and transformational leadership.

Charismatic leadership is characterized by an emotional relationship between the leader and the group members in which the leader "inspires others by obtaining an emotional commitment from followers and by arousing strong feelings of loyalty and enthusiasm" (Marriner-Tomey, 2000, p. 139). A charismatic relationship exists when the leader can communicate a plan for change and the followers adhere to the plan because of their faith and belief in the leader's abilities. The followers of a charismatic leader may be able to overcome extreme hardship to achieve the goal because of their faith in the leader.

In *authoritarian leadership,* the leader makes the decisions for the group. This style of leadership has also been referred to as *directive* or *autocratic leadership.* Authoritarian leadership is likened to a dictatorship and presupposes that the group is incapable of making its own decisions. The leader determines policies, giving orders and directions to the group members. Authoritarian leadership generally has negative connotations and often makes group members dissatisfied. Because of the differences in status between the leader and group members, the degree of openness and trust between leader and group members is minimal or absent. Under this type of leadership, procedures are well defined, activities are predictable, and the group may feel secure. Although productivity is usually high, the group members' needs for creativity, autonomy, and self-motivation are not met (Tappen, 2001, p. 26). Authoritarian leadership may, however, be most effective in situations requiring immediate decisions, such as cardiac arrest, fire on the unit, airplane crash, or other emergency, when one person must assume responsibility without being challenged by other team members. Similarly, when group members are unable or unwilling to participate in making a decision, the authoritarian style effects resolution of the problem and enables the individual or group to move on. This style can also be effective when a project must be completed quickly and efficiently.

In *democratic, or participative leadership,* the leader acts as a catalyst or facilitator, actively guiding the group toward achieving the group goals. Providing constructive criticism, offering information, making suggestions, and asking questions become the focus of the participative leader. This type of leadership demands that the leader have faith in the group members to accomplish the goals. Democratic leadership is based on the following principles (Tappen, 2001, p. 26):

1. Every group member should participate in decision making.

2. Freedom of belief and action is allowed within reasonable bounds that are set by society and by the group.

3. Each individual is responsible for himself or herself and for the welfare of the group.

4. There should be concern and consideration for each group member as a unique individual.

Although democratic leadership has been shown to be less efficient and more cumbersome than authoritarian leadership, it allows for more self-motivation and more creativity among group members. Democratic leadership calls for a great deal of cooperation and coordination among group members. This style of leadership can be extremely effective in the health care setting (Tappen, 2001, p. 26).

The *laissez-faire, or nondirectional, leader* is described as inactive, passive, and permissive; offering few commands, questions, suggestions, or criticism (Tappen, 2001, p. 27). Although there are various degrees of nondirectional leadership, leadership participation is, in general, minimal. The group's members may act independently of each other and suffer from a lack of cooperation or coordination. Apathy, chaos, and frustration may arise. The laissez-faire approach works best when group members have both personal and professional maturity, so that once the group has made a decision, the members become committed to it and have the required expertise to implement it. Individual group members then perform tasks in their area of expertise, with the leader acting as a resource person. Table 9–2 compares the authoritarian, democratic, and laissez-faire leadership styles.

In *situational leadership,* levels of direction and support vary according to the level of maturity of the employees or group. The leader assumes one of four styles (Hellriegel, Jackson, and Slocum, 1999, pp. 514–515):

Table 9–2 Comparison of Authoritarian, Democratic, and Laissez-Faire Leadership Styles

	Authoritarian	Democratic	Laissez-Faire
Degree of freedom	Little freedom	Moderate freedom	Much freedom
Degree of control	High control	Moderate control	No control
Decision making	By the leader	Leader and group together	By the group or by no one
Leader activity level	High	High	Minimal
Assumption of responsibility	Primarily the leader	Shared	Abdicated
Output of the group	High quantity, good quality	Creative, high quality	Variable, may be of poor quality
Efficiency	Very efficient	Less efficient than authoritarian	Inefficient

Source: Nursing Leadership and Management: Concepts and Practice, 4th ed., by R. M. Tappen, Philadelphia: F. A. Davis, 2001, p. 26. Reprinted with permission.

1. *Directive.* A leadership style characterized by the giving of clear instructions and specific direction to immature employees.
2. *Coaching.* A leadership style characterized by expanding two-way communication and helping maturing employees build confidence and motivation.
3. *Supporting.* A leadership style characterized by active two-way communication and support of mature employees' efforts to use their talents.
4. *Delegating.* A hands-off leadership style in which the highly mature employees are given responsibilities for carrying out plans and making task decisions.

The situational leadership model poses some questions. First, can leaders actually choose one of these four leadership styles when faced with a new situation? Second, how do such factors as personality traits and the leaders' power base influence the leader's choice of style? Third, what should the leader choose for a group whose members are at different levels of maturity?

An important issue in situational leadership is the value placed on the accomplishment of tasks and on the interpersonal relationships between leader and group members and among group members. For example, the nurse-manager encourages input from staff members when planning daily work assignments so that the needs of both staff and clients are met. The nurse-manager may also solicit input from staff members when doing both short-range and long-range planning for the unit. However, when a new staff member is being oriented to the unit, the nurse-manager may be more directive in making assignments until the staff member develops experience and professional maturity. In emergency situations or situations in which the task needs to be completed quickly, the nurse-manager may be more authoritative in directing the actions of all staff members.

Transactional leadership represents the traditional manager focused on the day-to-day tasks of achieving organizational goals. The transactional leader understands and meets the needs of the group. Relationships with followers are based upon an exchange for some resource valued by the follower. These incentives are used to promote loyalty and performance. For example, in order to ensure adequate staffing on the night shift, the nurse-manager negotiates with a staff nurse to work the night shift in exchange for a weekend shift off.

In contrast, *transformational leadership* theory, which was developed in the 1980s, "reconsiders the characteristics of the leader-manager, reemphasizes the vision that the leader-manger shares with the group, and stresses the importance of preparing people for change (Tappen, 2001, p. 44). This model combines elements of earlier theories and recognizes the influence of the leader, workers, tasks, and environment. Transformational leadership is characterized by four primary factors (p. 44):

1. *Charisma.* Charismatic leaders are highly respected and are viewed with reverence, dedication, and awe. They set high standards, challenging their staff to go beyond the expected level of effort.
2. *Inspirational motivation.* The leader shares visions with the staff that appeal to both their emotions and their ideals.

Research Box

Stordeur, S., Vandenberghe, C., and D'hoore, W. 2000. **Leadership styles across hierarchical levels in nursing departments.** *Nursing Research* 49(1):37–43.

The purpose of this study was to examine the cascading effect of leadership styles across hierarchical levels in a sample consisting of 464 respondents working on 41 nursing units in 12 divisions at eight hospitals in Belgium. The study also examined whether the relationship between leader behavior and outcome variables is stronger at the upper levels of the organization. The Multifactor Leadership Questionnaire was used to measure leadership in the participants. The correlations between nurses' evaluation of their head nurse and the head nurses' evaluations of their associate directors showed no significant correlation between leadership behaviors across hierarchical levels. However, scores on transformational leadership and passive management by exception (MBEP) varied significantly (p > .0001). The study provides evidence for the impact of transformational leadership and of transactional components on nurses' satisfaction with their leader, extra effort, and perceived unit effectiveness. Transformational leaders provide a significant and positive impact on nurses' perceptions by encouraging nurses' autonomy, transforming staff into leaders, and providing a sense of mission and future vision. Leaders who use transformational leadership strategies may contribute to the quality of care beyond their clinical expertise.

3. *Intellectual stimulation*. The leader stimulates followers to question the status quo: to question critically what they are doing and why.

4. *Contingent reward*. The leader recognizes mutually agreed-upon goals and rewards the employee's achievements.

It is expected that transformational leadership will become critically vital in the creation of a health care system that embodies community well-being, basic care for all, cost-effectiveness, and holistic nursing care. The transformational leader is a mythmaker and storyteller, painting vivid descriptions of an inspiring, uplifting future everyone will build together. A survey of 2500 health care leaders identified six factors in transformational leadership that will effect these changes in the 21st century: (1) mastering change, (2) systems thinking, (3) shared vision, (4) continuous quality improvement, (5) an ability to redefine health care, and (6) a commitment to serving the public and community (Trofino, 1995, p. 45).

Caring leadership is a concept that is an extension of transformational leadership. The term *caring leadership* was introduced in 1991 by a Fortune 500 executive, who stated: "Good management is largely a matter of love. Or if you're uncomfortable with the word call it caring, because proper management involves caring for people, not manipulating them" (Brandt, 1994, p. 68). Caring leadership recognizes the importance of caring in the practice of nursing, combining concepts from both caring and leadership theories.

Effective leadership is a learned process requiring an understanding of the needs and goals that motivate people, the knowledge to apply the leadership skills, and the interpersonal skills to influence others. Much has been written about effective leadership and style; some descriptive statements about effective leaders are listed in the accompanying box. Humanistic leadership can serve as a means of creating an environment "that is stimulating, motivating, and empowering to the professional nurse" (Glennon, 1992, p. 41). Strategies for humanistic and caring leadership are identified in the box on page 157.

Consider . . .

■ nursing leaders you admire. What characteristics of leadership do they have that you admire? Are there characteristics that you don't like? What leadership style or styles do they employ to influence others? Do they emphasize one style or several styles? Are the nursing leaders you admire well liked by other colleagues and health professionals? Is it important to be liked when you are a leader?

■ nursing heroes past and present. What qualities of leadership do they share? How important is risk taking to effective leadership?

■ your own leadership activities. What characteristics of leadership do you have? What leadership style or styles are you most comfortable with? How might you improve your abilities as a leader?

NURSING MANAGEMENT

As a manager and provider of client care, the nurse coordinates various health care professionals and their services to help the client meet desired outcomes.

Theories of Management Style

Concern with management practices began in the latter part of the nineteenth century, as the United States

Characteristics of Effective Leaders

- Use a leadership style that is natural to them
- Use a leadership style appropriate to the task and the members
- Assess the effects of their behavior on others and the effects of others' behavior on themselves
- Are sensitive to forces acting for and against change
- Express an optimistic view about human nature
- Are energetic
- Are open and encourage openness, so that real issues are confronted

- Facilitate personal relationships
- Plan and organize activities of the group
- Are consistent in behavior toward group members
- Delegate tasks and responsibilities to develop members' abilities, not merely to get tasks performed
- Involve members in all decisions
- Value and use group members' contributions
- Encourage creativity
- Encourage feedback about their leadership style

Strategies for Putting Humanistic and Caring Leadership into Action

- Praise or positively recognize staff and colleagues.
- Always think good thoughts about yourself and others.
- Work on discovering group members' unique personal and professional needs.
- Always give before you get—give colleagues and staff a reason for doing whatever it is that you are asking of them.
- Smile often—it generates enthusiasm and goodwill.
- Recognize the expertise of others.
- Remember the names of the people you work with.
- Think, act, and look successful.
- Always greet others with a positive, affirmative statement.

- Foster an atmosphere of collegiality and mutual trust.
- Write informal appreciation notes; this shows appreciation and reinforces positive performance.
- Get out of the nurse's station or office; make a point of circulating among those who work in your circle of influence.
- Foster creativity, independence, and professional growth.
- Talk less and listen more; encourage communication and the sharing of ideas and information.
- Don't condemn, criticize, or complain; instead, work on ways to improve the situation or solve the problem.
- Accept responsibility.

Sources: Adapted from "Empowering Nurses through Enlightened Leadership" by T. K. Glennon, *Revolution: The Journal of Nurse Empowerment,* **2:** 40–44, Spring 1992; and "Caring Leadership: Secret Path to Success" by M. A. Brandt, *Nursing Management* **25:** 68–72, August 1994.

began emerging as a leading industrial nation. Early management theory focused on how to get as much work as possible from each worker. The oldest and most widely accepted viewpoint on management is called the *traditional, or classical, viewpoint.*

The traditional style stresses the manager's role in a strict hierarchy and focuses on efficient and consistent job performance. Traditionalists are concerned with the formal relations among an organization's departments, tasks, and structural elements, and they stress the manager's role in a hierarchy. Superiors are assumed to have greater expertise and are therefore to be obeyed by subordinates. Time-and-motion studies, Gantt charts, and the development of early management principles were the work of the traditionalists. Characteristics of traditional management include adherence to routines and rules, impersonality, division of labor, hierarchy, financial motivation, and authority structure. The benefits of the traditional style include efficiency, consistency, clear structure, and an emphasis on productivity (Hellriegel, Jackson, and Slocum, 1999, pp. 44–55). Although most traditionalists today recognize the emotional and humanistic component of management, the focus on efficient and effective job performance remains overriding. Many managers and health care organizations still use the traditional management style today.

The expansion of labor unions in the 1930s, the Great Depression, and World War II heralded another era in management theory. Against the backdrop of change and reform, managers were forced to focus on the humanistic side of managing organizations. *Behavioral theory* moves beyond the traditionalists' mechanical view of the work world and stresses the importance of group dynamics and the leadership style of the manager. The behavioral viewpoint includes the following four basic assumptions (Hellriegel, Jackson, and Slocum, 1999, p. 60):

1. Workers are motivated by social needs and get a sense of identity through their associations with one another.

2. Workers are more responsive to the social forces exerted by their peers than to management's financial incentives and rules.

3. Workers respond to managers who can help them satisfy their needs.

4. Managers need to coordinate the work of their subordinates democratically in order to improve efficiency.

These assumptions really do not hold true for the workforce of the new century. Today's work world is more complex than the work world of the traditionalist and behaviorist. The post–World War II years brought a new management theory, *systems theory*. Just as the human body is a system consisting of organs, muscles, bones, and a circulatory system that links all the parts together, an organization is a system consisting of many departments that are linked by people working together. Systems theory approaches problems by looking at inputs, transformation processes, outputs, and feedback. Inputs are the physical, human, material, financial, and information resources that enter the system and leave as outputs. The technology used to convert the inputs are the transformation processes. Outputs are the original physical, human, material, financial, and information resources that are now in the form of goods and services. A vital part of systems theory is the feedback loops, which provide ongoing information about a system's status and performance. Another vital component of the systems theory is the interaction of the system with the environment. The manager who uses systems theory "makes decisions only after identifying and analyzing how other managers," units, clients, or others might be affected by the decisions (Hellriegel, Jackson, and Slocum, 1999, p. 60).

Contingency theory emerged in the mid-1960s in response to managers' unsuccessful attempts to apply traditional, behavioral, and systems concepts to managerial problems. Contingency theory is a blend of these concepts. Using contingency theory, the manager is expected to determine which method or combination of methods will be most effective in a given situation. To apply the contingency viewpoint effectively, the manager must be able to diagnose and understand a situation thoroughly, determine the most useful approach, and recognize the impact of the external environment, technology, and the people involved prior to acting (Hellriegel, Jackson, and Slocum, 1999, pp. 64–65).

The contingency theory of management moves the manager away from the "one size fits all" approach. Managers are encouraged to analyze and understand the differences in each situation, selecting the solution that best suits the organization and individual in each situation.

Management Competencies

Hellriegel, Jackson, and Slocum (1999, pp. 16–28) describe six competencies essential for successful managers: communication, planning and administration, teamwork, strategic action, global awareness, and self-management:

1. *Communication competency.* This competency is the most fundamental of managerial competencies. Effective managers are able to communicate so that the exchanged information is clearly understood by the managers and those with whom they communicate. Communication can involve information communication, formal communication, and negotiation. Communication is not only face-to-face discussion; it also includes effective use of the many means of communicating verbally and in writing, including telephone, individual or group conferences, written communications (such as memos and newsletters), electronic communications, and the effective use of body language.

2. *Planning and administration competency.* The effective manager must be able to decide which tasks need to be done, how they should be done, and what resources need to be allocated; then the manager must follow through to make sure that the tasks are accomplished. This competency includes information gathering and analysis, planning and organizing projects, time management, and budgeting and financial management.

3. *Teamwork competency.* Effective managers must be able to accomplish tasks through teams of people. This competency requires that managers be able to design work teams properly, create a supportive team environment, and manage team dynamics appropriately. Nurse-managers in the hospital or institutional environment have a team of registered nurses and other care providers who must work together to provide quality care to their patients.

4. *Strategic action competency.* Managers must understand the overall mission and values of the organization. They must then ensure that their actions and those of the people they manage are consistent with the organization's mission and values. For nurses, the mission and values may reflect not only the organization where they work but also those of the nursing profession.

5. *Global awareness competency.* Contemporary nurse-managers must have an awareness of the multicultural beliefs, values, and practices of their clients and their staff. In addition to cultural awareness, nurse-managers must be culturally sensitive and culturally competent in their interactions with clients and staff.

6. *Self-management competency.* Finally, effective nurse-managers must be able to take responsibility for their life at work and outside of work. This competency includes integrity and ethical conduct, personal drive and resilience, balancing life and work issues, and being aware of self and personal development needs.

The relative importance and skill mix at each level of management change as one moves from first-line managers to middle and top management. Interpersonal and communication skills are of equal importance to all levels of management. The professional nurse may be promoted into a middle management position because of excellent technical nursing skills. These new managers often rely on their nursing expertise, unaware that they also need to develop other skills associated with business and finance. Duffield (1994, p. 64) explored the responsibilities of first-line managers. She found consensus that the first-line manager is required not only to maintain the technical skills associated with managing client care but also to master the technical skills of finance and business management, such as budget and finance, human resource management, and development of policies and procedures.

The higher a manager's position in the organization, the greater the need for conceptual and interpersonal skills. Many of the responsibilities of top nurse-managers, such as allocating resources and developing overall strategies, require a broad outlook and ability to see the "big picture." The ability to provide visionary leadership will become an even more highly valued managerial skill in the coming years. This means creating a vision with which people can identify and to which they can commit (Hellriegel, Jackson, and Slocum, 1999, p. 521). Offering educational programs such as workshops, seminars, and mentor programs is one way the organization and profession can help the new nurse-manager build on their nursing knowledge. Nurse-managers may also choose to take classes in budgeting and finance, human resource development, conflict management, and other business-related areas.

Management Roles

Nurses function differently in various types of organizations. An autocratic organization confers primary knowledge and power to one person and places other persons in subordinate roles. Bureaucratic organizations exert control through policy, structured jobs, and compartmentalized actions. Other organizations decentralize control and emphasize self-direction and self-discipline of members. Still another type of organization is the component of a system that interacts interdependently with other components and adapts dynamically to change. This type of organization is particularly beneficial for the nurse who manages the care of individuals, families, and communities. On a larger scale, the nurse-manager must work in the organizational framework of the employing agency.

Authority is the official power given by the organization to direct the work of others. It is an integral component of managing. Authority is conveyed through leadership actions; it is determined largely by the situation, and it is always associated with responsibility and accountability.

Accountability is the ability and willingness to assume responsibility for one's actions and to accept the consequences of one's behavior. Accountability can be viewed within a hierarchic systems framework, starting at the individual level, through the institutional/professional level, and then to the societal level. At the individual or client level, accountability is reflected in the nurse's ethical integrity. At the institutional level, it is reflected in the statement of philosophy and objectives of the nursing department and nursing audits. At the professional level, accountability is reflected in standards of practice developed by national or provincial nursing associations. At the societal level, it is reflected in legislated nurse practice acts.

To be successful, the nurse-manager must exert authority and assume accountability in implementing the managerial functions of planning, organizing, leading and delegating, and controlling. These functions help to achieve the goal of quality client care.

Planning

Planning is often considered the first and most basic management function. Planning is a process that includes the following steps (Hellriegel, Jackson, and Slocum, 1999, pp. 218–222):

- Choosing the organization's mission and vision. The mission describes the purpose or reason for the existence of the organization. The vision "expresses the organization's fundamental aspirations and purpose. A vision statement adds soul to the mission statement."
- Devising departmental goals. The nursing unit should reflect the more global goals of the nursing department and the health care agency.
- Selecting strategies to achieve the goals. Strategies are the courses of action the unit staff will take in order to achieve the unit's goals.
- Deciding on the allocation of resources. Distribution of money, personnel, equipment, and physical space is included in resource allocation.

Nurse-managers must keep in mind that plans are the means, not the ends. Quick fixes may cause one to neglect the big picture. Planning can help the nurse-manager (1) identify future opportunities, (2) anticipate and avoid future problems, and (3) develop strategies and courses of action.

Organizing

Organizing is the formal system of working relationships. The nurse-manager is responsible for identifying particular tasks and assigning them to individuals or teams who have the training and expertise to carry them out. Along with organizing, the nurse-manager is responsible for coordinating activities to meet the unit's objectives. Health care reform, downsizing, and restructuring have all impacted the management role of organizing.

Leading and Delegating

The beginning of this chapter discussed many of the elements of effective leadership. These elements, even when combined with the motivation to lead and basic leadership skills, will not necessarily make an effective leader; power is also an essential component of leading.

Power, in this context, is defined as "the ability to influence or control individual, departmental, team, or organizational decisions and goals" (Hellriegel, Jackson, and Slocum, 1999, p. 275).

Another component of leading is *delegating*. Delegation is defined as "transferring to a competent individual authority to perform a selected nursing task in a selected situation" (Hansten and Washburn, 1994, p. 1). The delegation function in the health care field is often complex because of the number and diversity of caregivers, the amount of different knowledge and skills needed to provide care, and the intricacy of the relationships among staff, client, and environment (Tappen, 1995, p. 307).

Delegation is a major tool in making the most efficient use of time. Delegation is a high-level implementation skill. To delegate effectively, the nurse must be aware of the needs and goals of the client and family, the nursing activities that can help the client meet the goals, and the skills and knowledge of various nursing and support personnel.

In delegating, the nurse must also determine how many and what type of personnel are needed. Decisions about delegation may be based on information from the client's records, the client, the charge nurse, other nursing personnel, and the nurse's own judgment.

After establishing that assistance is required, the nurse must identify what type of help is needed, how long help will be required, when it will be required, and what assistance is available. Before beginning the nursing activity, the nurse must arrange for assistance, usually by asking the appropriate person on the unit. Delegation does not require that the nurse have the personal knowledge and expertise to perform a specific nursing activity, but it does require that the nurse know who does have the knowledge and expertise and can recognize when it is needed. For example, a nurse may call a dietitian to assist a client in choosing foods from a menu or request a social worker to assist a client who needs financial assistance and homemaker services after discharge.

An important aspect of delegation is the development of the potential of nursing and support personnel. By knowing the background, experience, knowledge, skill, and strengths of each person, a nurse can delegate responsibilities that help develop each person's competence. Nursing personnel to whom aspects of care have been delegated need to be supervised and evaluated. The amount of supervision required is highly variable and depends on the knowledge and skills of each person. As the person who assigns the activity and observes the performance, the nurse contributes to the evaluation process. Because individual motivation varies, the nurse needs to realize that not all persons perform equally. Thus, the nurse must evaluate standards of performance against written job descriptions, rather than by comparing one person's performance to that of another. It is essential, too, for the nurse to realize that people require ongoing feedback about their performance and to give feedback, including both positive and negative input, in an objective manner.

Controlling

Controlling is a method to ensure that behaviors and performances are consistent with the planning process. Control is not something managers do *to* employees, but rather *with* them. Formal, structured, bureaucratic controls, such as tightly written job descriptions, extensive rules and procedures, and top-down authority, are familiar control mechanisms. Increasingly in health care agencies, more flexible controls such as continuous quality improvement (CQI), shared governance, and team building help make control an easier and integral part of the management process.

The discussion of management roles would be incomplete without a few words on "the games people play" within the world of work. A lack of understanding of the politics of work can cause even the most competent and committed nurse to feel helpless and frustrated.

Many nurses feel that being politically astute is a genetic trait, that they have neither the ability nor desire to "get involved in that political mess." These nurses soon discover that power and politics are inevitable in today's workplace. First, there will always be those people who will do anything to obtain and hang on to power. Second, hard work is usually measured by the manager in charge, not by the rules and regulations on the top shelf. Menke and Ogborn (1993, pp. 35–37) describe the following behaviors that nurses should develop to negotiate the politics of the workplace.

1. *Read the environment.* Observe where the power lies in the organization. Historically, power has rested in those who bring in the money and those who supply the resources for those in power.

2. *Listen.* Listen to everyone, everywhere. Move slowly, and don't be anxious to exhibit everything you know.

3. *Read.* Read organizational charts, policies and procedure statements, and professional journals. Learn to identify what is acceptable and what is not.

4. *Detach.* Don't hook up with people who are on the losing side. Detach and stay independent until you know the political ropes.

5. *Analyze.* Identify your own unique characteristics that may be seen as being "different." For example, are you the only male, the only nurse with a baccalaureate degree, or the only newcomer? If so, you may have to work a little harder to achieve your goal.

6. *Create competence.* A firm handshake, offering your name, and politeness never go out of style. Summarizing your project status with your manager while sharing credit for success when due keeps your manager aware of what is going on.

7. *Never gossip about the manager.* Keep the manager from being blindsided and embarrassed. Don't whine!

8. *Always roll with the punches.* Remain enthusiastic! The nurse may never like being in the political game, but being knowledgeable will make it easier to understand and survive it.

Characteristics of effective nurse-managers as described by Tappen (2001, pp. 221–222) are listed in the accompanying box.

Consider . . .

■ the organizational structure of your practice setting. How many levels of management are there? How many of these levels are managed by nurses? Identify advantages and disadvantages to having nurses in mid-level and high-management positions in health care organizations.

■ the activities of nurse-managers at the unit level of your practice setting. What management activities do they perform? What management activities do staff nurses perform? What management activities do you perform? How do the management responsibilities of the staff nurse differ from those of the nurse-manager? What is the relationship between good unit management and effective client care?

■ the experience and educational background of nurse-managers at all levels of your organization. What are their clinical nursing experiences? What is their education? Do they have formal or informal education in management or business? Do the experience levels and educational backgrounds differ among nurse-managers at different levels of organizational or unit management? How could you best prepare yourself for the management responsibility?

NURSING DELIVERY MODELS

Common configurations for the delivery of nursing care include the case method, the functional method, team nursing, primary nursing, case management, managed care, differentiated practice, and shared governance.

Characteristics of Effective Nurse-Managers

- Assume leadership of the group
- Actively engage in planning the current and future work of the group
- Provide direction to staff members regarding the way the work is to be done

- Monitor the work done by staff members to maintain quality and productivity
- Recognize and reward quality and productivity
- Foster the development of every staff member
- Represent both administration and staff members as needed in discussions and negotiations with others

---

Source: R. M. Tappen, *Nursing Leadership and Management: Concepts and Practice,* 4th ed. Philadelphia: F. A. Davis, 2001, pp. 221–222. Reprinted with permission.

Case Method

Case method nursing, also referred to as *total care,* is one of the earliest models of nursing care. This method was used by private-duty nurses in providing total care to the client. This method is client centered: one nurse is assigned to and is responsible for the comprehensive care of a group of clients during an 8- or 12-hour shift. For each client, the nurse assesses needs, makes nursing plans, formulates diagnoses, implements care, and evaluates the effectiveness of care. In this method, a client has consistent contact with one nurse during a shift but may have different nurses on other shifts. The case method, considered the precursor of primary nursing, continues to be used in a variety of practice settings, such as intensive care nursing. With the shortage of nursing personnel during World War II, the case method could no longer be the chief mode of care for clients. To meet staff shortages, managers hired personnel with less educational preparation than the professional nurse and developed on-the-job training programs for auxiliary helpers. The case method became unfeasible in such situations, and the functional method was developed in response.

Functional Method

The **functional nursing method,** which evolved from concepts of scientific management used in the field of business administration, focuses on the jobs to be completed. In this task-oriented approach, personnel with less preparation than the professional nurse perform less complex care tasks. The functional method is based on a production and efficiency model that gives authority and responsibility to the person assigning the work, for example, the nurse-manager. Clearly defined job descriptions, procedures, policies, and lines of communication are required. The functional approach to nursing is economical and efficient and permits centralized direction and control. Its disadvantages are fragmentation of care (the client receives care from several different categories of nursing personnel) and the possibility that nonquantifiable aspects of care, such as meeting the client's emotional needs, may be overlooked.

Team Nursing

In the early 1950s, Eleanor Lambertson (1953) and her colleagues proposed a system of team nursing to overcome the fragmentation of care resulting from the task-oriented functional approach and to meet the increasing demands for professional nurses created by advances in technologic aspects of care. **Team nursing** is the delivery of individualized nursing care to clients by a nursing team led by a professional nurse. A nursing team consists of registered nurses, licensed practical nurses, and, often, nursing assistants. This team is responsible for providing coordinated nursing care to a group of clients during an 8- or 12-hour shift. Compared to the functional system, team nursing emphasizes humanistic values and responds to the needs of both clients and employees. It emphasizes individualized client care on a personal level rather than task-oriented care on an impersonal level. The professional nurse leader motivates employees to learn and develop skills and instructs them, supervises them, and provides assignments that offer the potential for growth.

Primary Nursing

Primary nursing, a system in which one nurse is responsible for total care of a number of clients 24 hours a day, 7 days a week, was introduced at the Loeb Center for Nursing and Rehabilitation in the Bronx, New York. Primary nursing is a method of providing comprehensive, individualized, and consistent care.

Primary nursing uses the nurse's technical knowledge and management skills. The primary nurse assesses and prioritizes each client's needs, identifies nursing diagnoses, develops a plan of care with the client, and evaluates the effectiveness of care. Associates provide some care, but the primary nurse coordinates it and communicates information about the client's health to other nurses and health professionals. Primary nursing encompasses all aspects of the professional role, including teaching, advocacy, decision making, and continuity of care.

According to Tappen (2001, p. 247), "the primary nurse does all initial assessments and then develops care plans for assigned patients. They provide complex treatments, coordinate the nursing care plan with other disciplines, administer medications, prepare patients for discharge, provide needed education, and evaluate the efficacy of the interventions." The primary nurse may call upon other staff members to assist in the care of the assigned patients, but then he or she coordinates the work of the other staff members. Primary nursing has been implemented in various ways in different organizations to provide quality client care with the most effective use of personnel and other resources.

Case Management

Case management, a more recent model of nursing care delivery, was pioneered at the New England Medical Center in the 1980s. Initially, public health and psychiatric–mental health nurses served as case managers. Today, case management is used in insurance-based programs, employer-based health programs, worker's compensation programs, maternal-child health settings, mental health settings, and hospital-based practice. Case management is defined as "a collaborative process that assesses, plans, implements, coordinates, monitors, and evaluates options and services needed to meet a person's health needs" (Turner, 1999, p. 136). The American Nurses Credentialing Center (2001) further defines nursing case management as a "participative process to identify and facilitate options and services for meeting individuals' health needs, while decreasing fragmentation and duplication of care and enhancing quality, cost-effective clinical outcomes." Case managers assist clients through the complex health care system with the goal of increasing the quality of life in a cost-effective way. Case management enables patients, their families, and their health care providers to be actively involved in providing for ongoing care needs.

Nurse case managers combine their clinical knowledge, communication skills, and nursing process skills to assist clients in a variety of clinical settings. The activities of case management require the nurse to integrate a variety of disciplines and services in coordinating care throughout the client's span of illness. Collaboration, coordination, information processing, and information exchange are imperative in this role. The case manager must be familiar with eligibility criteria for the different services that the client requires. Turner (1999, p. 140) states that "case management requires skills in critical thinking, communication, negotiation, and collaboration." Case managers serve as patient advocates because they provide the link between the client, the health care provider, and the payer. Case managers also function as client advocates by providing for client education, wellness, and prevention services. They also work to obtain resources, improve access, and achieve a smooth transition for clients along the care continuum. Functions of nurse case managers can be seen in the accompanying box.

The American Nurses Association (ANCC, 2001) recommends that case managers have a minimum educational preparation of a baccalaureate degree in nursing, have functioned as a registered nurse for 4000 hours, and have at least 2000 hours within the scope of practice during the last two years.

Shared Governance

Marquis and Huston (2000, p. 156) describe shared governance as organizational governance that is "shared among board members, nurses, physicians, and management." The focus of this model is to encourage nurses to participate in decision making at all levels of the organization, either at their own request or as part of their job criteria. More commonly, nurses participate through serving in decision-making groups, such as committees or task forces. The decisions they make may address employment conditions, cost-effectiveness, long-range planning, productivity, and wages and benefits. The underlying principle of shared governance is that employees will be more committed to an organization's goals if they have had input into planning and decision making. Marquis and Huston also state that "the number of health care organizations using shared governance models is increasing" (p. 156). In this model of delivery, the nurse-manager becomes a consultant, teacher, and collaborator; he or she creates the environment for shared decision making between the

---

Function of Nurse Case Managers

- Conduct case screening
- Identify target populations
- Validate clinical and demographic data
- Administer assessment tools and risk screens
- Identify barriers to availability, accessibility, and affordability of treatment
- Explore motivational and adherence issues
- Review client history and current status

- Identify opportunities for health promotion and illness prevention
- Identify educational needs and readiness to learn
- Evaluate support systems (individual, family, significant other, and community)
- Examine patterns of over- and/or underutilization of resources

Source: American Nurses Credentialing Center, *ANCC Board Certification,* 2001. www.ana.org/ancc.

nursing staff and administration. The nursing staff, in turn, must make a significant and long-term commitment to the organization.

Porter-O'Grady (1994, p. 187) sees shared governance as a tool that facilitates the maturing of the nursing professional: "It has facilitated the creation of a structure supportive of behaviors reflecting an adult, collaborative, and active decision-maker in any clinical partnership that will advance the integrative role of the nurse and the care of the patient."

Managed Care

Managed care is a method of organizing care delivery that emphasizes communication and coordination of care among health care team members. Managed care differs from case management in that it is unit based and designed to promote and support care at the client's bedside in the acute-care setting. Case management may be used as a cost-containment strategy in managed care. Managed care has gained popularity with the health care reform movement in the United States. "Managed care is viewed as a system that provides the generalized structure and focus when managing the use, cost, quality, and effectiveness of health care services" (Cohen and Cesta, 1993, p. 33).

Both case management and managed care use critical pathways to track the client's progress.

Critical Pathways are "written structured-care methodologies used to standardize care by mapping the time and activity sequence for an episode of care" (Huber, 2000, p. 524). Other structured-care methodologies are algorithms, protocols, standards of care, order sets, and clinical practice guidelines. Critical pathways are used by all health care providers to lay out the time and sequence of events for a diagnosis-specific episode of care delivery. Critical pathways often focus on high-cost, high-volume areas involving many physicians and specialties. They have become essential for the financial survival of a delivery system within a managed-care environment.

Providing the high-quality care within a highly regulated environment requires the identification and elimination of excessive, inefficient systems and a high degree of collaboration. The involvement of physicians, clinical nurse specialists, and a multidisciplinary staff are key to developing and implementing successful critical pathways.

More information about the impact of economics on health care can be found in Chapters 17, "Nursing in an Evolving Health Care Delivery System," and 18, "Health Care Economics."

Differentiated Practice

Differentiated nursing practice refers "to the sorting of the roles, functions, and work of registered nurses according to some identified criteria—usually education, experience, and competence—or some combination of these" (Huber, 2000, p. 584). Differentiated practice models recognize the broad domain of professional nursing, the multiple roles and responsibilities that nurses assume, and the contribution of all nursing personnel as valuable and unique. Differentiated practice can improve client care and contribute to client safety. Used effectively, differentiated practice models allow for the effective and efficient use of resources. Most important, if used properly, differentiated practice increases nurses' ability to provide safe, effective care based on their expertise and, in turn, increases their professional satisfaction (Koerner and Karpiuk, 1994, p. 10).

As early as 1967, a Harvard Business School research project identified the role of differentiated practice in nursing. Not only are technical tasks involved but also such factors as time frame, space, personal development, ethical action, interpersonal effectiveness, critical thinking, and commitment to lifelong learning. As the nursing paradigm changes, the areas of communication and critical thinking, rather than technical skills, expand. The American Hospital Association sees the need for differentiated practice in responding to change in the health care system, client acuity, payment systems, and reward systems (Allender, Egan, and Newman, 1995, p. 42). Differentiated practice models include nurses prepared at all educational levels: bachelor's degree, master's degree, and doctorate, recognizing the diversity of these roles.

The newer models of case management, managed care, differentiated practice, and shared governance may be the keys to meeting the demands of the future by (1) increasing demand for quality and excellence in service across the continuum of care; (2) facilitating the use of appropriate, efficient skill mix and delivery of client-centered care; (3) reducing health care costs; and (4) rewarding performance based on measured team outcomes, including the value of interdependent contributions (Wenzel, 1995, p. 62).

Consider . . .

- your own experience with the various nursing delivery models. Which models do you prefer, and why? Which models promote the value of the professional nurse? Are there models that tend to devalue the abilities of the professional nurse?
- key factors in determining the appropriateness of a

specific nursing delivery model for a specific practice setting. Are there models of nursing delivery that are more appropriate for some practice settings and less appropriate for others?
■ how you might implement a different model of nursing delivery in your current practice setting.

MENTORS AND PRECEPTORS

Mentoring has been widely used as a strategy for career development in nursing during the last 20 years. Mentors are "compentent, experienced professionals who develop a relationship with a novice for the purpose of providing advice, support, information, and feedback in order to encourage development of the individual" (Schutzenhofer, 1995, p. 487). Most nursing literature describes the nurse-mentor relationship as important for career development in nursing administration or nursing education. Through mentoring, the experienced nurse can also foster the professional growth of the new graduate, who may choose to mentor those who follow. Marriner-Tomey (2001, p. 313) describes three phases to the mentoring process:

1. *The invitational stage.* In this stage, the mentor must be willing to use time and energy to nurture an individual who is goal directed, willing to learn, and respectfully trusting of the mentor. The nurse-mentor invites the new nurse to share knowledge, skill, and personal experiences of professional growth.
2. *The questioning stage.* In this stage, the novice experiences self-doubt and fear of being unable to meet the goals. The mentor helps the protégé clarify goals and the strategies for achieving them, shares personal experiences, and serves as a sounding board and a source of support during times of doubt.
3. *The transitional stage.* In this stage, the mentor assists the protégé to become aware of the protégé's own strengths and uniqueness. The protégé now is able to mentor someone else.

Mentors provide support. Often, the mentor relationship is one of teacher-learner. The mentor instructs the protégé in the expected role, introduces the protégé to those who are important to the achievement of goals, listens to and helps the protégé evaluate ideas in light of institutional policy, and challenges the protégé to advance professional practice. Marriner-Tomey (2001, p. 313) describes a mentor as "a confidant who personalizes role modeling and serves as a sounding board for decisions."

Nurses who wish to improve and advance their professional practice, whether in education, administration, or clinical practice, should seek mentors to assist them. Mentors usually are of the same sex, 8 to 14 years older, and have a position of authority in the organization. Most are knowledgeable individuals who are willing to share their knowledge and experience. Mentors often choose protégés because of their leadership or managerial qualities. Mentoring is a process that can promote the personal and professional growth of both mentor and protégé.

A preceptor is "an experienced nurse who provides emotional support and is a strong clinical role model for the new nurse" (Marquis and Huston, 2000, p. 239). Preceptors are usually assigned to nurses who are new to the nursing unit to assist them in improving clinical nursing skill and judgment necessary for effective practice in their environment. They also assist new nurses in learning the routines, policies, and procedures of the unit. Preceptors must be patient and willing to teach new nurses, and they must be willing to answer questions and clarify the expectations of the nurse's role within the practice environment.

Although preceptors are usually assigned, mentors are more often sought out by the person being mentored. Mentors and preceptors are important for the successful development of a nurse from a beginning care provider to an expert practitioner and professional.

Consider . . .

■ your own mentoring experiences. Were you mentored or did you seek out a mentor as a new graduate or as a new employee in a new practice setting? What qualities would you seek in a mentor? If you were mentored, how did your mentor assist you in your socialization to your work setting, the organization, the nursing profession?
■ whether there are or should be differences between mentors and preceptors. If there are differences, what are they?
■ your own ability to mentor a new graduate or new employee. What knowledge, attitudes, and skills do you have that would make you an effective mentor? What knowledge, attitudes, and skills do you need to become an effective mentor? How will you develop the knowledge, attitudes, and skills needed?

NETWORKING

To function effectively in all nursing roles, but especially in leadership and management roles, the nurse needs to network with other professionals. Marriner-Tomey (1993, p. 175) describes **networking** as a process in which people communicate, share ideas and information, and offer support and direction to each other. Networking builds linkages with people throughout the profession, both within and outside the work environment. Getting to know people helps build a trust relationship that can facilitate the achievement of professional goals. It is easier to access people one knows than it is to access strangers.

Networking is a long-term, deliberate process, a powerful tool for building relationships. Networking requires time, commitment, and follow-through. Networking is an opportunity for nurses to develop their careers, share information, organize for political action, and effectively promote change (Strader and Decker, 1995, p. 481). Active membership in professional organizations may be the nurse's most important networking tool. Other networking opportunities include (1) continuing-education or university classes, (2) socializing with professional colleagues, and (3) keeping in touch with former professors and nursing associates. Strader and Decker (p. 482) offer a few important tips in networking: Be discreet, deliver on your promises, and don't burn bridges.

CHANGING TIMES

In the changing health care system, where cost-effectiveness is of equal importance to quality of care, health care agencies have instituted two measures: downsizing and restructuring patient-care delivery.

Downsizing

Downsizing is a polite term for layoffs: employer cuts in human resources in order to reduce expenses. Downsizing is not exclusive to health care: Virtually all industries, from manufacturing to service industries, have experienced some degree of downsizing in recent years. Russ (1994, pp. 66–67) offers the following strategies to help nurses prepare for potential downsizing:

1. *Network.* Reestablish your network by calling a colleague for career or personal advice. Participate in meetings of professional nursing organizations.
2. *Update your résumé.* Even if you have a secure job, an updated résumé reflecting your accomplishments and future goals is important. Occasionally "testing the waters" to brush up on your interview skills and seeing what positions are available in the market may also be advisable.
3. *Develop a portfolio.* Keep documentation of your previous work accomplishments. Reports, memos, completed projects, and published articles that reflect your achievements and potential should be neatly compiled for future employers.
4. *Compile a reference list.* Keep a list of people with whom you have worked and who will attest to your merits. Be sure to get permission to use a contact and always send written thanks.
5. *Remain active during the layoff period.* "Sleeping in" will not get you a new position. Rather, continue to attend professional meetings and social gatherings and to investigate employment agencies, want ads, and human resource departments.
6. *Fight depression, denial, and anger.* These are common responses to downsizing. Don't burn bridges and "bad mouth" your old employer. Remember to remain positive and keep your cup half full, not half empty!

Reengineering

Downsizing, reorganization, computerization, and decentralization of services may reshape business structure, but they do not necessarily reengineer how those services are delivered. Health care administrators view reengineering as a way to enter the 21st century with a flexible, lean, efficient corporation. The single largest reengineering program in the health care industry is called *patient-focused care.*

Health care consultants and analysts view the current model of service delivery as inefficient, fragmented, and expensive. Patient-focused care entails components that require reengineering of health care (Richardson, 1995, pp. 31–34).

1. *Hospital architecture.* Self-sufficient service units replace departments. The clients in these units have commonality of care, often reflecting DRG groupings.
2. *Teams.* Specialized self-governed teams responsible for delivery of services are organized. These self-directed work teams may be constructed or titled differently, but all focus on developing an intact work group responsible for the entire work process.
3. *Information technology.* To reduce the amount of time nurses spend writing, scheduling, and communicating, up-to-date technology is essential. Automated medication dispensers, bedside computers, voice messaging, pneumatic tubes, and fax machines are common in the reengineered environment.
4. *Multiskilling and cross-training.* In the most common form of multiskilling and cross-training, a staff member who is skilled in one discipline obtains the knowledge and skill of another discipline. The staff member goes through the process of obtaining licensure, if required. For example, many respiratory therapists are currently seeking licensure as registered nurses. A more cost-effective development is the creation of the

generic health care worker. Depending on the needs of the agency, the multiskilled worker would receive prescribed training. Currently, many colleges and universities have introduced programs for certification in multiskilled health care practitioners.

Much controversy surrounds patient-focused care. Clearly, there is a financial benefit: Estimates of a 40% decrease in personnel costs are commonly quoted. Health care consultants and administrators also maintain that patient-focused care increases satisfaction among clients, staff, and physicians alike. Some consultants, however, state that patient-focused care reduces the number of staff having contact with a patient during a stay by 75% (Clouten and Weber, 1994, p. 35).

Consider . . .

■ the role of the professional nurse in a changing health care system. What new knowledge, attitudes, and skills are essential for the nurse to prepare for the changes in health care? How can the nurse best prepare for changes in health and nursing care delivery?

■ the concept of the multiskilled worker and the historical work activities of nursing. Are there activities that other health care professionals or paraprofessionals currently do that previously were done by nurses? How might this merging of roles affect nursing? How might it affect the other health care professionals and paraprofessionals?

SUMMARY

Leadership and management are the responsibility of all professional nurses. Knowledge of the different, yet intertwined, roles of leader and manager are vital to nurses' ability to work within the health care system.

The ability of the professional nurse to advocate for clients is linked to leadership and management skills. As an individual, family, or community advocate, professional nurses may offer a wide variety of support and services.

Leadership styles include charismatic, authoritarian, democratic, laissez-faire, situational, transactional, and transformational. Effective leadership is a learned process involving understanding of the needs and goals that motivate others and interpersonal skills to influence others.

Management involves the basic functions of planning, organizing, leading, and delegating. The degree to which a nurse carries out these functions depends on the position the nurse holds in the organization. Regardless of degree, authority and accountability remain important to the process.

Nursing delivery models include the case method, the functional method, team nursing, primary nursing, case management, managed care, differentiated practice, and shared governance. Emphasis on efficiency, outcomes, cost-effectiveness, and client satisfaction have become buzzwords within the newer delivery models.

Mentors and preceptorships can have a positive impact. Mentoring and preceptorships can assist in the personal and professional growth of both the novice and professional nurse.

Personal integrity, honesty, and a concern for human dignity should guide all the nurse's leadership and management decisions.

Bookshelf

Covey, S. R. 1989. *The 7 habits of highly effective people: Powerful lessons in personal change.* **New York: Simon and Schuster.**

This national best-seller presents a paradigm of seven habits, starting with three self-mastery habits that move a person from dependence to independence (private victories), and followed by other habits that move a person toward effective interdependence (public victories). The seven habits become the basis of a person's character, "creating an empowering center of correct maps from which an individual can effectively solve problems, maximize opportunities, and continually learn and integrate other principles in an upward spiral of growth." (p. 52). Covey inspires readers to integrate personal, family, and professional responsibilities into their lives. He emphasizes the need to restore the "character" ethic in our society. The character ethic is based on the idea that there are *principles* that govern human effectiveness.

Ulrich, B. T. 1992. *Leadership and management according to Florence Nightingale.* **Norwalk, Conn.: Appleton-Lange.**

This pocket-sized book analyzes the writings of Florence Nightingale and points out the relevancy of her thoughts for nurses today. For example, it is still true today that "whoever is in charge keep this simple question in her head (not, how can I always do this right thing myself, but) how can I provide for this right thing to always be done?" (p. 38). It is a historical approach to the contemporary issue of delegation.

REFERENCES

Allender, C. D., Egan, E. C., and Newman, M. A. 1995. An instrument for measuring differentiated nursing practice. *Nursing Management* **26**(4): 42–45.

American Nurses Association. 1991a. *Nursing's agenda for health care reform*. Washington, D.C.: ANA.

American Nurses Association. 1991b. *Standards of clinical nursing practice*. Washington, D.C.: ANA.

American Nurses Credentialing Center. 2001. *ANCC Board Certification*. www.ana.org/ancc.

Bower, K. A. 1992. *Case management by nurses*. Washington, D.C.: American Nurses Association.

Brandt, M. A. 1994. Caring leadership: Secret and path to success. *Nursing Management* **25**(8): 68–72.

Christensen, P., and Bender, L. 1994. Models of nursing care in a changing environment: Current challenges and future directions. *Orthopaedic Nursing* **13**(2): 64–70.

Clouten, K., and Weber, R. 1994. Patient-focused care: Playing to win. *Nursing Management* **25**(2): 34–36.

Cohen, E. L., and Cesta, T. G. 1993. *Nursing case management: From concepts to evaluation*. St. Louis: Mosby-Year Book.

Duffield, C. 1994. Nursing unit managers: Defining a role. *Nursing Management* **25**(4), 63–67.

Glennon, T. K. 1992, Spring. Empowering nurses through enlightened leadership. *Revolution: The Journal of Nurse Empowerment* **2**: 40–44.

Hansten, R. I., and Washburn, M. J. 1994. *Clinical delegation skills: A handbook for nurses*. Gaithersburg, Md.: Aspen Publishers, Inc.

Hellriegel, D., Jackson, S. E., and Slocum, J. W. 1999. *Management*, 8th ed. Cincinnati, Ohio: South-Western.

Hellriegel, D., and Slocum, J. W. 1993. *Management*, 6th ed. Reading, Mass.: Addison-Wesley.

Huber, D. 2000. *Leadership and nursing care management*, 2d ed. Philadelphia: W. B. Saunders.

Koerner, J. G., and Karpiuk, K. L. 1994. *Implementing differentiated nursing practice*. Gaithersburg, Md.: Aspen.

Lambertsen, E. C. 1953. *Nursing Team—Organization and Functioning*. Published for the Division of Nursing Education by the Bureau of Publications, Teachers College, Columbia University.

Lyon, J. C. 1993. Models of nursing care delivery and case management: Clarification of terms. *Nursing Economics* **11**(3): 163–169.

Marquis, B. L., and Huston, C. J. 2000. *Leadership roles and management functions in nursing: Theory and application*, 3d ed. Philadelphia: Lippincott.

Marriner-Tomey, A. 1993. *Transformational leadership in nursing*. St. Louis: Mosby-Year Book.

Marriner-Tomey, A. 2000. *Guide to nursing management*, 6th ed. St. Louis: Mosby-Year Book.

Menke, K., and Ogborn, S. E. 1993. Politics and the nurse manager. *Nursing Management* **23**(12): 35–37.

Porter-O'Grady, T. 1994. Whole systems shared governance: Creating the seamless organization. *Nursing Economics* **12**(4): 187–195.

Richardson. T. 1995, Summer. Patient focused care. *Revolution: The Journal of Nursing Empowerment*, 31–34, 37–38.

Russ, A. 1994. Downsizing: A survival kit for employees. *Nursing Management* **25**(8): 66–67.

Schutzenhofer, K. K. 1995. Power, politics and influence. In P. S. Yoder-Wise, *Leading and managing in nursing*. St. Louis: Mosby-Year Book.

Simms, L. M., Price, S. A., and Ervin, N. E. 2000. *Professional practice of nursing administration*, 3d ed. Albany, N.Y.: Delmar.

Stordeur, S., Vandenberghe, C., and D'hoore, W. 2000. Leadership styles across hierarchical levels in nursing departments. *Nursing Research* **49**(1): 37–43.

Strader, M. K., and Decker, P. J. 1995. *Role transition to patient care management*. East Norwalk, Conn.: Appleton and Lange.

Tappen, R. M. 1995. *Nursing leadership and management: Concepts and practice*, 3rd ed. Philadelphia: F. A. Davis.

Tappen, R. M. 2001. *Nursing leadership and management: Concepts and practice*, 4th ed. Philadelphia: F. A. Davis.

Trofino, J. 1995. Transformational leadership in health care. *Nursing Management* **26**(8): 42–47.

Turner, S. O. 1999. *The nurse's guide to managed care*. Gaithersburg, Md.: Aspen.

Wenzel, K. 1995. Redesigning patient care delivery. *Nursing Management* **26**(8): 60–62.

Yoder-Wise, P. S. 1995. *Leading and managing in nursing*. St. Louis: Mosby-Year Book.

The Nurse as Research Consumer

Objectives

- Discuss the trend toward evidence-based practice in nursing.
- Describe the nurse's role in research.
- Analyze ethical concerns in nursing research.
- Differentiate approaches in nursing research.
- Identify the criteria for using research in nursing practice.
- Identify available resources for evidence-based practice in nursing.

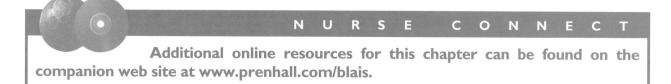

N U R S E   C O N N E C T

Additional online resources for this chapter can be found on the companion web site at www.prenhall.com/blais.

Nursing practice based on scientific evidence poses unique challenges for today's nursing care provider. It is a rather recent phenomenon. During the 1970s, research utilization became a buzzword and a focus for translating research findings into practice. This was slow to happen in part because there was a limited nursing research data base from which to practice and also in part because nurses were not comfortable enough with research to apply it to practice. Nurse researchers and nurses in practice were not a tightly meshed group, and there was limited communication between them.

The term evidence-based practice has been applied to nursing in recent years. It brings together theory, clinical decision making and judgment, and knowledge of the research process; it incorporates them into the evaluation of research and scientific evidence. Resulting from this process is the application of clinically meaningful evidence to nursing practice and applying the best available research evidence to a specific clinical question. The evidence-based practice movement began in medicine during the 1970s but has developed within nursing since that time. In 1998 the journal *Evidence-Based Nursing* was established to advance evidence-based nursing practice, thus facilitating the highest quality of care and the best client outcomes.

CHALLENGES AND OPPORTUNITIES

Closing the gap between research and practice is a continuing challenge because nursing has more often based practice upon tradition, authority, or past experience. Looking to research to provide answers represents a change in thinking for many. Implementing practice changes based upon research is also a challenge.

Opportunities for providing high-quality care with accountability to clients and families are presented when practice decisions are based upon scientific evidence and data. Confidence in that decision making can be founded upon information that has been tested and has demonstrated effectiveness in providing the best strategies to care for those needing nursing.

EVIDENCE-BASED PRACTICE

Nursing research represents a systematic search for the knowledge needed to provide high-quality care. It is one of the requirements for professionalism and supplies a foundation for accountability. A sound knowledge base is necessary for decision making in practice.

The knowledge base for practice in nursing has relied on information from a number of sources, representing varying degrees of rigor. Tradition as a source of knowledge has provided a substantial amount of the foundations for practice. Nursing has developed ways of doing things that have continued in practice simply because "that is the way it has always been done." One such example of this is the routine monitoring of vital signs at specified times during a shift, regardless of the client's condition. Another source of nursing knowledge is authority. Things are done a certain way because a physician or other person with a perceived higher level of knowledge has prescribed a particular way of providing care. Experience and trial and error have also provided an impetus for decision making and procedure development. As nurses become more grounded in a scientific rationale for practice, logical reasoning and the application of research findings become the focus when care is planned.

Consider . . .

- how nurses apply research in daily practice.
- what happens when problems related to care are identified by nurses.
- how solutions to problems are developed. What sources of information are used?

Empirical Nursing Knowledge

In Chapter 6, "Theoretical Foundations of Professional Nursing," the ways of knowing were discussed as they apply to nursing. Empirical knowledge comes from scientific evidence and is developed through research. It is a characteristic of the scientific approach that includes order and control and allows generalization of results. The purposes of scientific research are description, exploration, explanation, and prediction and control. The findings are then applied to practice.

One way for a nurse to access empirical knowledge is to learn about research methods and be able to assess strengths and weaknesses of studies when he or she reads them in professional journals. Another mechanism is to use systematic reviews that are conducted by expert groups for the purpose of critiquing studies and providing recommendations to guide practice. The Agency for Healthcare Research and Quality (formerly the Agency for Health Care Policy and Research) is a federal agency that has developed clinical practice guidelines. As nurses move toward evidence-based care, they must be involved in decision making and protocol development that strive to incorporate the best information available. Strategies for implementing evidence-based practice are presented in Table 10–1.

RESEARCH IN NURSING

Research is directed toward building a body of nursing knowledge about "human responses to actual or potential health problems" (ANA, 1980, p. 9) and to the effects of nursing action on human responses. The human responses may be (1) reactions of individuals, groups, or families to actual health problems, such as the caregiving burden on the family of an older individual with Alzheimer's disease; and (2) concerns of individuals and groups about potential health problems, such as accident prevention or stress management in a factory or assembly plant.

- Nursing research also reflects the traditional nursing perspective. In this view, the client is seen as a whole

Table 10–1 Strategies for Implementing Evidence-Based Practice

1. Assess the extent to which your practice is evidenced-based.

2. Review literature that provides evidence to strengthen your belief that EBP results in better patient outcomes.

3. Ask questions about your current practice strategies (e.g., Is use of distraction really effective in reducing children's distress during intrusive procedures? Does nonnutritive sucking alleviate pain in infants?).

4. Determine whether other colleagues at your practice site have an interest in the same clinical question so that you can form a collaboration to search for and review the evidence.

5. Conduct a search for studies or systematic reviews in the specific area of your clinical question (Remember that randomized clinical trials are typically the "gold standard" for producing the best evidence).

6. Critique the studies from your search to determine whether you have the "best evidence" to guide your practice.

7. Develop a practice guideline using the "best evidence."

8. Establish measurable outcomes that you can use to determine the effectiveness of your guideline.

9. Implement the practice guideline.

10. Measure the established outcomes.

11. Evaluate the effectiveness of the practice guideline and determine whether you should continue the practice guideline as established or whether there is a need for revision.

12. Develop a mechanism for routinely disseminating and discussing evidence-based literature upon which decisions can be made to improve practice at your clinical site (e.g., EBP rounds).

Used by permission from B. M. Melnyk, P. Stone, E. Fineout-Overhold, and M. Ackerman. Evidence-Based Practice: The Past, the Present, and Recommendations for the Millennium. *Pediatric Nursing* **26**(1): 77–80, 2000.

person with physiologic, psychologic, spiritual, social, cultural, and economic aspects:

For example, when a person has a head injury, the nurse needs to understand the body's processes for dealing with the increased pressure within the head and the changes this brings about in the patient's condition. At the same time, the nurse focuses on care that can maintain the person's cognitive, that is, thinking and feeling, processes. A nurse would also examine the person's life patterns that could lead to other head injuries. (Roy, 1985, pp. 2–3)

In addition to reflecting the concern for the whole person, a nursing perspective implies 24-hour responsibility. Thus, this viewpoint encompasses all of the factors in a client's environment, such as fatigue, noise, sensory deprivation, nutrition, and positioning, that may influence coping patterns. Diers (1979, pp. 13–15) identifies three distinguishing properties of nursing research:

1. The final focus of nursing research must be on a difference that matters for improving client care.

2. Nursing research has the potential for contributing to developing theory and the body of scientific knowledge.

3. A research problem becomes a nursing problem when nurses have access to and control over the phenomena being studied.

The information revolution that is transforming the present and shaping the future has made reading, understanding, and using nursing research as fundamental to professional practice as the knowledge of asepsis, application of the nursing process, and communication skills. Polit and Hungler (1999, pp. 3–4) cite four reasons why research is important in nursing:

1. As a profession, nursing needs research to evolve and expand a scientific body of knowledge that is unique and separate from other disciplines.

2. Research is important to maintain nursing's scientific accountability to clients, families, and the public in general.

3. The current concerns regarding the economics and efficacy of health care require nursing to document

through research how its services contribute to health care delivery.

4. When multiple interventions are possible in a given client-care situation, nursing research is essential to the clinical decision-making process.

Roles in Research

According to the American Nurses Association *Position Statement on Education for Participation in Nursing Research* (1994), all nurses share a commitment to the advancement of nursing science. The responsibility for assuming various activities and roles is related to level of education. Research-based practice is seen as essential for effective and efficient patient care. The development and utilization of research depends upon the interaction between researchers and clinicians. Nurses in clinical practice identify the problems in need of investigation and collaborate with nurse-researchers, who design studies to address the problems identified and analyze the data. It is again up to the clinicians to determine the appropriate application of those findings to practice.

Nurses are sometimes employed on care units or in services where research is conducted by a variety of disciplines. It is the nurse's responsibility to support the research protocol and uphold the scientific rigor of the study by carefully maintaining the research protocol. At the same time, it is the right of the nurse to be informed of the purpose of the study and to understand the protocol. Likewise, the nurse has a right to know that human subjects are being protected, that the study has been reviewed by an Institutional Review Board (IRB), and that the researchers are qualified to do the research.

Preparation for these research roles begins at the undergraduate level as the student learns about research and develops practice that is based on the critical analysis of research findings. The preparation of nurse scientists who have primary responsibility for the conduct of research occurs in graduate education. It begins at the master's level and is concentrated at the doctoral and postdoctoral level. Table 10–2 lists the roles identified as appropriate for the varying levels of education.

With regard to the role of the nurse prepared at the baccalaureate level, the ANA makes this statement:

> . . . education for research prepares nurses to read research critically and to use existing standards to determine the readiness of research for utilization in clinical practice.

Promoting understanding of the ethical principles of research, especially the protection of human subjects and other ethical responsibilities of investigators, is an essential objective of research preparation for baccalaureate students (ANA, 1994).

During the curriculum of the BSN program, students will have a course in research that provides the tools needed for implementing the role in practice. It is not the purpose of this chapter to present research in that depth, but a brief overview will be given to provide a context for the discussion of evidence-based practice. See the box on page 173.

Historical Perspective

As early as 1854, Florence Nightingale demonstrated the importance of research in the delivery of nursing care. When Nightingale arrived in the Crimea in November of 1854, she found the military hospital barracks overcrowded, filthy, rat- and flea-infested, and lacking in food, drugs, and essential medical supplies. As a result of these conditions, men died from starvation and such diseases as dysentery, cholera, and typhus (Woodham-Smith, 1950, pp. 151–167). By systematically collecting, organizing, and reporting data, Nightingale was able to institute sanitary reforms and significantly reduce mortality rates from contagious disease.

Although the Nightingale tradition influenced the establishment of American nursing schools in 1873, the research approach did not take hold until the beginning of the 20th century. Recognizing the need, nursing leader Isabel Stewart integrated research into the graduate nursing curriculum at Teachers College, Columbia University, and published the first research journal in nursing, the *Nursing Education Bulletin,* in the late 1920s. The journal *Nursing Research* was established in 1952 to serve as a vehicle to communicate nurses' research and scholarly productivity. The publication of many other nursing research journals followed, some dedicated to research and others combining clinical and research publications.

The National Institute of Nursing Research (NINR) was established as a Center at the NIH in 1986. In 1993, it was elevated to an Institute, placing it among 25 Institutes and Centers within NIH and adding a clinical and nursing perspective to the mainstream of the biomedical and behavioral research in the United States. According to its mission statement:

> The Institute supports clinical and basic research to establish a scientific basis for the

Table 10–2 Research Roles at Various Levels of Nursing Education According to the ANA Position Statement on Education for Participation in Nursing Research

Associate Degree in Nursing
- Help to identify clinical problems in nursing practice
- Assist in the collection of data within a structured format
- In conjunction with nurses holding more advanced credentials, appropriately use research findings in clinical practice

Baccalaureate Degree in Nursing
- Identify clinical problems requiring investigation
- Assist experienced investigators gain access to clinical sites
- Influence the selection of appropriate methods of data collection
- Collect data and implement nursing research findings

Master's Degree in Nursing
- Be active members of research teams
- Assume the role of clinical expert collaborating with experienced investigators in proposal development, data collection, data analysis and interpretation
- Appraise the clinical relevance of research findings
- Help create a climate that supports scholarly inquiry, scientific integrity, and scientific investigation of clinical nursing problems
- Provide leadership for integrating findings in clinical practice

Doctoral Education
- Conduct research aimed at theory generation or theory testing
- Design studies independently as well as collaborate with other clinicians and researchers
- Acquire funding for research
- Disseminate their research findings

Postdoctoral Education
- Develop a systematic program of research
- Become a sustaining member of the scientific community

Based on the ANA Position Statement: *Education for Participation in Nursing Research,* originated by the Council of Nurse Researchers and Council of Nursing Practice and adopted by the ANA Board of Directors, April, 1994.

American Nurses Association's Standard of Professional Performance Pertaining to Research

Standard VII. Research
THE NURSE USES RESEARCH FINDINGS IN PRACTICE.
Measurement Criteria

1. The nurse utilizes best available evidence, preferably research data, to develop the plan of care and interventions.

2. The nurse participates in research activities as appropriate to the nurse's education and position. Such activities may include

- Identifying clinical problems suitable for nursing research
- Participating in data collection
- Participating in a unit, organization, or community research committee or program
- Sharing research activities with others
- Conducting research
- Critiquing research for application to practice
- Using research findings in the development of policies, procedures, and practice guidelines for patient care

Source: Standards of Clinical Nursing Practice by the American Nurses Association, Washington, D.C., 1998.

care of individuals across the life span—from management of patients during illness and recovery to the reduction of risks for disease and disability and the promotion of healthy lifestyles. According to its mandate, the Institute seeks to understand and ease the symptoms of acute and chronic illness, to prevent or delay the onset of disease or disability or slow its progression, to find effective approaches to achieving and sustaining good health, and to improve the clinical settings in which care is provided. The NINR's research extends to problems encountered by patients, families, and caregivers. It also emphasizes the special needs of at-risk and underserved populations with an emphasis on health disparities. These efforts are crucial in translating scientific advances into cost-effective health care that does not compromise quality (NINR, 1997).

NINR has established the following goals for the 5-year period 2000–2004 (NINR Strategic Plan, 2000):

1. Identify and support research opportunities that will achieve scientific distinction and produce significant contributions to health.
2. Identify and support future areas of opportunity to advance research on high-quality, cost-effective care and to contribute to the scientific base for nursing practice.
3. Communicate and disseminate research findings resulting from NINR-funded research.
4. Enhance the development of nurse-researchers through training and career development opportunities.

The overall focus is to provide leadership in emphasizing the inclusion of cultural and ethnic considerations throughout the research, encompassing culturally sensitive interventions to decrease disparities among groups in health and health care. In doing this, nurse-researchers will focus on health promotion and chronic illness–management strategies and an interdisciplinary and collaborative effort.

Sigma Theta Tau International is the honor society for nursing, and its mission is to provide leadership and scholarship in practice, education, and research to enhance the health of all people. *Strategic Plan 2005* contains a goal for research support to "advance the scientific base of nursing practice through the scholarship of research." According to the strategic plan:

The scientific base of nursing practice is strengthened through the promotion of research studies and the dissemination of findings—particularly the findings that are readily integrated into practice. The diverse society membership has expressed a critical need for research support and innovations for clinical applications. The society is uniquely qualified to fill this need. Technological innovation, expansion of the Virginia Henderson International Nursing Library, development of systems to support evidence-based practice, and the provision of research funding are continued priorities of the society (STTI, 2000).

Ethical Concerns

Because nursing research usually focuses on humans, a major nursing responsibility is to be aware of and to advocate on behalf of clients' rights. All clients must be informed about the consequences of consenting to serve as research subjects. In other words, there must be informed consent to participate. The client needs to be able to assess whether an appropriate balance exists between the risks of participating in a study and the potential benefits, either to the client or to the development of knowledge.

Research ethics not only protect the rights of human subjects but also encompass a broader range of principles. Most of these principles are reflected in the ANA's *Human Rights Guidelines for Nurses in Clinical and Other Research* (1975). These guidelines are based on historic documents, such as the Nuremberg Code (1949) and the Declaration of Helsinki (adopted in 1964 by the World Medical Assembly and revised in 1975), and on United States federal regulations, all of which set standards governing the conduct of research involving human subjects. The notorious Tuskegee study in Alabama, begun in 1932 and ended in 1972, illustrates how subjects' human rights were violated for a period of 40 years while a research study was being conducted.

All nurses who practice in settings where research is being conducted with human subjects or who participate in such research as data collectors or collaborators play an important role in safeguarding the following rights.

Right Not to Be Harmed

The Department of Health and Human Services defines **risk of harm** to a research subject as exposure to the possibility of injury going beyond everyday situations. The risk can be physical, emotional, legal, financial, or social. For instance, withholding standard care from a client in labor for the purpose of studying the course of natural childbirth clearly poses a potential physical danger. Risks can be less overt and involve psychologic factors, such as exposure to stress or anxiety, or social factors, such as loss of confidentiality or loss of privacy.

Right to Full Disclosure

Even though it may be possible to collect data about a client as part of everyday care without the client's particular knowledge or consent, to do so is considered unethical. **Full disclosure** is a basic right. It means that deception, either by withholding information about a client's participation in a study or by giving the client false or misleading information about what participating in the study will involve, violates ethical principles.

Right of Self-Determination

Many clients in dependent positions, such as people in nursing homes, feel pressured to participate in studies. They feel that they must please the doctors and nurses who are responsible for their treatment and care. The **right of self-determination** means that subjects should feel free from constraints, coercion, or any undue influence to participate in a study. Masked inducements, for instance, suggesting to potential participants that by taking part in the study they might become famous, make an important contribution to science, or receive special attention, must be strictly avoided. Nurses must be assertive in advocating for this essential right.

Right of Privacy and Confidentiality

Privacy enables a client to participate without worrying about later embarrassment. The anonymity of a study participant is ensured when even the investigator cannot link a specific subject to the information reported. **Confidentiality** means that any information a subject relates will not be made public or available to others without the subject's consent. Investigators must inform research subjects about the measures that provide for these rights. Such measures may include the use of pseudonyms or code numbers or reporting only aggregate or group data in published research.

Approaches in Nursing Research

There are two major approaches to investigating phenomena in nursing research. These approaches originate from different philosophical perspectives and use different methods for collection and analysis of data.

Quantitative research uses precise measurement for data collection and analyzes numerical data. The design is rigorously controlled, and statistical analysis is used to summarize and describe findings or to test relationships among variables. The quantitative approach is most frequently associated with a philosophical doctrine called *logical positivism*, which asserts that scientific knowledge is the only kind of factual knowledge. It is viewed by some as "hard" science and tends to use deductive reasoning and emphasize *measurable* aspects of the human experience. The following are examples of research questions that lend themselves to a quantitative approach:

- What are the differential effects of continuous versus intermittent application of negative pressure on tracheal tissue during endotracheal suctioning?
- Is the therapeutic touch effective in reducing pain perception postoperatively?
- Are there differences in skin breakdown in premature infants bathed with plain water and with bacteriostatic soap?

Qualitative research investigates phenomena through narrative data that describe the phenomena in an in-depth and holistic fashion. The research design is typically more flexible and less controlled than quantitative designs. The data may be the transcription of an unstructured interview, and the analysis looks for patterns and themes that come from the data by using an inductive approach. This allows exploration of the subjective experiences of human beings and can provide nursing with a better understanding of phenomena from the client's perspective. The qualitative approach is appropriate for the following types of questions:

- What is the nature of the bereavement process in spouses of clients with terminal cancer?
- What is the nature of coping and adjustment after a radical prostatectomy?
- What is the process of family caregiving for older family relatives with Alzheimer's dementia as experienced by the caregiver?

There are several important steps in the conduct of research, and each of these requires decision making by the researcher. The first step is identification of the problem. Ideally, this is the step at which the nurse in clinical practice makes known the information needs. Once the problem is clearly identified and a statement is formulated, the next step is a search of existing literature, especially related research. Before the researcher designs a study to answer the question, the state of the art of current knowledge should be known.

A literature review will identify other studies related to the topic, and this can serve several purposes. It can provide an answer or partial answer to the question and may even eliminate the need to conduct further research, or it may change the problem focus. Gaps in the literature will support the need for the research. In performing a literature review, the focus should be on **primary** rather than **secondary** sources. A primary source is a publication authored by the person who conducted the research. A secondary source is a description of a study or studies prepared by someone other than the person who conducted the research. Review articles describing a number of studies on a particular topic are considered secondary sources. The secondary sources are helpful in identifying studies that are related to the topic of interest, but a researcher needs to rely on the primary source when designing a study.

One of the challenges in conducting a literature review is identifying the sources to be included. Electronic databases and computer searches have become the mainstay of literature searches. The *Cumulative Index of Nursing and Allied Health* (CINAHL) is one of the most common databases accessed by nurses. Medline also references nursing journals. Hard copies or CD ROM indexes are also available in most libraries and include such sources as *The Cumulative Index to Nursing and Allied Health, International Nursing Index,* and *Cumulative Index Medicus.* These sources give bibliographical references. Other databases provide abstracts for review; some of these are *Annual Review of Nursing Research, Dissertation Abstracts International,* and *Nursing Research Abstract.*

Once the researcher has identified the problem, reviewed the literature, and identified specific research questions or hypotheses, an appropriate study can be designed to answer the questions or test the hypotheses. Decisions need to be made regarding who should be included in the study. The researcher needs to select a sample that is representative of the population of interest so that findings from the study are applicable or generalizable to that group. Data-collection methods will determine the quality of the data being analyzed in the study. The researcher will have to decide on a reasonable way to either observe or measure the concepts in the study; this is referred to as **operational definition** of the variable. Data collection can be done according to three categories: **biophysiologic measures, observation,** and **self-report by the study participants or subjects.** Decisions need to be made

about the amount of control over outside influences (extraneous variables) and timing of data collection. The tools selected for data collection need to be evaluated for reliability and validity, i.e., how well they measure what they claim to measure and how consistently they do so. A procedure or protocol must be developed, clearly spelled out, and consistently adhered to during the study. An appropriate method of data analysis must be selected, whether the study is quantitative (descriptive or inferential statistics) or qualitative (content analysis). Once the data are analyzed and results are known, the researcher must be very careful about the interpretation of those results and be certain that any conclusions are supported by the study data. It is at this point that the practicing nurse is again a valuable team member. The utilization of research in practice and the development of evidence-based practice need a close partnership between the nurse scientist and the nurse in clinical practice.

USING RESEARCH IN PRACTICE

Critiquing Research Reports

If professional nurses are to use research, they must first learn to conduct a critical appraisal of research reports published in the literature. A research critique enables the nurse as a research consumer to evaluate the scientific merit of the study and decide how the results may be useful in practice. Critiquing involves intensive scrutiny of a study, including its strengths and weaknesses, statistical and clinical significance, as well as the generalizability of the results.

Polit and Hungler (1999, pp. 625–639) proposed that the following elements be considered in conducting a research critique: substantive and theoretical dimensions, methodologic dimensions, ethical dimensions, interpretive dimensions, and presentation and stylistic dimensions.

■   *Substantive and theoretical dimensions.* For these dimensions, the nurse needs to evaluate the significance of the research problem, the appropriateness of the conceptualizations and the theoretical framework of the study, and the congruence between the research question and the methods used to address it.
■   *Methodologic dimensions.* The methodologic dimensions pertain to the appropriateness of the research design, the size and representativeness of the study sample as well as the sampling design, validity and reliability of the instruments, adequacy of the research procedures, and the appropriateness of data analytic techniques used in the study.

- *Ethical dimensions.* The nurse must determine whether the rights of human subjects were protected during the course of the study and whether any ethical problems compromised the scientific merit of the study or the well-being of the subjects.
- *Interpretive dimensions.* For these dimensions, the nurse needs to ascertain the accuracy of the discussion, conclusions, and implications of the study results. The findings must be related back to the original hypotheses and the conceptual framework of the study. The implications and limitations of the study should be reviewed, together with the potential for replication or generalizability of the findings to similar populations.
- *Presentation and stylistic dimensions.* The manner in which the research plan and results are communicated refers to the presentation and stylistic dimensions. The research report must be detailed, logically organized, concise, and well written.

Consider . . .

- resources (libraries, colleges and universities, schools of nursing and so on) that are available in your practice setting and in your community to assist you in researching nursing practice problems.

Research Utilization

Research utilization is the process in which study findings are used to initiate and support innovations in the delivery of nursing care. In the 1970s, the lag between publication of research and the transfer of findings into actual practice was recognized. This gap was demonstrated in Ketefian's study (1975, p. 91), in which she found that despite widely published research about the optimal placement time for oral glass thermometers (9 min), only 1 of 87 nurses surveyed was aware of the correct placement time.

The Western Interstate Commission for Higher Education (WICHEN) and the Conduct and Utilization of Research in Nursing (CURN) projects were developed to promote the dissemination and utilization of nursing research (Horsley, Crane, and Bingle, 1978; Krueger, Nelson, and Wolanin, 1978). As a result, research-utilization training programs and research-based innovations were implemented.

Studies by Brett in 1987 and by Coyle and Sokop in 1990 revealed that the process of adoption of research-based innovations was consistent with the stages of Rogers' (1983) theory of diffusion innovation. According to this theory, a nurse passes through four stages before adopting research-based ideas or practices:

1. *Knowledge stage*—when a nurse learns about an innovation.

2. *Persuasion stage*—when a nurse develops a positive or negative attitude about the innovation.
3. *Decision stage*—when a nurse determines whether to adopt or reject the innovation.
4. *Implementation stage*—when the nurse uses the innovation regularly.

Inhibitors and Facilitators of Research Utilization

Factors that inhibit and facilitate the process of using research in clinical settings have been identified. The availability of research findings and nurses' attitudes toward research are related to research utilization. The factors inhibiting the use of research in practice are the nurses' perceived lack of authority to change client care procedures; insufficient time to implement new ideas; lack of support and cooperation from physicians, administrators, and other staff; inadequate facilities for implementation; and lack of time to read research. Facilitators of research utilization are enhanced administrative support and encouragement, improved accessibility of research reports, advanced nurses' research knowledge base, and colleague support networks (Champion and Leach, 1989; Funk et al., 1991).

The factors facilitating research utilization are those that provide nurses with information about research developments. These factors include monthly research newsletters, research meetings, continuing education programs, computer networks, and research study guides. Factors inhibiting research utilization are lack of time, lack of interest among the nursing staff, lack of support from other health care disciplines, and prior negative experience in research activities (Pettengill, Gillies, and Clark, 1994).

To be able to integrate research as part of day-to-day practice, nurses must work to overcome the inhibitors and perpetuate the facilitators of research utilization. Key strategies for success follow:

- Nurses must develop a positive attitude toward research utilization, viewing it as a tool to attain clinical excellence.
- Nursing administrators need to provide time, facilities, equipment, and support personnel needed for research utilization activities.
- Administrators of hospitals and clinical agencies must create an environment that is conducive to research-based innovation.

Criteria for Research Utilization

If a nurse reads in a research journal that teaching guided imagery to clients was found to be effective in enabling clients to deal with postoperative pain, can the nurse utilize the intervention in his or her own clients? How would a nurse know that the research he or she reads is ready for use in practice?

Haller, Reynolds, and Horsley (1979) formulated criteria for utilization of research in nursing practice, based on the CURN project. These criteria are replication, scientific merit, risk, clinical merit, clinical control, feasibility, cost, and potential for clinical evaluation.

REPLICATION The criterion of replication requires that the results of a study be replicated a number of times before its findings are accepted as credible and applicable to practice. A change in current practice or procedure cannot be based solely on one study. Establishing a research base of three or more studies confirms that the findings are true and prevents nurses from committing a type I error. A **type I error** is the rejection of a null hypothesis that is true, that is, concluding that the intervention was effective when in reality it was not.

SCIENTIFIC MERIT The scientific merit of a study is probably the single most important criterion in judging its readiness for application in practice. Scientific rigor is evident in all steps of the research project—the clarity of the research problem, adequacy of the literature review, and the appropriateness of the design, sampling, data collection procedures, and data analytic techniques. The validity and reliability of the instruments used must also be evaluated.

Internal validity and external validity are key concerns in this area. **Internal validity** is the degree to which the independent variable influences the dependent variable. A classic monograph by Campbell and Stanley (1963) discussed factors that threaten internal validity. An example is selection bias if subjects in a study are not randomly assigned to the experimental or control groups. If a statistically significant difference is found, it would be difficult to conclude whether the change in the dependent variable is truly attributable to the independent variable (the intervention) or whether it is related to some preexisting differences between the groups.

External validity pertains to the degree to which the findings of the study can be generalized to similar settings and populations. Even if statistically significant differences are demonstrated, findings can be generalized to other settings or populations only if these settings and populations are similar to those of the study.

RISK The degree or risk involved in using the findings of a study is another criterion to be considered. Nursing

Research Box

Retsas, A. 2000. Barriers to using research evidence in nursing practice. *Journal of Advanced Nursing* **31(3): 599–606.**

The purpose of this study was to (1) establish the extent to which research use and research expertise existed at a particular medical center in Melbourne, Australia, (2) identify barriers the nursing staff believe interfere with their ability to use research findings in clinical practice, and (3) establish the extent to which nursing staff perceived that they were supported in these efforts. A self-administered questionnaire was used to collect data on demographics, education background, and research access habits of the full-time nursing staff. The questionnaire incorporated items from the Barriers to Research Utilization Scale (Funk et al. 1991) and qualitative questions about what helps in the use of research.

Two-thirds of the 400 participants read a journal monthly or more frequently. Barriers were classified by four factors: accessibility of research findings, anticipated outcomes of using research, organizational support to use research, and support from others to use research. The most outstanding finding was considered to be the significance participants gave to the need for organizational support to use research. The most significant barrier to using research evidence was having insufficient time to implement new ideas on the job and insufficient time to read research.

The researcher concluded that staff nurses have a high level of research readiness and value the contribution that research can make to improve practice. The organizational change that needs to occur is increasing the time available for nurses to achieve this goal.

interventions that have been found effective through research may be readily implemented if they carry little risk. According to Haller, Reynolds, and Horsley (1979), risk must be evaluated along with scientific merit. If a protocol entails serious risks, then the evaluation of scientific merit must be applied more stringently.

CLINICAL MERIT This criterion evaluates the degree to which research findings have the potential to

Research Box

Kajermo, K. N., Nordstrom, G., Krusebrant, A., and Bjorvell, H. 2000. Perceptions of research utilization: Comparisons between health care professionals, nursing students and a reference group of nurse clinicians. *Journal of Advanced Nursing* 31(1): 99–109.

This study conducted in Sweden was done to investigate perceptions of barriers to and facilitators of nurses' use of research findings in clinical practice. Five comparison groups were surveyed with a Barriers Scale and a demographic questionnaire; the five groups were (1) teachers of nursing, (2) nursing students, (3) nursing administrators, (4) physicians, and (5) registered nurses in clinical practice.

The organization and communication of research were seen as barriers by all of the groups except the physicians. Education to increase the nurses' knowledge of research and to develop their competence to evaluate research results, increased resources for education, more staff, support from the administration, and research presented in a user-friendly way were the most frequently suggested facilitators. The nurses' isolation from knowledgeable colleagues with whom to discuss the research was seen as a barrier by the majority of the participants.

These findings among the Swedish population were similar to findings in the United States and other countries.

solve an existing problem in the clinical setting. Nurses working in a neonatal nursery may be concerned about the pain that infants experience during blood drawing for laboratory tests or during surgical procedures. For nurses working in this unit, a published study by Campos (1994) that reported the effects of rocking and pacifiers on relieving heelstick pain in infants would be rated high for clinical merit.

CLINICAL CONTROL Clinical control refers to the degree to which nurses are in control of the circumstances related to the implementation and evaluation of the research-based innovation. Nurses may not be able to exert clinical control if a research-based protocol requires collaboration or decision making by a team of health professionals. There may also be instruments or methods documented to be effective in research but unavailable to nurses in certain settings.

FEASIBILITY This is defined as the degree to which resources—time, personnel, expertise, equipment—are available to implement the innovation. For instance, the introduction of a new intervention may require the ordering and purchasing of equipment or supplies and inservice training for nursing staff.

COST In this era of downsizing and restructuring, cost is always a vital consideration. Cost is closely related to feasibility. A cost-benefit analysis would be important in order to weigh the costs against the benefits of implementing a new intervention. Benefits may include improved client outcomes or improved staff satisfaction.

POTENTIAL FOR CLINICAL EVALUATION Potential for clinical evaluation pertains to the degree to which the department variables in the original research base can be evaluated by nurses in the clinical setting. Specifically, this criterion requires that nurses have control over the variables in the protocol and that they possess the knowledge and skills needed to measure the outcome of the innovation.

Mechanisms for Research Utilization

Research utilization in the clinical setting may occur through a number of mechanisms. There are situations in which research utilization takes place through individual action by nurses. In other cases, research-based protocols are developed by groups of nurses for a unit or hospital and may require changes in existing hospital or agency procedure.

INDIVIDUAL ACTION According to the ANA *Standards of Clinical Nursing Practice,* nurses are expected to use interventions that are based on research. Low-risk, low-cost interventions that have potential to improve client outcomes may be readily implemented by individual nurses. One example is an innovation listed in the Coyle and Sokop (1990, p. 177) study—internal rotation of the femur during dorsogluteal intramuscular injection to reduce client discomfort.

RESEARCH-BASED PROTOCOLS AND PROCEDURES Many hospitals and clinical agencies follow a compendium of policies, procedures, and protocols in specific client care situations. For example, there are procedures to be followed when irrigating a Foley catheter, administering nasogastric tube feeding, or performing wound care. Current research literature must be the basis for developing or revising these procedures or protocols.

Resources for Research Utilization
Clinical Practice Guidelines

The implementation of research-based clinical practice guidelines from the Agency for Health Care Policy and Research (AHCPR) is another mechanism to use research in the management of specific clinical conditions. The AHCPR guidelines were developed by multidisciplinary panels of experts to assist practitioners and clients in making decisions regarding the efficacy and appropriateness of health care. The guidelines were based on an exhaustive search and analysis of published research and, in areas where research is lacking, used expert opinion and consensus.

Key nursing researchers and clinicians have been members and sometimes chairpersons of these panels. For example, Nancy Bergstrom of the University of Nebraska Medical Center School of Nursing chaired the expert panel that drafted the AHCPR guideline on the prevention of pressure ulcers. The accompanying box shows some recently published AHCPR clinical practice guidelines.

These and other guidelines are available free of cost from AHCPR (1-800-358-9525, or at the Center for Research Dissemination and Liaison, AHCPR Clearinghouse, P.O. Box 8547, Silver Spring, MD 20907).

Product Evaluation

The systematic application of research findings may also be helpful in the evaluation of new products before they are adopted for use in a clinical setting. Janken, Rudisill, and Benfield (1992, p. 188) described how the research utilization strategy was used in their institution to examine a new closed-system catheter for use in the endotracheal suctioning of mechanically ventilated patients. A group of staff nurses, clinical nurse specialists, the director of nursing, and the nurse-researcher reviewed recent research literature on endotracheal suctioning. The research findings noted that decreased oxygen saturation was a significant adverse effect for clients who are being suctioned. Thus, the effect of the new closed-system catheter on oxygen saturation was one of the main outcomes that needed to be evaluated.

Triggers

Factors called *triggers,* arising from various sources, may serve as a strong stimulus for change in clinical practice. Titler and colleagues (1995, p. 307) reported that triggers are used in the Iowa Model of Research in Practice for infusing research into practice to improve the quality of care.

Triggers may be *problem focused* or *knowledge focused.*

Agency for Healthcare Research and Quality Clinical Practice Guidelines

Each guideline has several versions: Clinical Practice Guidelines, Quick Reference Guides for Clinicians, and Consumer Versions. Each of these is available in English and Spanish.

Acute Pain Management: Adult/Pediatric
Urinary Incontinence in Adults
Pressure Ulcer Prevention
Cataract in Adults
Depression in Primary Care
Sickle Cell Disease
Early HIV Infection
Benign Prostatic Hyperplasia

Unstable Angina
Heart Failure
Otitis Media with Effusion
Quality Mammography
Acute Low Back Problems in Adults
Pressure Ulcer Treatment
Post-Stroke Rehabilitation
Cardiac Rehabilitation
Smoking Cessation
Early Alzheimer's Disease

New guidelines are always under development. The reader is advised to check with the agency for new listings. They may be obtained online.

Problem-focused triggers are clinical problems that are repeatedly encountered in practice, risk management, quality improvement (QI) data, and total quality management (TQM) programs. By contrast, knowledge-focused triggers proceed from new or freshly recognized information from credible sources such as standards and practice guidelines from national agencies and organizations, philosophies of care, recent research publications, and nurse experts within the organization.

Research Utilization Groups

The formation of research utilization groups—composed of researchers and nurses—is another mechanism that may be used to promote research utilization. Beckstrand and McBride (1990, p. 170) reported how novice researchers (staff nurses) and experienced researchers (nursing faculty) working together successfully addressed the problem of estimating the insertion length of nasogastric tubes (NGT) in children through a review of the research literature and, later, through completed research projects. Research utilization groups may be organized to address specific clinical problems or conditions encountered in the practice setting.

Bookshelf

Laurence, L., and Weinhouse, B. 1994. *Outrageous practices.* **New York: Fawcett Columbine.**
This book focuses on the lack of research studies related to women's health issues, such as hormone-replacement therapy, breast cancer, heart disease in women, menopause, premenstrual syndrome (PMS), and other disease processes that have a higher incidence in women than men. In many cases, research has been done on exclusively male populations, and women have been purposely excluded because of female-specific hormone changes, physiologic differences, and the potential for pregnancy during the study. The authors also discuss how women are treated differently from men in the health care system. These differences in treatment are grounded in assumptions by both physicians and researchers about women—assumptions based on studies that have been done exclusively in men.

Moore, T.J. 1995. *Deadly medicine.* **New York: Simon and Shuster.**
This book chronicles the history of multiple studies over approximately 10 years in the effectiveness of cardiac arrhythmia suppressant therapy (CAST) in the treatment of clients diagnosed with cardiac dysrythmias. It points out how inaccurate assumptions and errors in study design can cause errors in conclusions that can have fatal results in client populations.

Palmer, M. 1998. *Miracle cure.* **New York: Bantam Doubleday.**
The political pressures in biomedical research form the backdrop for this novel presenting the story of the phase II clinical trial and FDA decisions about a drug under investigation as a cure for cardiovascular disease.

SUMMARY

Nursing research refers to research directed toward building a body of nursing knowledge about "human responses to actual or potential health problems." Research is important in nursing to expand the scientific body of knowledge, to maintain specific accountability to the public, to document nursing's contribution to health care delivery, and to provide the bases for sound clinical decision making in client care.

The information revolution that is transforming the present and shaping the future has made reading, understanding, and using nursing research as fundamental to professional practice as are knowledge of asepsis, application of the nursing process, and communication skills. *The Cumulative Index to Nursing and Allied Health Literature,* the *International Nursing Index,* and the *Cumulated Medical Index* are excellent resources for locating published research on a phenomenon of interest.

The quantitative and qualitative approaches are both valid approaches to investigations of nursing phenomena, although they proceed from different philosophic perspectives and use different methods of data collection and analysis.

If nursing is to develop evidence-based practice, the clinical nurse must know the process and language of research, be sensitive to protecting the rights of human subjects, participate in identifying significant researchable problems, and be a discriminating consumer of research findings.

All nurses who practice in settings where research is conducted with human subjects or who participate in research as data collectors or collaborators play an important role in safeguarding the rights of human subjects.

REFERENCES

American Nurses Association. 1975. *Human rights guidelines for nurses in clinical and other research.* Kansas City, Mo.: ANA.

American Nurses Association. 1980. *Nursing: A social policy statement.* Kansas City, Mo.: ANA.

American Nurses Association, Council of Nurse Researchers and Council of Nursing Practice. 1994. *Position statement on education for participation in nursing research.* Washington, D.C.: ANA.

American Nurses Association. 1998. *Standards of clinical nursing practice.* Washington, D.C.: ANA.

Beckstrand, J., and McBride, A. B. 1990. How to form a research interest group. *Nursing Outlook* **38**(4): 168–171.

Brett, J. L. L. 1987. Use of nursing practice research findings. *Nursing Research* **36**(6): 344-349.

Brink, P. J., and Wood, M. J. 1988. *Basic steps in planning nursing research,* 3d ed. Boston: Jones and Bartlett.

Campbell, D. T., and Stanley, J. C. 1963. *Experimental and quasi-experimental designs for research.* Boston: Houghton Miflin.

Campos, R. G. 1994. Rocking and pacifiers: Two comforting interventions for heelstick pain. *Research in Nursing and Health* **17**(5), 321–331.

Caplan, A. L. 1992. When evil intrudes. *Hastings Center Report* **22**(6): 29–32.

Carlson, D. S., and Rouse, C. L. 1999. Staff nurses: Using research in everyday practice. *Journal of Emergency Nursing* **25**(6): 564-568.

Carper, B. A. 1978. Fundamental patterns of knowing in nursing. *Advances in Nursing Science* **1**(1): 13–23.

Champion, V. L., and Leach, A. 1989. Variables related to research utilization in nursing: An empirical investigation. *Journal of Advanced Nursing* **14**(9): 705–710.

Cohen, I. B. 1984. Florence Nightingale. *Scientific American* **250**(3): 128–137.

Coyle, L. A., and Sokop, A. G. 1990. Innovation adoption behavior among nurses. *Nursing Research* **39**(3): 176–180.

Coyne, C., Baier, W., Perra, B., and Sherer, B. K. 1994. Controlled trial of backrest elevation after coronary angiography. *American Journal of Critical Care* **3**(4): 282–288.

Diers, D. 1979. *Research in nursing practice.* Philadelphia: Lippincott.

Ellis, R. 1970. Values and vicissitudes of the scientist nurse. *Nursing Research* **19**(5): 440–445.

Fawcett, J., and Downs, F. 1992. *The relationship of theory and research.* Norwalk, Conn.: Appleton-Century-Crofts.

Funk, S. G., Champagne, M. T., Wiese, R. A., and Tornquist, E. 1991. Barriers: The barriers to research utilization scale. *Applied Nursing Research* **4**(1): 39–45.

Good, M. 1995. A comparison of the effects of jaw relaxation and music on postoperative pain. *Nursing Research* **44**(1): 52–57.

Gortner, S. 2000. Knowledge development in nursing: Our historical roots and future opportunities. *Nursing Outlook* **48**(2): 60–67.

Grossman, D. G. S., Jorda, M. L., and Farr, L. A. 1994. Blood pressure rhythms in early school-age children of normotensive and hypertensive parents: A replication study. *Nursing Research* **43**(4): 232–237.

Haller, K. B., Reynolds, M. A., and Horsley, J. A. 1979. Developing research-based innovation protocols: Process, criteria, and issues. *Research in Nursing and Health* **2**(2): 45–51.

Horsley, J. A., Crane, J. and Bingle, J. D. 1978. Research utilization as an organizational process. *Journal of Nursing Administration* **8**(7): 4–6.

Janken, J. K., Rudisill, P., and Benfield, L. 1992. Product evaluation as a research utilization strategy. *Applied Nursing Research* **5**(4): 188–193.

Ketefian, S. 1975. Application of selected nursing research findings into nursing practice. *Nursing Research* **24**(2): 89–92.

Krueger, J. C., Nelson, A. H., and Wolanin, M. O. 1978. *Nursing research: Development, collaboration, and utilization.* Germantown, Md.: Aspen Systems.

Melnyk, B. M., Stone, P., Fineout-Overholt, E., and Ackerman, M. 2000. Evidence-based practice: The past, the present, and recommendations for the millennium. *Pediatric Nursing* **26**(1):77–80.

Munro, B. H., Visintainer, M. A., and Page, E. B. 1986. *Statistical methods for health care research.* Philadelphia: Lippincott.

National Institute of Nursing Research. 2000. *Mission statement and strategic planning for the 21st century.* http://www.nih.gov/ninr/a_mission.html.

Nativio, D. G. 2000. Guidelines for evidence-based clinical practice. *Nursing Outlook* **48**(2): 58–59.

Orem, D. E. 1971. *Nursing: Concepts of practice.* New York: McGraw-Hill.

Pettengill, M. M., Gillies, D. A., and Clark, C. C. 1994. Factors encouraging and discouraging the use of nursing research findings. *Image: Journal of Nursing Scholarship* **26**(2): 143–147.

Polit, D. F., and Hungler, B. P. 1999. *Nursing research: Principles and methods,* 6th ed. Philadelphia: Lippincott.

Retsas, A. 2000. Barriers to using research evidence in nursing practice. *Journal of Advanced Nursing* **31**(3): 599–606.

Rogers, E. 1983. *Diffusion of innovations,* 3d ed. New York: Free Press.

Roy, C. 1985. Nursing research makes a difference. *Nurses' Educational Funds Newsletter* **4**(1): 2–3.

Sigma Theta Tau International. 1995. Listing of doctoral programs in the United States. *Reflections* **21**(3): 18–19, 22–23.

Sigma Theta Tau International. 2000. *Strategic Plan 2005.* http://www.nursingsociety.org/stratplan/man. html.

Stetler, C. B., and DiMaggio, G. 1991. Research utilization among clinical nurse specialists. *Clinical Nurse Specialist* **5**(3): 151–155.

Titler, M. G., Kleiber, C., Steelman, V., Goode, C., Rakel, B., Barry-Walker, J., Small, S., and Buckwalter, K. 1995. Infusing research into practice to promote quality care. *Nursing Research* **43**(5): 307–313.

Woodham-Smith, C. 1950. *Florence Nightingale.* London: Constable & Co.

Youngblut, J. M., and Brooten, D. 2000. Moving research into practice: A new partner. *Nursing Outlook* **48**(2): 55–56.

The Nurse as Political Advocate

Objectives

- Discuss the role that power plays in nursing practice.
- Discuss the relevance of political action to nursing.
- Explain various strategies used to influence political decision making.
- Identify skills that are essential to political action.
- Identify ways in which nurses can participate in the political arena.

NURSE CONNECT

Additional online resources for this chapter can be found on the companion web site at www.prenhall.com/blais.

Nurses are actively participating in political processes to promote change within the profession and to influence policymaking regarding nursing and health care policy issues. The realities of the health care scene, such as more government regulation and increasingly scarce resources, demand that nurses become knowledgeable about and capable of influencing the development of health care policy and the delivery of care to clients.

Although political action is ordinarily associated with governmental concerns, Mason and Leavitt (1998) identify four spheres of political action. These spheres are interconnected and overlapping; they include the workplace, government, professional organizations, and community. In the workplace, policies and procedures may be the focus of political action, and government and professional organizations as well as the community may influence these workplace policies. Professional organizations play a key role in influencing the practice of nursing through standards of practice, lobbying, and collective action. Nursing has become increasingly focused on the community, particularly through the American Nurses Association's agenda for health care reform (See Chapter 17, "Nursing in an Evolving Health Care Delivery System").

CHALLENGES AND OPPORTUNITIES

Political power is a concept that has not been traditionally associated with nursing. In fact, nursing has been seen as powerless with regard to decisions about clinical practice, stemming from the fact that nurses are predominantly female working in a male-dominated setting. Nursing is challenged to change that perception and assume more power over its own practice.

In recent years, more nurses have been appointed to senior administrative positions and elected to public office, and the image is gradually changing. These changes create opportunities for nurses to influence policy and assume power commensurate with their knowledge and expertise as care providers.

POWER

Power is described as one of the most difficult concepts to define and measure (Mason and Leavitt 1998). One definition is "power is the potential capacity to influence events, cause change, initiate action, and control outcomes" (Lee, 2000, p. 26). Often, the terms *power, influence,* and *authority* are used interchangeably, but they need to be differentiated. Power is the source of influence, whereas influence is the result of the use of power. Authority is the official or legitimized right to use a given amount or type of power, i.e., the right to act and the right to command (Claus and Bailey, 1977, p. 21). Authority may be either delegated or acquired.

Empowerment

The concept of empowerment has been applied since the 1970s to promote the rights of ethnic and sexual minorities in training and education programs and organizational development (Kuokkanen and Leino-Kilpi, 2000). It is associated with attempts to increase power and influence of oppressed groups. Recently the concept has been more broadly applied to varying groups and the individual. The basic element of empowerment is taking action to generate positive results at both the individual and organizational level.

A useful theoretical framework for application of empowerment to practice is Kanter's (1993) theory of organizational empowerment. Assumptions of this theory are that people react rationally to their situations and that situations structured to support employee's feelings of empowerment result in benefit to the organization in effectiveness and employee attitude. The organizational structures that benefit the growth of empowerment are (1) having access to information, (2) receiving support, (3) having access to resources necessary to do the job, and (4) having the opportunity to learn and grow. Management should create conditions for work effectiveness by ensuring that employees have the access they need to information, support, and resources in order to do their job and that they have opportunity for employee development. This results in employees being more productive and effective in meeting the organization's goals. A model of Kanter's theory is shown in Figure 11–1.

Conger and Kanungo (1988) pose additions to the Kanter model by arguing that managers or leaders need to eliminate situations fostering powerlessness and use motivation strategies. They further pose that task accomplishment builds a sense of competence and self-determination. Attempts at empowerment without consideration of employee capability may not result in empowerment of people who are incapable or overwhelmed or unmotivated.

Sources of Power

Power theorists describe a variety of sources from which a person derives power. Understanding these sources of power is prerequisite to formulating a plan for developing one's own power and recognizing it in others. French and Raven (1960, pp. 607–623) identified five sources of power: legitimate, reward, coercive, referent, and expert powers. Hershey, Blanchard, and Natemeyer (1979) added two more: connection (association) and information powers. Most leaders use all types of power at different times, depending on the particular situation.

- *Legitimate (or positional) power* derives from one's formal position or title in an organization. It is associated with the authority that the position gives its holder to make and enforce decisions. The title "vice president for nursing" implies that the holder has power by virtue of the position, regardless of who holds that position or how effective that person is.
- *Reward power* is derived from the perception of one's abilities to bestow rewards or favors on others.
- *Coercive power,* by contrast, arises from the perception of one's ability to threaten, harm, or punish others.

Figure 11–1

Relationship of Concepts in Rosabeth Kanter's (1979) Structural Theory of Power in Organizations

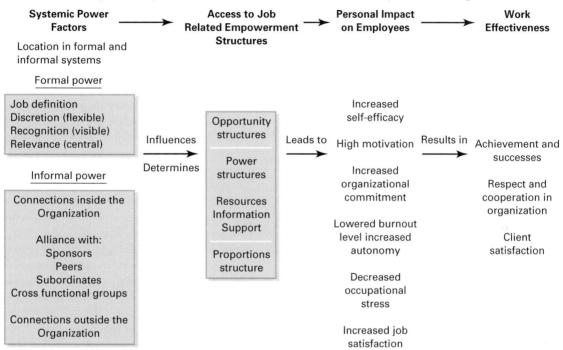

Used by permission from H. K. S. Laschinger, J. Finegan, J. Shamian, and S. Casier. Organizational trust and empowerment in restructured healthcare settings: Effects on staff nurse commitment, *Journal of Nursing Administration* **30**(9): 415, 2000.

■ *Information power* is associated with persons who are perceived to control key information.

Reward, coercive, and informational power all relate to the degree an individual can control the distribution of resources.

■ *Referent (charismatic or personal) power* is power derived from an individual's own vision, sense of self, and ability to communicate these so that others regard the person with admiration and are motivated to follow.

■ *Connection (associative) power* derives from the perception that one has important contacts or relationships with others. These connections can be an aspect of both formal and informal networks.

■ *Expert (or knowledge) power* is power derived from one's expertise, talents, and skills. One can include in this category Benner's (1984) vision of power, i.e., the positive power the nurse brings to the nurse-client relationship. This power enables the nurse to transform the client's life through advocacy and other means of caring.

Some feminist scholars believe this framework of power to be based upon masculine norms. They prefer to see sources of power available to women as based on structural, individual, organizational, interpersonal, and symbolic factors (Kelly and Duerst-Lahti, 1995).

Caring Types of Power

Benner (1984), in her classic work on clinical nursing excellence, describes six types of power that nurses can use when dealing with clients and significant others. These are powers that are associated with caring: transformative, integrative, advocacy, healing, participative/affirmative, and problem-solving powers.

Transformative Power

Transformative power represents the ability of the nurse to assist clients to change their views of reality or their own self-images. Nurses display this type of power in caring for clients who have long-term illness. Providing compassionate care to clients who are unable to perform their normal hygienic care can help transform their self-image from one of worthlessness to one of value.

Integrative Power

Integrative power is the nurse's ability to assist a client to return to a normal life. In this process, the nurse helps clients integrate any disabilities into their lives and assists them back into the family and society.

Research Box

Laschinger, H. K. S., Finegan, J., Shamian, J., and Casier, S. 2000. Organizational trust and empowerment in restructured healthcare settings. *Journal of Nursing Administration* 30(9): 413–425.

A predictive, nonexperimental design was used to test Kanter's theory linking staff-nurse work empowerment to organizational trust and organizational commitment. A random sample of 412 Canadian staff nurses was surveyed, with five self-report scales used to measure work empowerment. The overall work-empowerment score suggests that nurses perceived only moderate empowerment in their work settings. They did not believe that they had a high degree of formal power in their jobs but did perceive a moderate amount of informal power. The nurses reported higher confidence and trust in their peers than in management. The results of the study support the proposition that staff nurses' empowerment affects their trust in management and ultimately influences affective commitment. Staff nurses believed that their sense of workplace empowerment strongly affected their trust in management and subsequently their belief and acceptance of organizational goals and values, their willingness to exert effort in the workplace, and their desire to stay in the organization (affective commitment). The strongest relationships were found between trust in management and perceived access to information and support. The authors believe that the findings stress the importance of creating environments that provide access to structures that empower nurses to accomplish their work.

Research Box

Laschinger, H. K. S., Wong, C., McMahon, L., and Kaufmann, C. 1999. Leader behavior impact on staff nurse empowerment, job tension, and work effectiveness. *Journal of Nursing Administration* 29(5): 28–39.

This study tested a model linking leader-empowering behaviors to staff-nurse perceptions of workplace empowerment, occupational stress, and work effectiveness in a Canadian acute-care hospital. A sample of 537 nurses was surveyed with six self-report questionnaires developed to test an integration of Kanter's organizational-empowerment theory and Conger and Kunungo's model of the leader-empowerment process. Leader-empowering behaviors significantly influenced employees' perceptions of formal and informal power and access to empowerment structures (information, support, resources, and opportunity). Higher perceived access to empowerment structures were likely to result in lower levels of job tension and increased work effectiveness. Support for the integrated model highlights the importance of managers' leadership behaviors in health care organizations.

Research Box

Ellefsen, B., and Hamilton, B. 2000. Empowered nurses? Nurses in Norway and the USA compared. *International Nursing Review* 47: 106–120.

This comparative study investigated the degree to which nurses from two major university hospitals in two different countries experienced empowerment. Five hundred ninety Norwegian nurses and 135 North American nurses responded to five self-report questionnaires based upon Kanter's theory of empowerment. Formal power explained 51% of the variance in the overall empowerment score, and the combination of formal and informal power explained 65%. The Norwegian nurses experienced slightly more informal power, whereas the North American nurses experienced more formal power. The small difference in reported experience of the nurses in two different countries is an interesting finding.

Advocacy Power

Advocacy power enables the nurse to help a client and significant others deal with a health care bureaucracy. The nurse can explain to the client what services are available. In addition, the nurse can act as an "interpreter" between the client and physician. For example, a client may hesitate to express a concern to a busy physician. Recognizing that the physician may be able to ease the client's mind, the nurse may act as a liaison between the two.

Healing Power

Nurses can establish a healing relationship and a healing climate with a client. According to Benner, nurses can do this by mobilizing hope in themselves, the staff, and the client; finding an interpretation or understanding of a specific situation; and assisting the client to use social, emotional, and/or spiritual support. Benner writes that an affirming and caring nurse-client relationship provides a basis for healing. A healing relationship empowers the client by bringing hope, confidence, and trust (1984, p. 213).

Participative/Affirmative Power

Participative/affirmative power is the nurse's ability to draw strength by investing it in others. Benner disputes the more traditional view that nurses have only so much emotional strength to draw on and suggests that involvement and caring permit the nurses to obtain strength (1984, p. 214).

Problem Solving

A committed person is more sensitive to cues than a less committed person; thus, a caring and involved nurse is able to solve problems at a higher level than a less involved nurse. Commitment and caring enhance the nurse's receptivity to cues and enables the nurse to recognize solutions that are not obvious. These abilities are due partly to intuition and feeling.

Traditional Types of Power

It is also important for nurses to be aware of the traditional types of power: physical, position, expert, and economic powers.

Physical power has been traditionally looked upon as the main source of power. Traditional male roles were based on men's superior physical strength: Men were responsible for providing food and shelter for the family because they were stronger. Now, as a result of technologic changes, many positions that formerly were available only to men because the job required physical strength are also available to women.

Position power is the power that results from an individual's title or position. For example, a nursing supervisor has specific responsibilities and power that other nurses do not have. Position power alone is not as strong as position power that is supported by expert or economic power.

Expert power is the result of demonstrated knowledge and competence. Nurses who have expert power and share it with others gain credibility and a sense of

authority. Nurses who refuse to share their expertise lose power and are often considered selfish and unprofessional.

Economic power is the power people gain through providing or withholding resources. When nurses are involved in budget development, for example, they gain power through financial decision making. Traditionally, management controlled economic power in health care agencies; now, however, the advent of shared governance has distributed economic power more widely.

Laws of Power

Berle describes power as a "universal experience and human attribute of man with five discernable natural laws" (1969, p. 32).

Law 1 Power invariably fills any vacuum. People generally prefer peace and order and are usually willing to give power to someone who will restore order and thereby reduce their discomfort. When a problem arises, an individual will usually show the initiative to handle the problem and thus will exert power. Nurses should be aware that these are opportunities to assume power.

Law 2 Power is invariably personal. In many instances, people who effect change find common ground and come together committed to that change. To be successful, nurses must develop personal power, that is, the power one develops in oneself: self-esteem, self-respect, and self-confidence. Through their professional organizations, nurses can then exert personal power in the health care field.

Law 3 Power is based on a system of ideas and philosophy. When people demonstrate behaviors that indicate power, they reflect a personal belief or philosophy. It is this belief or philosophic system that gains followers and their respect. Nurses, however, have traditionally been comfortable "taking orders" and accommodating a hospital hierarchy rather than taking the initiative in such spheres as clients' rights and preventive care. Current problems in the health care system, such as increasing technology and cost, offer nurses an opportunity to fill a vacuum for change in the health care system and thereby offer solutions to these problems.

Law 4 Power is exercised through and depends on institutions. Individuals can feel powerless and unable to deal with many situations in a hospital, community agency, government agency, or other institution. By banding together with others through a state or provincial nursing organization, nurses can magnify their power and support changes in health care.

Law 5 Power is invariably confronted with, and acts in

the presence of, a field of responsibility. Nurses in power positions act on behalf of other nurses or clients. Power is communicated to people observing the situation and is reinforced by positive responses. If group members believe that their beliefs or ideals are not represented, the vacuum will be filled by another person who can carry out the role and is supported by the organization.

Consider . . .

■ sources of power available to you as a clinical nurse. How can you enhance your expert power, your advocacy power, your healing power, your connection power, and your participative/affirmative power?

■ how a nurse's self-image can affect that nurse's referent power.

■ how expert power can enhance position power.

POLITICS

Politics can also be defined as "influencing—specifically, influencing the allocation of scarce resources" (Mason and Leavit, 1998, p. 9). Defined in this way, the word denotes more than action in the governmental arena; it is also applicable to every sphere of life where resources are limited and more than one person or group competes for them. "It is a process by which one influences the decisions of others and exerts control over situations and events. It is a means to an end" (p. 9). *Resources* may refer not only to money but also to any number of cherished assets that are limited, such as personnel, programs, time, status, and power.

The allocation of scarce resources involves everyone in some way. Consider the following examples:

■ A student applying for a college loan or competing with other students for his or her fair share of a teacher's time and attention.

■ A client advocate competing for hospital education funds in order to provide more preoperative teaching.

■ A citizen lobbying against the school board's proposal to divide one RN's time between two large schools.

■ A member of a professional association seeking association action on a practice issue, such as care of clients with acquired immune deficiency syndrome (AIDS).

Nurses have always been involved in politics. For example, the founder of modern nursing, Florence Nightingale, used her contacts with powerful men in government to obtain needed personnel and supplies for wounded soldiers in the Crimea. Subsequent nursing leaders such as Lavinia Dock, Lillian Wald, Harriet Tubman, and Margaret Sanger—who were all skilled politicians and made significant contributions to the profession and society—may have been influenced by these wise words of Nightingale:

> When I entered service here, I determined that, happen what would, I *never* would intrigue among the Committee. Now I perceive that I do all my business by intrigue. I propose in private to A, B, or C the resolution I think A, B, or C most capable of carrying in Committee, and then leave it to them, and I always win. (Huxley, 1975, p. 53)

Political action refers to action by a group of individuals that is designed to attain a purpose through the use of political power or through the established political process. **Policy** is shaped by politics and has been defined as the principles that govern actions directed toward given ends; policy statements outline a plan, direction, or goal for action. Policy encompasses the choices that a society, segment of society, or organization make regarding its goals and priorities and how it will allocate its resources. Governmental bodies form public policy. Social policy pertains to directives that promote the welfare of the public. Institutional policies govern the workplace. Organizational policies govern professional organizations. Policies may be laws, guidelines, or regulations that govern behavior in government, workplaces, organizations, and committees.

Strategies to Influence Political Decisions

Many of the strategies used to influence political decisions will serve the nurse well in everyday professional activities.

Negotiating

Negotiation is a give-and-take process between individuals and groups to work out differences of opinion regarding the best solution to an issue. Guidelines to consider in negotiations are shown in the accompanying box. Two basic forms of negotiation are problem-solving negotiation and trade-off negotiation. In *problem-solving negotiation,* both parties confer to resolve a complex situation together. In *trade-off negotiation,* one party gives some concessions, or "points," to the other party in exchange for other concessions, or points. Negotiating demands good communication skills of all participants. Before beginning negotiation, the nurse needs to know all the essential facts of the issue and conduct research to support a particular viewpoint. A familiar example of the negotiating process for nurses

Guidelines for Negotiation

- Obtain all of the essential facts of the issue beforehand.
- Explore the other party's viewpoint. If the other party is a legislator, for example, obtain information about his or her views from news media and congressional records.
- Consider the consequences of the issue and how you can deflect those consequences in order to support your viewpoint.

- Verify the strength of your own viewpoint and ways to strengthen it further; then consider ways to counteract or weaken the other party's viewpoint.
- Determine any limitations surrounding your viewpoint, such as time constraints or other resources.
- Consider other groups that support your viewpoint or that of the other party.

---

is the collective bargaining (contract negotiations) process between employees and employers. Guidelines for negotiation are found in the accompanying box.

Networking

Networking refers to a process in which people with similar interests and goals communicate, share ideas and information, and offer support and direction to each other. Network development builds linkages with people throughout the profession, both within and outside the work environment. Getting to know people helps build a trust relationship that can facilitate the achievement of professional goals: It is easier to access people one knows than it is to access strangers.

Nurses can develop networks by (1) attending local, regional, and national conferences; (2) taking classes for continuing education or toward an academic degree; (3) joining alumni associations and attending alumni meetings; (4) joining and participating in professional organizations; (5) keeping in touch with former teachers and coworkers; and (6) socializing with professional colleagues.

Political networks generally have three functions: (1) to provide information about legislative activities on particular issues, (2) to increase political action and awareness, and (3) to promote issues through the legislative process. These networks may be formal, with signed agreements and fee structures, or informal, requiring minimal monetary contributions.

Preparing Resolutions

Resolutions are formal statements expressing the opinion, will, or intent of an individual or group. Most nurses will be familiar with the specific format used to present resolutions at annual association meetings or conventions about nursing and health care concerns.

Resolutions are an effective means of writing concise reasons and proposed recommendations for action, particularly for areas where services are inadequate. Nurses who present resolutions must, however, be well informed about the data presented, be prepared to offer additional data others might request, and be willing to consider amendments to the recommendations.

Establishing Political Action Committees

Political action committees (PACs) endorse candidates for public office, such as the senate and the house of representatives. Because tax laws limit nonprofit professional organizations from participating in various types of political activities, PACs provide an avenue for professional political action activities. Groups such as nursing organizations, women's groups, church groups, and civic groups may form PACs. Members of a PAC provide additional donations or pay dues to support the organization's activities because general membership fees in any nonprofit organization cannot be used to support such activity. Because they are used for political purposes, donations made to a PAC are not tax deductible.

The ANA Political Action Committee (ANA-PAC) is a political organization formed by the ANA. Many state nursing organizations also have political action organizations that serve similar functions on the state level as ANA-PAC does on the national level. PACs support legislative candidates based on their stands on key issues. For example, ANA-PAC would consider a candidate's stand on such specific health and nursing issues as national health insurance, third-party reimbursement for nurses, funding for biomedical and nursing research, elder abuse, and so on. Although nursing PACs have not created power equal to that of such groups as labor, education, and medicine, nurses are becoming more sophisticated in the political process and are gaining increased power.

Communicating with Legislators

Nurses can communicate with legislators through telephone calls, telegrams, face-to-face meetings, e-mail, fax, and written letters. For each method, the nurse needs to identify clearly the issue and the bill (by number if possible), explain reasons for interest in the issue, and provide constructive information and ideas. Telephone calls are usually received by a legislative assistant who keeps a record of all calls and the positions of the callers. In many regions, a toll-free number is available during the legislative session.

For visits to legislative officials, the nurse first needs to contact the local offices, which will provide assistance in arranging the visit and may additionally arrange other activities, such as tours of the legislature, attendance at committee hearings, and visits to a legislative session. Before the visit, the nurse should obtain information about the legislators's background, such as the legislator's occupation, previous professional and civic activities, political affiliation, voting record, and interests. Because only a few minutes may be allotted to the visit, the nurse should be prepared to be succinct in presenting personal ideas and facts, allow time for the legislator to answer questions, and leave a summary of facts and recommendations with the legislator to add to the perspective of the visit.

Letters are probably the most common mode of communicating with elected officials. Personal letters that reflect thoughtful and informed comments about an issue often receive more attention from legislators than form letters or postcards. When writing to legislators, the nurse should use a professional letterhead and address the public official appropriately. For example, in written communication, the president, vice president, senators, and state representatives are cited as The Honorable (full name) followed by their position (e.g., President of the United States) and the specific address. Salutations in letters are written as Dear Mr. (or Madame) President/Vice President or Dear Senator (full name), or Dear Representative (last name). When communicating in person it is appropriate to say the following: Mr. or Madame President/Vice President or President (last name); Senator (last name); and Representative or Mr./Ms. (last name). Elements to include in the letter follow:

- A statement of the request in the first sentence (e.g., "I request that you support Bill XY604") and a brief summary of the issue.

- A brief rationale for the request (e.g., "The bill is vital to improving . . ." or "the bill will adversely affect . . .").
- Factual data that support your viewpoint.
- A closing statement thanking the legislator for his or her concern and continuing support or attention.
- Appropriate closing. For a letter to the president of the United States, the appropriate closing is "Very respectfully yours"; for all other letters, "Sincerely yours."

In general, e-mail messages and faxed copies are useful when time constraints exist, but they tend to have less impact.

Building Coalitions

Coalitions are alliances that distinct bodies, persons, or states form in order to achieve a common purpose. Coalitions are like networks in function but differ in that the members of the coalition represent groups with numerous purposes and issues. The groups negotiate, compromise, and merge to achieve specific goals. Groups or organizations may be in coalition on one issue but adversaries on another. Building coalitions is a strategy to empower oneself; thus, nurses solicit organizations whose power is greater than their own. Groups with whom nurses may form coalitions are as diverse as the topics that are of concern to nurses; women's issues, child care, and the environment are only a few examples.

Professional specialty organizations frequently form coalitions for areas of common interest. For instance, the American Association of Critical Care Nurses is building coalitions with the American Nurses Association, the Emergency Nurses Association, and the American Hospital Association.

Lobbying

Lobbying is a process in which individuals or groups attempt to influence legislators to support or oppose particular legislation. Lobbyists monitor legislative activities and communicate the group's position to members of the legislature. Professional lobbyists may be employed by groups from various sources: public relations firms, management relation firms, legal firms, legislative consultants, and independent lobbyists, many of whom are former legislators. Which source is used depends on the issue. Law firms, for example, can provide legal advice as well as lobbying; public relations firms generally provide media resources for campaigns. Individuals and groups can lobby independently, but such efforts require considerable time, personnel, and funding. Lobbyists must follow various legal guidelines. Lobbying techniques include negotiating, media and letter-writing campaigns, testifying, endorsements, and donations.

Testifying

Decisions related to health care and nursing are often made by committees and commissions of various levels of government. These committees frequently conduct hearings to obtain information before making a decision. Hearings generally include people or groups with opposing views. **Testifying** refers to the presentation of information at a committee hearing, usually about controversial aspects of a proposed bill. Nurses may testify either as independent individuals or as official representatives of an organization. Opportunities to testify may be found in professional publications or newspapers. Guidelines for testifying are shown in the accompanying box. Most committees will accept written testimony if the individual cannot be present.

Developing Political Astuteness and Skill

By contributing to political activities in various ways, nurses can develop their political astuteness and skills. All nurses, as citizens and employees, can join and participate in organizations and participate in election processes. However, nurses who are employed by a governmental agency, such as the Veterans Administration or a public health department, must follow restrictions defined in the Hatch Act regarding their po-

litical activity. These restrictions do not apply to the general public and include serving as an officer or spokesperson of a particular political party. The major objective of the Hatch Act initiated in the 1930s was to prevent government workers from being forced to support political activities. Although these restrictions remain controversial, attempts to modify and repeal the Hatch Act have failed. Because each state has its own version of this act, nurses who are employed by state governmental agencies are advised to investigate specific limitations in their state of employment.

A discussion of when and where to engage in political action must be prefaced by a statement of three key assumptions:

1. *Individuals who are deeply concerned about a particular issue or cause are most likely to identify ways to take action.* Before becoming politically involved, an individual must make choices, including the conscious decision to set aside the necessary resources. For example, a student who wants her or his school to offer evening or weekend clinical practice hours may decide to seek election to the student council to work for this change from within.

2. *Political action in any sphere is best carried out by a group.* Individual activism is laudable, but group action is much more effective. It provides change agents with the collegiality and support necessary to sustain a vision for change and fosters creative thinking and planning.

Guidelines for Testifying

- Confirm the time to register. In some instances, registration occurs at the meeting place on the day of testifying; in others, you must notify the committee of your visit to testify at a specified time before the hearing.

- Prepare your testimony concisely and clearly in advance. Avoid the use of professional terminology that may not be understood by the legislators, or explain any technical term used.

- Dress appropriately to convey your professional status, and introduce yourself. Make your position clear so that legislators know whether you are representing an organization.

- Maintain a courteous, professional composure throughout the hearing. Adhere to the rules of the proceedings.

- Verify any time limits to your presentation so that you can present essential facts and arguments first.

- Provide copies of your written testimony, including any graphs or other illustrations, to each committee member.

- Present your material without reading it to make the presentation more interesting for the listeners. Summarize the main ideas. Convey knowledge of the subject.

- Answer any questions completely. Be prepared to support any facts and figures you present with appropriate sources.

- Thank the committee for allowing your testimony.

3. *Successful political action requires the thoughtful application of change theory.* Before embarking on a project, the politically astute nurse will review the principles of change theory. Achieving goals for change requires thoughtful planning. Effective political activists plan strategy, much as nurses use the nursing process to evaluate clients' needs for care.

Seeking Opportunities for Political Action

Workplace

The workplace for nurses may be a public or a private (for-profit or nonprofit) organization and that can influence who sets policies and the values underlying the policies. These can have a profound influence on a nurse's professional life, and it is therefore important to examine ways to influence those policies. It is up to nurses to see that a nursing perspective is available, listened to, and incorporated into decisions about the administration of the organization (Mason and Leavitt, 1998). Nurses can exert expert, position, and economic power by negotiating the presence of nurse members on standing committees and the board of trustees and by becoming involved in the collective bargaining process. The accompanying box gives tips on effective committee involvement.

In most hospitals, nursing homes, and public health agencies, a system of committees exists to deal with specific issues. For example, a nursing department has an equipment evaluation committee that selects and evaluates client care products used by the nursing staff. A pharmacy committee in the same hospital has representatives from nursing, medicine, and the pharmacy. In addition to formal standing committees, ad hoc committees or task forces can be appointed to deal with particular issues or problems. For example, a task force on a nursing unit might examine the best way to initiate a case management program and critical pathways.

Nurses who have an idea or problem they want addressed are advised to look for existing committees that might already be dealing with the concern or are likely to do so. For example, nurses concerned about staff safety in the parking lot may find that a hospital security committee is already looking into the problem.

Another way to generate interest in an issue is to write an article for the hospital or nursing department newsletter. Nurses who are present at nursing grand rounds also have the opportunity to inform their colleagues of an issue of mutual concern and enlist their aid in dealing with it. If there are no newsletters or grand rounds, a nurse can form a task force of concerned nurses and, using a model for change, plan a strategy to establish ways of helping nurses communicate with one another through a newsletter, grand rounds, or possibly a support group.

Nurses need certain knowledge and skills to increase their political astuteness and activity (Skaggs, 1994, p. 239; Ellis and Hartley, 1992, p. 359):

■ *Keeping informed about health care issues.* Obtain information from sources such as the daily newspaper; television and radio news reports; professional journals (space about current legislative issue is routinely

Tips on Committee Involvement

- The person who chairs a committee and sets the meeting agenda has a major influence on the direction of the committee's work.

- The person who takes minutes influences the manner in which the committee activities are recorded.

- The committee secretary can keep the participants focused on the agenda by alerting the chair when the group's attention strays. She might also offer to summarize the discussion to help the committee determine a plan of action.

- A committee member can influence action on an item of concern by lobbying other members before the meeting.

- Sometimes a member's initial efforts to influence action fail, but will be successful the second time.

- A member who wants to work on a particular committee should seek out the chair to find out details of the committee's work and then ask to be appointed.

Used by permission from D. J. Mason and J. K. Leavitt, *Policy and Politics in Nursing and Health Care,* 3d ed. Philadelphia: W.B. Saunders, 1998, p. 146.

provided in both national and state and provincial nursing journals); open meetings of nursing organizations or other health-related organizations, which often sponsor speakers who are knowledgeable about the issue.

■ *Ability to analyze an issue.* Identify all the relevant facts about the issue, look at the issue from all angles, and recognize how the issue fits into the larger picture.

■ *Ability to speak out and voice an opinion.* Obtain knowledge of both the issue and the best person to whom to voice the opinion. After studying the dynamics of the organization, the nurse may choose a head nurse or supervisor who is a good listener and is concerned about the issue.

■ *Ability to participate constructively.* Be a team player who encourages creative brainstorming and offers positive feasible alternative solutions to an issue, rather than offering only criticism.

■ *Ability to use power bases.* Through discussion with colleagues and other professional experiences, identify people who influence decision making. It is important to remember that power does not always follow the hierarchical lines on the organizational chart and that the source of information is sometimes considered as powerful as the information itself. The nurse who uses many different channels of information gains power to choose among them.

The politics of client care impinges on the practice of every nurse. For example, the prospective payment system has drastically shortened hospital stays in efforts to reduce hospital costs. Preparing clients for earlier discharge has brought about the need for nurses to be "faster and smarter" in delivering client care and client education.

How can nurses ensure that cost-containment measures do not impair the quality of nursing care? One way is for nurses to collaborate with each other and other providers to delegate nonnursing tasks, such as answering the telephone, emptying the garbage, and transporting nonacute clients. Developing a demonstration project that compares cost and quality of care issues under different hospital unit structures can provide the necessary data and generate support from other providers and administrators for changing the role of staff nurses. This sort of "proactive" planning can empower nurses to take charge of nursing practice in ways that benefit clients and health professionals while conserving scarce resources such as money, time, and supplies.

Nursing Organizations

Powerful and influential professional associations, such as the American Nurses Association and Canadian Nurses Association and their affiliated state/province and district associations, provide a collective voice for promoting nursing and quality health care. As such, these associations exert influence on the individual nurse as well as in the spheres of government, the workplace, the community, and the profession. Associations monitor and influence laws and regulations affecting nursing and health care. Their role in workplace matters ranges from studying practice issues to acting as the collective bargaining agent for nurses. Additionally, the professional nursing organization is often a visible presence in the community because it presents the nursing perspective on health care issues.

Professional organizations—including the ANA, CNA, NLN, and NSNA—publish articles on legislative matters and encourage nurses to take action on behalf of health care consumers and the nursing profession. Nursing lobbyists at the state and national level work to influence the development of health policy and legislation, but their success depends on the active support of nurses who back up these paid lobbyists by doing personal lobbying among their own elected officials.

The collective efforts of nurses influence the federal government through the political action committees such as the American Nurses Association Political Action Committee (ANA-PAC). ANA-PAC also counts on nurses at the grassroots level to work for these candidates and to serve as congressional district coordinators (CDCs). CDCs are responsible for organizing nurses in their congressional districts for lobbying and campaigning. This effort has provided a mechanism for nurses to influence governmental politics collectively at the federal level.

Individual nurses can become politically active in local, state or provincial, and national organizations by participating in the activities of their professional associations, by serving as delegates at conventions, by becoming members of commissions, and by supporting national association efforts such as the ANA's Nursing Agenda for Health Care Reform. Student nurses can benefit from participation in the National Student Nurses Association (NSNA) by learning about the politics of professional associations.

Community

The community in which the nurse lives and works can include the local neighborhood, the corporate world, the nation, and the international community. The community encompasses the workplace, professional organizations, and government. Many nurses, including Lillian Wald, founder of the Henry Street Settlement and modern public health nursing, view the community as more than a practice setting. Nurses who live in the community where they work can understand and influence the complex interplay among individuals and groups that compete for scarce resources.

Many communities depend on expert nurses to help with a wide variety of health and social policy decisions, such as environmental pollution and health care for the homeless. For example, a nurse who serves as an elected member of the community school board can influence decisions that affect the health and health care of students, such as the hiring of nurses for the school system. Nurses' opinions on matters of public health are frequently sought, and the enterprising nurse looks for opportunities to promote a positive image of nursing while serving the community.

Political involvement in the community often arises out of one's own interest in living and working in a community that is supportive of the health and well-being of its citizens. For instance, a nurse may become involved with an ad hoc committee to stop unlawful dumping of hazardous wastes in the neighborhood. As a member of such a group, the nurse wears two hats: She or he is both a concerned citizen and an expert on health issues. At the same time, the nurse's position in the group enables the nurse to extend networks and expand a support base for nursing.

As the self-help movement continues to expand, nurses are realizing how influential consumer groups can be. In many instances, such groups are founded by nurses who realize that customers, often their own clients, have a need for a self-help group. Sometimes nurses who have been clients themselves start postmastectomy support groups or similar groups. Nurses contribute their leadership skills to many organizations, including the National Alliance for the Mentally Ill (NAMI). The personally devastating experience of having a child with schizophrenia can be a powerful motivating force toward working in behalf of others through a group such as NAMI. The political power of groups with particular health concerns—including the Gray Panthers, the American Association of Retired Persons, and the Juvenile Diabetes Association—can generate extraordinary political influence on elected and appointed officials. Such groups offer nurses a variety of ways to learn about grassroots political activism. These groups can also be a community support base for nursing.

A variety of other opportunities for community involvement exist for nurses. Since many nurses are also parents, they can work on health issues through their school board. Those who ultimately run for government office have frequently begun their careers by running for the school board. Other nurses volunteer for community action groups, such as a community planning board or a fund-raising committee for the city's art museum. Or, a nurse may get involved in the tenant's organization in her or his apartment building. Regardless of the issue, the same opportunity to organize and plan for change exists in the community as it does in the workplace, government, or professional association.

The Government

Numerous ways to influence governments personally are open to nurses. Of course, the most basic step is registering to vote. Voter-registration drives are sponsored by a variety of organizations, including NSNA, which has developed a kit for nursing students to hold such drives. By voting, responsible citizens convey their opinions to elected and appointed officials on matters of concern.

The laws and regulations of local, state, and federal governments greatly influence nursing practice and health care. For example, federal laws and regulations establish funding of health care for the elderly, poor, and disabled (Medicare and Medicaid), authorize care services for special groups (including Native Americans, migrant workers, and veterans), set policies and formulas for reimbursement of health care services (as with prospective payment), and appropriate funding for special health care and social services (such as community health centers, the food stamp program, and the school lunch program).

State and provincial laws are responsible for defining and regulating nursing practice. Nurse practice acts in some states prohibit nurses from providing a broad range of services and can effectively limit nurses' ability to compete with other health care professionals in providing primary care services.

Nurses can become involved with political parties and local political clubs, work with elected officials, and accept political appointments as a means to influence health policy as well as nursing practice. Involvement in political parties and local political clubs enables the nurse to have some influence over affairs in the community and to develop a nonnursing support base for nursing and health care issues.

Nurses can also actively participate in campaigns of politicians who support nursing and health care, can become candidates for legislative offices, and act as information sources for legislative representatives. The box on page 197 lists ways to influence the legislative process for nursing and become politically active.

How to Influence Legislative and Regulatory Processes

- Become informed about the public policy and health policy issues that are currently under consideration at the local, state, and federal levels of government.

- Become acquainted with the public officials and elected officials that represent you in the legislative arena at the local, state, and federal levels of government. Communicate with them regularly to share your expertise and perspective on health care and nursing issues.

- Call, write, or send a fax or e-mail message to your legislator, stating briefly the position you wish him or her to take on a particular issue. Always remember to mention that you are a registered nurse and that you live and vote in the legislator's district.

- Request that legislation be introduced or a regulatory change made. Offer your expertise to assist in developing new legislation or in modifying existing legislation/rules.

- Become active in your professional association and work to activate a strong grassroots network of

- members who are prepared to contact their elected representatives on key health care issues.

- Attend a public hearing on a bill or regulation to show support for an issue, or actually testify yourself.

- Build your own political resumé—become active in local politics in your area.

- Volunteer to work on the campaigns of candidates who are knowledgeable and supportive of nursing's perspective on health care issues.

- Seek appointment to a government task force or commission and have the opportunity to make legislative, regulatory, and public policy changes.

- Seek election to public office or employment in an administrative or executive agency.

- Explore opportunities to be involved with the policy and legislative process through internships, fellowships, and volunteer experiences at the local, state, and federal levels.

Used by permission from D. J. Mason and J. K. Leavitt, *Policy and Politics in Nursing and Health Care,* 3d ed. Philadelphia: W.B. Saunders, 1998, p. 395.

Consider . . .

- ways in which you have participated in political activities in the past—in the work setting, in professional organizations, in the community, and in government.
- how you would like to increase your participation in political activities.
- whether you believe nurses have an obligation to be politically active. Why or why not?

- selected political issues affecting nursing:
  a. Reimbursement of nursing services
  b. Equal pay for work of comparable value
  c. National health insurance
  d. Health care reform
  What sources would you use to obtain information about these issues? What political actions would you like taken in regard to these issues?

SUMMARY

Power is an invaluable instrument, the effects of which can be positive or negative depending on the way it is used and the ends to which it is applied. Power is assumed by a person; it is a skill that can be learned and effectively practiced. Sources or bases of power are described as reward, coercive, legitimate, referent, expert, connection, and information powers. An understanding of these sources helps nurses formulate a plan to develop their own power and to recognize it in others. Benner describes six types of power that nurses use when caring for clients: transformative power, integrative power, advocacy power, healing power,

participative/affirmative power, and problem-solving power. Empowerment enables individuals and groups to participate in actions and decision making in a context that supports an equitable distribution of power.

Politics is the process of influencing the allocation of scarce resources in the spheres of government, workplace, organizations, and community. Political action in one sphere often affects other spheres. Strategies to influence political decisions include negotiating, networking, establishing political action committees, communicating with legislators, building coalitions, lobbying, and testifying.

As citizens, parents, and members of the nursing profession, all nurses can contribute to political activities in numerous ways—by voting, joining organizations, becoming members of committees, supporting deserving candidates, and so on. To make any effective contribution, nurses must keep themselves informed about health care and nursing issues, be able to analyze an issue, voice an opinion, participate constructively, use power bases, and communicate clearly. Nurses who value the nursing perspective on health issues recognize that a powerful voice for nurses is a powerful voice for health care consumers, the profession, and the nation.

SELECTED REFERENCES

Backer, B. A., Costello-Nickitas, D. M., Mason, D. J., McBride, A. B., and Vance, C. 1993. Feminist perspectives on policy and politics. In D. J. Mason, S. W. Talbott, and J. K. Leavitt, *Policy and politics for nurses: Action and change in the workplace, government, organizations, and community,* 2d ed. Philadelphia: W. B. Saunders.

Benner, P. 1984. *From novice to expert: Excellence and power in clinical nursing practice.* Menlo Park, Calif.: Addison-Wesley Nursing.

Berle, A. A. 1969. *Power.* New York: Harcourt, Brace, and World.

Boykin, A., ed. 1995. *Power, politics and public policy: A matter of caring.* New York: National League for Nursing. Pub. no. 14-2684.

Claus, K. E., and Bailey, J. T. 1977. *Power and influence in health care: A new approach to leadership.* St. Louis: Mosby.

Conger, J. A., and Kanungo, R. N. 1988. The empowerment process: Integrating theory and practice. *Academic Management Review* 13(3): 471–482.

Davidhizar, R., and Giger, J. N. 1994, Sept./Oct. You have power, too! *NSNA/Imprint* 41(4): 64–66.

Dennis, K. E. 1991. Empowerment. In J. L. Creasia and B. Parker, eds., *Conceptual foundations of professional nursing practice.* St. Louis: Mosby-Year Book.

Ellefsen, B., and Hamilton, G. 2000. Empowered nurses? Nurses in Norway and the USA compared. *International Nursing Review* 47: 106–120.

Ellis, J. R., and Hartley, C. L. 1992. *Nursing in today's world: Challenges, issues, and trends,* 4th ed. Philadelphia: Lippincott.

Ferguson, V. D. 1993. Perspectives on power. In D. J. Mason, S. W. Talbott, and J. K. Leavitt, *Policy and politics for nurses: Action and change in the workplace, government, organizations, and community,* 2d ed. Philadelphia: W.B. Saunders.

French, J. R., and Raven, B. H. 1960. The bases of social power. In D. Cartwright & A. Zanders, eds., *Group dynamics: Research and theory,* 2d ed. New York: Harper and Row.

Gilbert, T. 1995, May. Nursing: Empowerment and the problem of power. *Journal of Advanced Nursing* 21: 865–871.

Hershey, P., Blanchard, K. and Natemeyer, W. 1979. Situational leadership: Perception and impact of power. *Group Organizational Studies* 4: 418–428.

Huxley, E. 1975. *Florence Nightingale.* New York: Putnam.

Kanter, R. M. 1993. *Men and women of the corporation,* 2d ed. New York: Basic Books.

Kelly, R. M., and Duerst-Lahti, G. 1995. The study of gender power and its link to governance and leadership. In G Duerst-Lahti and R. N. Kelly, eds., *Gender power, leadership and governance* (pp. 39–64). Ann Arbor: University of Michigan Press.

Kuokkanen, L., and Leino-Kilpi, H. 2000. Power and empowerment in nursing: Three theoretical approaches. *Journal of Advanced Nursing* 31(1): 235–241.

Laschinger, H. K. S., Wong, C., McMahon, L., and Kaufmann, C. 1999. Leader behavior impact on staff nurse empowerment, job tension, and work effectiveness. *Journal of Nursing Administration* 29(5): 28–39.

Laschinger, H. K. S., Finegan, J., Shamian, J., and Casier, S. 2000. Organizational trust and empowerment in restructured healthcare settings: Effects on staff nurse commitment. *Journal of Nursing Administration* 30 (9): 413–425.

Lee, L. 2000, Oct. Buzzwords with a basis. *Nursing Management:* 10, 25–27.

Mason, D. J., and Leavitt, J. K. 1998. *Policy and politics in nursing and health care,* 3d ed. Philadelphia: W.B. Saunders.

Milstead, J. A. 1999. *Health policy and politics: A nurse's guide.* Gaithersburg, Md.: Aspen Publications.

Skaggs, B. 1994. Political action in nursing. In J. Zerwekh and J. C. Claborn, *Nursing today: Transitions and trends* (pp. 236–256). Philadelphia: W.B. Saunders.

The Nurse as Colleague and Collaborator

Objectives

- Explain the essential aspects of collaborative health care.
- Discuss the nurse's collaborative role.
- Describe the competencies in collaborative practice.
- Analyze factors that impact collaboration in health care.

NURSE CONNECT

Additional online resources for this chapter can be found on the companion web site at www.prenhall.com/blais.

Changing models of health care have created a need for modification of traditional roles. Nurses and physicians have been especially affected by these changes and work more collaboratively. According to the ANA (1995):

The boundaries of each health care professional are constantly changing, and members of various professions cooperate by exchanging knowledge and ideas about how to deliver high-quality health care. Collaboration among health care professionals involves recognition of the expertise of others within and outside one's profession and referral to those providers when appropriate. Collaboration also involves some shared functions and common focus on the same overall mission.

Traditionally, models of health care have shown a one-sided distribution of power in provider-client relationships. The system has been physician dominated and has focused on cure of illness. Recently, however, the health care system has moved toward more collaborative efforts and initiatives in which provider and client become partners in care. Many advance the idea that care is client centered and client directed and involves collaboration between provider and client.

With the restructuring of health care, the old systems and practices have changed health jobs in ways designed to improve care and control costs. This restructuring has changed roles and created new ways of interacting among the members of the health care team.

CHALLENGES AND OPPORTUNITIES

Resistance to change is inevitable when the traditional ways of providing care have been so drastically disrupted by the changes in health care that were outside the control of those affected by the change. Changes in power structure are particularly difficult to manage. Nurses need to develop the ability to assume a new place in health care and work with those members of the team who are not fully accepting of the new structure.

Opportunities to create new practice models and redefine relationships are now abundantly available to nurses. The time is ripe for a reshaping of practice under the direction of those willing to assume leadership.

COLLABORATIVE HEALTH CARE

During the early years, the nurse was seen as providing assistance to the physician in caring for patients. The term handmaiden has been used to describe the role. However, during wars and times of crisis, nurses worked in a more collegial and autonomous manner. As early as the American Civil War, there is documentation of a more independent practice (Nursing Trends and Issues 1998). The emergence of advanced practice nursing roles provided impetus to the emerging concerns about collegiality and collaboration. In 1992 the ANA held a Congress on Nursing Practice and adopted the following operational definition of collaboration:

"**Collaboration** means a collegial working relationship with another health care provider in the provision of (to supply) patient care. Collaborative practice requires (may include) the discussion of patient diagnosis and cooperation in the management and delivery of care. Each collaborator is available to the other for consultation either in person or by communication device, but need not be physically present on the premises at the time the actions are performed. The patient-designated health care provider is responsible for the overall direction and management of patient care" (ANA 1992).

Characteristics and Beliefs Basic to Collaborative Health Care

- Clients have a right to self-determination: that is, the right to choose to participate or not to participate in health care decision making.

- Clients and health care professionals interact in a reciprocal relationship. Instead of making decisions about the client's health care, health care professionals foster joint decision making. Client dependence and professional dominance are minimized; client participation in the health care process is maximized.

- Equality among human beings is desired in health care relationships. The ideas of both clients and health care professionals receive an equal hearing.

- Responsibility for health falls on the client rather than on health care professionals.

- Each individual's concept of health is important and legitimate for that individual. Although clients lack expert knowledge, they have their own ideas about health and illness. Health care professionals need to understand these ideas to be able to effectively help the client.

- Collaboration involves negotiation and consensus seeking rather than questioning and ordering.

ANA Standard of Clinical Nursing Practice for Collaboration

STANDARD VI. COLLABORATION

THE NURSE COLLABORATES WITH THE PATIENT, FAMILY, AND OTHER HEALTH CARE PROVIDERS IN PROVIDING PATIENT CARE.

Measurement Criteria

1. The nurse communicates with the patient, family, and other health care providers regarding patient care and nursing's role in the provision of care.

2. The nurse collaborates with the patient, family, and other health care providers in the formulation of overall goals and the plan of care and in decisions related to care and the delivery of services.

3. The nurse consults with other health care providers for patient care, as needed.

4. The nurse makes referrals, including provisions for continuity of care, as needed.

Virginia Henderson (1991, p. 44), one of the pioneers of nursing, defines collaborative care as "a partnership relationship between doctors, nurses, and other health care providers with patients and their families." It is a process by which heath care professionals work together with clients to achieve quality health care outcomes. Mutual respect and a true sharing of both power and control are essential elements. Ideally, collaboration becomes a dynamic, interactive process in which clients (individuals, groups, or communities) confer with physicians, nurses, and other health care providers to meet their health objectives. Effective collaboration requires cooperation and coordination between client(s) and various health care providers across the continuum of care. See the accompanying boxes.

More recently, a published executive summary from ANA (1998) released in *Nursing Trends and Issues* described collaboration as intrinsic to nursing:

> Nurses and physicians working together and independently assessing, diagnosing, and caring for consumers by preparing patient histories, conducting physical and psychosocial assessments, and reviewing and discussing their cases with other health professionals to determine the changing health status of each client.
>
> To provide effective and comprehensive care, nurses, physicians, and other health care professionals must collaborate with each other. No group can claim total authority over the other. The different areas of professional competence exhibited by each profession, when combined, provide a continuum of care that the consumer has come to expect (www.nursingworld.org/readroom/nti/9805nti.htm).

Research Box

Higgins, L. W. 1999. Nurses' perceptions of collaborative nurse-physician transfer decision making as a predictor of patient outcomes in a medical intensive care unit. *Journal of Advanced Nursing* **29(6): 1434–1443.**

Using a prospective correlation design, a convenience sample of 175 patient-transfer decisions was examined. Medical records and electronic databases were used to collect patient information and a questionnaire was developed to gather demographic data from 42 nurses working in a medical intensive care unit. These nurses also completed an adapted version of the Decision about Transfer scale to measure perceptions of collaboration and satisfaction with regard to the decisions. The Acute Physiology and Chronic Health Evaluation was utilized to adjust for patient risk.

Nurses in this study perceived their involvement in decision making to be at a very low level. There was a positive correlation between nurses' perception of collaboration and their satisfaction with the decision to transfer. However, the perceptions were not significant predictors of patient outcomes. Furthermore, analysis of decision complexity and years of nursing experience did not moderate the prediction of outcomes. The findings of this study are in conflict with other similar studies. The researchers believe that this is due to the lower level of perceived collaboration in this group of nurses. This validates the need for research related to differences in outcomes related to varying levels of collaboration between nurses and physicians.

Collaborative Practice

The overall objectives of collaborative initiatives are high-quality client care and client satisfaction. In addition, many health care professionals believe that a multidisciplinary, collaborative framework can limit costs as well as enhance quality. Collaborative practice models propose to achieve several objectives:

- Provide client-directed and client-centered care using a multidisciplinary, integrated, participative framework.
- Enhance continuity across the continuum of care, from prehospitalization through an acute episode of illness to transfer or discharge and recuperation.
- Improve client(s) and family satisfaction with care.
- Provide quality, cost-effective, research-based care that is outcome driven.
- Promote mutual respect, communication, and understanding between client(s) and members of the health care team.
- Create a synergy among clients and providers, in which the sum of their efforts is greater than the parts.
- Provide opportunities to address and solve system-related issues and problems.
- Develop interdependent relationships and understanding among providers and clients.

See the accompanying box.

Collaborative practice can include nurse-physician interaction in joint practice, nurse-physician collaboration in care giving, or interdisciplinary teams or committees.

Interdisciplinary collaborative practice teams may consist of a single unit or a group of units with similar client populations. Most committees consist of physicians, nurses, social workers, pharmacists, and other health care professionals (Velianoff, Neely, and Hall 1993). Such multidisciplinary teams address clinical practice guidelines and clinical issues so as to ensure cost-effective, quality outcomes. Committees such as these may provide the foundation for establishing a truly collaborative practice setting.

The ability to collaborate becomes particularly important when nurses implement advanced-practice roles; it has been designated as a core competency for advanced-practice nurses. The drivers for this have been health care reform, leading to group practice and managed care as well as certification and practice standards. A continuum of collaboration begins with parallel communication, whereby everyone is communicating with the client independently and asking the same questions. Parallel functioning may have more coordinated communication, but each professional has separate interventions and a separate plan of care. Information exchange involves planned communication, but decision making is unilateral, involving little, if any, collegiality. Coordination and consultation represent midrange levels of collaboration seeking to maximize the efficiency of resources. Comanagement and referral represent the upper levels of collaboration, where providers retain responsibility and accountability for

A Practice Exemplar of Collaboration

The Heart Center of Excellence of the North Broward Hospital District has developed a practice model based on collaboration, problem solving, and reevaluation, referred to as CPR techniques. Using this model has resulted in drastically reducing postoperative intubation time and the out-of-bed interval following extubation. Same-day admissions, first-day postoperative transfers, and length of stay following cardiac surgery also declined.

The key players in the team included medical staff, nursing, respiratory therapists, perfusionists, radiology technicians, exercise physiologists, case managers/social services, and pharmacy personnel. Collaboration was considered an essential component of success in the team effort.

As the model was implemented, some barriers to collaboration emerged, including the perspectives of the

multiple disciplines. A second was the multicultural nature of this diverse staff group; cultural influences were apparent in practice and communication. Beliefs and traditional practices were challenged, which created tension. To build a collaborative team, cultural awareness and education were approached with a variety of techniques, including role playing, cross-cultural experiences, exploration of personal beliefs and values, and evaluating communication styles.

Self-directed work teams (SDWT) were implemented and made accountable for outcomes. This improved the teamwork and resulted in increased resilience, with a direct effect on patient outcomes. It provided for a best-practice model for successfully improving outcomes in heart centers.

Figure 12–1

Continuum of Collaboration

Highest Level

┌-- Referral

├-- Comanagement

├-- Consultation

├-- Coordination

├-- Information exchange

├-- Parallel functioning

└-- Parallel communication

Lowest Level

their own aspects of care and patients are directed to other providers when the problem is beyond their expertise. Figure 12–1 illustrates this continuum.

Characteristics of effective collaboration include the following:

1. Common purpose and goals identified at the outset

2. Clinical competence of each provider
3. Interpersonal competence
4. Humor
5. Trust
6. Valuing and respecting diverse, complementary knowledge

Processes associated with these characteristics include recurring interactions among the providers of health care that bridge professional boundaries and develop connections. Interpersonal skills and respect for the competence of collaborators are essential to the outcome. Successful consultation comes about when there is recognition of the unique contribution that each person can make so that a unified plan can be implemented.

The Nurse as a Collaborator

Nurses collaborate with clients, peers, and other health care professionals. They frequently collaborate about client care but may also be involved, for example, in collaborating on bioethical issues, on legislation, on health-related research, and with professional organizations. The accompanying box outlines selected aspects of the nurse's role as a collaborator.

Collaboration is important in professional nursing

The Nurse as a Collaborator

With Clients:

- Acknowledges, supports, and encourages clients' active involvement in health care decisions.

- Encourages a sense of client autonomy and an equal position with other members of the health care team.

- Helps clients set mutually agreed-upon goals and objectives for health care.

- Provides client consultation in a collaborative fashion.

With Peers:

- Shares personal expertise with other nurses and elicits the expertise of others to ensure quality client care.

- Develops a sense of trust and mutual respect with peers that recognizes their unique contributions.

With Other Health Care Professionals:

- Recognizes the contribution that each member of the interdisciplinary team can make by virtue of his or her expertise and view of the situation.

- Listens to each individual's views.

- Shares health care responsibilities in exploring options, setting goals, and making decisions with clients and families.

- Participates in collaborative interdisciplinary research to increase knowledge of a clinical problem or situation.

With Professional Nursing Organizations:

- Seeks out opportunities to collaborate with and within professional organizations.

- Serves on committees in state (or provincial) and national nursing organizations or specialty groups.

- Supports professional organizations in political action to create solutions for professional and health care concerns.

With Legislators:

- Offers expert opinions on legislative initiatives related to health care.

- Collaborates with other health care providers and consumers on health care legislation to best serve the needs of the public.

practice as a way to improve client outcomes. To fulfill a collaborative role, nurses need to assume accountability and increased authority in practice areas. Education is integral to ensuring that the members of each professional group understand the collaborative nature of their roles, specific contributions, and the importance of working together. Each professional needs to understand how an integrated delivery system centers on the client's health care needs rather than on the particular care given by one group.

Collaboration in practice is not yet a reality for most nurses. However, because nurses are now more highly educated and have a defined area of expertise, nurses increasingly are functioning more as autonomous health professionals.

Benefits of Collaborative Care

A collaborative approach to health care ideally benefits clients, professionals, and the health care delivery system. Care becomes client centered and, most important, client directed. Clients become informed consumers and actively participate with the health care team in the decision-making process. When clients are empowered to participate actively and professionals share mutually set goals with clients, everyone—including the organization and health care system—ultimately benefits. When quality improves, adherence to therapeutic regimens increases, lengths of stay decrease, and overall costs to the system decline. When professional interdependence develops, collegial relationships emerge, and overall satisfaction increases. The work environment becomes more supportive and acknowledges the contributions of each team member. "Because authority is shared, this effort results in more integrated and comprehensive care, as well as shared control of costs and liability" (Miccolo and Spanier, 1993, p. 447).

COMPETENCIES BASIC TO COLLABORATION

Key features necessary for collaboration include effective communication skills, mutual respect, trust, giving and receiving feedback, decision making, and conflict management.

Communication Skills

Collaborating to solve complex problems requires effective communication skills. Initially the health care team needs to define collaboration clearly, establish its goals and objectives, and specify role expectations.

Effective communication can occur only if the involved parties are committed to understanding each other's professional roles and appreciating each other as individuals. Additionally, they must be sensitive to differences among communication styles. Instead of focusing on distinctions, each professional group needs to center on their common ground: the client's needs.

Communication styles are especially important to successful collaboration. Norton's theory of communicator style (1983) defines style as the manner in which one communicates and includes the way in which one interacts. Therefore, what is said and how it is said are both important. This theory describes nine specific communicator styles that are commonly used and impact the nature of the relationship between communicants. Three of these communicator styles (dominant, contentious, and attentive) have been used in a nursing study of collaboration styles as they relate to degree of collaboration and improved quality of care (Van Ess Coeling and Cukr 2000). Using attentive style and avoiding contentious and dominant styles made a significant difference in nurse-physician collaboration, positive patient outcomes, and nurse satisfaction. The researchers assert that attentive style can be taught by modeling the behavior of obvious listening, such as making eye contact while communicating and refraining from participating in other activities that interrupt communication while someone is trying to communicate. Verbal feedback and repeating back offers the opportunity to reflect on what was said and to correct misunderstanding. Questioning provides an opportunity to share concerns and initiate dialogue. Developing a noncontentious style means developing judgment in recognizing when it is necessary to stop a conversation and insist on clarification because it is an important point and when it is better to ignore a comment that is disagreed with because it is not essential to the goal. Developing a nondominant style involves controlling behavior of monopolizing the conversation or speaking so forcefully that others feel pushed back and unwilling to respond. Role playing followed by discussion and role modeling have been identified as effective strategies for developing positive communicator styles.

Mutual Respect and Trust

Mutual respect occurs when two or more people show or feel honor or esteem toward one another. **Trust** occurs when a person is confident in the actions of another person. Both mutual respect and trust imply a mutual process and outcome. They must be expressed both verbally and nonverbally. Sometimes professionals may verbalize respect or trust of others but demonstrate by their actions a lack of trust and respect. The health care system itself has not always created an environment that promotes respect or trust of the various health care providers. Although progress has been made toward creating more collegial relationships, past attitudes may continue to impede efforts toward collaborative practice.

Giving and Receiving Feedback

One of the most difficult challenges for professionals is giving and receiving timely, relevant, and helpful **feedback** to and from each other and their clients. When professionals work closely together, it may be appropriate to address attitudes or actions that affect the collaborative relationship. Feedback may be affected by each person's perceptions, personal space, roles, relationships, self-esteem, confidence, beliefs, emotions, environment, and time.

Negative feedback implies not negative content but rather a negative communication style, such as an attitude of condescension; positive feedback is characterized by a communication style that is warm, caring, and respectful. A review of basic communication skills and an opportunity to practice listening and giving and receiving feedback can enhance any professional's ability to communicate effectively (Ferguson, Howell, and Batalden, 1993, p. 5). Giving and receiving feedback helps individuals acquire self-awareness, while assisting the collaborative team to develop an understanding and effective working relationship.

Decision Making

The decision-making process at the team level involves shared responsibility for the outcome. Obviously, to create a solution, the team must follow each step of the decision-making process beginning with a clear definition of the problem. Team decision making must be directed at the objectives of the specific effort. Factors that enhance the process include mutual respect and constructive and timely feedback (Mariano, 1989, p. 287).

Decision making at the team level requires full consideration and respect of diverse viewpoints. Members must be able to verbalize their perspectives in a nonthreatening environment. Group members effectively use communication skills and give and receive feedback in the decision-making process. Interdependent relationships are actualized as members focus on client care issues (Velianoff, Neely, and Hall, 1993, p. 28).

An important aspect of decision making is the interdisciplinary team focusing on the client's priority needs and organizing interventions accordingly. The discipline best able to address the client's needs is given priority in planning and is responsible for providing its interventions in a timely manner. For example, a social worker may first direct attention to a client's social needs when these needs interfere with the client's ability to respond to therapy. Nurses, by the nature of their holistic practice, are often able to help the team identify priorities and areas requiring further attention.

Conflict Management

Role conflict can occur in any situation where individuals work together. **Role conflict** arises when people are called on to carry out roles that have opposing or incompatible expectations. In an interpersonal conflict, different people have different expectations about a particular role. Interrole conflict exists when one person's or group's expectations differ from the expectations of another person or group. Any one of these types of conflict can affect interdisciplinary collaboration.

To reduce role conflict, team members can also conduct interdisciplinary conferences, take part in interdisciplinary education in basic programs, and, most important, accept personal responsibility for team work (Benson and Ducanis, 1995, p. 211). Ongoing research exploring how professionals relate and how teams function will help professionals better understand ways to reduce role conflict when they collaborate with others.

Consider . . .

- what barriers to collaborative care you experience in your practice setting.
- what characteristics support collaborative practice in your practice setting.
- approaches you might implement to enhance collaboration.
- how your values, beliefs, and work experiences influence your abilities to be a collaborative member of a health care team.

It has been suggested that the failure of professionals to collaborate is due not to intent, but rather to lack of necessary skills (Van Ess Coeling and Cukr 2000). Expertise in collaboration and education in collaborative skills have been overlooked. Historically, nursing has been interested in identifying and valuing "nursing" as a unique entity and concentrating on nursing theory, nursing research, and nursing practice. Now the attention is shifting toward interdisciplinary collaboration and recognition of alternative perspectives. This requires not only the ability to articulate one's own perspective, but also the ability to engage in mutual give and take in order to determine the best approach to the specific situation.

Organizational structure contributes to the success of interdisciplinary collaboration. Structures that maintain a hierarchical authoritarian structure do not support interdisciplinary collaboration. The organization can be particularly effective in the promotion of collaboration between physicians and nurses where the tradition of an authority figure has been particularly strong. The relationship among participants must be one of trust and respect. The failure on anyone's part to either assume or yield power appropriately can block collaboration.

Conflict is inevitable in organizations, and that conflict can be functional, serving to generate positive changes, or dysfunctional, serving to choke the organization's efforts. There are five stages, or levels, of conflict. *Latent conflict* is always present when there is a complex organization or when roles are differentiated and may come into conflict. *Perceived conflict* is when awareness begins. The conflict may or may not progress beyond a latent or perceived level. When it does progress, *felt conflict* occurs, and hostilities, anxieties, and stress erupt. *Overt conflict* results when the conflict is acted out and battle lines are drawn. *Conflict aftermath* comes about with a resolution, and it may or not be optimal. The results may range from full cooperation to active or passive resistance. Although the conflict is resolved, the behaviors may still be affected There may be difficulty "letting go" once there is resolution.

The conflicts may be interpersonal between or among individuals, or the conflicts may involve groups. Intergroup conflicts may occur between nurses and laboratory personnel or between nurses and physicians, for example. Intragroup conflicts may occur within a group, such as when nurses on a care unit disagree about policies governing practice, such as a plan or policy for floating to another unit.

Whatever the conflict, resolution strategies are important to success. *Problem solving or confrontation* can be applied through open discussion and a thorough investigation of the dimensions of the conflict. When the goal is a win-win outcome in which each side is satisfied with the outcome, success is more likely. *Negotiating, or bargaining,* entails identifying one's bottom line as well as one's optimal result and then making trade-offs to get a final agreement that is as close as possible to one's optimal position. For this approach to be successful, both parties must be sincere in the desire to negotiate. Negotiation can be either cooperative or competitive; characteristics of each are found in Table 12–1. *Smoothing over* is a short-term resolution focused on minimizing the felt conflict without resolving it. With this approach, the felt conflict is likely to reemerge. *Avoidance* may be used when one side makes the decision to cease discussion and withdraw. *Forcing* uses power or influence to impose a preference; this often involves "going over someone's head" and using a higher authority to enforce the resolution.

FACTORS LEADING TO THE NEED FOR INCREASED COLLEGIALITY AND COLLABORATION

Collaboration is necessary to effectively meet the current problems facing the health care system. Among

Table 12–1 Characteristics of Negotiation

Cooperative Negotiation	Competitive Negotiation
The tangible goals of the negotiation are seen as fair and reasonable to each side.	The tangible goals are for each side to get as much as possible.
There are sufficient resources for a win-win resolution.	There are insufficient resources for each side to attain the desired goal.
Each side believes they can attain their desired goal.	Each side believes it is not possible for each side to attain the desired goal.
The sides work together to maximize joint outcomes.	The goal is to win against the other side.

those problems are unmet health care needs of the older adult, the increased number of people who have chronic illnesses, and poverty and homelessness. These health problems are complex and involve diverse needs requiring expertise across disciplines.

Worldwide, there are a number of significant influences on health and health care that will require international collaboration. The World Health Organization (WHO) set an objective that they hoped all persons would achieve by the year 2000, a level of health that would permit them to lead socially and economically productive lives. The report *Healthy People 2000* focused on national health promotion and disease prevention goals for U.S. citizens. *Healthy People 2010* (USDHHS 2000) continues the objective of improving health and well-being worldwide.

Increasingly, governments and society are striving to reduce health risks, minimize the incidence of chronic illness, and improve the health and quality of life for all. The overall goal is to provide health care for all individuals, but health and health care are not guaranteed. Today, the most pressing question for the health care system remains how to provide quality health care that is in line with the socioeconomic realities of society. A number of factors influence the provision of health care; they are described here.

Consumer Wants and Needs

Although the diagnosis and treatment of illness are still necessities, the focus of health care is changing. Health care consumers are demanding comprehensive, holistic, and compassionate health care that is also affordable. Clients expect that health care providers will view each person as a biopsychosocial whole and respond to his or her individual needs. They want wellness-related care that focuses on the quality of life, not the quantity of life. They want expert care that humanistically integrates that available technology and provides information and services related to health promotion and illness prevention.

Today's health care consumers have greater knowledge about their health than in previous years and they are increasingly influencing health care delivery. Formerly, people expected a physician to make decisions about their care; today, however, consumers expect to be involved in making any decisions.

Consumers have also become aware of how lifestyle affects health. As a result, they desire more information and services related to health promotion and illness prevention.

Increasingly people are actively assuming responsibility for their level of health and are willing to participate in health-promoting activities. They are beginning to view health care professionals as a resource to guide these activities. Many health plans already provide participants with memberships to physical fitness clubs and nutrition classes or offer free attendance at smoking-cessation classes.

Self-Help Initiatives

Responsibility for the self is a major belief underlying holistic health that recognizes the interdependency of body, mind, and spirit. Increasingly people are adopting the view that the self is empowered with the ability to create or maintain health or disease.

Today many individuals seek answers for acute and chronic health problems through nontraditional approaches to health care. Alternative medicine and support groups are among two of the most popular self-help choices. Each year, more adults are using alternative or unconventional therapies to treat numerous health problems. The most commonly used therapies include relaxation techniques, chiropractic treatments, massage, imagery, spiritual healing, weight-loss programs, and herbal medicine. Back problems, fibromyalgia, cancer, allergies, arthritis, insomnia, chronic fatigue syndrome, strains or sprains, headache, high blood pressure, digestive problems, anxiety, and depression are the most common conditions for which individuals seek unconventional therapy.

In addition to alternative therapies, many adults participate in one or more self-help groups during their lifetime. In North America, there are more than 500 different mutual support or self-help groups that focus on nearly every major health problem or life crisis people experience. These groups developed, in part, because people felt such organizations could meet needs not addressed by the traditional health care system. Alcoholics Anonymous (AA), which formed in 1935, serves as a model for many of these groups. The National Self-Help Clearinghouse in the United States provides information on current support groups and guidelines about how to start a self-help group. Groups vary in effectiveness, but most provide education to encourage self-care as well as offering social and emotional support.

Changing Demographics and Epidemiology

It is predicted that by the year 2020, there will be more than 50 million adults over the age of 65 years living in the United States (Abrams, Beers, and Berkow, 2000). The growing number of older adults, combined with the fact that the average older adult has three or more chronic health conditions, will greatly impact the health care system and insurers in the future.

Closely related is the major epidemiological influence posed by chronic illness. One of these is HIV/AIDS, a problem that is growing each year. The Centers for Disease Control and Prevention report that a total of 733,374 Americans have been diagnosed with AIDS and 59% of that group have died. Worldwide, it is estimated that 32.4 million adults and 1.2 million children are living with HIV/AIDS (Centers for Disease Control and Prevention, 1999).

According to the National Coalition for the Homeless (1999), homelessness and poverty are inextricably linked. Limited resources result in difficult choices when trying to pay for housing, food, childcare, health care, etc. The number of poor in the United States has remained fairly stable in recent years; however, the number of people living in extreme poverty has increased dramatically. In the two-year span from 1995–1997, the number increased by 500,000 (U.S. Bureau of the Census, 1998). Limited access to health care services significantly impacts the health of the poor and the homeless.

Health Care Costs

Expenditures for health care in the United States were more than $1.1 trillion in 1998, an increase of 5.6% from 1997 (HCFA, 1998). Despite these tremendous expenses, a number of Americans have limited access to health care. However, in the United States there are not accurate data about how many individuals are underinsured or uninsured.

The health care system in the United States is thought to be in financial distress. For example, since its inception, Medicare has repeatedly increased monthly premiums, deductibles, and related taxes.

Several alternative health delivery systems have been implemented to control costs. These include health maintenance organizations (HMOs), preferred provider organizations (PPOs), physician/hospital organizations (PHOs), and so on. Additionally, the development of prospective payment systems significantly influenced the health care system. Concerns remain, however, about ways to further reduce health care costs and at the same time achieve the desired goal of improving the quality of health care delivery.

Employers, legislators, insurers, and health care providers continue to collaborate in efforts to resolve these concerns. Ethical issues such as rationing of health care, access to health care, the use of health care technology and extraordinary interventions, and organ transplantation can be resolved only through collaboration.

Technological Advances

Technology has had a major influence on health care costs and services. In fact, available technology often influences decisions about the level of care and intervention. With advances in medicine and technology, an individual's life span can in many cases be extended. However, that same technology may result in fragmentation of care and acceleration of health care costs. New medical devices, technological advances, and new medications frequently are introduced with limited consideration to the associated costs or the efficacy of their use. For example, the vital functions of circulation and breathing of a client who has no measurable brain activity can be maintained through advanced life support. In the United States, it is estimated that more than 25% of Medicare dollars are expended for the last year of life (Abrams, Beers, and Berkow, 2000). At the societal level, the difficult questions of when and how life should be extended through use of technology have not been answered.

Consider . . .

- which demographic factors most affect your practice setting.
- how you would advise a client who asks you about the use of a nontraditional approach to health care.

Bookshelf

Schrage, M. 1995. *No more teams! Mastering the dynamics of creative collaboration.* **New York: Currency Doubleday.**
In this follow-up book to *Shared Minds,* the author discusses communication in organizations and the optimum use of modern technology.

Schrage, M. 1990. *Shared minds: The new technologies of collaboration.* **New York: Random House.**
This book discusses business management with a focus on communication using new technologies.

SUMMARY

Collaborative health care is a concept that addresses many existing problems in the health care system. Its multidisciplinary, integrated, and participative approach focuses on client-centered and client-directed care. Collaborative care involves mutual goal setting and care planning between the client, physicians, nurses, and other involved health care providers.

Key competencies necessary for collaborative practice include effective communication skills, mutual respect and trust, giving and receiving feedback, decision-making ability, and conflict management. In addition, each health team member needs knowledge about the roles, views, and unique contributions of the other team members.

Several factors are currently impacting health care delivery. These include (1) the World Health Organization's objective for all people to achieve by the year 2000 a level of health that will permit them to lead socially and economically productive lives; (2) consumers of health care, who are insisting on comprehensive, holistic, compassionate, and affordable health care that includes services related to health promotion and illness prevention; (3) increasing recognition by consumers of self-help initiatives such as alternative or nontraditional health care and self-help groups; (4) changing demographics, such as an increase in the older, homeless, and AIDS populations; (5) economic issues related to health care, in particular, the exorbitant costs of health care and inequities in people covered by insurance in the United States; and (6) technological advances.

Health care systems remain challenged to provide cost-efficient care and, at the same time, to ensure quality care to all. *Nursing's Agenda for Health Care Reform* emphasizes a basic "core" of essential health care services for everyone and a restructuring of the health care system to focus on consumers and their health needs.

REFERENCES

Abrams, W. B., Beers, M. H., and Berkow, R. eds. 2000. *The Merck manual of geriatrics,* 3d ed. Whitehouse Station, N.J.: Merck.

Alspach, G. 1999. When the "evidence" in evidence-based practice is ignored: A time for advocacy. *Critical Care Nursing* 19(4): 10, 12, 14.

American Nurse Association. 1992. *House of delegates report: 1992 convention, Las Vegas, Nev.* (pp. 104–120). Kansas City, Mo.: ANA.

American Nurses Association. 1995. *Nursing's policy statement.* Washington, D.C.: ANA.

American Nurses Association. 1998. Collaboration and independent practice: Ongoing issues for nursing. *Nursing Trends and Issues* 3(5).

Angelucci, P. 1999. Advocate for your patients—and your nurses, *Nurse Manager* 30(11): 14.

Benson, L., and Ducanis, A. 1995. Nurses' perceptions of their role and role conflicts. *Rehabilitation Nursing* 20: 204–211.

Centers for Disease Control and Prevention. 1995. First 500,000 AIDS cases—United States, 1995. *Morbidity and Mortality Weekly Report* 44(46): 849–853.

Centers for Disease Control and Prevention. 2000. Basic statistics. *Division of HIV/AIDS Prevention.* www.hivmail@cdc.gov.

Dickenson-Hazard, N. 1999. Inquiry, insights, and history. *Journal of Professional Nursing* 15(5): 261.

Ferguson, S., Howell, T., and Batalden, P. 1993. Knowledge and skills needed for collaborative work. *Quality Management in Health Care* 1: 1–11.

Foley, B. J., Minick, P., and Kee, C. 2000. Nursing advocacy during a military operation. *Western Journal of Nursing Research* 22(4): 492–507.

Hamric, A. B. 2000. What is happening to advocacy? *Nursing Outlook* 48(3): 103–104.

Health Care Financing Administration. 1998. *Highlights—national health expenditures, 1998.* http://www.hcfa.gov/stats.

Henderson, V. A. 1991. *The nature of nursing: Reflections after 25 years.* New York: National League for Nursing.

Higgins, L. W. 1999. Nurses' perceptions of collaborative nurse-physician transfer decision making as a predictor of patient outcomes in a medical intensive care unit. *Journal of Advanced Nursing* 29(6): 1434–1443.

Mariano, C. 1989. The case for interdisciplinary collaboration. *Nursing Outlook* 37: 285–288.

Meadors, A. C. 1993. The United States healthcare system and quality of care. In A. F. Al-Assaf and J. A. Schmele, eds., *The textbook of total quality in healthcare.* Delray Beach, Fla.: St. Lucie Press.

Miccolo, M. A., and Spanier, A. H. 1993. Critical care management in the 1990s. *Critical Care Unit Management* **9**(3): 443–453.

Morra, M. E. 2000. New opportunities for nurses as patient advocates. *Seminars in Oncology Nursing* **16**(1): 57–64.

National Coalition for the Homeless. 1999. *NCH fact sheet #1: Why are people homeless?* Washington, D.C.: NCH.

National Coalition for the Homeless. 1999. *NCH fact sheet #2: How many people experience homelessness?* Washington, D.C.: NCH.

Norton, R. W. 1983. *Communicator style: Theory, applications, and measures.* Beverly Hills, Calif.: Sage Publications.

Smith-Love, J., and Carter, C. 1999, Fall. Collaboration, problem-solving reevaluation: Foundation for the Heart Center of Excellence. *Progress in Cardiovascular Nursing:* 143–149.

U.S. Bureau of the Census. 1998. Poverty in the United States: 1997. *Current Population Reports,* Series P 60–201.

U.S. Department of Health and Human Services, Public Health Service. 1990. *Healthy People 2000: National Health Promotion and Disease Prevention Objectives.* DHHS Pub no. (PHS) 91-50212. Washington, D.C.: U.S. Government Printing Office.

U.S. Department of Health and Human Services, Public Health Service. 2000. *Healthy People 2010 Goals.* www.health.gov/healthy people.

Van Ess Coeling, H., and Cukr, P. L. 2000. Communication styles that promote perceptions of collaboration, quality, and nurse satisfaction. *Journal of Nursing Care Quality* **14**(2): 63–74.

Velianoff, G. D., Neely, C., and Hall, S. 1993. Development levels of interdisciplinary collaborative practice committees. *Journal of Nursing Administration* **23:** 26–29.

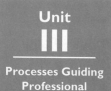

Unit
III
Processes Guiding
Professional
Practice

C H A P T E R   1 3

Communication

Objectives

■ Define communication.

■ Describe the four components of the communication process.

■ Analyze factors influencing the communication process.

■ Discuss the types of communication and their characteristics.

■ Differentiate between therapeutic and nontherapeutic communication.

■ Identify barriers to effective communication.

■ Differentiate between nursing documentation and other forms of written communication.

■ Discuss technology as a form of communication.

N U R S E   C O N N E C T

Additional online resources for this chapter can be found on the companion web site at www.prenhall.com/blais.

Nursing is an interaction between nurses and clients, nurses and other health professionals, and nurses and the community. The process of human interaction occurs through communication: verbal and nonverbal, written and unwritten, planned and unplanned. Communication between people conveys thoughts, ideas, feelings, and information. For nurses to be effective in their interactions, they must have good communication skills. They must be aware of what their words and body language are saying to others. As nurses assume leadership roles they must be effective in both verbal and written communication skills. And as nurses practice in the 21st century, they must have effective computer communication skills.

CHALLENGES AND OPPORTUNITIES

Clear and appropriate communication is essential for providing effective nursing care, and this is a unique challenge in the current health care scene. Overcoming barriers to communication is necessary in a society where many languages are spoken and the population is multicultural. Individual nurses cannot be fluent in each language that will be encountered, nor can they be fully informed of the cultural contexts of words and phrases that may have multiple meanings. Nonverbal communication also has cultural meaning. Not only is this a challenge in providing care to clients, it is also a challenge in working with colleagues when there is diversity of cultures and languages. Clear communication about care and about client information is equally important, whether it is in the form of verbal interactions with coworkers, written records, or publications in professional journals. A challenge for nurses in the 21st century is to become proficient with communicating via technology, including telephone communication such as telephone triage and communication using computers such as nursing-documentation systems and e-mail.

Finding effective ways to overcome communication barriers provides the opportunity for nurses to bridge cultural gaps in delivering health care. Nurses who can use available resources and solve problems when there are communication difficulties will be better able to assist clients and families to access care and benefit from health care services. Clear communication will help the health care team provide effective care. It is essential in interdisciplinary teams. When nurses are able to communicate well in verbal and written form, the quality of professional publications benefits, and nurses can provide better resources to the profession. Nurses can use technology to enhance communication with clients and other health care providers, to improve access to care for people in remote areas, and to increase their own knowledge using the information resources available on the Internet.

DEFINITIONS OF COMMUNICATION

Communication can be defined as the giving or exchanging of information through verbal or written means. Kozier and colleagues (2000, p. 1389) define communication as "a two-way process involving the sending and receiving of messages." Sherman (1994) defines communication as the sharing of experience and the sharing of feelings and emotions. This suggests a broader concept of communication that goes beyond the simple transfer of information to the establishment of a relationship between people. Such relationships are founded upon effective communication skills.

Most definitions of communication suggest that it is a process between two or more individuals or interpersonal communication. However, people can communicate within themselves—intrapersonal communication—as they reflect upon their own knowledge, ideas, and feelings.

Nurses who communicate effectively are better able to establish successful relationships between themselves and others, including clients and their families, other nurses and health care professionals, health care administrators, and the lay public. Effective communication can also prevent many of the errors that lead to legal incidents associated with nursing practice.

THE COMMUNICATION PROCESS

The communication process involves a sender, message, channel, receiver, and response or feedback. (See Figure 13–1.) In its simplest form, communication involves the sending and receiving of a message between two people. The sender defines the original message and transmits it to the receiver through a selected channel. The receiver then interprets the message and provides a response to the sender. This enables the sender to determine if the receiver understood or interpreted the message correctly. If the message was not interpreted correctly or if additional information is needed, the process starts again. Therefore, communication is an ongoing process, where the roles of sender and receiver transact as each transmits new information or understandings to the other.

Communication can also be an exchange of information between an individual and a group of people (e.g., by giving a lecture or teaching a class) or an ex-

Figure 13–1

The communication process.

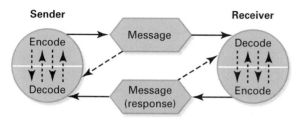

The dashed arrows indicate intrapersonal communication (self-talk). The solid lines indicate interpersonal communication.

Source: B. Kozier, G. Erb, A. J. Berman, and K. Burke. *Fundamentals of Nursing,* 6th ed. Upper Saddle River, N.J.: Prentice Hall Health, 2000. Reprinted with permission.

change of information between several people (e.g., a change-of-shift report or a group meeting). The components of the communication process are sender, message, channel, receiver, and feedback.

Sender

The **sender** is the person or group who wishes to transmit a message to another. Another term for sender is *source encoder.* This means that the originator of the message, or source, has a purpose for the message and determines its content. The content of the message must be put in a form that is understandable to the receiver, called *encoding.* Encoding involves "the selection of specific signs or symbols (codes) to transmit the message" (Kozier et al., 2000, p. 432). Encoding includes the choice of specific words and the language of the message. It also includes the speech inflection and body language used to accompany the message. For example, when nurses are communicating with other nurses about a client's condition, they may use medical terminology (e.g., hypertension); however, when they are talking with the client or family, they may use lay terminology (e.g., high blood pressure).

Message

The second part of the communication process is the encoded **message** itself—the information or feelings to be transmitted and the content and context of the message. Messages between nurses and clients include verbal and written discharge instructions, interactions of support and caring, and information gathering.

Channel

The **channel** is the method selected to convey the message, including whether the message is spoken or written, the choice of words or language, and the choice of accompanying body language. A change-of-shift report between nurses may be verbal in a face-to-face interaction or it may be recorded on audiotape. Client-discharge instructions may be written or verbal. Communications with physicians may be face to face, via telephone, or through the client record. The channel can be visual, auditory, or through touch. Some of the most effective communication interactions use more than one sensory channel.

Receiver

The **receiver,** also called the *decoder,* is the one who receives the message, interprets (decodes) it, and makes a decision about how to respond. If the message is aural, the receiver must be able to hear or attend to the message and the sender. If the message is written or visual, the receiver must be able to see and read. The receiver decodes or interprets the message in relation to his or her past experiences, knowledge, and personal characteristics. If the receiver interprets the message congruently with the intent of the sender, then communication has been effective. Ineffective communication occurs when the message is not understood or is interpreted inaccurately. For example, a nurse may instruct the client to take his medication three times a day with meals. The client, however, eats only twice a day. This difference could result in the client not taking the medication as required. Feedback, or response, from the client is essential to validate interpretation and understanding of the message.

Response

The receiver's **response** is the feedback that enables the sender to know if the message was received and interpreted correctly. Feedback is the message that the receiver returns to the sender. Failure to obtain a response or feedback can result in ineffective communication. Feedback can also be verbal or nonverbal. Feedback may be verbal clarification or acceptance or rejection of the information or feelings. It may also be nonverbal. Examples of nonverbal feedback are nodding of the head, a facial expression of confusion or understanding, or signs of boredom, such as yawning. It is important to use verbal feedback to be sure that nonverbal language has not been misinterpreted. For example, clients may nod their head indicating understanding, but further questioning might show that they misunderstood the message.

The response is the message back to the sender. The receiver has changed roles and becomes the sender. And so the process continues until the communication is ended.

FACTORS INFLUENCING THE COMMUNICATION PROCESS

Many factors influence the communication process. These include the developmental stage, gender, roles and relationships, sociocultural characteristics, values and perceptions, space and territoriality, environment, congruence, and interpersonal attitudes.

Developmental Stage

As individuals grow and develop, language and communication skills develop through various stages. It is important for a nurse to understand the developmental processes related to speech, language, and communication skills. Knowledge of the client's developmental stage enables the nurse to select appropriate communication strategies. For example, when communicating with infants and toddlers whose language skills are not well developed, the nurse may rely more on the child's nonverbal communications to assess comfort and pain. For older children, nurses may use pictures as an adjunct to verbal language to communicate. For adolescents and adults, nurses are more able to rely on verbal language for communication. With older adults, physical changes associated with the aging process may affect communication. For example, it may be more effective to use visual communication methods for clients who are hearing impaired or aural communication methods for clients who are visually impaired. Also, intellectual processes develop across the life span as people acquire knowledge and experience. The knowledge and experiences that people have influence their understanding and acceptance of transmitted information and feelings.

Gender

Males and females tend to communicate differently. They may give different meanings to transmitted information or feelings. This may be the result of differences during psychosocial development, because boys use communication to establish independence and negotiate status within a group, whereas girls use communication to seek confirmation, minimize differences, and establish or reinforce intimacy. It is important

Research Box

Sudia-Robinson, T. M., and Freeman, S. B. 2000. **Communication patterns and decision making: Parents and health care providers in the neonatal intensive care unit: A case study.** *Heart and Lung: The Journal of Acute and Critical Care* 29(2): 143–148.

The purpose of this study was to examine patterns of communication and decision making among NICU health care providers and the parents of a premature infant who required neonatal intensive care. A descriptive design was used for data collection to answer the question: What patterns of communication and decision making are evident in the interactions of parents of an infant in the NICU and the NICU professionals providing care? A parent-professional conference was videotaped, and audiotapes were used for interviews with the parents and the professionals directly involved in care (two nurses, a neonatologist, a resident, and a social worker). The parents and the professionals reviewed the videotape individually, and each was interviewed about feelings, impressions, and concerns.

The audiotapes of the interviews were transcribed and analyzed by content analysis. The parents were found to have four areas of concern regarding their infant's routine care: parental visitation, change of shift, the infant's transfer to the IMCU, and administration of immunizations. The parents indicated a desire to be involved in daily decisions and expressed a need for more information. They expressed a desire to have adequate time to establish a trusting relationship with the new set of caregivers at shift change. They felt they needed an opportunity to engage in additional conversation with the professionals before the transfer of the infant. Misinterpretation of information from the professionals was evident. Therapeutic communication techniques and spending time and sharing perceptions with parents were recommended.

that nurses, when working with clients or colleagues of the opposite gender, be aware that the same communication may be interpreted differently by a man and a woman.

Roles and Relationships

The roles and relationships between the sender and the receiver can influence communication. Roles such as nurse and client, nurse and colleague, nurse and physician, and nurse and administrator/supervisor can affect the content and response in communication. Roles may influence choice of message content, communication vehicle, tone of voice, and body language. For example, nurses may choose face-to-face communication for interaction with clients or health providers on the nursing unit, whereas they may use e-mails or telephones to communicate with physicians or administrators. Nurses may choose a more informal or comfortable stance when communicating with clients or colleagues and a more formal stance when communicating with physicians or administrators. The length of the relationship may also affect communication. For example, nurses may use more formal language and a more formal stance when meeting clients or colleagues for the first time but use a more relaxed stance when interacting with clients or colleagues with whom they have an established relationship.

Sociocultural Characteristics

Sociocultural characteristics such as culture, education, or economic level can influence communication. Nonverbal communication characteristics such as body language, eye contact, and touch are influenced by cultural beliefs about appropriate communication behavior. Some cultures may believe direct eye contact is disrespectful, whereas other cultures believe that direct eye contact shows trustworthiness. In some cultures, touch would be appropriate to communicate caring and concern, but in other cultures physical touch would be offensive. Verbal communication may be difficult for the receiver whose primary language is not that of of the sender.

A person's level of education may affect the extent of their vocabulary or their ability to read written communication. Economic level may affect a person's ability to access written communication. Today, when many people are using e-mail to communicate or the Internet to obtain health information, people who cannot afford a computer or who do not have access to one will not be able to communicate using that means.

Values and Perceptions

Communication is influenced by the values people hold about themselves, others, and the world in which they live. Because all people have values and perceptions based on their own experiences and characteristics, people who hold different values may send, receive, and interpret messages differently. For example, a client who values stoicism in managing his or her pain may not tell the nurse about the pain and may be offended when the nurse inquires about pain or offers pain medication.

Space and Territoriality

Space involves the distance at which an interaction takes place. Territoriality involves the space and contents of the space that the individual considers belonging to him or her.

Hall (1969) describes four distances at which interactions take place: intimate distance, personal distance, social distance, and public distance. Intimate distance ranges from physical contact to 1½ feet. Nurses interact with clients within the intimate range when they assess and provide some direct care activities for clients. Taking blood pressure, listening to body sounds with a stethoscope, assessing pulse, changing a dressing, or giving an injection are all performed with physical contact. The manner in which the tasks are performed and the conversation during these activities communicate to the client in various ways. If the nurse is brusque when changing a dressing, the client may interpret the nurse's behavior as uncaring. If the nurse is gentle and shows concern, the client may perceive that the nurse is caring and feel comforted. Clients may feel uncomfortable when others enter their intimate space, especially if a trusting relationship has not been established. Nurses can alleviate this discomfort by telling the client before moving into the intimate distance range.

Personal distance ranges from 1½ to 4 feet. Most one-to-one communication takes place within this range. Nurses interact with clients in the personal distance range when they sit with a client to obtain a health history or when they teach clients self-care. Nurses also interact with colleagues in the range of personal distance when they exchange information with a nursing colleague or physician.

Social distance ranges from 4 to 12 feet. Interactions with clients and family members or groups of clients are more likely to occur in the range of social distance. This is also the range of distance within which nurses interact with groups of colleagues, such as during a group change-of-shift report. It is important to note that usually the voice is louder when communicating in this range; therefore, a nurse must be aware of issues of client confidentiality. Communication with a client who is in a semiprivate room may be compromised if the nurse asks personal questions at this range while in the presence of other clients or caregivers.

Public distance starts at 12 feet and goes beyond that distance. This is the distance at which interactions with larger groups take place. There is less individual interaction or awareness of individual needs when communicating at this distance. Nurses communicate in public distance when they conduct community health education classes.

It is human nature to establish a boundary or territory that is considered to be one's own. Whether clients are being cared for in their own home, their own room in a long-term care facility, or in a hospital room, they create a personal environment that gives them comfort. They may have photographs, religious materials, or other personal items on a nearby table or bed tray. If the nurse attempts to change or rearrange furniture or objects in the client's environment, the client may perceive this as not caring or devaluing. Similarly, nurses who have their own desk or locker often have personal objects that create their personal work territory or environment.

Environment

The nature of the environment can also affect communication. Communication occurs best in an environment that supports the exchange of information, ideas, or feelings. Loud noises, poor lighting, noxious odors, or an uncomfortable temperature can all interfere with effective communication. The arrangement of furniture can affect communication. For example, communicating across a desk conveys a more formal interaction than when the nurse sits in a chair next to the client. When interacting with clients, their families, or others, nurses should try to create an environment that is conducive to effective communication and minimizes environmental distractions.

Congruence

When communication is congruent, the nonverbal behaviors match the verbal message. Nurses may state that they want clients to call if they have any questions or need anything. However, if a nurse appears to be rushed or distracted, a client may be unsure about calling the nurse when he or she has a question or is experiencing pain.

Interpersonal Attitudes

Positive attitudes of respect, acceptance, trust, and caring facilitate communication, whereas negative attitudes of mistrust, rejection, and condescension inhibit effective communication. When one person is interacting with another, attitudes are conveyed by facial expression, tone of voice, the choice of words, and other body language. It is important to convey a nonjudgmental attitude during interactions. If the client feels that the nurse disapproves of some aspect of his or her lifestyle (e.g., smoking, promiscuity, addiction to drugs or alcohol), the client might not share the information.

TYPES OF COMMUNICATION

There are two types of communication, verbal and nonverbal. Verbal communication may be spoken or written and involves words. Verbal communication is mainly conscious because people choose the words they use. Verbal communication depends on language mastery. Language mastery includes vocabulary and grammar and is dependent upon one's culture, educational level, socioeconomic background, and age. Because of these factors, information can be given, ideas discussed, and feelings exchanged using many different words and word configurations. Nonverbal communication uses other forms such as facial expression, gestures, touch, or other types of body language. Nonverbal communication also includes the use of pictures to communicate. Although both verbal and nonverbal communication occur simultaneously, the majority of communication during face-to-face interactions is nonverbal.

Oral Communication

Oral communication is a spoken exchange of information, ideas, or feelings using words. Words can have different meanings for different people. Wilson and Kneisl (1996) describe four concepts related to word meanings: (1) denotative meaning, (2) connotative meaning, (3) private meaning, and (4) shared meaning. Denotative meaning is the way in which the word is generally used by people who share a common language. Connotative meaning is the meaning of a word that derives from one's personal experiences; for example, the word love may have different meanings when used with a parent, a child, a spouse, or a lover or to describe one's favorite flavor of ice cream. Private meanings are those held by the individual. Shared meanings are the mutual understanding of the word or words between people who are trying to communicate effectively.

Kozier et al. (2000) state that when choosing words for oral communication, nurses must consider (1) pace and intonation, (2) simplicity, (3) clarity and brevity, (4) timing and relevance, (5) adaptability, (6) credibility, and (7) humor.

1. *Pace and intonation.* Pace is the speed or rapidity of speech. Intonation is its tone, accent, or inflection.

Pace and intonation can express a variety of states, including interest, happiness, anxiety, boredom, anger, fear, or depression. For example, when people speak in a monotone, not changing the pace or tone of their speech, they may be expressing boredom or apathy.

2. *Simplicity.* Simplicity in communication is the choice of commonly understood words. Nurses must remember to use language that is clearly understood when communicating with clients. This may mean avoiding complex medical terminology when discussing a client's illness or injury. It also means that the nurse must clarify that the client understands the word meanings in the same way that the nurse does.

3. *Clarity and brevity.* Clarity means choosing words that say unmistakably what is meant. Brevity is using the fewest words necessary to convey a message. It is important to communicate clearly so that the message is understood.

4. *Timing and relevance.* Timing is an important aspect of effective communication. If the client is experiencing pain or is otherwise distracted, it is not an appropriate time to give complex instructions in self-care. Communication must also be relevant to the receiver. If the receiver is not interested in the information at the time it is being given, he or she may be less attentive.

5. *Adaptability.* When speaking with clients and others, nurses must be cognizant of verbal and nonverbal cues from the receiver and adapt their communication accordingly. If the receiver appears confused after instructions have been given, the nurse must clarify understanding by restating or rephrasing the instructions.

6. *Credibility.* Credibility means being believable and trustworthy. To be credible when communicating, nurses must be consistent, dependable, and honest. Nurses must give accurate information and be willing to say when they don't know something or don't have information. It is more credible to state, "I don't know, but I'll find out for you" than to give inaccurate information that must be corrected later. Consistency is important when communicating to avoid confusion or misunderstanding. When a nurse is consistent and accurate in communicating, he or she is more believable or credible.

7. *Humor.* Humor can be effective in communication when used appropriately. It can help people adjust to difficult situations and decrease tension. Laughter can release endorphins that promote a sense of well-being. However, one must be careful in using humor, especially when communicating with people whose primary language is different or who are from a different culture. For example, jokes may seem funny only when used within a particular culture; they may be offensive to or not understood by people of a different culture.

Nonverbal Communication

Nonverbal communication is also referred to as body language. It is the way in which one uses one's body to reinforce or contradict verbal, specifically oral, communication. Nonverbal communication includes (1) eye contact, (2) facial expressions, (3) body movements, (4) gestures, (5) touch, and (6) physical appearance.

1. *Eye contact.* Eye contact may initiate interaction and communication. Often when a person is trying to get another's attention, he or she does so by trying to make eye contact. However, before making judgments about the importance of eye contact, the nurse must know the meaning of eye contact within the client's culture. In many Western cultures, eye contact is interpreted as attentiveness, interest, understanding, or trustworthiness. In some cultures, however, direct eye contact is considered disrespectful. Knowing the cultural meaning of eye contact can help a nurse assess its meaning in a specific interaction.

2. *Facial expression.* Facial expressions provide the emotion or feeling underlying the verbal communication. The face can express feelings of surprise, fear, concern, disgust, happiness, anger, confusion, and sadness. As with eye contact, facial expression can have a cultural meaning. Some cultures are more expressive than others. It is important that one's facial expression is congruent with the verbal message. An expression of concern when inquiring about a client's pain is congruent, whereas an expression of boredom or anger would be incongruent and could lead the client to believe that the nurse does not care.

3. *Body movements.* The way in which people stand, sit, or move their bodies also communicates to others. Posture and gait can communicate one's feelings about self, one's mood, and one's current state of health. When interacting with a client, a nurse demonstrates interest and concern by leaning toward the client or by reaching out his or her hands and arms toward the client. Leaning away from the client or crossing his or her arms and legs may indicate distance or withdrawal. Standing over a client during interaction may be intimidating to the client. Agitated movements may convey fear or anx-

iety. Lack of movement may indicate pain, discomfort, or depression.

4. *Gestures.* Hand and body movements may emphasize or clarify verbal communication, such as when separating fingers or hands to indicate the size of something or to point to a part of the body where one has pain. When the client is asked to describe chest pain, a different meaning could be attributed to the gesture of a clenched fist in the center of the chest as opposed to an open hand waived vaguely in front of the chest. Some people use their hands as part of their verbal speech and may find difficulty in expressing themselves if they are unable to use their hands. For people who are hearing impaired or unable to speak, sign language may be their primary means of communicating.

5. *Touch.* Physical touch can convey concern, comfort, and caring or it can convey anger or agitation. Like eye contact, touch has cultural meaning. In some cultures, touch is inappropriate between people of the opposite gender or between people of different classes. It is important that the nurse determine the meaning of touch in the client's culture. When touch is inappropriate, clients may withdraw if a nurse reaches out toward them.

6. *Appearance.* How people present themselves, their dress, and their grooming can convey information about them. People who are physically or mentally ill may not be as attentive to their dress and grooming. Dress may indicate a person's position or status. For example, physicians, some nurses, and therapists may wear lab coats over business clothes; administrators may wear suits; and nursing assistants and dietary personnel may wear required uniforms or smocks. Jewelry may provide information about a person. Religious jewelry provides important information about a client or colleague. Nurses often wear pins or other insignia that indicate their position or accomplishments, such as their school pin or a pin indicating they are a member of Sigma Theta Tau, the nursing honor society.

It is important that nurses be aware of their verbal and nonverbal communication patterns and characteristics. How they speak, their mannerisms, and their gestures may be effective tools for communication or they may impede communication.

Consider . . .

■ your speech patterns when communicating verbally with others, such as colleagues, clients, and friends. What feedback do you receive?

■ mannerisms and gestures you use when communicating nonverbally with others. What feedback do you receive?

■ role playing with a colleague or classmate. Ask them to comment on your verbal and nonverbal communication patterns.

■ videotaping an interaction with a colleague or client. (You must first obtain permission to videotape.) Analyze the videotape to identify inconsistencies between your verbal and nonverbal communication. In what ways would you improve your verbal and nonverbal communication behaviors?

Therapeutic Communication

Therapeutic communication is defined as "an interactive process between nurse and client that helps the client overcome temporary stress, to get along with other people, to adjust to the unalterable, and to overcome psychological blocks which stand in the way of self-realizations" (Kozier et al., 2000, p. 1409). Therapeutic communication differs from social communication in that there is always a specific purpose or direction to the communication; therefore, therapeutic communication is planned communication. Communication is most therapeutic when an attitude of respect that considers the individuality and self-esteem of both the client and the nurse is conveyed (Frisch and Frisch 1998). There are specific verbal and nonverbal techniques of communication that express such an attitude.

Presence, or an attitude of being wholly there for the client, is part of therapeutic communication. A nurse cannot appear to be distracted; rather, a client must feel that he or she is the primary focus of the nurse during the interaction. Being there for a client is conveyed by presenting an open and relaxed posture and leaning toward the client. The nurse faces the client directly and maintains eye contact.

Listening, sometimes referred to as attentive listening, is active listening. Frisch and Frisch (1998) and Kozier et al. (2000) describe listening as the most important communication technique. To be therapeutic, listening must be active and involve all the senses rather than passively involving only the ear. Silence is a part of attentive listening. Nurses need to become comfortable with silence. Silence allows clients to think about or reflect upon what has been said. Sometimes silence can communicate more than words; it can enable the expression of feelings or emotions.

Therapeutic communication techniques facilitate effective communication and enhance the nurse-client interaction. This communication focuses on the client's thoughts and concerns. Therapeutic communication techniques are described in Table 13–1.

Table 13–1 Therapeutic Communication Techniques

Technique	Description	Examples
Using silence	Accepting pauses or silences that may extend for several seconds or minutes without interjecting any verbal response.	Sitting quietly (or walking with the client) and waiting attentively until the client is able to put thoughts and feelings into words.
Providing general leads	Using statements or questions that (a) encourage the client to verbalize; (b) choose a topic of conversation; and (c) facilitate continued verbalization.	"Perhaps you would like to talk about . . . ." "Would it help to discuss your feelings?" "Where would you like to begin?" "And then what?" "I follow what you are saying."
Being specific and tentative	Making statements that are specific rather than general, and tentative rather than absolute.	"You scratched my arm." (specific statement) "You are as clumsy as an ox." (general statement) "You seem unconcerned about Mary." (tentative statement) "You don't give a damn about Mary and you never will." (absolute statement)
Using open-ended questions	Asking broad questions that lead or invite the client to explore (elaborate, clarify, describe, compare, or illustrate) thoughts or feelings. Open-ended questions specify only the topic to be discussed and invite answers that are longer than one or two words.	"I'd like to hear more about that." "Tell be about . . ." "How have you been feeling lately?" "What brought you to the hospital?" "What is your opinion?" "You said you were frightened yesterday. How do you feel now?"
Using touch	Providing appropriate forms of touch to reinforce caring feelings. Because tactile contacts vary considerably among individuals, families, and cultures, the nurse must be sensitive to the differences in attitudes and practices of clients and self.	Putting an arm over the client's shoulder. Placing your hand over the client's hand.
Restating or paraphrasing	Actively listening for the client's basic message and then repeating those thoughts and/or feelings in similar words. This conveys that the nurse has listened and understood the client's basic message and also offers clients a clearer idea of what they have said.	*Client:* "I couldn't manage to eat any dinner last night—not even the dessert." *Nurse:* "You had difficulty eating yesterday." *Client:* "Yes, I was very upset after my family left." *Client:* "I have trouble talking to strangers." *Nurse:* "You find it difficult talking to people you do not know?"
Seeking clarification	A method of making the client's *broad overall* meaning of the message more understandable. It is used when paraphrasing is difficult or when the communication is rambling or garbled. To clarify the message, the nurse can restate the basic message or confess confusion and ask the client to repeat or restate the message.	"I'm puzzled." "I'm not sure I understand that." "Would you please say that again?" "Would you tell me more?"
	Nurses can also clarify their own message with statements.	"I meant this rather than that." "I guess I didn't make that clear—I'll go over it again."

Table 13–1 (Cont.)

Technique	Description	Examples
Perception checking or seeking consensual validation	A method similar to clarifying that verifies the meaning of *specific words* rather than the overall meaning of a message.	*Client:* "My husband *never* gives me any presents." *Nurse:* "You mean he has *never* given you a present for your birthday or Christmas?" *Client:* "Well—not *never*. He does get me something for my birthday and Christmas, but he never thinks of giving me anything at any other time."
Offering self	Suggesting one's presence, interest, or wish to understand the client without making any demands or attaching conditions that the client must comply with to receive the nurse's attention.	"I'll stay with you until your daughter arrives." "We can sit here quietly for a while; we don't need to talk unless you would like to." "I'll help you to dress to go home."
Giving information	Providing, in a simple and direct manner, specific factual information the client may or may not request. When information is not known, the nurse states this and indicates who has it or when the nurse will obtain it.	"Your surgery is scheduled for 11 AM tomorrow." "You will feel a pulling sensation when the tube is removed from your abdomen." "I do not know the answer to that, but I will find out from Mrs. King, the nurse in charge."
Acknowledging	Giving recognition, in a nonjudgmental way, of a change in behavior, an effort the client has made, or a contribution to a communication. Acknowledgment may be with or without understanding, verbal or nonverbal.	"You trimmed your beard and mustache and washed your hair." "I notice you keep squinting your eyes. Are you having difficulty seeing?" "You walked twice as far today with your walker."
Clarifying time or sequence	Helping the client clarify an event, situation, or happening in relationship to time.	*Client:* "I vomited this morning." *Nurse:* "Was that after breakfast?" *Client:* "I feel that I have been asleep for weeks." *Nurse:* "You had your operation Monday, and today is Tuesday."
Presenting reality	Helping the client to differentiate the real from the unreal.	"That telephone ring came from the program on television." "That's not a dead mouse in the corner; it is a discarded washcloth." "Your magazine is here in the drawer. It has not been stolen."
Focusing	Helping the client expand on and develop a topic of importance. It is important for the nurse to wait until the client finishes stating the main concerns before attempting to focus. The focus may be an idea or a feeling; however, the nurse often emphasizes a feeling to help the client recognize an emotion disguised behind words.	*Client:* "My wife says she will look after me, but I don't think she can, what with the children to take care of, and they're always after her about something—clothes, homework, what's for dinner that night." *Nurse:* "You are worried about how well she can manage."
Reflecting	Directing ideas, feelings, questions, or content back to clients to enable them to explore their own ideas and feelings about a situation.	*Client:* "What can I do?" *Nurse:* "What do you think would be helpful?" *Client:* "Do you think I should tell my husband?" *Nurse:* "You seem unsure about telling your husband."

Table 13–1 (Cont.)

Technique	Description	Examples
Summarizing and planning	Stating the main points of a discussion to clarify the relevant points discussed. This technique is useful at the end of an interview or to review a health teaching session. It often acts as an introduction to future care planning.	"During the past half hour we have talked about . . . ." "Tomorrow afternoon we may explore this further." "In a few days I'll review what you have learned about the actions and effects of your insulin."

Source: B. Kozier, G. Erb, A. J. Berman, and K. Burke. *Fundamentals of Nursing,* 6th ed. Upper Saddle River, N.J.: Prentice Hall Health, 2000. Reprinted with permission.

WRITTEN COMMUNICATION

Nurses have many opportunities for written communication. The most common form of written communication in nursing are the notes made in the medical record about a client's status. Nurses also write discharge instructions for clients and their families, memos to nursing colleagues and other health professionals, and client educational materials. Nurse-managers write employee evaluations, policies and procedures, and other communications to administrators, colleagues, and nursing staff. Nurse-educators write educational handouts and course syllabi. An important consideration in written communication is that decoding often occurs when the writer is not present and may occur long after the document is written. Therefore, clarity is important because it may not be possible to ask questions or clarify areas of confusion.

Characteristics of Effective Written Communication

In addition to simplicity, brevity, clarity, relevance, credibility, and humor (characteristics of effective oral communication), written communication must contain (1) appropriate language and terminology; (2) correct grammar, spelling, and punctuation; (3) logical organization; and (4) appropriate use and citation of resources.

1. *Appropriate language and terminology.* Language and terminology must be appropriate for the age, education and reading level, and culture of the reader. Materials written for children should be different than health education materials written for adults. For people whose primary language is other than English, it may be more effective to have written materials translated into their primary language by a professional translator. Appropriate lay terminology may be substituted for medical terminology; for example, high blood pressure may be used instead of hypertension. See Chapter 8, "The Nurse as Learner and Teacher," for more information about reading level of written materials.

2. *Correct grammar, spelling, and punctuation.* Using correct grammar, spelling, and punctuation provides clarity for the reader. Misspelled words, misplaced punctuation, or incorrect grammar can change the intended meaning and lead to confusion on the part of the reader. Most computer word-processing programs have spelling- and grammar-checking features that assist writers in improving their writing.

3. *Logical organization.* Written materials are well organized when they are "logical and easy for readers to follow" (Hacker, 1994, p. 46). Consider what the reader needs to know first. Simple and foundational information is usually provided first, followed by more complex information. Using examples can also assist readers.

4. *Appropriate use and citation of resources.* Information taken from other sources must always be credited to the original source. Failure to reference work taken from another writer is called plagiarism and is considered unethical. There are various styles of referencing, including the Modern Language Association (MLA) and the American Psychological Association (APA). Another benefit of citing references is that readers who want additional information have references to read.

Consider . . .

■   your professional activities other than charting on client records that require written communication.

What professional activities of you and your colleagues require written communication?

■ your own comfort and ability at written communication. What strategies would you implement to improve your ability at written communication? How would you assist your colleagues to improve their written communication?

BARRIERS TO COMMUNICATION

Just as there are characteristics of effective communication, there are identified barriers to effective communication. Nurses need to be cognizant of these barriers and avoid them. Nurses also need to recognize them when they occur so that they can change to more effective communication. Kozier et al. (2000, p. 439)

identify "failure to listen, improperly decoding the client's intended message, and placing the nurse's needs above the client's needs as major barriers to communication." Additional barriers to effective communication are given in Table 13–2.

NURSING DOCUMENTATION

Documentation of clients' care and their responses to that care is essential for effective communication of clients' status between health care providers. When such documentation is complete, accurate, and clearly understood by all health care professionals involved in providing the care, the quality of clients' care is improved. Although the primary purpose of

Table 13–2 Barriers to Communication

Technique	Description	Examples
Stereotyping	Offering generalized and oversimplified beliefs about groups of people that are based on experiences too limited to be valid. These responses categorize clients and negate their uniqueness as individuals.	"Two-year-olds are brats." "Women are complainers." "Men don't cry." "Most people don't have any pain after this type of surgery."
Agreeing and disagreeing	Akin to judgmental responses, agreeing and disagreeing imply that the client is either right or wrong and that the nurse is in a position to judge this. These responses deter clients from thinking through their position and may cause a client to become defensive.	*Client:* "I don't think Dr. Broad is a very good doctor. He doesn't seem interested in his patients." *Nurse:* "Dr. Broad is head of the Department of Surgery and is an excellent surgeon."
Being defensive	Attempting to protect a person or health care services from negative comments. These responses prevent the client from expressing true concerns. The nurse is saying, "You have no right to complain." Defensive responses protect the nurse from admitting weaknesses in the health care services, including personal weaknesses.	*Client:* "Those night nurses must just sit around and talk all night. They didn't answer my light for over an hour." *Nurse:* I'll have you know we literally run around on nights. You're not the only client, you know."
Challenging	Giving a response that makes clients prove their statement or point of view. These responses indicate that the nurse is failing to consider the client's feelings, making the client feel it necessary to defend a position.	*Client:* "I felt nauseated after that red pill." *Nurse:* "Surely you don't think I gave you the wrong pill?" *Client:* "I feel as if I am dying." *Nurse:* "How can you feel that way when your pulse is 60?" *Client:* "I believe my husband doesn't love me." *Nurse:* "You can't say that; why, he visits you every day."

Table 13–2 (Cont.)

Technique	Description	Examples
Probing	Asking for information chiefly out of curiosity rather than with the intent to assist the client. These responses are considered prying and violate the client's privacy. Asking "why" is often probing and places the client in a defensive position.	*Client:* "I was speeding along the street and didn't see the stop sign." *Nurse:* "Why were you speeding?" *Client:* "I didn't ask the doctor when he was here." *Nurse:* "Why didn't you?"
Testing	Asking questions that make the client admit to something. These responses permit the client only limited answers and often meet the nurse's need rather than the client's.	"Who do you think you are?" (forces people to admit their status is only that of client) "Do you think I am not busy?" (forces the client to admit that the nurse really *is* busy)
Rejecting	Refusing to discuss certain topics with the client. These responses often make clients feel that the nurse is rejecting not only their communication but also the clients themselves.	"I don't want to discuss that. Let's talk about . . ." "Let's discuss other areas of interest to you rather than the two problems you keep mentioning." "I can't talk now. I'm on my way for coffee break."
Changing topics and subjects	Directing the communication into areas of self-interest rather than considering the client's concerns is often a self-protective response to a topic that causes anxiety. These responses imply that what the nurse considers important will be discussed and that clients should not discuss certain topics.	*Client:* "I'm separated from my wife. Do you think I should have sexual relations with another woman?" *Nurse:* "I see that you're 36 and that you like gardening. This sunshine is good for my roses. I have a beautiful rose garden."
Unwarranted reassurance	Using clichés or comforting statements of advice as a means to reassure the client. These responses block the fears, feelings, and other thoughts of the client.	"You'll feel better soon." "I'm sure everything will turn out all right." "Don't worry."
Passing judgment	Giving opinions and approving or disapproving responses, moralizing, or implying one's own values. These responses imply that the client *must* think as the nurse thinks, fostering client dependence.	"That's good (bad)." "You shouldn't do that." "That's not good enough." "What you did was wrong (right)."
Giving common advice	Telling the client what to do. These responses deny the client's right to be an equal partner. Note that giving *expert* rather than common advice is therapeutic.	*Client:* "Should I move from my home to a nursing home?" *Nurse:* "If I were you, I'd go to a nursing home, where you'll get your meals cooked for you."

Source: B. Kozier, G. Erb, A. J. Berman, and K. Burke. *Fundamentals of Nursing,* 6th ed. Upper Saddle River, N.J.: Prentice Hall Health, 2000. Reprinted with permission.

documenting care in clients records is for communication between health care providers so that they can plan appropriate care, there are other uses of the information provided in clients' records: (1) auditing for quality assurance, (2) research, (3) education, (4) reimbursement, (5) legal documentation, and (6) health care analysis (Kozier et al., 2000).

■ *Auditing for quality assurance.* The client record is used by accrediting organizations to review and evaluate the quality of care given in health care institutions.

- *Research.* Information in a client record can be used as a source of data for health care research. Data gathered from the medical records of numerous clients with the same health problem may yield information about (1) the effectiveness of specific treatment methods, (2) the effectiveness of specific nursing interventions, or (3) specific client characteristics that enhance or impede the effectiveness of a specific treatment or intervention.
- *Education.* Client records are used by students in the health professions as educational tools. Although textbooks provide generalized information about pathophysiology, signs and symptoms, usual treatment, and outcomes of a specific health problem, client records provide a comprehensive view of specific clients, their health problems, their medical treatments and nursing interventions, and their responses to the treatment and interventions. A client record provides a case study of the unique experience of one client with a specific health problem. This helps students understand the individual experience of the client with the health problem.
- *Reimbursement.* Documentation of care helps the health care organization receive reimbursement from third-party payors, including private insurance companies and governmental sources of reimbursement such as Medicare and Medicaid. Medicare requires that the client record must contain the correct diagnosis-related group (DRG) codes and document that the appropriate care was given for the health care provider to receive payment.
- *Legal documentation.* The client's record is considered a legal document that can be used as evidence in a legal action. Such a record is a major source of information about the care that a client received when there is an accusation of negligence or malpractice against a health care provider.
- *Health care analysis.* In addition to being used by accrediting organizations to review the quality of care in a health care agency, client records can also help the health care agency analyze and plan the agency's needs. For example, analysis of client records can help the agency identify services that are underutilized or overutilized such as specific diagnostic studies or medications. This analysis can help the agency determine which services generate revenue and which cost the agency money.

Methods of Documentation

There are several methods of organizing the client record, including the traditional source-oriented narrative record, problem-oriented medical record, focus charting, charting by exception (CBE), and CORE documentation. Table 13–3 provides a brief descrip-

Table 13–3 Methods of Documentation

Method	Organization	Advantages	Disadvantages
Source-oriented narrative record	Each provider documents in a separate section or sections of the client's record (e.g., Progress Notes, Nurses Notes, etc.). Information is written in chronological order in the appropriate section.	Each discipline can easily locate the forms on which to document their data. Easy-to-follow information specific to one's discipline.	Information scattered throughout the record. Difficult to find chronological information.

Problem-oriented medical record (POMR) or problem-oriented record (POR)
 	
  S—Subjective data
  O—Objective data
  A—Assessment
  P—Plan
  I—Interventions
  E—Evaluation
  R—Revision
	Consists of baseline data, a problem list at the front of the record, a plan of care for each problem, and progress notes written in SOAP, SOAPIE, SOAPIER, or PIE format.
	
	Data are organized according to the client problems identified.
		Encourages collaboration between health care providers.
		
		The problem list in front alerts caregivers to client's needs.
		
		Easier to track the status of each problem.
			Caregivers differ in their ability to use the required format.
			
			Requires constant vigilance to maintain up-to-date problem list.
			
			Inefficient because assessments and interventions that apply to more than one problem must be repeated.

Table 13–3 (Cont.)

Method	Organization	Advantages	Disadvantages
Focus Charting	Client concerns and strengths are the focus of care. Data are organized according to data (D), nursing action (A), and client response (R); often uses flowsheets.	Allows charting on any significant area, not just problems. Flexible.	Not multidisciplinary. Difficult to identify chronological order. Notes may not relate to care plan.
CORE	Focuses on nursing process—the core of documentation. Consists of data base (D), plan of action (A), and evaluation (E).	Incorporates the entire nursing process in one system. Groups nursing diagnoses and functional status assessments together. Promotes concise documentation with minimal repetition.	Does not always present information chronologically. Notes may not always relate to the plan of care.
Charting by exception (CBE)	Only significant findings or exceptions to norms are recorded.	Efficient—uses flowsheets. Rapid detection of changes. Can take place of plan of care.	Expensive to institute. Not prevention focused.
FACT	Incorporates elements of charging by exception (CBE). Consists of: F—Flowsheets for specific services. A—Assessment. C—concise, integrated progress notes and flowsheets. T—Timely entries recorded when care is given.	Computer ready. Eliminates duplication. Encourages consistent language and structure. Outcome oriented. Permits immediate recording of current data. Readily accessible at the client's bedside. Eliminates the need for different forms.	Narrative notes may be too brief. Nurse's perspective may be overlooked. Nursing process framework may be difficult to identify.

Source: Adapted from *Mastering Documentation.* Springhouse, Pa.: Springhouse Corporation, 1995; B. Kozier, G. Erb, A. J. Berman, and K. Burke. *Fundamentals of Nursing: Concepts, Process, and Practice,* 6th ed. Upper Saddle River, N.J.: Prentice Hall Health, 2000; R. F. Craven and C. J. Hirnle. *Fundamentals of Nursing: Human Health and Function,* 2d ed. Philadelphia: Lippincott, 1996.

tion of the various methods of documentation and their advantages and disadvantages.

Consider . . .

- nursing documentation systems in your health care agency. What are the advantages and disadvantages of the documentation system used in your health care agency? Are there areas that need improvement? How might you go about making needed changes?

COMMUNICATION THROUGH TECHNOLOGY

Nurses are increasingly using computers to enhance their communication. Nurses use e-mail to communicate with other nurses, other departments in their employment setting, and resources outside the employment setting. Nurses can use computers to access health information through websites and literature databases.

Many health care agencies are implementing computer programs for client record systems. Computers may be found at nurses' stations, the clients' bedsides, or as handheld models in nurses' pockets. Computers at the bedside enable nurses to check orders immediately before administering a treatment or medication. Data from bedside monitors can be incorporated readily into clients' records through bedside computers. Computerized client information can be transmitted rapidly from one health care setting to another to facilitate consultation with other health care providers. Computer documentation systems decrease the time spent in charting and increase the legibility and accuracy of information.

More information about the use of computers and technology is provided in Chapter 16, "Technology and Informatics."

SUMMARY

For nurses to be effective in their interactions with clients, they must have effective communication skills. They must be aware of what their words and body language are saying to others. Professional nurses must be effective in both verbal and written communication, and they need to possess good computer skills in order to communicate with clients and other health care providers and to increase their knowledge through Internet resources.

Communication involves the sending and receiving of messages between two or more people. The communication process involves a sender, message, channel, receiver, and response, or feedback. The sender defines the original message and transmits it to the receiver through the channel or method of communication. The receiver then interprets the message and provides a response to the sender. By responding, the receiver becomes the sender of a new message. Thus, communication is an ongoing process, where the roles of sender and receiver are exchanged as each transmits new information or understandings to the other.

There are many factors that influence the communication process. These include developmental stage, gender, roles and relationships, values and perceptions, sociocultural characteristics, space and territoriality, environment, congruence, and interpersonal attitudes.

Types of communication include verbal and nonverbal. Verbal communication includes both spoken

---

Bookshelf

Arnold, E.N., and Boggs, K. U. 1999. *Interpersonal relationships: Professional communication skills for nurses,* **3d ed. Philadelphia: Saunders.**

This text covers all aspect of nursing interaction and communication, including communication with clients, families, and colleagues.

Luckmann, J. 1999. *Transcultural communication in nursing.* **New York: Delmar.**

This text provides a resource for better communication with clients, interpreters, and colleagues whose primary language is other than English. It also provides resources of books, novels, videos and other media that demonstrate communication between cultures.

Springhouse. 1999. *Mastering documentation,* **2nd ed. Springhouse, Pa.: Springhouse Publishing.**

This text covers all aspects of documentation in nursing, including documentation in acute care, long-term care, and home-care settings. A significant amount of content focuses on the legal and ethical aspects of nursing documentation.

and written words. Nonverbal communication uses facial expression, gestures, touch, or other types of body language. Therapeutic communication is an interactive process between the nurse and the client that helps the client overcome temporary stress, to get along with other people, to adjust to the unalterable, and to overcome psychological blocks that stand in the way of self-realizations.

Documentation of clients' care and their responses to that care is essential for effective communication of the clients' status between health care providers. Additional uses of nursing documentation are in auditing for quality assurance, research, education, reimbursement, legal documentation, and health care analysis.

Nurses are increasingly using computers to enhance their communication. They use e-mail to communicate with other nurses, other departments in their employment setting, and resources outside the employment setting. Nurses can use computers to access health information through websites and literature databases.

SELECTED REFERENCES

Bradley, J. C., and Edinberg, M. A. 1990. *Communication in the nursing context,* 3d ed. Norwalk, Conn.: Appleton and Lange.

Craven, R. F., and Hirnle, C. J. 1996. *Fundamentals of nursing: Human health and function,* 2d ed. Philadelphia: Lippincott.

Fontaine, K. L., and Fletcher, J. S. 1995. *Essentials of mental health nursing,* 3d ed. Redwood City, Calif.: Addison-Wesley.

Frisch, N. C., and Frisch, L. E. 1998. *Psychiatric mental health nursing.* Albany, N.Y.: Delmar.

Hacker, D. 1994. *The Bedford handbook for writers,* 4th ed. Boston: St. Martin's Press.

Hall, E. T. 1969. *The hidden dimension.* Garden City, N.J.: Doubleday (Classic).

Kozier, B., Erb, G., Berman, A. J., and Burke, K. 2000. *Fundamentals of nursing: Concepts, process, and practice,* 6th ed. Upper Saddle River, N.J.: Prentice Hall Health.

Luckmann, J. 1999. *Transcultural communication in nursing.* New York: Delmar Publishers.

Mosby. 1999. *Surefire documentation: How, what, and when nurses need to document.* St. Louis: Mosby.

Sherman, K. 1994. *Communication and image in nursing.* Albany, N.Y.: Delmar.

Sieh, A., and Brentin, L. K. 1997. *The nurse communicates.* Philadelphia: Saunders.

Smith, S. 1992. *Communications in nursing,* 2d ed. St. Louis: Mosby.

Springhouse. 1995. *Mastering documentation.* Springhouse, Pa.: Springhouse Corporation.

Wilson, H. S., and Kneisl, C. R. 1996. *Psychiatric nursing,* 5th ed. Menlo Park, Calif.: Addison-Wesley.

Change Process

Objectives

- Differentiate spontaneous, developmental, and planned change.

- Explain the empirical-rational, normative-reeducative, and power-coercive approaches to change.

- Compare the change process models of Lewin, Lippitt, Havelock, and Rogers.

- Discuss types and characteristics of change agents.

- Identify ways to manage change by enhancing motivating forces and decreasing resistive forces.

- Identify steps in the change process.

N U R S E   C O N N E C T

Additional online resources for this chapter can be found on the companion web site at www.prenhall.com/blais.

To be effective and influential in today's world, nurses need to understand change theory and apply its precepts in the workplace, in government and professional organizations, and in the community. Change is a part of everyone's life; it is the way in which people grow, develop, and adapt. Change can be positive or negative, planned or unplanned.

Even though change is inevitable, it is not always welcome because it produces anxiety and fear even when it is planned. There is a sense of loss of the familiar, and a grief reaction may occur. The intensity can be worse when the change is unplanned. In the words of Tiffany and Lutjens (1998, p. 3), "Change is difficult. It helps. It hurts. It helps and hurts at the same time. Change is inevitable. We ignore change at our own peril."

The process of change is integral to many areas of nursing, such as teaching, client care, and health promotion. It involves individual clients, families, communities, organizations, nursing as a profession, and the entire health care–delivery system. Change can involve gaining knowledge, obtaining new skills, or adapting current knowledge in the light of new information. It can be particularly difficult when presenting challenges to one's values and beliefs, ways of thinking, or ways of relating.

CHALLENGES AND OPPORTUNITIES

The experience of change always presents some level of challenge to the person who must adapt. The rapidity and amount of change experienced in recent decades in health care has been particularly challenging for the nursing profession. New administrative structures, new technology, new professional roles, and new ways of providing care have challenged nurses to change the way they have practiced in the past. Assisting clients to make changes in lifestyle to enhance their health and well-being is a challenge for nurses.

With these challenges come opportunities to adapt to the new demands in a positive way. There are opportunities to incorporate the demands of change into improved ways of providing care. Nursing can meet the challenges of changing times with resistance and hang on to what is familiar or with acceptance and help create improved environments of care and improved ways of delivering health care. There is an opportunity for nursing to be proactive and manage planned change, thus emerging as a more autonomous and recognized profession.

MEANINGS AND TYPES OF CHANGE

Change is the process of making something different from what it was (Sullivan and Decker, 2001, p. 249). Change disrupts equilibrium, and it involves endings, transitions, and beginnings. People grieve when they lose something or are threatened with the loss of something. If they go through the steps of grieving, they may come to acceptance. Those who do not reach acceptance may experience disengagement or withdrawal, disidentification, with sadness and worry, disorientation and confusion, or disenchantment, accompanied by anger. Disengaged workers quit or retire in place doing only the bare minimum. People with disidentification are vulnerable, and they tend to sulk and dwell in the

past and resist new tasks. Disoriented workers no longer know where they fit in the organization and often do incorrect things because they do not know the new priorities. Disenchanted people become angry and negative and engage in destructive behavior (Tomey, 2000).

Changes are disturbing to those affected, and resistance often develops. Change is most threatening in the presence of insecurity. Causes of resistance to change include threats to self-interest, embarrassment, insecurity, habit, complacency, loss of power, and objective disagreement. Careful planning, appropriate timing of communication, adequate feedback, and employee confidence can reduce resistance to change. Informing personnel of reasons for change can help reduce resistance. Helping them cope and recognizing their contributions also minimize resistance (Tomey, 2000).

The noun and verb forms of the word *change* have different meanings. The noun form denotes substitution of one thing for another, an alteration in the state or quality of a thing, or permutations constituting varied arrangements of a set or series of things. Used as a verb, *change* means to make a thing other than it was (outward directed change) or to become different, to undergo alterations, or to vary (inward directed change). Synonyms for the verb *change* include *alter, transform, convert,* and *vary.* All these terms suggest that a fundamental difference or substitution is the outcome of change.

Change is not always the result of rational decision making. It generally occurs in response to three different activities: (a) spontaneous reactions, (b) developmental activities, and (c) consciously planned activities. Both individuals and organizations can undergo change.

Spontaneous Change

Spontaneous change is also referred to as reactive or unplanned change because it is not fully anticipated, it cannot be avoided, and there is little or no time to plan response strategies. Examples of spontaneous change affecting an individual include an acute viral infection, a spinal cord injury, and the unsolicited offer of a new position.

On a larger scale, spontaneous change can be either short term or long term. Examples of short-term spontaneous change include an earthquake or other natural disaster, a major airplane crash that is near a small hospital, or a wildcat strike that closes a tertiary health care facility. The impact of human immunodeficiency virus (HIV) on the policies and practices of health care facilities is an example of change with long-term consequences.

Responses to spontaneous change can be either

positive or negative. For example, the cold virus may create only minor inconveniences for one person but may lead to life-threatening illness in another. Likewise, an organization may respond successfully to the injuries resulting from a natural event if a well-developed disaster plan is in place; conversely, without such a plan the organization may experience disorganization, confusion, and major difficulties. The result of spontaneous change can be unpredictable. To ensure a successful response, spontaneous change demands flexibility and cohesiveness.

Developmental Change

Developmental change refers to physiopsychologic changes that occur during an individual's life cycle or to the growth of an organization as it becomes more complex. Examples of developmental change of individuals include the increasing size and complexity of a human embryo and fetus and the decreasing physical capability of an older person. These changes are not consciously planned; they just happen. However, the individual may make plans for dealing with the changes. For example, an older person may make plans for dealing with the physical changes, such as moving to a smaller, one-floor residence that is easier to care for and in which it is easier to move around.

Organizations often grow and develop in unpredictable ways. A once-successful small health organization may no longer meet the increasing demands and needs of a community. As the organization evolves into a larger, more complex entity, it may undergo such unwanted change as overwork, task changes, less personalized service, and more formalized staff communication patterns. Such unavoidable changes necessitate development of organizational charts, revised job descriptions, and, often, formal staff meetings to meet the defined needs.

Planned Change

According to Lippitt (1973), **planned change** is an intended, purposive attempt by an individual, group, organization, or larger social system to influence the status quo of itself, another organism, or a situation. Problem-solving skills, decision-making skills, and interpersonal skills are important factors in planned change. An example of planned change is an individual who decides to improve his or her health status by attending a smoking-cessation program or carrying out an exercise program. Organizations are continually involved in planned changes. In health care agencies changes are made in policies, in methods of care delivery, in staffing, and so on. Bringing about planned change is a major part of any nurse-manager's role.

From a personal perspective, Alfaro-LeFevre (1999, p. 1) addresses four ways people change. See the accompanying box.

Four Ways We Change

1. Pendulum change: "I was wrong before, but now I'm right."
2. Change by exception: "I'm right, except for . . ."
3. Incremental change: "I was *almost* right before, but now I'm right."
4. Paradigm change: "What I knew before was *partially* right. What I know now is more right, but only part of what I'll know tomorrow."

PARADIGM CHANGE IS TRANSFORMATIONAL

Paradigm change combines what's useful about *old* ways with what's useful about *new* ways and keeps us open to looking for *even better* ways.

We realize

- Our previous views were only part of the picture.
- What we now know is only part of what we'll know later.
- Change is no longer threatening: It enlarges and enriches.
- The unknown can then be friendly and interesting.
- Each insight smoothes the road, making the change process easier.

Sources: Aquarian Conspiracy: Personal and Social Transformation in Our Time by M. Ferguson, New York: Putnam, 1980; *Critical Thinking in Nursing: A Practical Approach* by R. Alfaro-LeFevre, 2nd ed, Philadelphia: W.B. Saunders, 1999, p. 1. Reprinted with permission.

Consider . . .

- spontaneous changes that have occurred in your personal and professional life. How did those changes affect you or your organization? What personal or professional strategies helped you or your organization adjust to the spontaneous changes?
- developmental changes that might be identified in the clients seen in your practice setting. Do the policies, procedures, and plans of care accommodate the identified developmental changes that are routinely occurring in your clients?
- developmental changes that are occurring in your organization. What are the staff reactions to these changes? How might the professional nurse cope with or assist colleagues to cope with organization change?
- planned changes that have occurred in your personal or professional life during the last year. Do planned professional changes result in planned personal changes? Is it possible that planned professional changes might result in spontaneous personal changes?

CHANGE THEORY

Approaches to Planned Change

Three broad strategies or approaches to planned change have been identified; they represent a contin-uum of least coercive (empirical-rational) through middle ground (normative-reeducative) to the most obtrusive (power-coercive). They are compared in Table 14–1. Each is appropriate in different situations and at different times. It is important to carefully select the appropriate strategy.

Empirical-Rational

The *empirical-rational approach* is based on two beliefs: that people are rational and that they will change if it is in their self-interest. Therefore, change will be adopted if the change can be rationally justified and shown to be advantageous to the people involved (Bennis, Benne, and Chinn, 1985).

However, people do not always act rationally, and therein can be the shortcoming. This strategy is most effective when there is little resistance to the change and the change is perceived as reasonable. Staff development in this strategy is through education and systems analysis (Tomey, 2000). The power ingredient is knowledge, and the flow of influence is from those who know to those who do not know. The style can be compared to marketing. Once people are informed, they will accept or reject the idea based upon its merits and consequences (Sullivan and Decker, 2001, p. 257).

Table 14–1 Change Approaches

Approach	Characteristics
Power-coercive	• Based on the application of power from a legitimate source. • Power is often economic or is political. • Minimal participation by target members. • Resistance may occur and morale may decrease. • Feelings and values of opposing forces are not a factor. • Model is nonparticipative and undemocratic.
Empirical-rational	• Knowledge is power. • Influence moves from those with knowledge to those without. • Once members of the target group have knowledge, they will accept or reject the idea. • Is a noncoercive model. • Appropriate for new technology. • Works well when the target group is discontented. • Fully participative and democratic.
Normative-reeducative	• Recognizes that change must deal with feelings, values, and needs. • Recognizes that not all responses of people to change are rational. • Information and rational arguments are often insufficient to bring about change. • Model is partially participative and democratic.

Normative-Reeducative

The *normative-reeducative approach* is based on the assumption that human motivation depends on the sociocultural norms and the individual's commitment to these norms. The sociocultural norms are supported by the attitudes and value systems of the individuals. In this instance, change occurs if the people involved develop new attitudes and values by acquiring new information. In this approach, knowledge is the power for change, but it may be a lengthy process because attitudes and values are difficult to change. People's roles and relationships, perceptual orientations, attitudes, and feelings will influence their acceptance of change.

The communication is participative and two-way (Baird, 1998). Staff development is through more individual means, such as personal counseling, small groups, and experiential learning. People participate in their own reeducation. The change agents are usually internal to the organization, and their relationship to other personnel is important (Tomey, 2000). The power ingredient is interpersonal relationships, and the change agent uses collaboration.

This approach can be effective in reducing resistance and stimulating creativity. It is well suited to nursing because nurses are well versed in behavioral science and communication skills (Sullivan and Decker, 2001, p. 258).

Power-Coercive

With the *power-coercive approach,* power lies with one or more persons of influence. The influence may come through political power, wealth, status, or ability. This approach does not deny the intelligence or rationality of people or the importance of their attitudes or values, but it recognizes the need to use power to attain change. It is a command and control approach in which positions of authority enforce the change. As a strategy, it can provoke resistance. The communication style is telling people what to do (Baird, 1998).

This approach is sometimes appropriate in large-scale changes or when consensus is unlikely to be achieved, time is short, resistance is anticipated, and the change is critical for the organization's survival. It tends to be better received when combined with the other two approaches. Strikes, sit-ins, and conflict resolutions are sometimes employed. These strategies should be used cautiously if there is a desire to foster a climate of openness to change (Sullivan and Decker, 2001, p. 257).

Change Strategies

Tiffany and Lutjens (1998) have identified seven change strategies that fit on a continuum from most neutral to most coercive.

1. *Educational.* This strategy provides a relatively unbiased presentation of fact that is intended to serve as a rational justification for the planned action.
2. *Facilitative.* This strategy provides resources critical to change. It assumes that people are willing to change but need the resources to bring it about.
3. *Technostructural.* This strategy alters the technology to access the social structure in groups or alters the social structure to get at technology. It assumes a relationship among technology, space, and structure. The use of space might be altered to affect the social structure.
4. *Data-based.* This strategy collects and uses data to make social change. Data are used to find the best innovation to solve the problems at hand.
5. *Communication.* Communication strategies spread information over time through channels in a social system.
6. *Persuasive.* The use of reasoning, arguing, and inducement are employed to bring about a change.
7. *Coercive.* There is an obligatory relationship between planners and adopters. Power is used to bring about change.

Frameworks for Change

Frameworks such as those of Lewin, Lippitt, Rogers, and Havelock follow the normative-reeducative approach. They are compared in Table 14–2.

Lewin

Kurt Lewin (1948) originated change theory. He saw change as having three basic stages: unfreezing, moving, and refreezing. See Figure 14–1. During the *unfreezing* stage, the motivation to establish some sort of change occurs. The individual becomes aware of the need for change. This stage is a cognitive process in which the person becomes aware of a problem or of a better method of accomplishing a task and hence of the need for change. Having identified this need, the individual must also identify restraining and driving forces. For example, a nurse who is instructing an adolescent client and his mother in dietary management of type I (juvenile-onset) diabetes may see the client's mother as a driving force and the client's father and siblings, who don't want to change their sugar-loaded diet, as restraining forces.

Table 14–2 Comparison of Change Models

Lewin	Lippitt	Havelock	Rogers
1. Unfreezing	1. Diagnose problem 2. Assess motivation 3. Assess change agent's motivations and resources	1. Building a relationship 2. Diagnosing the problem 3. Acquiring resources	1. Knowledge 2. Persuasion 3. Decision
2. Moving	4. Select progressive change objects 5. Choose change agent role	4. Choosing the solution 5. Gaining acceptance	4. Implementation
3. Refreezing	6. Maintain change 7. Terminate helping relationship	6. Stabilization	5. Confirmation

In the second stage, *moving,* the actual change is planned in detail and then started. Information is gathered from one or several sources. At this stage, it is important that the people involved agree that the status quo is undesirable. In this example, the nurse needs to help the family understand the importance of dietary management for diabetics and to enlist their support for the client. The nurse could ask the dietitian to meet with the client and his family to demonstrate how a diabetic diet can be nutritious and tasty. The nurse might also provide printed food exchange lists, sample menus, and recipes, as well as resources for diabetic information. As change agent, the nurse should work with the family to create an environment that is conducive to the change, including, perhaps, rewards to reinforce desired behaviors.

In the third stage, *refreezing,* the changes are integrated and stabilized. Those involved in the change integrate the idea into their own value system. Thus, in the example, the client and his family would come to value the importance of family involvement in dietary management of their diabetic son and sibling. The family may develop their own strategies for assisting their loved one to comply with the plan.

These three stages are described in Lewin's *force field theory.* Lewin recommended that before a change is begun, the forces operating for and against the change be analyzed. The forces for change are the *driving forces* and the forces against change are *restraining forces.* When the driving forces predominate, change occurs; when restraining forces predominate, change does not occur. It then becomes the responsibility of the change agent to use strategies to reduce the restraining forces and increase the driving forces. Reducing restraining forces usually is more effective than increasing the driving forces. This *unfreezing* is directed at the target system, that is, the individual, family, or group. See Figure 14–2 and the box on page 235.

Lippitt

Gordon Lippitt and his colleagues described planned change as having seven phases, as shown in Table 14–2 (Lippitt, Watson, and Westley, 1958). This extended Lewin's theory and focused more on what the change agent must do rather than on the evolution of the change. These seven phases begin with the recognized need for change. The manager can stimulate awareness and present the idea that a more desirable state is possible. Assessment can be made of the motivation and capacity to change as well as the resources for change. In Lewin's theory, this would be comparable to unfreezing.

Figure 14–1

Process of Change

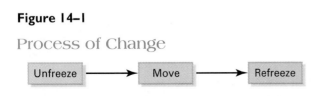

Figure 14–2

Status Quo

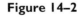

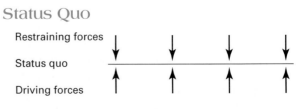

Common Driving and Restraining Forces

Motivating Forces

- Perception that the change is challenging
- Economic gain
- Perception that the change will improve the situation
- Visualization of the future impact of change
- Potential for self-growth, recognition, achievement, and improved relationships.

Restraining Forces

- Fear that something of personal value will be lost (e.g., threat to job security or self-esteem)
- Misunderstanding of the change and its implications
- Low tolerance for change related to intellectual or emotional insecurity
- Perception that the change will not achieve goals; failure to see the big picture
- Lack of time or energy

In order for the process to move, a helping relationship must begin. The success or failure of the planned change will often depend upon the quality and workability of the client and change agent relationship. Problems must be identified and analyzed, alternative possibilities must be examined, and goals and objectives must be planned. Resources will be examined and strategies developed. This corresponds to moving in Lewin's theory.

Generalization and stabilization correspond to Lewin's refreezing process. These are necessary to prevent slipping back into old ways. The change needs to spread and stabilize. A change in momentum, positive evaluation of the change, reward for change, and procedural and structural change are each important factors (Tomey, 2000).

Havelock

Ronald Havelock (1973) modified Lewin's theory regarding planned change by emphasizing planning the change process. He described the six-step process shown in Table 14–2. More attention is paid to the unfreezing stage, which he defines as building a relationship, diagnosing the problem, and acquiring resources. In the moving stage, the solution is chosen and acceptance is gained. Refreezing is referred to as stabilization and self-renewal.

Rogers

Everett Rogers (1983) developed a *diffusion-innovation theory* rather than a planned change theory. He defines *diffusion* as the process by which an innovation is communicated through certain channels over time among the members of a social system. Diffusion that involves innovation becomes *social change* when the diffusion of new ideas results in widespread consequences. His framework, diffusion of innovation, emphasizes the reversible nature of change. Participants may initially adopt a proposal and later discontinue it, or they may initially reject it and adopt it at a later time. Rogers thus introduced the idea that an adopted change is not necessarily permanent. Rogers' three phases in the diffusion of innovation follow (Rogers and Shoemaker, 1971; Rogers, 1995):

1. *Invention.* Collecting information about the proposed change. Data are collected and analyzed.

2. *Diffusion.* Communicating information or the idea to others. It includes disseminating information and estimating the case or difficulty of diffusing the new idea or information.

3. *Consequences.* The dissemination of information may result in the adoption or rejection of the change.

Rogers wrote that the factors associated with successful planned change are relativity, advantage, compatibility, complexity, divisibility, and communicability. His five steps to the diffusion of innovations, referred to as the *innovation-decision process*, follow:

1. *Knowledge.* The individual, called the decision-making unit, is introduced to change and begins to comprehend it.

2. *Persuasion.* The individual develops a favorable or unfavorable attitude toward the change.

3. *Decision.* The person makes a choice to adopt or not to adopt the change.

4. *Implementation.* The person acts on the choice. At this time, alterations may take place.

5. *Confirmation.* The individual looks for confirmation that the choice was right. If the person encounters mixed messages, the choice may be changed.

Rogers emphasized that for change to succeed, the people involved must be interested in the change and committed to implementing it. His theory is particularly useful for individuals who wish to track the adoption of technologic innovations. (Tiffany and Lutjens, 1998).

Consider . . .

- a nursing situation in which a client is presented with the need to change a behavior in order to better manage a health problem. Apply one of the frameworks discussed and identify how a nurse might assist with this change.
- a need for change you have identified in your community. Apply one of these frameworks and identify steps you could take to facilitate this change.

MANAGING CHANGE

There are internal and external forces that affect change. Internal forces originate inside the organization, but they may be due to external forces. There may be an internal force for changing the organization of health care delivery related to low staffing levels, but these low staffing levels may be caused by external forces such as the shortage of nurses or changing health care economics.

The change manager must be able to identify the source of the problem, assess motivations and capacity for change, determine and examine alternatives, and then determine and implement a helping relationship. Havelock (1973) believes change agents facilitate planned change by being a catalyst, solution giver, process helper, and resource linker. In using Lewin's theory, change agents identify the restraining and driving forces and assess the relative strengths of each. Driving forces could include desire to please authority figures or a desire to improve a situation. Restraining forces could include such things as conformity or threats to prestige. Strategies are then planned to reduce the restraining forces and strengthen the driving forces.

Change Agent

A **change agent** is one who works to bring about a change (Sullivan and Decker, 2001, p. 249). The change agent is the person or group who initiates, motivates, and implements the change. Change agents are lead-

Bookshelf

Johnson, S., and Blanchard, K. 1998. *Who moved my cheese? An amazing way to deal with change in your work and in your life.* **New York: Putnam Publishing.** This book presents a parable of four not-so-blind mice who learn to accept and adapt to change to get what they need. They live in a maze and look for cheese but are faced with an unexpected change. One of them learns to deal with it successfully and writes what he has learned on the maze walls.

Vance, M., and Deacon, D. 1997. *Think out of the box.* **New York: Career Press.** Written by the former dean of Disney University, this book uses a nine-dot matrix to plot the nine necessary points of a creative culture: people, place, product, involving, informing, inspiring, cooperation, and creativity.

Driegel, R. J., and Brandt, D. 1997. *Sacred cows make the best burgers: Developing change-ready people and organizations.* **New York: Warner Books, Inc.** Outdated and costly practices exist in every organization, and they slow down innovative ideas. This book provides a guide to why people hold on to the old and how to inspire them to bring on the new.

ers. The nurse uses critical thinking and knowledge of change theory to act as an effective change agent in a variety of health care settings.

An effective change agent must be highly skilled. As the nurse moves through the process of change with clients, families, groups, communities, or institutions, the nurse assumes a variety of roles, depending on the type of change and the needs of the individuals involved in the change. It is also important for the change agent to be accessible to all people involved in the change process. The change agent should be honest and straightforward about goals and problems. The box on page 237 describes effective change agent skills.

A key element in the change process is trust. The change agent must trust the participants in the change, and they in turn must trust the change agent. One of the greatest risks of change is that it can disrupt the system or even render it nonfunctional. For example, changing the method of nurse assignments could result in gaps and missed care for some clients. To avoid this problem, the change agent must closely observe the situation during the change process.

Change Agent Skills

- The ability to combine ideas from unconnected sources
- The ability to energize others by keeping the interest level up and demonstrating a high personal energy level
- Skill in human relations; well-developed interpersonal communication, group management, and problem-solving skills
- Integrative thinking; the ability to retain a "big picture" focus while dealing with each part of the system
- Sufficient flexibility to modify ideas when modifica-

tions will improve the change, but persistent enough to resist nonproductive tampering with the planned change
- Confidence and the tendency not to be easily discouraged
- Realistic thinking
- Trustworthiness; a track record of integrity and success with other changes
- Ability to articulate a "vision" through insights and versatile thinking
- Ability to handle resistance

Source: Effective Management in Nursing, 5th ed., by E. J. Sullivan and P. J. Decker, Redwood City, Calif.: Addison-Wesley Nursing, 2001, p. 258. Reprinted with permission.

A change agent may be formally or informally designated. A *formally designated change agent* is one who has the role and responsibility for change, such as a clinical nurse-specialist expected to make changes beneficial to specified clients. This person has the authority to plan and implement change. An *informally designated change agent* does not have the authority to make change by virtue of a position but does have the leadership skills and respect of others and therefore can serve an important function in the change process. A change agent who has formal status carries authority, whereas an informal change agent can operate only through persuasion (Ehrenfeld, Bergman, and Ziv, 1992, p. 23).

Change agents may also be internal or external. An *internal change agent* is a person who is part of the situation or system, for example, a charge nurse on a hospital unit or a public health nurse providing school health services to a specific school or within a school system. Internal change agents are familiar with the situation and the organization. However, they may have vested interests in the present system as well as biases. An *external change agent* comes to the situation from the "outside," for example, a nursing administrator from another hospital, a nurse-specialist from another health care facility, or a nurse-educator from a local college. External change agents are able to view the problem and the situation objectively and usually have no biases; they are often viewed as experts and are called consultants. However, they may not have per-

sonal knowledge of the situation and the problems. They may not be viewed as openly as an "insider"; therefore, they must develop a cooperative working relationship with the people involved in the change. A third option is to pair the external agent with the internal person to serve together as change agents. There are advantages and disadvantages to each of these options, and it is important for any change agent to be aware of both in each situation.

The American Nurses Association, in *Standards of Clinical Nursing Practice* (1998, p. 11), identifies measurement criteria for the nurse's role in change: Nurses use "the results of quality of care activities to initiate changes in practice" and "to initiate change throughout the health care delivery system."

Coping with Change

Although change is inevitable and necessary for growth, it is not always welcome and often produces anxiety. Even when change is well planned, it can be threatening because the process renders something different from the status quo. Change evokes emotional reactions, consumes considerable internal resources and energy, and often is associated with feelings of loss, grief, and pain. Various models have been proposed to explain the psychologic problems associated with change. Seven stages of change are identified and can be used as a framework for navigating transitions (Manion, 1998). These seven stages are depicted in Figure 14–3.

Figure 14–3

The Seven Stages of Change

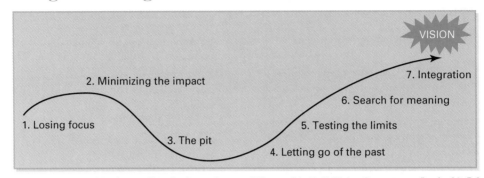

Used by permission from J. Manion, "Understanding the Seven Stages of Change," in E. C. Hein, *Contemporary Leadership Behavior Selected Readings,* 5th ed., Philadelphia: Lippincott, 1998, p. 237.

Stage 1: Losing focus. Confusion and disorientation occur and decisions are difficult. On the positive side, this stage is usually short and may not require specific interventions.

Stage 2: Minimizing the impact. Some denial is used to reduce the significance and portray the event as no big deal. Often the person feels the need to "put on a good face." If it is prolonged, productivity and commitment can disintegrate.

Stage 3: The pit. This represents the lowest point on the mood curve shown in Figure 14–3. There is anger, discouragement, resentment, and resistance. Morale suffers, and people often have difficulty dealing with the emotions in this stage.

Stage 4: Letting go of the past. This is a more positive stage; energy starts to return and people begin to see the end of the change process. There are two main tasks during this stage, letting go of the past and looking ahead. People begin to prepare for the future. There is optimism and renewed energy. It is not unusual to be dragged back to the pit from this stage, because things do not always unfold in a perfectly linear fashion, but the time is usually much shorter.

Stage 5: Testing the limits. Optimism is more energizing; people try new coping skills and deal with the situation in more creative ways.

Stage 6: Search for meaning. At this stage, there is an ability to look back and realize that even though the change was painful, meaning can be seen in the experience. There is a newly found confidence and freedom and sometimes a desire to reach out to others who are still experiencing difficulty.

Stage 7: Integration. By this stage, the transition is complete. The change has been integrated into life, and people are oriented toward the future.

Unfortunately, people often are called upon to deal with another change before they have reached full integration of a previous change. In today's rapidly changing health care environment, coping with change may be one of the biggest challenges. It calls for resilience, adaptability, and flexibility. The box on page 239 shows some tips for getting through each of the seven stages of change.

Resistance to Change

Resistance to change is not merely lack of acceptance but rather behavior intended to maintain the status quo—i.e., to prevent the change. The change agent should anticipate some resistance to change, no matter how beneficial the change may seem. Resistance to change is often greatest when the idea is not concurrent with existing trends, such as trying to change from primary nursing to functional nursing when primary nursing is the current trend. Resistance is also usually great when a proposed change would alter a situation with which people are comfortable.

Accepting change often takes time, particularly when it does not fit into a person's attitudinal frame of reference; in such a case, change may not occur at all. For example, stopping smoking may not be accepted as a desirable change by a person who enjoys smoking and does not believe that it is harmful. Optimally, this belief changes before the person tries to change the behavior.

A change agent should anticipate resistance to change. It is important to listen to what people are say-

Tips for Getting Through the Stages of Change

1. Losing focus
   - Expect some forgetfulness.
   - Use to-do lists.
   - Ask for clarification of expectations and temporary lines of authority.
2. Minimizing the impact
   - Tell yourself the truth about what's happening. List the gains and losses associated with the change. Be honest about what you're losing or giving up.
   - If others offer help but you're not ready to accept it, respond in a way that leaves the door open for their support at a later date.
   - Take one step at a time.
   - Don't stay in this stage too long—but don't try to end it precipitously either. Start gathering your courage for the next stage, which is the most difficult.
3. The pit
   - Expect to feel angry, discouraged, and resentful. If you know what's happening inside you, you're more likely to keep your equilibrium.
   - Let yourself experience the feelings. Suppressing or denying them will make it more difficult for you to deal with change in the future.
   - Find a safe place to express your feelings, preferably with someone who can listen comfortably without taking them on or trying to talk you out of them.
   - Develop a positive vision of what things will be like when you've finished this transition, then think of it often. People with a clear vision have an easier time getting through the pit.
4. Letting go of the past
   - Say good-bye to the past, either formally or informally. You might do this with a "letting-go" ritual. An example of such a ritual would be to review what was positive about the past, recount good memories, and then bury it. Or it may be more appropriate to have a graduation party.
   - Allow some sadness and longing for the way things used to be.
   - As you look ahead, think of what you'll need to adjust to the change—new skills and new approaches, for example. Consider specific ways to obtain them.
   - Take care of yourself. Celebrate the small successes.
5. Testing the limits
   - Seek new experiences and ways to use the skills you've gained.
   - Spend time with people who have experienced the same change or loss.
   - Talk about the past only with those who will listen and not become impatient.
   - Associate with people who are encouraging and supportive.
6. Search for meaning
   - Spend time reflecting on your experiences since the change occurred. Sort through your feelings. Ask yourself: "What have I learned that I didn't know before?"
   - Look back to how you handled the different emotional stages. Notice which were particularly difficult and give yourself a pat on the back for getting through them.
   - Find others going through the same experience. Listen carefully to see if you can offer any support.
7. Integration
   - Appreciate reaching this final stage. (It doesn't always happen.)
   - Recognize how far you've come and the skills you've learned along the way.

Used by permission from J. Manion, "Understanding the Seven Stages of Change," in E. C. Hein, *Contemporary Leadership Behavior Selected Readings*, 5th ed., Philadelphia: Lippincott, 1998, p. 239.

ing and under what circumstances. There are often nonverbal signs of resistance and perhaps passive aggression, including poor work habits and lack of effort in assigned tasks. Open resisters are easier to deal with than the more passive resisters.

Resistance to change is not always a bad thing; it can prevent the unexpected and provide a barrier to change that may not be desirable for the institution. Some degree of resistance to change is a natural response. Resistance may help people adapt to the proposed change as they try to understand the meaning on a personal level, establish a thread of continuity, and then accept and grow with the change. It forces the change agent to be clear and convincing about the need and to provide motivation. On the other hand, persistent resistance can wear down supporters and use up energy that could be directed to implementation. Morale can suffer. It then becomes necessary for the change agent to minimize the resistance.

To manage resistance, the leader (change agent) can analyze the field forces operating in the change (see the discussion on Lewin). After the analysis, three kinds of tactics can be used to "unfreeze" the system: (1) create discomfort, (2) induce guilt or anxiety, (3) provide psychological safety (Tappen, 2001, p. 207). To create discomfort, the change agent can confront the target system with conflicting evidence that challenges the status quo. Often the change agent meets with defensive responses that attempt to protect the individuals. By inducing guilt—for example, by pointing out that accepted goals are not being met—the change agent often upsets the balance of the driving and restraining forces. Then, by providing psychologic safety, the change agent can help the target system feel more comfortable and less threatened about the change. See the accompanying boxes.

The change agent needs to be aware of the sources of power that can energize change. This often means being politically astute within an organization. The following four political strategies may be helpful:

1. Analyze the organizational chart and be aware of the formal and informal lines of authority.

2. Identify the key people affected by the change. In an organizational hierarchy, the people immediately above and below those directly affected should be given attention.

3. Find out as much as possible about what makes these key people tick. It is important to know their likes and dislikes and with whom they usually align on decisions.

4. Begin to build a coalition of support before the change begins by identifying those individuals who are most likely to support the effort and those most likely to be persuaded easily. Their counsel on costs and benefits and objections can be used to make modifications that make the innovation more appealing (Sullivan and Decker, 2001, p. 259).

The successful change agent has a good sense of timing and can effectively adapt a time table to facilitate the process and gain support. Unfreezing can best be accomplished during coalition building when interest is high and resistance has not yet consolidated.

If resistance continues for a prolonged period of time, the change agent must consider two possibilities.

Managing Resistance

1. Communicate with those who oppose the change. Get to the root of their reasons for opposition.

2. Clarify information and provide accurate feedback.

3. Be open to revisions but clear about what must remain.

4. Present the negative consequences of resistance (threats to organizational survival, compromised client care, and so on).

5. Emphasize the positive consequences of the change and how the individual or group will benefit. However, do not spend too much energy on rational analysis of why the change is good and why the arguments against it do not hold up. People's resistance frequently flows from feelings that are not rational.

6. Keep resisters involved in face-to-face contact with supporters. Encourage proponents to empathize with opponents, recognize valid objections, and relieve unnecessary fears.

7. Maintain a climate of trust, support, and confidence.

8. Divert attention by creating a different "disturbance." Energy can shift to a "more important" problem inside the system, thereby redirecting resistance. Alternatively attention can be brought to an external threat to create a "bully phenomenon." When members perceive a greater environmental threat (such as competition or restrictive governmental policies), they tend to unify internally.

9. Follow the "politics of change."

Source: Effective Management in Nursing, 5th ed., by E. J. Sullivan and P. J. Decker, Redwood City, Calif.: Addison-Wesley Nursing, 2001, p. 259. Reprinted with permission.

Examples to Unfreeze a Target System

Producing discomfort
- Meet with small groups of nurses (target system) to discuss the inadequacies of the system of concern (e.g., staffing).

Inducing guilt and anxiety
- Demonstrate how the system is not meeting clients' needs for care.
- Explain that the administration wants the new system.
- Provide examples of how the old system has endangered client safety.

Providing psychologic safety
- Assure nurses (target system) that adequate numbers of nurses will be provided.
- Point out that sufficient time will be provided to implement the new system.
- Express confidence in the nurses' abilities to implement the change.
- Assure the nurses that there will be regular meetings to discuss progress.

One is that the change is not workable and must therefore be modified, and compromise is necessary to meet the strongest objections. The other possibility is that the change is appropriate and the plan is sufficiently developed but must proceed through more coercive means so resistance can be overcome.

Examples of Change

It is exciting to realize how effective nurses can be when they determine the need for change and plan strategies to bring it about. The following examples outline changes initiated by nurses who have identified a need to "do something" in each of four spheres of influence: the workplace, organizations, government, and the community.

THE WORKPLACE At each of three shift meetings Nurse Hawkins, head nurse, listened to nurses complain about problems with getting clients' laboratory work done and reported to the unit in a timely manner. She conferred with other head nurses and with the attending and resident physicians on her unit. It appeared that similar complaints were widespread.

At the next meeting of head nurses, Nurse Hawkins described the problem. The group appointed a task force, with Nurse Hawkins as chair, and asked it to present a plan to solve the problem at the next meeting. After gathering more data, the task force invited representatives from the attending and resident staff and the laboratory director to meet with them to review the data, consider alternative solutions, and select a plan to solve the problem.

By the next meeting of head nurses, a preliminary plan to alter the system of laboratory reporting had

Research Box

Ardern, P. 1999. Safeguarding care gains: A grounded theory study of organizational change. *Journal of Advanced Nursing* 29(6): 1370–1376.

A grounded theory approach examined the changes experienced by a group of staff working in an English day hospital for people with dementia. Interviews and observations took place over a two-year period of time, supplemented by diaries, workshops, documents, and organizational meetings, which were recorded and transcribed. The qualitative data were analyzed by a constant comparative technique to identify patterns, develop categories, and create links. Staff members experienced a period of prolonged change and loss of their model of care, with resulting perception of support differing from that of the organization. When threats to the future and low support were perceived, defensiveness and risk containment were evident in the responses. These responses were identified as *safeguarding care gains* or protecting the project and care gains that the staff members had established. Staff members were less able to accept changes when they threatened the traditional balance and support within the team at the social and group interaction level. A key element was found to be the influence of organizational support. When this was experienced as lacking, staff members experienced increasing isolation with disempowerment and defensiveness, eventually resulting in disintegration of the team and collapse of the gains.

Research Box

Ingersoll, G. L., Kirsch, J. C., Merk, S. E., and Light-foot, J. 2000. Relationship of organizational culture and readiness for change to employee commitment to the organization. *Journal of Nursing Administration* 30(1): 11–20.

This study was done to determine the influence of organizational culture and organizational readiness on employee commitment to the work of the institution. A longitudinal survey design was used, and questionnaires were distributed through the hospital's internal mailing system. Subjects were selected from all nursing, administrative, and ancillary support personnel using a systematic, stratified sample-selection plan. Two questionnaires were used for data collection, the Organizational Culture Inventory and the Pasmore Sociotechnical Systems Assessment Survey. Two tertiary hospitals undergoing the implementation of a patient-focused redesign were the sites of the study. The focus of the redesign was on bringing services closer to the patient, reducing the number of persons interacting with patients and families, and improving the efficiency and quality of services to consumers. Data were collected approximately 6 months after planning began and immediately before implementation. A sample size of 684 was analyzed by multiple regression. Organizational readiness was the strongest predictor of commitment. The researchers conclude that organizations in which change is seen as a positive characteristic of the environment and employees are reinforced for their contribution are more likely to develop work groups committed to the work of the institution.

been devised, and all concerned were working cooperatively to implement the plan.

THE PROFESSIONAL ORGANIZATION Nurses on the Education Committee of a district nurses' association recognized the need to make a public policy statement concerning the care of clients with AIDS. Since the board of directors had recently expressed interest in promulgating such policy statements, the committee sensed the timing was right and that the board would welcome its draft despite the controversial subject matter.

Members of the committee researched and drafted a statement. The full committee offered a critique and selected an articulate spokesperson to present the statement to the association president and seek support before asking to have the statement presented to the board. Once the president had approved the statement, it was placed on the agenda for the next board meeting.

After making minor additions, the board approved it for distribution to the lay and nursing press and asked the Education Committee to suggest a nurse to present the statement at a local hearing of the City Council Health Committee.

THE GOVERNMENT Although the pressure to contain health care costs escalated through the first half of the 1980s, a coalition representing the shared interests of the ANA, the National League for Nursing (NLN), and the American Association of Colleges of Nursing (AACN) mounted a campaign to convince Congress of the cost-effectiveness of a center for nursing research within the National Institutes of Health (NIH). Despite incredible odds, including a presidential veto and opposition from the American Medical Association, the American Association of Medical Colleges, and the NIH administrations, the proposal was passed by Congress in the fall of 1985. The success of this effort demonstrates the effectiveness of carefully planned change including the collaboration of nursing organizations. It also illustrates the clout organized nurses can wield on any level and in any sphere.

THE COMMUNITY Every nurse plays several roles besides that of registered nurse. Each resides in a community, and many are parents. Some serve on school boards, belong to the League of Women Voters, or participate in religious, club, or scouting activities. There are numerous opportunities for nurses to contribute to the health and welfare of the communities in which they live. A group of nursing students recognized a health problem within their community and developed a plan to intervene. Many of the students were parents of children in local elementary schools where a high percentage of children were being sent home daily with head lice. Because of previously enacted budget cuts, the district's school nurses were each responsible for between three and five schools. The students volunteered to work with the district nurses to provide screening and health teaching at each of the elementary schools, thereby helping to resolve the community's problem.

All nurses are affected by change; nobody can avoid it. Knowledgeable nurses make rational plans to deal with both opportunities to initiate and guide needed change as well as to respond to change that affects them in the workplace, government, organizations, and the community. To recognize these opportunities for change and respond to the factors that influence nursing from without, it is helpful to consider the history of nursing, current trends in nursing, and present political, social, technologic, and economic issues.

Consider . . .

■ what changes are needed in your professional skills and abilities to help you to become a more effective change agent. How will you approach these changes?

■ a change that is needed in policy at your workplace. What are the different driving and restraining forces involved in the proposed change? What strategies might you implement to reduce the restraining forces? What strategies might you implement to enhance the driving forces? How might you obtain the assistance of formal and informal change agents in your practice setting to facilitate the change?

SUMMARY

To be effective and influential in current and future health care delivery systems, nurses need to understand and apply change theory. Change generally occurs in response to three different activities: spontaneous reactions or events, developmental activities, and consciously planned activities. These three types of change can occur on an individual or organizational level.

The three most commonly used approaches to change are the empirical-rational approach, the power-coercive approach, and the normative-reeducative approach. In reality, all three of these approaches may operate in a situation of change simultaneously.

Lewin's theory of change has three stages: unfreezing, moving, and refreezing. His force-field analysis is a means of examining the driving forces for change and the restraining forces that would limit change. The analysis of the opposing forces is done in the unfreezing stage. Reducing restraining forces is usually more effective in accomplishing change than is increasing the driving forces.

Lippitt proposed a seven-stage process beginning with diagnosing the problem and ending with terminating the helping relationship. Havelock modified Lewin's theory to emphasize the planning stage of the change process. His six-stage theory begins with building a relationship and ends with stabilization and generating self-renewal. Rogers introduced the idea that

adopted change is not necessarily permanent. He developed a five-step diffusion-innovation process.

A change agent seeks to facilitate the processes of change. An effective change agent uses an understanding of the change process to plan and implement any change. To be effective change agents, nurses require excellent skills of communication, problem solving, decision making, and teaching and must be able to project expertise, know how to use available resources, be able to inspire trust in themselves and others, and have a good sense of timing. A change agent may be formally or informally designated, internal or external. Nurses frequently act as formal or informal change agents in relation to clients, families, work settings, and communities. The change agent works to alter the driving and restraining forces and facilitates the acceptance of change by encouraging the participation of all involved in the change process. Effective communication is vital to the success of planned change.

Change is stressful, and the individuals experiencing change need to be supported and empowered. The stress is often associated with emotional reactions of denial, anger, feelings of loss, grief, and pain. An understanding of these responses enables both change agents and those experiencing the change to minimize the trauma associated with it. Managing change requires adaptability, flexibility, and resilience.

SELECTED REFERENCES

Alfaro-Lefevre, R. 1999. *Critical thinking in nursing: A practical approach,* 2d ed. Philadelphia: W.B. Saunders.

American Nurses Association. 1998. *Standards of clinical nursing practice.* Washington, D.C.: ANA.

Ardern, P. 1999. Safeguarding care gains: A grounded

theory study of organizational change. *Journal of Advanced Nursing* **29**(6): 1370–1376.

Baird, A. 1998. Change theory and health promotion. *Nursing Standard* **12**(22): 34–36.

Bennis, W. G., Benne, K. D., and Chin, R. eds. 1985. *The*

planning of change, 4th ed. New York: Holt, Rinehart & Winston.

Ehrenfeld, M., Bergman, R., and Ziv, L. 1992, Jan./Feb. Academia—a stimulus for change. *International Nursing Review* **39**: 23–26.

Havelock, R. 1973. *The change agent's guide to innovations in education.* Englewood Cliffs. N.J.: Educational Technology Publications.

Hein, E. C. 1998. *Contemporary leadership behavior: Selected readings,* 5th ed. Philadelphia: Lippincott.

Ingersoll, G. L., Kirsch, J. C., Merk, S. E., and Lightfoot, J. 2000. Relationship of organizational culture and readiness for change to employee commitment to the organization. *Journal of Nursing Administration* **30**(1): 11–20.

Knox, S., and Irving, J. A. 1997. An interactive quality of work life model applied to organizational transition. *Journal of Nursing Administration* **27**(1): 39–47.

Lewin, K. 1948. *Resolving social conflicts.* New York: Harper and Brothers.

Lewin, K. 1951. *Field theory in social science.* New York: Harper and Row.

Lippitt, G. L. 1973. *Visualizing change: Model building and the change process.* La Jolla, Calif.: University Associates.

Lippitt, R., Watson, J., and Westley, B. 1958. *The dynamics of planned change.* New York: Harcourt Brace.

Manion, J. 1998. Understanding the seven stages of change. In E. C. Hein, *Contemporary Leadership Behavior: Selected Readings,* 5th ed. Philadelphia: Lippincott, pp. 236–240.

Miller, C. E. 1999. Stages of change theory and the nicotine-dependent client: Direction for decision making in nursing practice. *Clinical Nurse Specialist* **13**(1): 18–22.

Rogers, E. 1983. *Diffusion of innovations,* 3d ed. New York: Free Press.

Rogers, E. M. 1995. *Diffusion of innovations,* 4th ed. New York: Free Press.

Rogers, E., and Shoemaker, F. 1971. *Communication of innovations: A crosscultural approach.* New York: The Free Press of Glencoe.

Sullivan, E. J., and Decker, P. 2001. *Effective leadership and management in nursing,* 5th ed. Upper Saddle River, N.J.: Prentice Hall.

Tappen, R. M. 2001. *Nursing leadership and management: Concepts and practice,* 4th ed. Philadelphia: F. A. Davis Company.

Tiffany, C. R., and Lutjens, L. R. J. 1998. *Planned change theories for nursing: Review, analysis, and implications.* Thousand Oaks, Calif.: Sage Publications.

Tomey, A. M. 2000. *Guide to nursing management and leadership,* 6th ed. St. Louis: Mosby.

Group Process

Objectives

- Differentiate between different types of groups.

- Discuss the stages of group development.

- Describe characteristics of effective groups.

- Describe the essential characteristics of group dynamics.

- Analyze group interactions to determine effective and ineffective group processes.

- Discuss the purposes of different types of health care groups.

N U R S E   C O N N E C T

Additional online resources for this chapter can be found on the companion web site at www.prenhall.com/blais.

A group is defined by Huber (2000, p. 253) as "any collection of interconnected individuals working together for some purpose. Nurses belong to a variety of professional groups, ranging from the smallest group, consisting of two people, also called dyads, to large professional associations. In these groups the nurse may fill a variety of roles, including leader, advisor, elaborator, and encourager.

- People are usually born into a family group and interact with other groups at all stages of their lives through social, cultural, religious, and professional socialization.
- A group consists of two or more people who share needs and goals and who take each other into account in their actions.
- Groups are important in people's lives. The family provides for socialization, whereas other groups (e.g., peer, social, religious, work, political) are vehicles for learning and satisfaction.
- Group dynamics, or group process, is the way in which groups function. For group work to be accomplished and group goals to be achieved, group dynamics must be effective.

CHALLENGES AND OPPORTUNITIES

The changing health care system presents challenges for health care professionals if they are to be actively involved in decisions about health care policy and health care practice. Such decisions are rarely made by one person in isolation but rather by groups of people at all levels of society: think tanks, advocacy groups, professional groups, and politicians at local, regional, state, national, and international levels.

These challenges provide opportunities for nurses to participate as active members of the various decision-making groups. In order to be effective members of these groups, nurses must be knowledgeable about the dynamics of group work in addition to providing expert knowledge about nursing and health care.

GROUPS

Groups exist to help people achieve goals that might be unattainable by individual effort alone. By pooling the ideas and expertise of several individuals, groups can often solve problems more effectively than one person. Information can be disseminated to groups more quickly and with more consistency than to individuals. In addition, groups often take greater risks than do individuals. Just as responsibilities for actions are shared by group members, so are the consequences of actions.

In the clinical setting, nurses work in groups as they collaborate with other nurses, other health care professionals, clients, and support persons when planning and providing care. Nurses also work in groups when joining professional and specialty organizations and civic and community groups to promote the goals of nursing on professional, civic, and political levels. Group skills are therefore important for nurses in all settings.

Types of Groups

Groups are classified as either primary or secondary, according to their structure and type of interaction. A **primary group** is a small, intimate group in which the relationships among members are personal, spontaneous, sentimental, cooperative, and inclusive. Examples are the family, a play group of children, informal work groups, and friendship groups. Members of a primary group communicate with each other largely in face-to-face interactions and develop a strong sense of unity, or "oneness." What belongs to one person is often seen as belonging to the group. For example, a success achieved by one member is shared by all and is seen as a success of the group.

Primary groups set standards of behavior for the members but also support and sustain each member in stresses he or she would otherwise not be able to withstand. Expectations are informally administered and involve primarily internal constraints imposed by the group itself. To its members, the primary group has a value in itself, not merely as a means to some other goal. The group has a sense of "we" and "our" to it, in contrast to "I" and "mine." Affective relationships are stressed.

The role of the primary group, particularly the family, in health care is increasingly recognized. It is to the primary group that people turn for help and support when they have health problems. Treatment and health care of individuals therefore are developing an expanded focus that includes the family.

A **secondary group** is generally larger, more impersonal, and less sentimental than a primary group. Examples are professional associations, task groups, ad hoc committees, political parties, and business groups. Members view these groups simply as a means of getting things done. Interactions do not necessarily occur in face-to-face contact and do not require that the members know each other in any inclusive sense. Thus, there is little sentiment attached to such relationships. Expectations of members are formally administered through impersonal controls and external restraints imposed by designated enforcement officials. Once the goals of the group are achieved or change, the interaction is discontinued.

Functions of Groups

Sampson and Marthas (1990, pp. 3–21) describe eight functions of groups. See Table 15–1. Any one group generally has more than one function, and it may serve different functions for different group members. For example, for one member a group may provide support; for another, information.

Levels of Group Formality

Groups may be classified as formal, semiformal, or informal.

Formal Groups

The most common example of the formal group is the work organization. People become familiar with many different formal work groups during their lifetimes and spend a major part of their working hours in such groups. Formal groups usually exist to carry out a task or goal rather than to meet the needs of group members. Traditional features of formal groups are shown in the box on page 248.

Semiformal Groups

Examples of semiformal groups include churches, lodges, social clubs, PTAs, and some labor unions. Many of an individual's social and ego needs are often satisfied by membership in these groups. The groups are similar in form to formal groups, but exhibit slight differences. Features of semiformal groups are shown in the box on page 248.

Informal Groups

Most people, from childhood on, have membership in numerous informal groups. These groups provide

Table 15–1 Functions of Groups

Function	Description
Socialization	Primary socialization in growth and development. Professional socialization into nursing or to a change in position. Socialization into the culture of an organization (i.e., new customs and beliefs) when a hospital is taken over by a corporate organization.
Support	Provision of social support for the members, a source of collegiality, and a source of help when needed.
Task completion	Complete tasks that are beyond the scope of any one individual. Each person may bring specialized knowledge and skills. Cooperation is important in task completion.
Camaraderie	Provision of goodwill among the members, thereby providing moments of pleasure.
Information	Provide a context for defining social reality, for setting performance goals, for establishing priorities, and for sharing special knowledge.
Normative function	Develop definitions and standards and enforce those standards, thereby encouraging compliance and discouraging deviations.
Empowerment	Empowering people and thereby encouraging change. A group often has more power than any individual.
Governance	Groups are often active in making decisions and serving as a source of governance within an organization.

Source: Adapted from *Group Process for Health Professions,* 3d ed., by E. E. Sampson and M. Marthas, Albany, N.Y.: Delmar, 1990.

Characteristics of Formal Groups

- Authority is imposed from above.
- Leadership selection is assigned from above and made by an authoritative and often arbitrary order or decree.
- Managers are symbols of power and authority.
- The goals of the formal group are normally imposed at a much higher level than the direct leadership of the group.
- Fiscal goals have little meaning to the members of the group.

- Management is endangered by its aloofness from the members of the work group.
- Behavioral **norms** (expected standards of behavior), regulations, and rules are usually superimposed. The larger the turnover rate of members, the greater the structuring of rules.
- Membership in the group is only partly voluntary.
- Rigidity of purpose is often a necessity for protection of the formal group in the pursuit of its objectives.
- Interactions within the group as a whole are limited, but informal subgroups are generally formed.

much of a person's education and develop most cultural values. Five types of groups are representative of the numerous informal groups in existence:

- *Friendship groups.* The first groups formed in life are friendship groups. They are often formed on the basis of common interests. Many arise out of semiformal group interactions or are formed spontaneously from the work organization.
- *Hobby groups.* Hobby groups bring together people from all walks of life. Differences in members' personalities and backgrounds are largely ignored in the interests of the hobby itself.
- *Convenience groups.* Many examples of convenience groups are found both in and out of the work setting. Two examples are the carpool and the childcare group organized by mothers.

- *Work groups.* Informal work groups can make or break an organization. Managers need to be sensitive to such groups and cultivate their cooperation and good will. Friendships often arise between a new member and the person who makes him or her feel a welcome addition to the group.
- *Self-protective groups.* Self-protective groups can be found anywhere but are particularly common in work organizations. They arise spontaneously out of a real or perceived threat. For example, a supervisor may approach a worker too strongly and find a group of workers organizing a united front against the threat. Such groups dissipate as soon as the threat has subsided.

The main features of informal groups are shown in the box on page 249.

Characteristics of Semiformal Groups

- The structure is formal.
- The hierarchy is carefully delineated.
- Membership is voluntary but selective and difficult to achieve.
- Prestige and status are often accrued from membership.
- Structured, deliberate activities absorb a large part of the group's meeting time.

- Objectives and goals are rigid; change is not recognized as desirable.
- In many cases, the leader has direct control over the choice of a successor.
- The day-to-day operating standards and methods (group norms) are negotiable. Because most people become bored at quibbling about norms, people can often "railroad" acceptance of a list of norms they desire.

Characteristics of Informal Groups

- The group is not bound by any set of written rules or regulations.
- Usually there is a set of unwritten laws and a strong code of ethics.
- The group is purely functional and has easily recognized basic objectives.
- Rotational leadership is common. The group recognizes that only rarely are all leadership characteristics found in one person.
- The group assigns duties to the members best qualified for certain functions. For example, the person who is recognized as outgoing and sociable will be assigned responsibilities for planning parties.
- Judgments about the group's leader are made quickly and surely. Leaders are replaced when they make one or more mistakes or do not get the job done.
- The group is an ideal testing ground for new leader-

ship techniques, but there is no guarantee that such techniques can be transferred effectively to a large, formal organization.
- Behavioral norms are developed either by group effort or by the leader and adopted by the group.
- Deviance by one member from the group's behavioral norms is more threatening to the perpetuation of small, informal groups than to large, formal, heterogeneous groups. Conformity and group solidarity are important for the protection and preservation of small groups.
- Group norms are enforced by **sanctions** (punishments) imposed by the group on those who violate a norm. Different values are placed on norms in accordance with the values of the leader. One leader may regard the action as a gross violation, whereas another leader may find it quite acceptable.
- Interpersonal interactions are spontaneous.

Group Development

The phases of group development have been variously described. Clark (1994, pp. 59–63) divides group development into three phases: orientation, working, and termination. In the *orientation phase,* group members seek to be accepted, and to find out how similar and different each one is from the other. Anxiety is often high during this period. The group is more likely viewed as a group of individuals than as a unified whole. Uncertainty and insecurity are often present in the group; safe topics are discussed.

In the *working phase,* group members feel more comfortable with one another, and group goals are established. Decisions are more likely to be made by consensus rather than by vote. Problem solving takes place, and frustration is often replaced by cautious optimism. Differences that are present are handled by adapting and problem solving rather than conflict. Disagreements are dealt with openly.

During the *termination phase,* the focus is on evaluating and summarizing the group experience. Feelings vary from frustration and anger to sadness or satisfaction, depending on whether the group has achieved its goals and attained group cohesion (group unity).

Tuckman and Jensen (1977) identified six stages

of group (team) development. Each group member should be aware of these stages and of the process of development. See Table 15–2.

Characteristics of Effective Groups

To be effective, a group must achieve three main functions: accomplish its goals, maintain its cohesion, and develop and modify its structure to improve its effectiveness.

See Table 15–3 for comparative features of effective and ineffective groups.

Consider . . .

- the number and types of groups to which nurses belong. Identify primary and secondary groups and formal, semiformal, and informal groups in which nurses commonly participate. How does membership in these groups enhance the individual nurse and the goals of professional nursing?
- your own involvements in groups. How many groups do you participate in? Which groups fulfill personal goals? Which groups fulfill professional goals? Which groups are specific to fulfilling work goals? How does the organization of your different groups relate to the characteristics of the various types of groups described in this chapter?

Table 15–2 Stages of Team Development

Stage	Team Behaviors	Leadership Behaviors
Orientation	Uncertainty Unfamiliarity Mistrust Nonparticipation	Directive style Outline purpose Negotiate schedules Define the team's mission
Forming	Acceptance of each other Learning communication skills High energy, motivated	Plan/focus on the problem Positive role modeling Actively encourage participation
Storming	Team spirit developed Trust developed Conflict may arise Impatience, frustration	Evaluate group dynamics Focus on goals Conflict resolution Establish goals and objectives
Norming	Increased comfort Identify responsibilities Effective team interaction Resolution of conflicts	Focus on goals Attend to process and content Supportive style
Performing	Clear on purpose Unity/cohesion Problem solve and accept actions	Act as a team member Encourage increased responsibility Follow up on action plans Measure results
Terminating	Members separate Team gains closure on objectives	Reinforce successes Celebrate and reward

Source: "Quality Work Improvement Groups: From Paper to Reality" by G. B. Smith and E. Hukill, *Journal of Nursing Care Quality* **8:** 5, July 1994. Used with permission.

Table 15–3 Comparative Features of Effective and Ineffective Groups

Factor	Effective Groups	Ineffective Groups
Atmosphere	Informal, comfortable, and relaxed. It is a working atmosphere in which people demonstrate their interest and involvement.	Obviously tense. Signs of boredom may appear.
Goal setting	Goals, tasks, and objectives are clarified, understood, and modified so that members of the group can commit themselves to cooperatively structured goals.	Unclear, misunderstood, or imposed goals may be accepted by members. The goals are competitively structured.
Leadership and member participation	Shift from time to time, depending on the circumstances. Different members assume leadership at various times, because of their knowledge or experience.	Delegated and based on authority. The chairperson may dominate the group, or the members may defer unduly. Members' participation is unequal, with high-authority members dominating.

Table 15–3 (Cont.)

Factor	Effective Groups	Ineffective Groups
Goal emphasis	All three functions of groups are emphasized—goal accomplishment, internal maintenance, and developmental change.	One or more functions may not be emphasized.
Communication	Open and two-way. Ideas and feelings are encouraged, both about the problem and about the group's operation.	Closed or one-way. Only the production of ideas is encouraged. Feelings are ignored or taboo. Members may be tentative or reluctant to be open and may have "hidden agendas" (personal goals at cross-purposes with group goals).
Decision making	By consensus, although various decision-making procedures appropriate to the situation may be instituted.	By the higher authority in the group, with minimal involvement by members; or an inflexible style is imposed.
Cohesion	Facilitated through high levels of inclusion, trust, liking, and support.	Either ignored or used as a means of controlling members, thus promoting rigid conformity.
Conflict tolerance	High. The reasons for disagreements or conflicts are carefully examined, and the group seeks to resolve them. The group accepts unresolvable basic disagreements and lives with them.	Low. Attempts may be made to ignore, deny, avoid, suppress, or override controversy by premature group action.
Power	Determined by the members' abilities and the information they possess. Power is shared. The issue is how to get the job done.	Determined by position in the group. Obedience to authority is strong. The issue is who controls.
Problem solving	High. Constructive criticism is frequent, frank, relatively comfortable, and oriented toward removing an obstacle to problem solving.	Low. Criticism may be destructive, taking the form of either overt or covert personal attacks. It prevents the group from getting the job done.
Self-evaluation of the group	Frequent. All members participate in evaluation and decisions about how to improve the group's functioning.	Minimal. What little evaluation there is may be done by the highest authority in the group rather than by the membership as a whole.
Creativity	Encouraged. There is room within the group for members to become self-actualized and interpersonally effective.	Discouraged. People are afraid of appearing foolish if they put forth a creative thought.

Source: Psychiatric Nursing, 5th ed., by H. S. Wilson and C. R. Kneisl, Redwood City, Calif.: Addison-Wesley Nursing, 1996, p. 736.

GROUP DYNAMICS

Group dynamics, or group processes, are related to how the group functions, communicates, sets goals, and achieves objectives ((Marriner-Tomey, 2000). Every group has its own characteristics and ways of functioning. Seven aspects of group dynamics follow.

Commitment

The members of effective groups have a commitment (agreement, pledge, or obligation to do something) to the goals and output of the group. Because groups demand time and attention, members must give up some autonomy and self-interest. Inevitably, conflicts arise

Bookshelf

Smith, K., and Berg, D. 1998. *Paradoxes of group life: Understanding conflict, paralysis, and movement in group dynamics.* **San Francisco: Jossey-Bass.**
This text approaches understanding groups by exploring the hidden dynamics that can prevent a group from functioning effectively and offers new ways of thinking about groups.

Donelson, R. F. 1998. *Group dynamics,* **3d ed. Stamford, Conn.: International Thomson Publishing.**
An introductory book to group processes integrating many areas of inquiry, including psychology, sociology, and other social sciences, this text features extended cases to illustrate applications.

Brown, R. 2000. *Group processes: Dynamics within and between groups,* **2d ed. Oxford, U.K.: Blackwell Publishers.**
The book presents three key ideas: Groups are a source of social identity. There is constant tension in group life between its task and the socioemotional aspects. Group dynamics are often governed by comparisons within and between groups.

Stewart, G. L., Manz, C. C., and Sims, H. P. 1998. *Team work and group dynamics.* **New York: Wiley.**
The authors blend theory and practice with a realistic view of how teams function in actual work settings. The book is organized around input, process, and output.

between the interests of individual group members and those of the group as a whole. However, members who are committed to the group feel close to each other and willingly work for the achievement of the group's goals and objectives. Some indications of group commitment are shown in the accompanying box.

Leadership Style

Leadership style refers to the different ways in which a leader combines task and relationship behaviors to influence others to accomplish goals (Huber, 2000). See Chapter 9, "The Nurse as Leader and Manager," for more information about leaders and leadership styles.

Decision-Making Methods

Making sound decisions is essential to effective group functioning. Effective decisions are made when

1. The group determines which decision method to adopt.
2. The group listens to all the ideas of members.
3. Members feel satisfied with their participation.
4. The expertise of group members is well used.
5. The problem-solving ability of the group is facilitated.
6. The group atmosphere is positive.
7. Time is used well; that is, the discussion focuses on the decision to be made.
8. Members feel committed to the decision and responsible for its implementation.

Three decision-making aids are described by McMurray (1994, pp. 62–65): brainstorming, the nominal group technique, and the Delphi technique. The idea behind **brainstorming** is that the interaction of several people in a group can generate more ideas about a subject than could the individuals by themselves. According to McMurray, there is evidence that brainstorming groups produce more ideas than individuals acting alone. For brainstorming, (1) the individuals in the groups must have a level of trust, (2) there must be

Indications of Group Commitment

- Members feel a strong sense of belonging.
- Members enjoy each other.
- Members seek each other for counsel and support.
- Members support each other in difficulty.
- Members value the contributions of other members.
- Members are motivated by working in the group and want to do their tasks well.
- Members express good feelings openly and identify positive contributions.
- Members feel that the goals of the group are achievable and important.

a criticism-free atmosphere that allows ideas to flow freely, and (3) all ideas receive initial approval and are critically examined thereafter.

Nominal group technique (NGT) is also an aid to decision making. In this instance the individuals meet as a group, but they write their responses without discussion. The ideas are then collected and open discussion proceeds.

The **Delphi technique** was originally used for technologic forecasting. It has been used for decisions that require more time or need responses from people in disparate locations. The participants maintain their anonymity, which eliminates peer pressure. Data are gathered through interviews or questionnaires in a series of rounds in which an initial question is posed. Once the responses are returned, they are compiled and redistributed. The participants do not know who said what: The comments or ratings are gathered for a compiled listing and are rated through averaging or statistical analysis. With the Delphi technique, agreement is reached as the process continues, either by consensus, voting, or mathematical average (McMurray, 1994, p. 64). See Table 15–4 for a comparison of brainstorming, nominal group technique, and the Delphi technique.

Member Behaviors

The degree of input by members into goal setting, decision making, problem solving, and group evaluation is related to the group structure and leadership style, but members also have responsibilities for group behavior and participation. Each member participates in a wide range of roles (assigned or assumed functions) during group interactions. Individuals may perform different roles during interactions in the same group or may vary roles in different groups. These roles have been categorized as (1) task roles, (2) maintenance or building roles, and (3) dysfunctional roles.

Task roles are related to the task or work of the group. Their purpose is to enhance and coordinate the group's movement toward achievement of its goals. Some behaviors may be seen in many group members and some may not be seen at all. Marriner-Tomey (2000) describes the following task roles that facilitate group work:

■ Initiator-contributors suggest new ideas or different approaches to achieving the goals. They usually act to identify the problem and clarify the goals. They may suggest items for discussion and set time limits.

■ Information seekers try to find factual data about the

Table 15–4 Comparison of Brainstorming, Nominal Group Technique, and Delphi Technique

Brainstorming	Nominal Group Technique	Delphi Technique
Group activity, open discussion.	Group activity; initial silent interaction with later discussion.	No personal interaction; input is anonymous.
Can be conducted in one session.	Can be conducted in one session.	Takes place over three to four rounds of data collection and analysis.
Relaxed, noncritical atmosphere is essential.	Noncritical atmosphere desirable in discussion stage.	No interaction; responses are anonymous.
Largely unstructured format.	Structured format; sequential steps or stages to be followed.	Structured format; requires "rounds" of interaction.
Easy to conduct; requires little preparation or understanding.	Easy to conduct; requires little preparation or understanding.	Requires coordination of responses, can be time-consuming.
Promotes more ideas than do individuals acting alone.	Promotes more and better quality ideas than does brainstorming.	Promotes many high-quality ideas.
Possible influence of results by peer pressure.	Peer influence likely only in discussion phase.	Little peer pressure noted.

Source: "Three Decision-Making Aids: Brainstorming, Nominal Group and Delphi Technique" by A. R. McMurray, *Journal of Nursing Staff Development* **10**: 62–65, March/April 1994. Used with permission.

task. Information givers present facts and share experiences related to the task. The focus of information seekers and givers is facts rather than values and beliefs.

- Opinion seekers clarify values associated with the problem or task and the possible solutions. Opinion givers state their own beliefs and thoughts about what they think the group values should be. The focus of opinion seekers and givers is on values and beliefs rather than facts.
- Elaborators develop the ideas or suggestions. They take an idea and give substance to it. They may predict outcomes related to a particular approach.
- Orienters summarize the discussion of the group and its work.
- Critics evaluate the problem, its proposed solutions, and the group's work toward the solution. They may measure the group's work against a set of standards.
- Energizers stimulate the group to increase its productivity in both quantity and quality.
- Recorders take minutes of group meetings, keeping an account of the group's discussion, suggestions, and decisions.

Marriner-Tomey (2000) also describes group-member roles that build and maintain the group continuity, cohesiveness, and stability. Group members who exhibit these roles are focusing on how group members treat each other while working together to achieve the goals. Some of these roles are as follows:

- Gatekeepers, who regulate communication to ensure that all members have an opportunity to be heard.
- Encouragers, who provide acceptance and support for group members' ideas and values. They are particularly helpful when a group member is reluctant to present or explore an idea that is controversial.
- Harmonizers, who try to maintain group cohesion. They may mediate group members' disagreements or use humor to relieve tension.
- Compromisers, who seek to achieve common ground within the group. They may modify their ideas to maintain group cohesiveness.

Group task roles and group maintenance roles are essential for the successful outcomes of group work. Group task roles provide the stimulus for achievement of the group goals; group maintenance roles serve the human needs for recognition and worth.

Other group-member behaviors can interfere with the work of the group. Such interference may delay the work of the group or result in the group being unsuccessful in achieving its goals. These behaviors or roles are referred to as self-serving or dysfunctional roles. Often, these behaviors are more about the group member meeting his or her own needs rather than the group's needs. Marriner-Tomey (2000) identifies some of these behaviors as follows:

- *Aggressors* show disapproval of other group members by body language or verbal statements. They may disparage the ideas of another group member.
- *Dominators* assert their superiority by interrupting others or giving authoritative directions. They may make statements such as, "There is only one way to proceed . . ." (usually meaning their way).
- *Blockers* are negative, resistant to change, and disagreeable without apparent reason. They may make statements such as, "This is the way we have always done it," "Why do we need to do something different when what we are doing works just fine?" or "This is just not going to work."
- *Special-interest pleaders* focus on the needs of a specific interest group rather than the overall group task or goal.
- *Playboys or playgirls* demonstrate a lack of involvement in the group process. They may joke inappropriately or use the meeting time to gossip.

Interaction Patterns

Interaction patterns can be analyzed by using a sociogram, a diagram of the flow of verbal communication within a group during a specified period, for example, 5 to 15 minutes. This diagram indicates who speaks to whom and who initiates the remarks. Ideally the interaction patterns of a small group would indicate verbal interaction from all members of the group to all members of the group (Figure 15–1). In reality, not all communication is a two-way process. In the sociogram shown in Figure 15–2, the lines with arrowheads at each end indicate that the statement made by one person was responded to by the recipient; a short cross-line drawn near one of the arrowheads indicates who initiated the remark. One-way communication is indicated by lines with an arrowhead at only one end. Remarks made to the group as a whole are indicated by arrows drawn to the middle of the circle only. By using a sociogram, nurses can analyze strengths and weaknesses in a group's interaction patterns. Used in conjunction with member behavior tools, this can offer considerable data about the group's dynamics.

Cohesiveness

Groups that have the characteristic of **cohesiveness** possess a certain group spirit, a sense of being "we," and a common purpose. Groups lacking cohesiveness are unstable and more prone to disintegration. See the box on page 255 for some of the attitudes and behaviors that reflect group cohesiveness.

Figure 15–1

An ideal interaction pattern of a small group. Each member interacts with all other members.

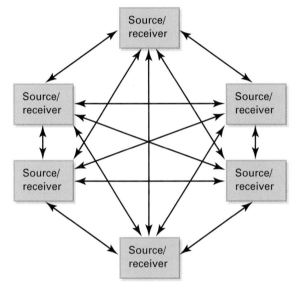

Figure 15–2

A sociogram indicating the flow of verbal communication within a group during a specific period. Note that five questions or comments calling for a response were directed at the leader.

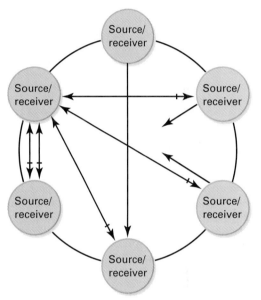

Attributes of Group Cohesiveness

Members' Attitudes and Behaviors

- Like each other, trust one another, and are friendly and willing to interact.
- Receive support from the group and praise one another for accomplishments.
- Have similar attitudes and beliefs.
- Are loyal to the group and defend it against outside criticism.
- Readily accept assigned roles and tasks.
- Influence each other and value being influenced by others.
- Feel satisfied and secure.
- Stay in the group and value group goals.

Group Characteristics

- Goals are valued and are consistent with the goals of individuals.
- Activities are handled by group action.
- Actions are interdependent and cooperative.
- Goals that are difficult to achieve are met by persistent efforts.
- Participation is high.
- Commitment is high.
- Communication is high.
- "We" is frequently heard in discussions.
- Productivity is high.
- Norms are adhered to and protected.

Power

Patterns of behavior in groups are greatly influenced by the force of power. **Power** can be defined as the ability to influence another person in some way or the ability to do something, whether it is to decide the fate of a nation or to decide that a certain change in policy or practice is necessary.

Many people have a negative concept of power, likening it to control, domination, and even coercion of others by muscle and clout. However, power can be viewed as a vital, positive force that moves people toward the attainment of individual or group goals. The overall purpose of power is to encourage cooperation and collaboration in accomplishing a task. For more about power, see Chapter 11, "The Nurse as Political Advocate."

Consider . . .

- groups in which you are a participant. What level of commitment do the various group members exhibit? How does the level of commitment exhibited by the individual group members affect the goal attainment of the group?
- the leaders of the various groups in which you are a participant. What are their leadership styles, and what decision-making methods do they use to achieve the group goals? How do the leader's style and decision-making method affect the goal attainment of the group?
- the interaction patterns demonstrated in groups in which you participate. How do the interaction patterns affect the goal attainment of the group? What strategies might have been used to improve the interaction of the group members?

FACILITATING GROUP DISCUSSION

A group leader can use certain techniques to facilitate group discussion. Smith and Hukill (1994, pp. 8–9) suggest the following:

- Ask open-ended questions to begin discussions and to probe for details from individuals and from the group.
- Encourage questions from group members.
- Respond with positive statements or a summary each time a participant makes a contribution.
- Reinforce participants' contributions by giving them your full attention.
- Avoid making negative comments about group members' contributions. Instead, summarize or restate them and ask other team members for their thoughts about the idea.
- Avoid taking sides on issues. Instead, summarize differences of opinion, stress that issues can be viewed from many different perspectives, and emphasize relative consensus.
- When monitoring small break-out work groups, avoid becoming involved in any of the groups. Participants tend to expect the group leader to intervene, rather than focusing on the task themselves or seeking input from each other.
- Seek equal contribution from all group members.

In order to conduct an effective group process, a leader needs to have certain skills. Some of these skills are listed in the box on page 257.

GROUP PROBLEMS

Problems that occur in groups include monopolizing, conflict, scapegoating, silence and apathy, and transference and countertransference.

Monopolizing

Because most group meetings have time restraints, domination of the discussion by one member seriously deprives others of their chances to participate. A sense of injustice develops, and ultimately members may direct their frustration and anger toward the group leader, who they think should do something to stop the monopolizer's behavior.

There may be several reasons for monopolizing behaviors, including anxiety, a need for attention, recognition, and approval. Whatever the reason, the goal of the leader is to assist the person to moderate his or her participation in the group. Often, compulsive talkers are unaware of their behavior and its effect on others and need help to recognize their behavior and its consequences.

Four strategies for dealing with monopolizing follow:

- *Interrupt simply, directly, and supportively.* This strategy is an initial attempt to get the person to hear others.
- *Reflect the person's behavior.* This strategy is an attempt to help the person become aware of the monopolizing behavior.
- *Reflect the group's feelings.* This strategy is an attempt to help the person become aware of the effects of his or her behavior on others.
- *Confront the person and/or the group.* This strategy can be directed toward the individual or toward the group to help members realize their own responsibility for the problem.

Conflict

Sampson and Marthas write that conflict is a normal stage in group development (1990, p. 242). Conflict

Group Process Skills

- Active listening.
- Focusing discussions on the purpose.
- Checking perceptions of the group.
- Reflecting—the ability to convey the essence of what a group member has said so that others can understand it.
- Clarifying—focusing on key underlying issues and sorting out confusing and conflicting feelings and thinking.
- Summarizing—restating, reflecting, and summarizing major ideas and feelings by pulling important ideas together and establishing a basis for further discussion. Summarize points of agreement and disagreement among group members.
- Facilitating—assisting the members to express their feelings and thoughts openly and actively working to create a climate of openness and acceptance in which members trust one another and therefore engage in a productive exchange of ideas, opinions, and perceptions.
- Interpreting—offering possible explanations.
- Questioning—if overused, members can become frustrated and annoyed with continued questions.
- Confirming—restating a member's basic ideas by emphasizing the facts and encouraging further discussion.
- Encouraging—as a leader, don't agree or disagree with a member's ideas. Use noncommittal words with a positive tone of voice. Examples: "I see . . ."; "Uh-huh . . ."; "That's interesting. . . ."

refers to disagreement, impatience, and argument among members. It can be either productive or nonproductive, and group leaders need to distinguish destructive conflict from constructive conflict. Conflict is productive and beneficial when members feel involved, when the issue being discussed is important to them, and when they are working intensively on a problem. Productive conflict contributes to problem solving as long as the goal is clearly understood.

Nonproductive conflict leads the group astray and hinders the achievement of group goals. There are three common reasons for this type of conflict (Bradford, Stock, and Horwitz, 1974, p. 38):

1. The group has been given an impossible task, or the task is not clear. Members are frustrated because they feel unable to meet the demands on them.

2. The main concern of members is to find status in the group and to deal with their personal and individual tasks rather than the group problem.

3. Members are operating from unique, unshared points of view and may have competing loyalties to and conflicting interests in outside groups.

The nurse-leader should intervene early rather than later. In some instances, the nonproductive conflict is best avoided or played down rather than confronted.

If the leader decides it is more beneficial for the group to face the issue directly, the leader can employ the following strategies (Sampson and Marthas, 1990, pp. 245–246):

- *Interpreting.* The leader explains her or his view of the problem. For example, the leader might say, "I think the group is having trouble making a decision because there are some distinct conflicts among several group members. Before we try to accomplish any other task I think we had better take some time and look at those conflicts."

- *Reflecting.* With this strategy, the leader points out certain behaviors of the members or points out his or her own feelings. To *reflect behavior* the leader may say, "I've noticed that several persons have been very quiet for some time, that others are talking a great deal but usually at cross-purposes, and that as a group we seem to be unable to focus our efforts on anything except disagreeing." To *reflect feeling* the leader may say, "I'm not sure how anyone else feels, but I'm feeling frustrated and annoyed over the constant bickering. I know we have a job to do, and I'd like to get on with it."

- *Confronting.* With this strategy, the leader calls the group's attention to what she or he perceives is taking place with one or more of the members. For example, the leader may say, "Mrs. Purple, I think you are angry because . . ., and you seem to feel. . . . Is that why you are so distressed?" or "I think that Mr. Black and Ms. White are each trying to gain some points in this discussion, but this is not helping us deal with the task at hand. I wonder if you two could listen for a while and let us get back to our task?"

- *Voicing the unmentionable.* Here the leader states a belief or feeling which will be uncomfortable for the listener, for example, "I think you are afraid of losing power on your unit, and that is why you are disagreeing with everything that is being said without listening to the others."

Scapegoating

Scapegoating is a process in which one or two members are singled out and agree, consciously or unconsciously, to be targets for group hostility or advice (Clark, 1994, p. 97). Scapegoating is a convenient method people use to negate any responsibility for what occurs in a group. By scapegoating, individuals can decrease their own anxiety. By also focusing on another's weakness, scapegoaters can minimize their own feelings of ineptitude.

For leaders to deal with scapegoating, they must be alert to its development and be prepared to accept anger when they confront the scapegoaters.

Silence and Apathy

Nonparticipation or **apathy** of one or more group members is sometimes best handled by nonintervention. Sometimes such silences are not a reflection of something in the immediate group setting but rather of some past experience. For example, after expressing an idea previously, this person may have been told, "That was a stupid thing to say." Having been hurt once in a group, such persons feel insecure about their views and are reluctant to express themselves again in groups.

Continued nonparticipation or apathy, however, needs to be dealt with by the leader, after a careful assessment of whether the apathy is a reflection of leadership style, task issues, or interpersonal conflicts.

For apathy reflecting the members' opinions that the task is unimportant, the leader may suggest, "I think there is general boredom with today's task. Do people feel that what we are doing is not really relevant or important?" After members have responded, the leader needs to ask, "What things would you prefer the group to do?"

For apathy related to members' feelings of inadequacy about handling the task or lack of the structure and organization needed for problem solving, the leader may ask, "Are people feeling generally that the group is not up to handling the task we are facing?" or "I think, because we're not really sure of what to do or how to go about dealing with the task facing us, that it may be helpful if we break up the task into smaller parts, decide what the important issues are, and develop a method for dealing with each part."

For apathy based on an interpersonal issue such as anger or fear and expressed by silence, the leader needs

to decide whether to let the silence simply pass or intervene. If generally responsive group members suddenly become silent, it is important to note which issue or topic immediately preceded the silence. Sometimes a conflict among a few members has been uncovered or the group has been pushed into discussing a topic considered irrelevant or threatening. In this situation the leader may say, "I am wondering whether people are angry at what I've done," or "Are some of you anxious about bringing up that topic, since it may bring out bad feelings?" For apathy in response to an autocratic leadership style, the leader must implement measures to change the style and assist the group to work through and change their relationship with the leader.

Transference and Countertransference

Transference is the transfer of feelings that were originally evoked by parents or significant others to people in the present setting. An example is a group member who acts toward the leader as she or he would act toward a parent. In addition, members of a group can transfer to others in the group personal feelings of love, guilt, or hate.

When leaders respond to group members because of reactions from earlier relationships, they are engaging in **countertransference.** For example, if a group member reminds a leader of a teacher who was menacing and demanding, the leader is likely to react with anxiety and may become unreasonably fearful. It is therefore important that leaders recognize the possibility of overreaction because of countertransference and that it is not an unusual reaction among nurses, who are highly involved in helping others.

Consider . . .

■ what personal goals may be achieved by a group member who exhibits monopolizing, scapegoating, or apathetic behaviors. How might the leader or other group members intervene to redirect such blocking behaviors?

■ the effect of problem behaviors in an individual group on the goals of the organization as a whole. How might such problem behaviors in groups composed of nurses be viewed by nonnurses within an organization? How might this affect the role of nursing in the organization?

TYPES OF HEALTH CARE GROUPS

Much of a nurse's professional life is spent in a wide variety of groups. As a participant in a group, the nurse may be required to fulfill different roles as member or leader, teacher or learner, adviser or advisee. Common types of health care groups include committees, teams, teaching groups, self-help groups, self-awareness/growth groups, therapy groups, work-related social support groups, and professional nursing organizations. There are similarities and differences among the characteristics of these various types of groups and the nurses' roles.

Committees or Teams

Committees are "relatively stable and formally composed" (Huber, 2000, p. 253). These are the most common types of work-related groups. They usually have a specific purpose that is part of the organizational structure and meet at defined intervals. Examples are policy committees, quality assurance committees, health care planning committees, nursing organization committees, and governmental affairs committees. Committees may also be referred to as teams, such as nursing care teams or wound-care teams. Teams are defined as "a small number of consistent people committed to a relevant shared purpose, with common performance goals, complementary and overlapping skills, and a common approach to their work" (Manion, Lorimer, and Leander, 1996, p. 6).

The leader of a committee or team, usually called the chairperson, must be accepted by the members as an appropriate leader and, therefore, should be an expert in the area of the committee's focus. The chairperson's role is to identify the specific task, clarify communication, and assist in expressing opinions and offering solutions. Committee or team members are generally selected in terms of their individual functional roles and employment status rather than in terms of their personal characteristics. Committee members may reflect diverse expertise in order to assist the committee to achieve its purpose. Committee or team members are accountable for the group's results or outcomes.

Task Forces

Task forces or ad hoc committees are work groups that usually have a defined task that is limited in duration. In other words, the task force is brought together to perform a specific activity, such as preparation for a joint commission (JCAHO) visit or Nurse Week. When the activity is accomplished, the task force is dissolved. Task forces and ad hoc committees function in the same way as committees or work teams. The difference is in the duration of their work.

Teaching Groups

The major purpose of teaching groups is to impart information to the participants. Examples of teaching

Research Box

Lin, M., Chang, Y., and Wang, C. 2000. The power of sharing groups: An exploration of nurse students' learning process in the clinical practice. *Journal of Nursing Research (China)* 8(5): 503–514.

The purpose of this qualitative study was to explore the learning process in a sharing group during nursing students' clinical practice and to determine its implications for interpersonal learning. The sample consisted of 14 senior baccalaureate nursing students in China. The students were invited to discuss their experiences in clinical practice during a focus interview process. All the interviews were recorded and transcribed. Narrative analysis was used to summarize the context of the learning process in the sharing group. Four categories were identified: (1) yielding to an open mind, (2) reflecting real self, (3) learning with regard for others, and (4) taking pleasure in learning. The interaction between the students in the sharing group provided a mechanism for self-understanding and change.

Using a sharing group process encourages more in-depth introspection and self-accommodation, which could help students better perform their professional roles. The findings may have implications for nurses working in stressful work areas, who may use the sharing group process to gain greater awareness and understanding about themselves and their coworkers.

groups include group continuing education and client health care groups. Numerous subjects are often handled via the group teaching format: childbirth techniques, exercise for middle-aged and older adults, and instructions to family members about follow-up care for discharged clients. A nurse who leads a group in which the primary purpose is to teach or learn must be skilled in the teaching-learning process discussed in Chapter 8, "The Nurse as Learner and Teacher."

Self-Help Groups

A **self-help group** is a small, voluntary organization composed of individuals who share a similar health, social, or daily living problem (Rollins, 1987, p. 403). These groups are based on the helper-therapy principle: those who help are helped most. A central belief

Positive Aspects of Self-Help Groups

- Members can experience almost instant kinship, because the essence of the group is the idea that "you are not alone."

- Members can talk about their feelings and listen to the concerns of others, knowing they all share this experience.

- The group atmosphere is generally one of acceptance, support, encouragement, and caring.

- Many members act as role models for newer members and can inspire them to attempt tasks they might consider impossible.

- The group provides the opportunity for people to help as well as to *be* helped—a critical component in restoring self-esteem.

Source: "Self-Help" by V. J. Gilbey, *Canadian Nurse* **83:** 25, April 1987.

of the self-help movement is that persons who experience a particular social or health problem have an understanding of that condition which those without it do not. Positive aspects of these groups are outlined in the accompanying box.

Self-Awareness/Growth Groups

The purpose of self-awareness/growth groups is to develop or use interpersonal strengths. The overall aim is to improve the person's functioning in the group to which they return, whether job, family, or community. From the beginning, broad goals are usually apparent, for example, to study communication patterns, group process, or problem solving. Because the focus of these groups is interpersonal concerns around current situations, the work of the group is oriented to reality testing with a here-and-now emphasis. Members are responsible for correcting inefficient patterns of relating and communicating with each other. They learn group process through participation and involvement in guided exercises.

Therapy Groups

Therapy groups work toward self-understanding, more satisfactory ways of relating or handling stress, and changing patterns of behavior toward health. Members are referred to as clients or, in some settings, as patients. They are selected by health professionals after extensive selection interviews that consider the pattern of personalities, behaviors, needs, and identification of group therapy as the treatment of choice. Duration of therapy groups is not usually set. A termination date is usually mutually determined by the therapist and members.

Research Box

Mok, E., and Martinson, I. 2000. Empowerment of Chinese patients with cancer through self-help groups in Hong Kong. *Cancer Nursing* 23(3): 206–213. The purpose of this study was to identify the process and outcomes of empowerment as experienced by Chinese Hong Kong patients with cancer through participation in cancer self-help groups. The sample consisted of 12 patients with cancer. Interviews of participants were conducted and observation of participants was done at self-help group meetings over a period of 6 months. Findings indicated personal empowerment through interconnectedness, confidence and hope, support and affirmation, and a feeling of usefulness. At a social level, participants reported expanded social network and opportunities to participate in more activities.

Nurses should strongly consider referral of cancer patients to self-help groups. Although the study was done in Hong Kong, China, the findings should be considered for nurses working with cancer patients in other parts of the world.

Work-Related Social Support Groups

Many nurses experience some of the high levels of vocational stress, for example, hospice, emergency, and critical care nurses. Social support groups can help reduce stress for such nurses if various types of support are provided to buffer the stress. Group members who know about the work of others can encourage and challenge members to be more creative and enthusiastic about their work and to achieve more. For example, a nurse may help another team member consider alternative strategies for intervention. Members also can share the joys of success and the frustration of failure through active listening without giving advice or making judgments. This type of social support is best given *outside* the work-related support group.

Professional Nursing Organizations

Professional nursing organizations function as groups, and through smaller groups composed of organization members promote quality health care for all and support the needs of nurses. Professional nursing organizations can serve as task groups, teaching groups, self-help groups, and support groups. The effectiveness of professional nursing organizations is related to the commitment and effectiveness of their members.

Consider . . .

■ the various health care groups in your practice setting. Identify specific committees, teams, teaching groups, self-help groups, self-awareness groups, therapy groups, and work-related groups in your practice setting. What are the purposes of these various groups? In what way are nurses actively involved in these groups? If nurses are not involved in the various groups, how might the lack of their participation affect the perception of professional nursing? How might nurses become involved in these groups?

■ the various health care groups in your community. Identify specific task groups, teaching groups, self-help groups, self-awareness groups, therapy groups, and work-related groups in your community. What are the purposes of these various groups? In what way are nurses actively involved in these groups? If nurses are not involved in the various groups, how might that affect the perception of professional nursing? How might nurses become involved in these groups?

■ the various professional nursing organizations in your community. How effective are these organizations in promoting quality health care for the community?

SUMMARY

Groups can be classified as primary or secondary, according to their structure or their type of interaction. Groups can assume any one or more of eight functions: socialization, support, task completion, camaraderie, information, normative function, empowerment, and governance. They can also be described according to their formality, that is, as formal, semiformal, or informal.

According to Clark (1994) groups develop in three stages: orientation, working, and termination. Tuckman and Jensen (1977) describe six states: orientation, forming, storming, norming, performing, and terminating. Effective groups produce outstanding results, succeed in spite of difficulties, and have members who feel responsible for the output of the group.

Group dynamics (group process) are forces in the group situation that determine the behavior of the group and its members. Factors in group dynamics include commitment, leadership style, decision-making methods,

member behavior, interaction patterns, cohesiveness, and power. Three decision-making aids are brainstorming, the nominal group technique, and the Delphi technique. Interaction patterns within a group can be assessed through the use of sociograms. Cohesive groups possess a common purpose and a group spirit. Groups lacking in cohesiveness are prone to disintegration.

Group discussion can be facilitated in eight ways, including asking open-ended questions and seeking equal contributions from all group members. Group leaders need certain skills to conduct an effective group process. A number of group problems commonly occur: monopolizing, conflict, scapegoating, silence and apathy, and transference and countertransference.

Nurses often serve as members of committees, teams, teaching groups, self-help groups, self-awareness groups, work-related social support groups, and professional nursing organizations.

SELECTED REFERENCES:

Bradford, L. P., Stock, D., and Horwitz, M. 1974. How to diagnose group problems. In L. P. Bradford, ed., *Group development.* La Jolla, Calif.: University Associates.

Clark, C. C. 1994. *The nurse as group leader,* 3d ed. New York: Springer.

Gilby, V. J. 1987, April. Self-help. *Canadian Nurse* **83:** 23, 25.

Huber, D. 2000. *Leadership and nursing care management,* 2d ed. Philadelphia: W. B. Saunders.

Lin, M., Chang, Y., and Wang, C. 2000. The power of

sharing groups: An exploration of nurse students' learning process in the clinical practice. *Journal of Nursing Research (China)* **8**(5): 503–514.

Manion, J., W. Lorimer, and Leander, W. J. 1996. *Team-based health care organizations: Blueprint for success.* Gaithersburg, Md.: Aspen.

Marriner-Tomey, A. 2000. *Guide to nursing management and leadership,* 6th ed. St. Louis: Mosby.

McMurray, A. R. 1994, March/April. Three decision-making aids: Brainstorming, nominal group and Delphi technique. *Journal of Nursing Staff Development* **10**: 62–65.

Mok, E., and Martinson, I. 2000. Empowerment of Chinese patients with cancer through self-help groups in Hong Kong. *Cancer Nursing* **23**(3): 206–213.

Rollins, J. A. 1987, Nov./Dec. Self-help groups for parents. *Pediatric Nursing* **13:** 403–409.

Sampson, E. E., and Marthas, M. S. 1990. *Group process for the health professions,* 3d ed. New York: Delmar.

Smith, G. B., and Hukill, E. 1994, July. Quality work improvement groups: From paper to reality. *Journal of Nursing Care Quality* **8:** 1–12.

Tuckman, B. W., and Jensen, M. A. 1977. Stages of small group development revisited. *Group and Organization Studies* **2:** 419–427.

Wilson, H. S., and Kneisl, C. R. 1996. *Psychiatric nursing,* 5th ed. Redwood City, Calif.: Addison-Wesley Nursing.

Technology and Informatics

Objectives

▪ Define nursing informatics and technology assessment.

▪ Describe current issues related to technology and informatics.

▪ Identify applications of information technology in health care.

▪ Discuss the role of nursing and health care informatics.

N U R S E   C O N N E C T

Additional online resources for this chapter can be found on the
companion web site at www.prenhall.com/blais.

Health care technologies and information management are two very important, closely related topics for professional nursing practice. For instance, when Fauquier Hospital installed point-of-care computers, nurses and other providers were given access to electronic patient records from any area in the facility. This was particularly important for error-free orders, capture and display of all current food and drug allergies, and documentation of medications to each electronic patient record. Acute care and outpatient services were subsequently linked, and departments such as physical therapy and respiratory therapy became paperless (Bishop, 2001).

With the availability of the Worldwide Web, nurses can instantly draw upon current research, industry experiences, and publications for all aspects of health care and nursing. Health care consumers likewise have greater access to information. The use of computers in nursing and health care and the nurse's responsibility in using technological advances in the delivery of care is the focus of this chapter. Several nursing and health care technology frameworks guide the presentation of three current issues: ethics, confidentiality of patient records, and caring for clients in an increasingly technical environment.

CHALLENGES AND OPPORTUNITIES

Nurses are continuously challenged to provide effective, efficient, and accessible care in a range of environments. New technologies, particularly information systems, are changing and improving nursing practice, education, research, and administration. Computers in health care have dramatically changed nursing practice and outcomes over the past several years. Indeed, they hold promise as important tools for caring for individuals, families, and groups. There are, however, challenges to overcome before the adoption of new technologies and information systems. Nurses who design and use information technologies must be aware of confidentiality and security concerns. In addition, nurses are challenged to manage information technologies in a manner that supports quality nursing care.

The opportunities provided by information technology are vast. Applications can change the face of practice, education, research, and administration by providing powerful tools for educating student nurses, continuing education, informing nurses about outcome management, storing and accessing patient records, teaching patients about wellness, and public education. Health care information systems continue to evolve and are providing effective and efficient means to support nursing care.

Many new applications will be developed in the near future and nursing should be instrumental in the design and application of systems for every aspect of patient care. Examples of four important applications are considered in this chapter: physician order entries, clinical information systems, wireless and portable devices, and computer-based patient records.

NURSING INFORMATICS, HEALTH CARE INFORMATICS, AND TECHNOLOGY

The term **informatics** is used to describe all aspects of computers and information systems. **Health care informatics** is the application of information technology to facilitate accountability, assist in cost containment, and enhance the quality of care (Ball and Douglas, 1997). According to Graves and Corcoran (1989), **nursing informatics** is the combination of computer and information science with nursing science. This combination assists in the management and processing of *nursing* data, information and knowledge in support of *nursing* practice, and the delivery of care. This definition is the historic one, and it remains relevant to the design, development, and implementation of health care information systems for nursing.

Since the introduction of information systems to acute care in 1965, a blend of consumer informatics and patient-centered information systems has evolved through the current wide use of the Internet (Staggers, Thompson, and Snyder-Halpern, 2001). Nursing information systems are now modules within larger integrated health care information systems. For example, the nursing documentation features for perioperative care may be part of a larger surgical information system that includes patient registration, orders management, inventory control, scheduling, billing, and postoperative patient-discharge instruction.

Nursing Roles and Education

A discussion of the role and educational preparation for nursing informatics will help apply these definitions. The informatics nurse, a specialty that requires baccalaureate preparation, or informatics nurse specialist, a specialty that requires graduate preparation, will generally find career opportunities in acute and ambulatory settings, academic institutions, application companies (vendors), and consulting firms. A recruiting advertisement for an informatics nurse might include the need for skills and experience to outline nursing functions to be automated, write technical manuals, manage projects, or train users. Informatics nurses design, develop, test, and evaluate new clinical applications and adapt existing systems to fit patient and provider requirements. Competencies vary and may include complex problem solving, database development, and application design and testing. In all cases, the prerequisite is clinical experience.

Nursing informatics is one of the newest specialties

in professional nursing. It was recognized by the American Nurses Association in 1992, and certification is available through the American Nurses Credentialing Center. The prerequisites for certification eligibility are shown in the accompanying box. A scope of practice and standards documents were developed under the direction of the American Nurses Association in 1995. New draft standards were reviewed in 2001 (ANA, 2001).

A wide variety of educational preparation is available for the nursing informatics role. Educational opportunities for the nursing informatics specialization may be found at the Ph.D. level, in post-master's certification, and in graduate nursing programs. The first two graduate programs in nursing informatics were established at the University of Maryland and University of Utah in 1988 and 1990, respectively. Undergraduate courses are often available as electives for nursing students. Conferences and weekend immersion programs are widely available (Newbold, 2001) to provide professional development and continuing education.

Nursing roles in informatics are continually evolving. The work of an informatics nurse can involve any aspect of information systems, including design, development, marketing, testing, implementation, training, and evaluation: Informatics nurses are engaged in clinical practice, education, consultation, research, administration, and pure informatics (ANA 2000). They may be entrepreneurs within start-up companies developing web-based products or have their own business as health database designers.

All nurses need informatics competencies, whether or not they are specialists in that area. All nurses must be information- and computer-literate. These competencies may be categorized as computer skills, information literacy skills, or overall informatics competencies. Basic computer skills include such things as using a word processor, being able to communicate by e-mail, and using applications to document patient care. Information literacy skills include the ability to retrieve bibliographic information from the Internet and the ability to evaluate and use the information appropriately. Overall informatics competencies include implementing policies to protect privacy and confidentiality and security of information and recording data relevant to the nursing care of patients. These skills are basic to the entry-level nursing role. Experienced nurses should have even greater proficiency in a particular area, such as administration, education, or public health.

Consider . . .

■ how the informatics nurse might be implemented in your work setting. How might this assist the practicing nurse? The patient? Administration and management?

Technology and Informatics

The leap in the development and use of information technologies calls for close examination of all aspects as they relate to quality of care. The purpose is to improve patient care through a comprehensive evaluation of the safety, effectiveness, cost/benefit, and social impact of a specific technology. Technologies are drugs, devices, procedures, and systems. Evaluation is essential to protect patients and diffuse safe, cost-effective technologies. Part of the role of informatics

---

Eligibility Requirements for Certification as a Nursing Informatics Specialist by the American Nurses Credentialing Center

- Baccalaureate or higher degree in nursing
- Active licensure as a registered nurse in the U.S. or territories
- Minimum of two years practice as an RN
- At least 2000 hours in informatics nursing within the past 5 years, *or*

- Completion of at least 12 semester hours of academic credits in a graduate program in informatics nursing *with* a minimum of 1000 hours in informatics nursing practice within the past 5 years; *and*
- 20 contact hours of continuing education applicable to informatics nursing within the past 2 years.

Source: American Nurses Credentialing Center, *Certification Catalog,* Washington, D.C.: ANCC, 2000.

nurses is to understand, apply, and disseminate the principles of health care technology assessment. The Health Care Technology Assessment (HCTA) framework was developed originally by the Office of Technology Assessment (OTA, 1982; Jacox, 1990) and may be used to evaluate health care information systems.

Telehealth technologies, a part of communication and information system technologies, are beginning to play a major role in delivering quality health care to patients at a distance. These technologies assist nurses in delivering quality care to remote patients in underserved areas or in prisons. Telehealth is "the removal of time and distance barriers for the delivery of health care services or related health care activities" (Milholland, 1997, p. 4).

Informatics Frameworks

A number of nursing and health care informatics models exist. Models or frameworks help clinicians understand how concepts are structured and operationalized. Four metastructures, or overarching concepts, are used in informatics theories and sciences:

- Data, information, and knowledge
- Sciences underpinning nursing informatics
- Concepts and tools from information science and computer science
- Phenomena of nursing

Data are discrete entities that are described objectively without interpretation. Information is data that have been interpreted, organized, or structured, and knowledge is synthesized information, whereby relationships are identified and formalized. Figure 16–1, developed by Graves and Corcoran in 1989, depicts the relationship among the three entities. As data are transformed into information and information into knowledge, increasing complexity requires greater application of human intelligence. The circles overlap in these three concepts because the concepts are blurred, and there are multiple feedback loops. Nurses are processors of information. They use informatics to manage and communicate data, information and knowledge to support patients, nurses, and other providers in making decisions. Informatics assists them in storing clinical data, translating clinical data into information, linking clinical data and knowledge, and aggregating clinical data.

The sciences underpinning nursing informatics are nursing science, information science, and computer science. They are used to manage and process nursing data, information, and knowledge to facilitate the delivery of health care. This combination of sciences creates a unique blend that can be used to solve information-management issues of concern to the dis-

Figure 16–1

Transformation of Data to Knowledge

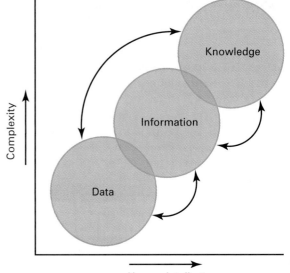

Used by permission of J. R. Graves and S. Corcoran, "The Study of Nursing Informatics," *Image: Journal of Nursing Scholarship* **21** (4): 227–231, 1989.

cipline. Informatics nurse specialists often collaborate with other informaticists and may borrow concepts from many sources, including linguistics, cognitive science, engineering, and a variety of others as needed.

The tools and methods derived from computer and information sciences include information technology, structures, management, and communication. Information technology includes computer hardware, software, communication, and network technologies. Human-computer interaction and ergonomics concepts are fundamental to the informatics nurse specialist. Ergonomics focuses on the design and implementation of the equipment related to human use. The goal is optimal task completion.

The metaconcepts of nursing are nurse, person, health, and environment. Decision making involves these four concepts, and nurses must make numerous decisions with important implications for quality of life and well-being of individuals, families, and communities. Nurses depend upon data that have been transformed into information to determine interventions.

Turley (1997) proposed a model to describe nursing informatics. His major contribution was adding cognitive science to the model of Graves and Corcoran. He acknowledged the growing interdisciplinary nature of health care and focused on the unique contribution provided by nursing.

Goossen (1996) illustrated a nursing information reference model to structure nursing data and information. Staggers, Thompson, and Happ (1999) proposed a pragmatic, patient-centered informatics model (PCIM) that is an interdisciplinary framework to guide clinicians and systems developers. See Figure 16–2. The model blends notions from prior conceptual models for a unique framework that enables users to evaluate the influencing factors in designing and implementing clinical systems. Influencing factors may be delivery methods, knowledge bases, and supporting technologies.

PCIM is important because it can be applied in the planning and integration of information systems. It also supports education and research by enabling technology assessment and critical thinking. PCIM is the only model that proposes a link to other disciplines. The Graves and Corcoran (1989) definition focuses on nursing phenomenon, but PCIM describes the relationship of nursing to other disciplines in planning and using information technologies. These models continue to evolve over time.

ISSUES RELATED TO INFORMATION TECHNOLOGY

As information technologies become basic tools for nurses, four issues need to be addressed: ethics, confidentiality, data integrity, and caring in a highly technical environment.

Ethical Concerns

The American Nurses Association code of ethics for nurses (1985) applies to the issues and dilemmas in informatics. Confidentiality, security, and privacy are of great concern. When medical data are stored electronically, special precautions are needed to be certain that unauthorized access is prevented.

Boykin (2000) elaborated on the basic principles that apply nursing ethics to the use of information technologies in health care. The concepts of autonomy, empowerment, accountability, and respect for the individual hold true for the practice of nursing informatics. Nurses have an ethical duty to protect patient confidentiality (ANA, 1985). All health care providers have a moral code that requires balancing the privacy of patients with the requirements for care, including access to patient records.

The expansion of guidelines for the ethical development of Internet sites has been ongoing since 1996, when Health On the Net Foundation (HON, www.hon.ch) became one of the very first websites to guide both patients and medical professionals to reliable sources of health care information on the Internet. HON's standards hold website developers to basic ethical standards in the presentation of information.

Figure 16–2

The Patient-Centered Informatics Model

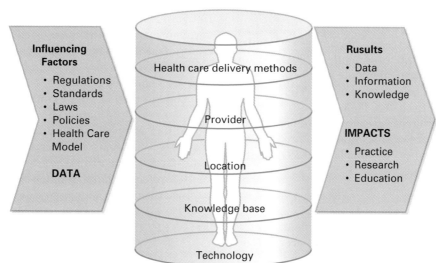

Patient-Centered Informatics Model

Used by permission of N. Staggers, C. B. Thompson, and B. A. Happ, "An Operational Model for Patient-Centered Informatics," *Computers in Nursing* **17** (6): 278–285, 1999.

The American Accreditation Healthcare Commission (2001) is also developing an accrediting process for health care websites.

Confidentiality of Medical Records and Data

An example of the blatant breach of the confidentiality of medical records and potential patient impact was reported in the February 12, 1999, *Detroit News* (Upton, 1999). Records with identifying information (names, social security numbers, diagnostic codes) of thousands of University of Michigan health system patients were inadvertently placed on the Internet. This is one of the perils of automation.

There are many laws addressing confidentiality and patient privacy. The first standard of the Health Insurance Portability and Accountability Act (HIPPA) of 1996 (August 21), Public Law 104–191, which amends the Internal Revenue Service Code of 1986 (also known as the Kennedy-Kassebaum Act) is expected to go into effect in the fall of 2002 (Phoenix Health Systems, 2001). However, the new administration and others in the nation are reexamining the law carefully and may revise the standards before they take effect.

In summary, HIPAA requires improved efficiency of health care delivery by standardizing electronic data interchange and protection of confidentiality and security of health data through setting and enforcing standards. Unique health identifiers for all providers and health plans and security standards to protect the individual's identifiable health information, past, present, and future, for all health organizations—physicians' offices, health plans, employers, public health groups, life insurance companies, and information systems vendors—are required.

Another important law (Gramm-Leach-Bliley Act), required by most states as of July 1, 2001, calls for health plans and insurers to handle member and subscriber data in special electronic formats. The new legislation is expected to change the way nurses work, access data, and communicate health information (Judy, 2001). For health care organizations, the preparation to provide for patient confidentiality is much like the Y2K efforts in past years.

Data Integrity

Health care providers should have confidence in the accuracy and quality of the data that they access. Data integrity procedures instill trust with controls that avoid incomplete or inaccurate entry of data. Although the term *data integrity* is often linked to data-bases, it also refers to ensuring that data are entered correctly and that there are data quality–management procedures in place. The correctness of patient information is always essential. The quality of the data input into the computer is critical to assuring quality output. Without processes and procedures in place, computers can replicate and speed up the communication of erroneous data. An example of a procedure to ensure the accuracy of data is when input fields are designed to check for correct data type. For example, if an alpha character is entered and a numeric character should have been entered, an error message appears on the screen.

Caring in a High-Tech Environment

Caring for patients in a highly technical environment confronts nursing with potential conflict between using effective tools and methods and providing professional nursing care. Rinard (1996) and Brennan (2000) describe the impact of the increased use of technologies and the provision of nursing care. Introduction of new technologies lead to a transformation of nursing, according to Rinard. The author attributes the massive waves of technological change and related funding in health care delivery over time in part to the deskilling (substitution of less trained people) and fragmentation of nursing tasks.

Brennan (2000), on the other hand, described innovation (technological change) as a partnership or compensatory relationship between the care-delivery system, the patient, the environment, and the patient's health goals. When designing information technologies to improve health outcomes, the author advocates a partnership model in delivering nursing care.

The title of the book *Nursing Informatics Where Caring and Technology Meet* (Ball, Hannah, Newbold, and Douglas, 2000) illustrates the related roles of nursing and informatics. Caring is an essential part of the provision of health. When technologies are introduced, informatics nurses may be the architects and bridges to improved patient outcomes.

The three issues ethics, confidentiality, and caring are important in a high-tech environment as the expansion of information technologies continues at a rapid pace. Informatics nurses are challenged to continue to research and apply the appropriate codes and laws to protect patients and to use information tools to improve the quality of patient care.

THE TECHNOLOGY EXPLOSION

Evolution of Technology

The growth of the Internet and information systems has been exponential. It has been predicted that by the year 2002, 490 million people around the world would have access to the Internet (Computer Industry Almanac, 2001). In April 2001, 57% of people using the Internet were searching for health-related information (Pew Foundation, 2001).

Nurses are often asked to verify information found on the Internet, and informatics nurses may be asked to explain and support research for more complex topics. Patients have come to expect health care information systems to provide services set by other industries. For instance, patient registration and billing should be as easy as the global ability to instantly authenticate accounts and access money online. Unfortunately, this may not always be the case. The evolution of new health care information technologies has not followed this pattern of revolutionary design and availability. Rather, traditional text-based health care records have been difficult to automate.

Managed-care funding for health care services has dwindled. New technologies have not only dramatically changed nursing and health care, but they have also added to the costs of patient care. Development of health care information systems generally is slower.

When the administration of a health care organization predicts physician and patient-care requirements, a study may be conducted and the system requirement may be added to the strategic plan. For example, when bedside computers were to be installed in a community hospital, a feasibility study was conducted and the system was tested on one unit. In addition, a cost-benefit study was undertaken. The board of trustees reviewed the new technology in light of the hospital strategic plan and recommended a phased approach, with careful analysis of patient outcomes and staff satisfaction.

The design of new patient-care systems has impacted staff in regard to workflow, efficiency, and effectiveness. Development of information systems is not simply automating a paper system. It involves studying and improving the processes. From intensive care to hospice and assisted living, the venue for automation initiatives continues to expand and improve health care.

Consider . . .

■ how the implementation of information technology has affected confidentiality in your work setting. Think of some ways that confidentiality could be enhanced.

■ what ethical concerns you have about the inclusion of information systems in health care. How might nurses address these ethical concerns?

■ whether increased uses of technology have affected the level of caring that nurses in your work setting have been able to deliver. What are some things nurses can do to increase caring in a highly technological care environment?

Computer Technology in Practice, Education, Research, and Administration

New technologies have significantly changed the way nurses practice, conduct research, manage and administrate, and advance their education. Automation in health care has assisted in defining a standardized nomenclature for all disciplines. Standardization of terminologies for nursing is essential for delivering appropriate care and managing outcomes.

Research Box

Larrabee, J. H., Boldreghini, S., Elder-Sorrells, K., Turner, A. M., Wender, R. G., Hart, J. M., and Lenzi, P. S. 2001. Evaluation of documentation before and after implementation of a nursing information system in an acute care hospital. *Computers in Nursing* **19(2): 56–65.**

The purpose of this quasi-experimental study was to evaluate the differences in documentation completeness, achievement of patient outcomes, and assessments before and after the implementation of a clinical computer system. The goal was to understand the relationship between quality of care and patient outcomes in order to improve both.

The study was conducted on two medical-surgical units and an intensive-care step-down unit in a 100-bed teaching facility in Tennessee. There were at least 90 records examined retrospectively at each of three points in time over 18 months. The tool used was the Nursing Care Plan Data Collection Instrument developed by Larrabee in 1992. Interrater reliability before and during the data collection was acceptable (ANOVA, $p < 0.05$).

Mean scores for nurse assessment and nurse-perceived patient outcomes did not improve until 18 months after implementation, when the staff was retrained on the computer system. Although the clinical information system did not seem to improve care early in this study, continued training on the system helped to improve nursing care quality and patient outcomes.

Nursing practice in an organization with an integrated clinical information system may include using an online kardex, care protocols, bedside computers, or a personal digital assistant (PDA) for patient care. Orders, procedures, and appointments are automatically updated and an online kardex may be used as a primary communications tool. The automated kardex shows allergies, interventions, specimens to be collected, current medications, diet, and patient weight. An automated rounds report allows providers to quickly view patient information, vital signs, intake and output, lab results, radiology reports, and patient-care notes. This increases accuracy and decreases redundancy and thus improves the efficiency and effectiveness of individual providers.

Orders-management systems streamline the entry, receipt, and monitoring of orders throughout the enterprise. Wireless bedside computers for patient documentation allow appropriate providers to enter and access patient records from anywhere at any time. For example, Rose Medical Center has been using wireless terminals successfully in the emergency room for several years.

Automated medication administration records that are integrated with orders-management, billing, and pharmacy systems proved effective and provided error-free access to drugs. Training for new applications and diverse equipment has become shorter and easier as nurses see the benefits and apply computer knowledge and skills from their everyday lives.

An informatics nurse's role in these new technologies is very important. It may involve examination and design of new workflow, development of an implementation plan, and training in and evaluation of the new technologies. Although patient access to the Internet may change the patient's level of knowledge, patient education and counseling must be augmented and mediated by trained nurses for full understanding and compliance and subsequent improved patient outcomes. Overall, new information systems improve the efficiency, productivity, safety, and quality of care in an organization, but this is not always the case. Investment in information systems must be tied to an organization's strategic plan, sufficient resources must be in place, and a change-management plan must be implemented to see the full benefits.

The influence of new technologies on nursing education is changing the basic philosophies about the tools and methods for pedagogy. From online courses to virtual-reality intravenous training systems, students have benefited from improvements in educational information technologies. At this time, you may be at a computer accessing an Internet-based course with a virtual instructor or working hands-on with an intravenous simulator.

Automated research tools and the Internet facilitate nursing research. Research databases such as the Cumulative Index for Nursing and Allied Health Literature (CINAHL) or MEDLINE provide nurses with effective methods to quickly find current relevant literature and access appropriate psychometric tools from the desktop. Statistical tools like the Statistical Package for the Social Sciences (SPSS) (http://www.SPSS.com/industries/health_care/) help nurse researchers organize and analyze data when conducting research.

Nurse-administrators use information technologies to manage under uncertain conditions, satisfy multiple stakeholders, and build and retain passionate workforces. Two elements moved nursing administration to embrace computers for decision making: the speed and accuracy needed and the financial constraints of managed care. Information systems enable nursing administration to manage budgets, collect and investigate staff and patient data to track and forecast resource needs, and anticipate quality-management interventions. Data from clinical and financial information systems allow nurse-administrators to analyze data for trends in patient problems and reimbursement gaps. The availability of appropriate data minimizes risk-taking. For instance, recruitment programs can be developed to improve staffing ratios when the seasonal influx of patients is higher than expected.

The introduction of information technologies continues to enhance nursing practice and to provide tools for research, administration, and nursing education. A survey of nursing informatics researchers identified ten priorities for research:

- Standardized language/vocabularies
- Technology development to support practice and patient care
- Database issues
- Patient use of information technologies
- Using telecommunications technology for nursing practice
- Putting technology into practice
- System-evaluation issues
- Information needs of nurses and other clinicians
- Nursing intervention innovations for professional practice
- Professional practice issues (Brennan et al., 1998)

Consider . . .

- how technology has changed nursing education since you were first introduced to nursing. What new skills do students need today compared to 5, 10, and 15 years ago?

CURRENT APPLICATIONS OF INFORMATION TECHNOLOGY IN PRACTICE

Four applications of information technology are of great importance to nursing: physician order entry, clinical information systems, wireless and portable devices, and the computer-based patient record.

Physician Order Entry

The Institute of Medicine (1999) report estimated that the number of deaths per year from medical errors is between 44,000 and 98,000. As part of the patient-safety strategy, strong consideration is being made for purchase and implementation of automated physician order–entry systems. These systems enable appropriate providers (physicians and, in some states, nurse practitioners) to enter, edit, schedule, track, and discontinue treatment and diagnostic services electronically. In this way, orders can be checked against patient allergies, interactions with other medications or tests, dosage levels, and standards of practice for the institution. With computerized physician order entry, adverse events and costs may be reduced and length of patient stay may be shortened.

Automated physician order entry is generally part of an integrated enterprise system that allows direct entry by the physician and reduces the likelihood of transcription errors. It is a complex system interfaced with many other systems; in the past it has not been available because of the cost and complexity of development. There is a current sense of urgency to purchase this application for patient safety, and companies are now developing such products.

Clinical Information Systems

Another publication from the Institute of Medicine and National Academy Press (Committee on Quality of Health Care in America, 2001) highlighted the need for implementation of improved clinical information systems. The authors recommended a fundamental change and redesign of the health care system to promote evidence-based practice, strengthen clinical information systems, and lead to the elimination of most handwritten clinical data by the end of the decade.

Clinical information and financial and administrative systems are found in most health care entities and are generally integrated to serve patients and providers. Clinical systems may include patient registration, orders, and departmental systems such as nursing, dietary, radiology, pharmacy, cardiology, laboratory, and physical therapy. Although there are many independent systems, integration helps to ensure coordination of care across patient conditions, services, and settings over time.

Wireless and Portable Devices

Wireless and portable devices are bringing patient records and provider services to the point of care. When bedside computers emerged in the early 1990s, advances enabled access to patient information anywhere and at any time. The location of patient care at home, in an office, in a church, in a community center, or in a hospital makes wireless and portable devices an attractive vehicle for documentation and record access.

One type of device is the personal digital assistant (PDA). Two PDA functions allow nurses wireless access to patient records and reference databases such as MedCalc (http://www.medcalc.be/page6.html) and ePocrates (http://www.epocrates.com/). RNpalm.com is a website dedicated to mobile computing for nurses. Wireless PDAs are being tested at Beth Israel Deaconess Medical Center to access medical records in the emergency room.

Computer-Based Patient Record

Interest in a computer-based patient record (CPR) or electronically maintained information about an individual's lifetime health status and health began more than ten years ago when Dick and Steen (1991) conducted an important study on the value of a complete and accurate patient record. The text was updated in 1997 (Dick, Steen, and Detmer, 1997) and remains the seminal study for CPRs. These systems are not yet in use but are being developed with testing in some places.

The ideal CPR (also called electronic patient record or electronic medical record) will support users with reminders and alerts, clinical decision-support systems, and links to medical knowledge. The intent of a CPR is to capture quality measurements and clinical outcome data to support the analysis of patient problems. A CPR will affect quality improvements in patient care through effective documentation and monitoring.

An excellent example of a CPR is the system used by the Department of Veterans Affairs (VA). By leveraging the best parts of an older system and integrating commercial software applications, the VA has developed an advanced system that captures patient data in a provider-friendly way. Clinical documentation is standardized, accurate, always available, and very reliable throughout the inpatient areas and clinics in the VA system.

Beth Israel Deaconess Medical Center in Boston has an integrated online CPR-type information system with ready access to electronic patient records via a web browser (Landro, 2000). This new system enables a clinician (with appropriate security clearance) in the emergency room to access patient records via the web. This can cut the time for intervention and treatment, saving money and improving patient conditions.

These four applications of information technology in health care are but a few of the many important developments to support providers and patients. New applications are developed and become cost effective as demand grows and system requirements are defined.

Consider . . .

■ the needs for changes in the technological environment of patient care in the future. What supports will nurses need to keep current with new technology applications? Are the current approaches to continuing education sufficient?

Bookshelf

Ball, M. J., Hannah, K. J., Newbold, S. K., and Douglas, J. V. 2000. *Nursing informatics where caring and technology meet,* 3d ed. **New York: Springer-Verlag.** This is an excellent reference on the topic of nursing and computers. It covers a wide scope of easy-to-read information including a chapter on tele-nursing and information system management. The references are very good and the indexing allows for quick scanning of selected topics.

Ellis, D., Campbell, M. L., Crandall, D. K., Peters, B. E., Ruff, C., and Seitz, K. 2000. *Technology and the future of health care: Preparing for the next 30 years.* **New York: Wiley.** The author projects the rate of technological development into the next three decades of the health care industry. The idea is presented that the most visible technological advances such as MRI, CAT, and PET scanners are less important in the long run than the technological advances in streamlining administration of health care agencies and doctor's offices. Processing and storage of medical records and billing technology will have a greater impact.

SUMMARY

Nursing informatics is the combination of computer and information science with nursing science. It is part of the larger health care informatics. Nurses are being prepared as specialists in this area, but every practicing nurse needs some level of expertise. Four current applications of information technology that are important for nursing are physician order entries, clinical information systems, wireless and portable devices, and computer-based patient records.

Several issues related to the increased use of technology in nursing include ethics, confidentiality, data integrity and caring. Nurses are concerned with the ethical practices used in information access, storage, and retrieval. Ethical practices have a direct effect on confidentiality. The changes in technology of care also raise concerns about the caring practices that nurses implement. Advocacy is needed on the part of the nurse to see that patients, rather than equipment, remain the focus of care.

The application of computer technology has changed practice, education, and research. The skills required to interface with information systems at the point of care, to participate in educational programs that further one's career, and to manage research data have changed and will continue to change. This challenges continuing education both in its own application and in providing the means to learn new skills.

The ability of nurses to manage and use information systems is critical in improving outcomes, decreasing costs, and improving access to care. The 21st century will bring more and better technologies to challenge and enhance professional nursing. The role of the informatics nurse will expand, and confounding technology issues will multiply.

SELECTED REFERENCES

American Accreditation Healthcare Commission. 2001. *Healthcare website accreditation.* http://www.urac.org/websiteaccreditation.htm.

American Nurses Association. 1985. *Code for nurses with interpretive statements.* Kansas City, Mo.: ANA.

American Nurses Association. 2000. Informatics Nurse Certification. www.nursingworld.org/ancc/certify/.

Ball, M. J., and Douglas, J. V. 1997 Winter. Health care informatics: Where caring and technology meet. *CommonHealth* **18.**

Ball, M. J., Hannah, K. J., Newbold, S. K., and Douglas, J. V. 2000. *Nursing informatics where caring and technology meet,* 3d ed. New York: Springer-Verlag.

Bishop, B. R. 2001, Jan. Informatics at the point of care: How one hospital integrated a new health information system with mobile documentation devices. *Advance for Nurses.*

Boykin, P. 2000. *Confidentiality and security.* Presented at the 10th Annual Summer Institute in Nursing Informatics. Baltimore, Md., July 20.

Brennan, P. F. 2000. *Partnering with patients: Creating new pathways for innovation in health care.* Presented at the 10th Annual Summer Institute in Nursing Informatics. Baltimore, Md., July 19.

Brennan, P. F., Zielstorff, R. D., Ozbolt, J. G., and Strombom, I. 1998. Setting a national research agenda in nursing informatics. In B. Cesnik, A. T. McCray, and J.-R. Scherrer, eds., Medinfo '98: Proceedings of the Ninth World Congress on Medical Informatics, (pp. 1188–1191). Amsterdam: IOS Press.

Committee on Quality of Health Care in America. 2001. *Crossing the quality chasm: A new health system for the 21st century.* Washington D.C.: National Academy Press.

Computer Industry Almanac. 2001. http://www.ITAlmanac.com/italmanac/index.html.

Dick, R., and Steen, E. 1991. *The computer-based patient record: An essential technology for health care.* Washington, D.C.: National Academy Press.

Dick, R., Steen, E., and Detmer, D. 1997. *The computer-based patient record: An essential technology for health care.* Washington, D.C.: National Academy Press.

Goossen, W. 1996. Nursing information management and processing: A framework and definition for systems analysis, design and evaluation. *International Journal of Biomedical Computing* **40:** 187–195.

Graves, J. R., and Corcoran, S. 1989. The study of nursing informatics. *Journal of Nursing Scholarship* **21:** 227–231.

Health On the Net Foundation. 2001. http://www.hon.ch/.

Institute of Medicine. 1999. *To err is human: Building a safer health system.* Washington, D.C.: National Academy Press.

Jacox, A. 1990. Nursing and technology, technology assessment in reducing costs and improving care. *Nursing Economics* **8**(2): 116, 118.

Judy, K. 2001. Nursing informatics: What does HIPAA mean to you? *Advance for Nurses.* http://www.advance-fornurses.com/feature4.html.

Landro, L. 2000. Deal with our doctors. *The Wall Street Journal.* November 13, R23.

Milholland, D. K. 1997. Telehealth: A tool for nursing practice. *Nursing Trends and Issues* **2:** 4.

Newbold, S. 2001. Nursing Informatics and Health Informatics Conferences. http://nursing.umaryland.edu/~snewbold/sknconf.htm.

Office of Technology Assessment. 1982. *Strategies for medical technology assessment.* Springfield, Va.: NTIS.

Pew Foundation. 2001. Internet and American Life. http://www.pewinternet.org/reports/toc.asp?Report=30.

Phoenix Health Systems. 2001. *HIPA Advisory.* http://www.hipaadvisory.com/.

Rinard, R. G. 1996. Technology, deskilling, and nurses: The impact of the technologically changing environment. *Advances in Nursing Science* **18**(4): 60–69.

Staggers, N., Thompson, C. B., and Happ, B. A. 1999. An operational model for patient-centered informatics. *Computers in Nursing* **17** (6): 278–285.

Staggers, N., Thompson, C. B., and Snyder-Halpern, R. 2001. History and trends in clinical information systems in the United States. *Journal of Nursing Scholarship* **First Quarter:** 75–81.

Turley J. 1997. Toward a model for nursing informatics. *Image* **28:** 309–313.

Upton, J. 1999. U-M medical records end up on web. *The Detroit News.* Friday, February 12. http://detnews.com/1999/metro/9902/12/02120114.htm.

Nursing in an Evolving Health Care Delivery System

Outline

Objectives

- Examine the issues of cost containment and access to health care as they affect nursing.
- Differentiate health, wellness, and well-being.
- Compare selected models of health.
- Identify factors affecting health status, beliefs, and practices.
- Discuss the initiatives of the World Health Organization for the promotion of *Health for All.*

N U R S E   C O N N E C T

Additional online resources for this chapter can be found on the companion web site at www.prenhall.com/blais.

Changes in the health care–delivery system have had a dramatic impact on the practice of nursing. In the early 1900s nurses made home visits and focused on personal care of sick individuals. As hospitals became the workplace where physicians provided medical and surgical care, nurses were employed to provide nursing care, and nursing followed common organizational patterns by establishing specialty areas of practice such as psychiatric, pediatric, obstetrical, medical, and surgical nursing. As nursing education evolved and nurses began to understand more about what constituted the practice of nursing, the boundaries expanded. During the 1970s and 1980s nurses began to seek more autonomy in the practice of nursing, particularly with regard to physicians and hospital administration. Simultaneously, health care costs were rising at an alarming rate, so there was a congressional demand for cost containment related to the government-funded Medicare program. This began with a demand for prospective payment through diagnosis-related groups (DRGs). Private insurance companies followed suit, and hospital administrators were forced to cut costs to survive. Care became focused on costs and profit, with less concern about quality. Health care providers were then forced to do more with fewer resources, and new models of care delivery emerged in response (Milstead, 1999). This resulted in major changes in the paradigm of health care, as shown in the box on page 277.

CHALLENGES AND OPPORTUNITIES

A commitment to high-quality care challenges nurses as never before to find ways of providing such care without resources from the administrative levels of the health care organization. Creative ways of doing more with less while avoiding undue stress and burnout are needed. Traditional values, such as advocacy for the individual client, holistic care, and meeting the health care needs of individuals and populations, are at stake in the new health care arena.

The continued evolution of nursing and its place in health care delivery provides a wide range of opportunities for the future. Nursing is in a position to create new roles and redefine nursing in a way that can have a positive impact upon health care now and in the future.

SELECTED ISSUES

Two issues at the forefront of the nursing profession's response to health care changes are cost containment and access to health care. Third-party payers have shaped much of the change in an attempt to control rapidly increasing health care costs that many believe to be out of control. Many people are not covered by third-party payers and have few options. For them, there is little availability of health care, and they have been a concern in shaping delivery of care in communities and in providing more primary and preventive care.

Cost-Containment Strategies

Many cost-containment strategies in health care have emerged in response to pressures from consumers and third-party payers. The resulting changes in the economic structure will be discussed in Chapter 18, "Health Care Economics." Some of the strategies used by nurses in an attempt to control costs and maintain quality include resource management, the development of critical pathways, and the utilization of assistive personnel.

Resource management is an important skill for successful, clinically competent nurses. It is of great importance that nurses be aware of limited resources and the consequences for health care delivery. Resource management uses cost-effective approaches to high-quality health care. The basic resources include financial, physical, and human, but others are organizational systems, information systems, and technical capabilities. Effective time management is an important resource-utilization skill consisting of the planned and organized assessment of when and how long it will take to complete an activity; consequently, control is exercised over what is responded to and the problems that are addressed. Responding to downsizing or the reduction in personnel has been a major challenge in resource allocation (Price, Koch, and Bassett, 1998).

The restructuring of care delivery has been a cost-containment response; one example of such an attempt has been the introduction of **critical pathways**. These are interdisciplinary plans for managing the care of clients that specify interdisciplinary assessments, interventions, treatments, and outcomes for specific health-related conditions across a time line. Critical pathways are also called critical paths, interdisciplinary plans, anticipated recovery plans, interdisciplinary action plans, and action plans. These plans can be developed for surgical procedures, medical diagnoses, emergency care, trauma care, and health-related interventions. They are generally used for high-volume case types or situations that have relatively predictable outcomes. The pathways are designed in collaboration with members of the health care team who are involved in managing the case type.

Nurses have been pivotal in the development of

Comparison of Old Health Care Paradigm with New Paradigm

OLD PARADIGM	NEW HEALTH CARE PARADIGM
Hospital-based, acute care	Short-term hospital: same-day surgery, 23-hour stays; prehospital testing and precertification; telehealth/telemedicine; home health; mobile vans; school and mall clinics
Specialty units	Cross-training (multiskilled workers): LDRP, OR/PACU, CCU/telemetry
Hierarchical management	Decentralization (unit budget, scheduling, variance); shared governance; strategic plan
Physician "captain of ship"; others are followers	Inter/multidisciplinary team, collaboration; case management (registered nurse/broker)
Nurse as employee: job-focused, "refrigerator nurse"	Nurse as professional: career focused; clinical ladder; continuing credentials; tuition reimbursement, paid certification exam
Medical condition, focus on segment	Holistic person in family/community; pastoral care, parish nurse
"Sick care," focus on cure	Health care, health promotion, prevention programs; care and continuity of care; complementary health alternatives
Cost containment, focus on billing	Focus on patient and accountability of caregivers/agency; electronic patient record, continuous quality improvement, care maps
Written medical record	Integrated electronic records: smart card, bedside computers
Fee for service	Managed competition (HMO, PPO, IPA)
Physician as employer	Physician as employee; capitation system
One insurance plan	Variety of insurance options ("covered lives"): basic plan plus dental, eye, long-term care, cancer, disability
80–100% insurance	Greater deductible, lower percentage coverage, or copayment

Reprinted by permission of J. A. Milstead, *Health Policy and Politics: A Nurse's Guide.* Gaithersburg, Md.: Aspen Publishers, 1999. p. 16.

critical pathways through the contribution of nursing content that is clinically sound and through collaboration with other disciplines. The nurse is often the one who facilitates the integration of interdisciplinary effort. The implementation of the pathway is dependent upon nurses providing the care. Evaluation of the pathway is the final phase of implementation and variances feed back into the development. Critical pathways are fluid documents that evolve as care is refined and advances in science emerge.

Critical pathways establish the sequence and timing of interdisciplinary interventions and incorporate education, discharge planning, assessments, consultations, nutrition, medications, activities, diagnostic testing, therapeutic measures, and so on.

Critical pathways strive to meet several goals: to achieve realistic, expected client and family outcomes; to promote professional, collaborative practice and care; to ensure the continuity of care; to guarantee the appropriate use of resources; to reduce costs and length of stay; and to provide the framework for continuous quality improvement.

When agencies use critical pathways, members of the health care team work together to set client goals

Research Box

Pillar, B., and Jarjoura, D. 1999. Assessing the impact of reengineering on nursing. *Journal of Nursing Administration* 29(5): 57–64.

This study assessed the impact of organizational reengineering on nursing in a hospital setting using an observational repeated-measures design. Mail surveys were used to collect data on nurses' perceptions of their authority and autonomy in a new nursing model and philosophy, that of patient-focused care. They also assessed the satisfaction with ability to deliver care. Patient satisfaction was assessed at the same time using a sample of 227 patients who had been hospitalized a minimum of 3 days. The study covered a one-year span and included both a cross-sectional and a longitudinal sample of 445 nurses. There were no differences in the perceptions of nurses or patients related to the reengineering. The authors report this as no positive effects of the reengineering, and they further state that the study reinforces the need to build evaluation research into organizational activities such as reengineering.

Research Box

Geddes, N., Salyer, J., and Mark, B. A. 1999. Nursing in the nineties: Managing the uncertainty. *Journal of Nursing Administration* 29(5): 40–48.

This study examined qualitative data on nurses' work lives as part of the National Institutes of Health Outcomes Research in Nursing Administration Project (ORNA). Fifty-three people at different institutions kept journal entries for 6 months, consisting of critical incidents and implications. Content analysis was done on the narrative data. The acute-care environment was characterized as turbulent and uncertain. Contributing factors included (1) workload related to fluctuating census, staff preparation, and turnover of staff; (2) loss of workplace identity coming from unit consolidation, hospital buyouts, and system mergers; and (3) reengineering related to skill mix, new equipment/system changes, new documentation systems, and rumored changes. The authors conclude that new initiatives are at risk unless personnel needs are attended to and seen as unique in each care setting.

and delineate professional roles, functions, and responsibilities. Once the critical pathway is developed, the collaborative team pilots the tool and revises it as indicated. If care for a specific case type is delivered using a critical pathway, a case manager may be assigned to the case type. Critical pathways may be used in managed care settings, traditional delivery systems, or patient-focused care models.

The use of clinical nursing assistants (CNAs), also called certified nursing assistants or nurse aides, has been a controversial attempt at resource utilization. The intent of using these individuals in providing care has been to relieve the professional nurse of tasks that can safely and effectively be delegated to someone with less educational preparation who can provide that level of care more cost-effectively. Criticism of this approach has been that individuals in the role were placed in situations of care that went beyond their limited preparation and thereby jeopardized the quality of care provided. In many instances, the CNAs were thrust upon nursing without sufficient planning for the implementation of the role and without sufficient input from the nurses who would be working with them. Some have

suggested that CNAs will be around for the foreseeable future because of the potential cost savings and because nursing needs to take charge of developing effective systems that maximize both the professional role of the nurse and the role of the CNA (Salmond 1999).

Consider . . .

- what are the wasted resources and wasted efforts found in health care today?
- what nurses can do to increase cost-effective, quality health care?

Access to Health Care

The issue of access to health care has been a major factor in shaping the changes in nursing. Without universal health care coverage, about 40 million Americans are estimated to be uninsured, and many more are underinsured and economically limited from accessing health care. Barriers to accessing health care have been identified as cost of care, lack of insurance, problems with insurance, difficulty getting appointments, difficulty finding services, and lack of transportation (Glick, 1999).

The American Nurses Association (ANA) published *Nursing's Agenda for Health Care Reform* in 1991. This document represented the efforts of the ANA, the National League for Nursing (NLN), the American Association of Colleges of Nursing (AACN), and the American Organization of Nurse Executives (AONE). It provides for cost-effective, community-based delivery of care in a restructured health care system.

A central objective of this reform is to provide a basic "core" of essential health care services for everyone. The statement calls for a restructuring of the health care system to focus on consumers and their health needs. It also recommends that health care be delivered in such diverse settings as schools, workplaces, and homes and that the health care system shift its focus from illness and cure to wellness and care. See the box on page 280.

The AONE (1992, p. 42) writes that effective health care must

1. Encourage consumer partnerships so that consumers can take an active role in their health and their care and in decisions about their care.
2. Allow all U.S. citizens and residents access to basic health care services.
3. Increase health care access through the use of physician and nonphysician providers.
4. Create incentives that promote health, wellness, and prevention; individuals with chronic illnesses will not be penalized.
5. Promote affordable, safe, and effective health care.
6. Make provisions for skilled and long-term care.
7. Make provisions for catastrophic care, with some limitation on extraordinary procedures.
8. Finance health care through a combination of public- and private-sector funding.

Community nursing centers are innovative health care–delivery models that represent a step in the paradigm shift from the centralized biomedical model of curing to the community-based and more holistic nursing model of caring (Glick, 1999). The purpose of these centers is to meet the needs of underserved populations by providing the public with direct access to a range of services that are not otherwise available in the community. Nursing centers provide a setting where patients' needs rather than medical diagnoses are the focus. They are located in places to which people have access, such as churches, mobile units, homeless shelters, and schools. Emphasis is on controlling costs by providing noninstitutional care through models that include community participation, care and case man-

agement, community health promotion, coordination of community resources, and referral.

This change in focus to prevention and community-based health care requires a shift in perspective from cure and treatment of illness to promotion of health, wellness, and well-being.

CONCEPTS OF HEALTH, WELLNESS, AND WELL-BEING

Nurses need to clarify their understanding of health and wellness because their definitions largely determine the scope and nature of nursing practice. Clients' health beliefs influence their health practices. Some people think of health and wellness (or well-being) as the same thing or, at the very least, as accompanying one another. However, health may not always accompany well-being: A person who has a terminal illness may have a sense of well-being; conversely, another person may lack a sense of well-being yet be in a state of good health.

For many years, the concept of disease was the yardstick by which health was measured. In the late nineteenth century, the "how" of disease (pathogenesis) was the major concern of health professionals. Currently, the emphasis on health and wellness (salutogenesis) is increasing.

Health

There is no consensus about any definition of health. There is knowledge of how to attain a certain level of health, but health itself cannot be measured.

Traditionally, **health** has been defined in terms of the presence or absence of disease. Nightingale defined health as a state of "being well and using every power the individual possesses to the fullest extent" (Nightingale, 1969 [1860], p. 334). At an international conference on global health issues in 1947, the World Health Organization (WHO) took a more holistic view of health. It defined health as "a state of complete physical, mental, and social well-being, and not merely the absence of disease or infirmity" (WHO, 1947, p. 1). This definition

■ Reflects concern for the individual as a total person functioning physically, psychologically, and socially. Mental processes determine people's relationship with their physical and social surroundings, their attitudes about life, and their interaction with others.

■ Places health in the context of environment. People's lives, and therefore their health, are affected by everything they interact with—not only environmental influences such as climate and the availability of nutritious food, comfortable shelter, clean air to breathe, and pure water to drink but also other

Nursing's Agenda for Health Care Reform (Executive Summary)

The basic components of nursing's "core of care" include

- A restructured health care system which
  - Enhances consumer access to services by delivering primary health care in community-based settings.
  - Fosters consumer responsibility for personal health, self-care, and informed decision making in selecting health care services.
  - Facilitates utilization of the most cost-effective providers and therapeutic options in the most appropriate settings.
- A federally defined standard package of essential health care services available to all citizens and residents of the United States, provided and financed through an integration of public and private plans and sources:
  - A public plan, based on federal guidelines and eligibility requirements, will provide coverage for the poor and create the opportunity for small businesses and individuals, particularly those at risk because of preexisting conditions and those potentially medically indigent, to buy into the plan.
  - A private plan will offer, at a minimum, the nationally standardized package of essential services. This standard package could be enriched as a benefit of employment, or individuals could purchase additional services if they so choose. If employers do not offer private coverage, they must pay into the public plan for their employees.
- A phase-in of essential services, in order to be fiscally responsible:
  - Coverage of pregnant women and children is critical. This first step represents a cost-effective investment in the future health and prosperity of the nation.
  - One early step will be to design services specifically to assist vulnerable populations who have had limited access to our nation's health care system. A "Healthstart Plan" is proposed to improve the health status of these individuals.
- Planned change to anticipate health service needs that correlate with changing national demographics.
- Steps to reduce health care costs include
  - Require usage of managed care in the public plan and encouraged in private plans.
  - Incentives for consumers and providers to utilize managed care arrangements.
  - Controlled growth of the health care system by planning and prudent resource allocation.
  - Incentives for consumers and providers to be cost efficient in exercising health care options.
  - Development of health care policies based on effectiveness and outcomes research.
  - Assurance of direct access to a full range of qualified providers.
  - Elimination of unnecessary bureaucratic controls and administrative procedures.
- Case management will be required for those with continuing health care needs. This will reduce the fragmentation of the present system, promote consumers' active participation in decisions about their health, and create an advocate on their behalf.
- Provisions for long-term care, which include
  - Public and private funding for services of short duration to prevent personal impoverishment.
  - Public funding for extended care if consumer resources are exhausted.
  - Emphasis on the consumers' responsibility to financially plan for their long-term care needs, including new personal financial alternatives and strengthened private insurance arrangements.
- Insurance reforms to improve access to coverage, including affordable premiums, reinsurance pools for catastrophic coverage, and steps to protect both insurers and individuals against excessive costs.
- Access to services assured by no payment at the point of service and elimination of balance billing in both public and private plans.
- Establishment of public/private sector review—operating under the federal guidelines and including payers, providers, and consumers—to determine resource allocation, cost reduction approaches, allowable insurance premiums, and fair and consistent reimbursement levels for providers. This review would progress in a climate sensitive to ethical issues.

Source: Nursing's Agenda for Health Care Reform, American Nurses Association, Washington, D.C.: ANA, 1991. PR-3 22M 6/91. Reprinted with permission.

people, including family, lovers, employers, coworkers, friends, and associates of various kinds.

■ Equates health with productive and creative living. It focuses on the living state rather than on categories of disease that may cause illness or death.

In 1953 the (United States) President's Commission on Health Needs of the Nation made the following statement about health:

> "*Health* is not a condition; it is an adjustment. It is not a state but a process. The process adapts the individual not only to our physical, but also our social environments" (President's Commission, 1953, p. 4).

This definition emphasizes health as an adaptive process rather than a state.

Health has also been defined in terms of role and performance. Parsons (1972, p. 107) wrote that health is "the state of optimum capacity of an individual for effective performance of his roles and tasks." Parsons further explained that when people feel well, they assume the health role; when they feel ill, in contrast, they assume the sick role. He describes four aspects of the sick role:

■ The person is not held responsible for the illness.
■ The person is exempt from the usual social tasks.
■ The person has an obligation to get well.
■ The person has an obligation to seek competent help to treat the illness.

Dubos (1968) viewed health as a creative process and described it as "a quality of life, involving social, emotional, mental, spiritual, and biological fitness on the part of the individual, which results from adaptations to the environment." (1968, p. 5) In Dubos's view, the individual must have sufficient knowledge to make informed choices about his or her health and also the income and resources to act on choices. Dubos (1978) believes that complete well-being is unobtainable, in contrast to the 1947 definition by the World Health Organization.

In 1980, the American Nurses Association (ANA) defined health in their social policy statement as "a dynamic state of being in which the developmental and behavioral potential of an individual is realized to the fullest extent possible" (ANA, 1980, p. 5). In this definition, health is more than a state or the absence of disease; it includes striving toward optimal functioning.

In recent years, the idea of health has come to include a more holistic approach and to encompass quality of life. Elements such as environmental, spiritual, emotional, and intellectual aspects have been included, and the term wellness has become more popular (Donatelle and Davis, 2000).

Wellness and Well-Being

Wellness is "a continual balancing of the different dimensions of human needs—spiritual, social, emotional, intellectual, physical, occupational, and environmental" (Anspaugh, Hamrick, and Rosata, 2000, p. v). It is a process of identifying needs for improvement and making choices that facilitate a higher level of health. Basic concepts of wellness include self-responsibility; an ultimate goal; a dynamic, growing process; daily decision making in the areas of nutrition, stress management, physical fitness, preventive health care, emotional health, and other aspects of health; and, most importantly, the whole being of the individual. See the accompanying box.

Concepts of Wellness

• Wellness is a choice—a decision you make to move toward optimal health.

• Wellness is a way of life—a lifestyle you design to achieve your highest potential for well-being.

• Wellness is a process—a developing awareness that there is no end point, but that health and happiness are possible in each moment, here and now.

• Wellness is an efficient channeling of energy—energy received from the environment, transformed within you, and sent on to affect the world outside.

• Wellness is the integration of body, mind, and spirit—the appreciation that everything you do, and think, and feel, and believe has an impact on your state of health.

• Wellness is the loving acceptance of yourself.

Source: Reprinted with permission, *Wellness Workbook,* Travis and Ryan, Ten Speed Press, Berkeley, Calif.: © 1981, 1988 by John W. Travis, MD.

Well-being is a *subjective* perception of balance, harmony, and vitality. It is a state that can be described objectively, occurs at levels, and can be plotted on a continuum (Leddy and Pepper, 1998, p. 230).

Illness and Disease

People may view illness and disease as the same entity; however, health professionals generally view them as completely separate. Emotions are not believed to cause disease, but they may create an environment in which disease can develop through their effect upon the immune system.

Illness is a highly personal state in which the person feels unhealthy or ill. Illness may or may not be related to disease. An individual could have a disease, for example, a growth in the stomach, and not feel ill. By the same token, a person can feel ill, that is, feel uncomfortable, yet have no discernible disease. Illness is highly subjective; only the individual person can say he or she is ill.

Disease is a term that can be described as an alteration in body functions resulting in a reduction of capacities or a shortening of the normal life span. Traditionally, intervention by physicians had the goal of eliminating or ameliorating disease processes. Primitive people thought disease was caused by "forces" or spirits. Later, this belief was replaced by the single-causation theory. Today, multiple factors are considered to interact in causing disease and determining an individual's response to treatment.

Another distinction needs to be made between disease and deviance. **Deviance** is behavior that goes against social norms. Some deviant behaviors may be considered diseases according to the earlier definition of disease. For example, alcoholism can result in an alteration of body functioning, a reduction in capacities, and a shortening of the life span. Other deviant behavior can be considered a disease, not because it alters the function of a body organ, but because it disrupts a family or a community. An example is drug addiction. However, differentiation between disease and deviance is not always clear and often depends on the perspective of the person observing the behavior.

Consider . . .

- what behaviors of others indicate to you that they are healthy or unhealthy.
- your own definition of health.
- whether you believe that your clients should agree with your definition of health.
- which factors you believe most affect your own sense of wellness.

Disease Prevention

Disease prevention is a part of health promotion. Health promotion is covered in greater detail in Chapter 7, "The Nurse as Health Promoter and Care Provider." Prevention is taking action to avoid a later illness and is conceptualized in three levels: primary, secondary, and tertiary. **Primary prevention** is directed toward avoiding health problems before they begin and includes such activities as getting immunized and practicing safe sex. **Secondary prevention** occurs with the recognition of risk and taking action to reduce risk before disease gets a foothold. An example would be stopping smoking. **Tertiary prevention** refers to treatment or rehabilitation, such as physical therapy following an injury to restore function.

Research Box

Stuifbergen, A. K., Seraphine, A., and Roberts, G. 2000. **An explanatory model of health promotion and quality of life in chronic disabling conditions.** *Nursing Research* 49(3): 122–129.

The objective of this study was to test an explanatory model of variables influencing health promotion and quality of life in persons living with multiple sclerosis. A sample of 786 completed a battery of instruments measuring severity of illness-related impairment, barriers to health-promoting behaviors, resources, self-efficacy, acceptance, health-promoting behaviors, and perceived quality of life. A causal model was created from the data using the software program LISREL8. The antecedent variables accounted for 58% of the variance in frequency of health-promoting behaviors and 66% of the variance in perceived quality of life. The effects of severity of illness on quality of life were mediated partially by health-promoting behaviors, resources, self-efficacy, and acceptance. The strength of the direct and indirect paths suggests the interventions to enhance social support, decrease barriers, and increase specific self-efficacy for health behaviors would result in improved health-promoting behaviors and quality of life.

MODELS OF HEALTH AND WELLNESS

Because health is such a complex concept, various researchers have developed models or paradigms to explain health and, in some instances, its relationship to illness or injury. Models can be helpful in assisting health professionals to meet the health and wellness needs of individuals. Nurses need to clarify their own understanding of health, wellness, and illness for the following reasons:

- Nurses' definitions of health largely determine the scope and nature of nursing practice. For example, when health is defined narrowly as a physiologic phenomenon, nurses confine themselves to assisting clients regain normal physiologic functioning. When health is defined more broadly, the scope of nursing practice increases correspondingly.
- People's health beliefs influence their health practices. Thus, a nurse's health values and practices may differ from those of a client. Nurses need to ensure that plans of care developed for individuals relate to the client's conception of health. Otherwise, clients may fail to respond to a health care regimen.

Leavell and Clark's Agent-Host-Environment Model

The *agent-host-environment model,* also called the *epidemiologic triangle,* is a traditional approach to health and disease developed to address communicable disease and is one of the early models (Leavell and Clark, 1965). It has been expanded to other health conditions as a more general model, but it is still used primarily to predict illness. The three variables in the model are depicted as a triangle when they are in their normal state of equilibrium. A change in any of the three sides results in disequilibrium. In a healthy state, equilibrium exists (Anderson and McFarlane, 2000). The three dynamic interactive elements in this model are described as follows:

1. *Agent.* Any environmental factor or stressor (biologic, chemical, mechanical, physical, or psychosocial) that by its presence or absence (e.g., lack of essential nutrients) can lead to illness or disease.
2. *Host.* Person(s) who may or may not be at risk of acquiring a disease. Family history, age, and lifestyle habits influence the host's reaction.
3. *Environment.* All factors external to the host that may or may not predispose the person to the development of disease. Physical environment includes climate, living conditions, noise levels, and economic

level. Social environment includes interactions with others and life events, such as the death of a spouse.

Because each of the agent-host-environment factors constantly interacts with the others, health is an ever-changing state. When the variables are in balance, health is maintained; when variables are not in balance, disease occurs.

Dunn's Levels of Wellness

Dunn described a health grid in which a health axis and an environmental axis intersect (1959a, p. 786). It demonstrates the interaction of the environment with the illness-wellness continuum (Figure 17–1).

The health axis extends from peak wellness to death, and the environmental axis extends from very favorable to very unfavorable. The intersection of the two axes forms four health/wellness quadrants:

1. *High-level wellness in a favorable environment.* An example of this is a person who implements healthy lifestyle behaviors and has the biopsychosocial, spiritual, and economic resources to support this lifestyle.
2. *Emergent high-level wellness in an unfavorable environment.* An example of this is a woman who has the knowledge to implement healthy lifestyle practices but does not implement adequate self-care practices because of family responsibilities, job demands, or other factors.

Figure 17–1

Dunn's Health Grid: Its Axes and Quadrants

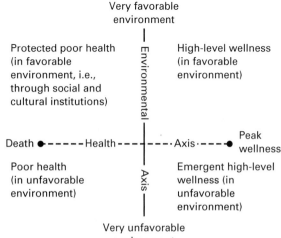

Source: "High-Level Wellness for Man and Society" by H. L. Dunn, *American Journal of Public Health,* **49:** 788, June 1959. Used with permission of the American Public Health Association.

3. *Protected poor health in a favorable environment.* An example of this is an ill person (e.g., one with multiple fractures or severe hypertension) whose needs are met by the health care system and who has access to appropriate medications, diet, and health care instruction.
4. *Poor health in an unfavorable environment.* An example of this is a young child who is starving in a drought-stricken country.

In his book about high-level wellness in the individual, Dunn (1973) explored the concept of wellness as it relates to family, community, environment, and society. He believed that family wellness enhances wellness in individuals. In a well family that offers trust, love, and support, the individual does not have to expend energy to meet basic needs and can move forward on the wellness continuum. By providing effective sanitation and safe water, disposing of sewage safely, and preserving beauty and wildlife, the community enhances both family and individual wellness. Environmental wellness is related to the premise that humans must be at peace with and guard the environment. Societal wellness is significant because the status of the larger, social group, affects the status of smaller groups. Dunn believed that social wellness must be considered on a worldwide basis.

Health and Wellness Continuum

Health and illness or disease can be viewed as the opposite ends of a health continuum. The continuum ranges from optimum wellness to premature death and includes the six dimensions of health that affect movement along the continuum. These dimensions are described as follows:

Physical health—Body size, sensory acuity, susceptibility to disease, body functioning, physical fitness, and recuperative abilities

Intellectual health—Ability to think clearly and analyze critically to meet life's challenges

Social health—Ability to have satisfying interpersonal relationships and interactions with others

Emotional health—Appropriate expression of and control of emotions; self-esteem, trust, and love

Environmental health—Appreciation of the external environment and the role one plays in preserving, protecting, and improving environmental conditions

Spiritual health—Belief in a supreme being or a way of living prescribed by religion; a guiding sense of meaning or value in life

Many people believe optimum wellness is best achieved by a holistic approach where there is a balance among the dimensions (Donatelle and Davis, 2000).

Consider . . .

■ how the models of health and wellness fit your views.
■ how the nurse might best care for a client with a belief in a model of health and wellness that differs from the nurse's.

HEALTH STATUS, BELIEFS, AND BEHAVIORS

The *health status* (state) of an individual is the health of that person at a given time. In its general meaning, the term may refer to anxiety, depression, or acute illness and thus describes the individual's problem in general. Health status can also describe such specifics as pulse rate and body temperature. The *health belief* of an individual is a perception of the relationship between things such as actions or objects and health. Beliefs may or may not be founded on fact. Some of these are influenced by culture, such as the "hot-cold" system of some Hispanic Americans. In this system, health is viewed as a balance of hot and cold qualities within a person. Citrus fruits and some fowl are considered cold foods, and meats and bread are hot foods. In this context, hot and cold do not denote temperature or spiciness but innate qualities of the food. For example, a fever is said to be caused by an excess of hot foods.

Health behaviors are the actions people take to understand their health state, maintain an optimal state of health, prevent illness and injury, and reach their maximum physical and mental potential. Behaviors such as eating wisely, exercising, paying attention to signs of illness, following treatment advice, and avoiding known health hazards such as smoking are all examples. Many factors contribute to health behaviors. Figure 17–2 shows a model of influences on these behaviors.

Consider . . .

■ what behaviors you consider to be the most likely to affect your own health.
■ how you would respond to a client who holds health beliefs that are contrary to the treatment that is prescribed.

HEALTH BELIEF MODELS

Several theories or health belief/behavior models have been developed to help determine whether an indi-

Figure 17–2

Factors Influencing Health Behavior Change

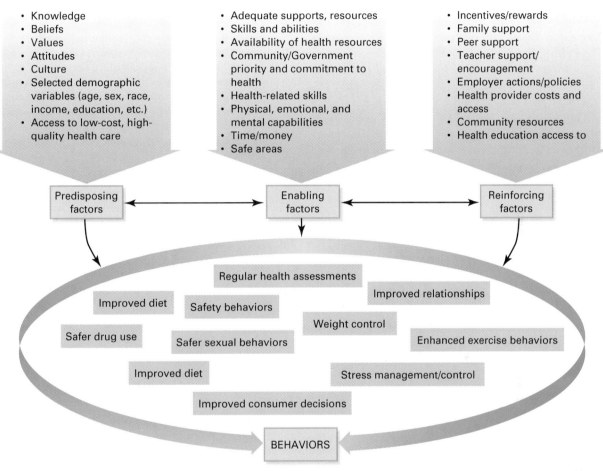

- Knowledge
- Beliefs
- Values
- Attitudes
- Culture
- Selected demographic variables (age, sex, race, income, education, etc.)
- Access to low-cost, high-quality health care

- Adequate supports, resources
- Skills and abilities
- Availability of health resources
- Community/Government priority and commitment to health
- Health-related skills
- Physical, emotional, and mental capabilities
- Time/money
- Safe areas

- Incentives/rewards
- Family support
- Peer support
- Teacher support/ encouragement
- Employer actions/policies
- Health provider costs and access
- Community resources
- Health education access to

Predisposing factors → Enabling factors → Reinforcing factors

Regular health assessments
Improved relationships
Improved diet
Safety behaviors
Weight control
Safer drug use
Safer sexual behaviors
Enhanced exercise behaviors
Improved diet
Stress management/control
Improved consumer decisions

BEHAVIORS

Source: R. J. Donatelle and L. G. Davis, *Access to Health,* 5th ed. Boston: Allyn and Bacon, Copyright © 1998. Reprinted by permission of Pearson Education, Inc.

vidual is likely to participate in disease prevention and health-promotion activities. These models can be useful tools in the development of programs for helping people change to healthier lifestyles and develop a more positive attitude to preventive health measures. See also Chapter 7, "The Nurse as Health Promoter and Care Provider."

Health Locus of Control Model

Locus of control is a concept from social learning theory that nurses may consider when determining who is most likely to take action regarding health, that is, whether clients believe that their health status is under their own or others' control. People who believe that they have a major influence on their own health status are internally controlled. They are more likely than others to take the initiative in their own health care, be more knowledgeable about their health, and adhere to prescribed health care regimens, such as taking medication, making and keeping appointments with physicians, and maintaining diets. By contrast, people who believe their health is largely controlled by outside forces (e.g., chance, luck, or powerful others) and is beyond their control are externally controlled and may need assistance to become more internally controlled if behavior changes are to be successful. Locus of control is a measurable concept that can be used to predict which people are most likely to change their behavior.

The results of a study by Lewis suggest that greater personal control over one's life is associated with higher levels of self-esteem, greater purpose in life, and decreased self-report of anxiety (Lewis, 1982, p. 113). Nurses can use this information about a client's locus of control in order to improve the client's self-care.

Rosenstock and Becker's Health Belief Model

In the 1950s, Rosenstock (1974) proposed a health belief model (HBM) intended to predict which individuals would or would not use such preventive measures as screening for early detection of cancer. Becker (1974) modified the health belief model to include these components: *individual perceptions, modifying factors,* and *variables likely to affect initiating action.*

The health belief model (Figure 17–3) is based on motivational theory. Rosenstock assumed that good health is an objective common to all people. Becker added "positive health motivation" as a consideration.

Individual Perceptions

Individual perceptions include the following:

- *Perceived susceptibility.* A family history of a certain disorder, such as diabetes or heart disease, may make the individual feel at high risk.
- *Perceived seriousness.* The question here is: In the perception of the individual, does the illness cause

death or have serious consequences? Concern about the spread of acquired immune deficiency syndrome (AIDS) reflects the general public's perception of the seriousness of this illness.

- *Perceived threat.* According to Becker, perceived susceptibility and perceived seriousness combine to determine the total perceived threat of an illness to a specific individual. For example, a person who perceives that many individuals in the community have AIDS may not necessarily perceive a threat of the disease; if the person is a drug addict or a homosexual, however, the perceived threat of illness is likely to increase because of the combined susceptibility and seriousness.

Modifying Factors

Factors that modify a person's perceptions include the following:

- *Demographic variables.* Demographic variables include age, sex, race, and ethnicity. An infant, for example, does not perceive the importance of a healthy diet; an adolescent may perceive peer approval as more important than family approval and participate as a

Figure 17–3

The Health Belief Model

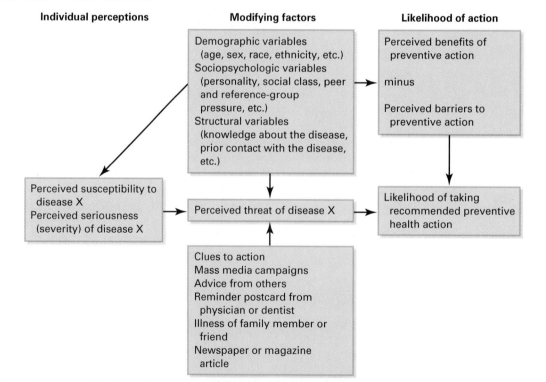

Source: "Selected Psychosocial Models and Correlates of Individual Health-Related Behaviors" by M. H. Becker, D. P. Haefner, S. V. Kasi, et al., *Medical Care* **15**: 27–46, 1977. Used with permission.

consequence in hazardous activities or adopt unhealthy eating and sleeping patterns.

■ *Sociopsychologic variables.* Social pressure or influence from peers or other reference groups (e.g., self-help or vocational groups) may encourage preventive health behaviors even when individual motivation is low. Expectations of others may motivate people, for example, not to drive an automobile after drinking alcohol.

■ *Structural variables.* Structural variables that are presumed to influence preventive behavior are knowledge about the target disease and prior contact with it. Becker found higher compliance rates with prescribed treatments among mothers whose children had frequent ear infections and occurrences of asthma.

■ *Cues to action.* Cues can be either internal or external. Internal cues include feelings of fatigue, uncomfortable symptoms, or thoughts about the condition of an ill person who is close.

Likelihood of Action

The likelihood of a person's taking recommended preventive health action depends on the perceived benefits of the action minus the perceived barriers to the action.

■ *Perceived benefits of the action.* Examples include refraining from smoking to prevent lung cancer, and eating nutritious foods and avoiding snacks to maintain weight.

■ *Perceived barriers to action.* Examples include cost, inconvenience, unpleasantness, and lifestyle changes.

Nurses play a major role in helping clients implement healthy behaviors. They help clients monitor health, supply anticipatory guidance, and impart knowledge about health. Nurses can also reduce barriers to action (e.g., by minimizing inconvenience or discomfort) and can support positive actions.

INTERNATIONAL INITIATIVE FOR HEALTH AND WELLNESS

Health for All has been proclaimed by the World Health Organization (WHO) as an international goal. The WHO constitution proclaims that the highest attainable standard of health is "one of the fundamental rights of every human being without distinction for race, religion, political belief, economic or social condition" (WHO, 1998, 2000). *Health for All* was adopted in 1977 and launched at the Alma Ata Conference in 1978. A renewal was launched in 1995 to ensure that individuals, countries, and organizations are ready to meet the world's health care needs in the 21st century.

WHO (2000) published a document titled *Health for All in the Twenty-first Century*. It describes global priorities and targets for the first two decades of the century that will create conditions worldwide for people to reach and maintain the highest level of health. The goals are to achieve an increase in life expectancy and quality of life, to improve equity in health between and within countries, and to ensure access for all to sustainable health services and systems. Key values underpin this effort:

■ Providing the highest attainable standard of health as a fundamental right
■ Strengthening application of ethics
■ Implementing equity-oriented policies and strategies
■ Incorporating a gender perspective to health policies and strategies

---

Global health targets

1. Healthy equity: childhood stunting
2. Survival: MMR,[1] CMR,[2] life expectancy
3. Reverse global trends of five major pandemics
4. Eradicate and eliminate certain diseases
5. Improve access to water, sanitation, food, and shelter
6. Measures to promote health
7. Develop, implement, and monitor national HFA policies
8. Improve access to comprehensive, essential, quality health care
9. Implement global and national health information and surveillance systems
10. Support research for health

[1]MMR—maternal mortality rate.
[2]CMR—child mortality rate.
Source: World Health Organization, *Health for All in the Twenty-first Century.* Geneva: WHO, 2000, executive summary, p. vi.

There are ten global targets that support *Health for All*, as shown in the box on page 287. Regional and national targets will be developed within the framework of the global policy reflecting the diversity of needs and local priorities. The actions by all member states are to be guided by two policy objectives: making health central to human development and developing sustainable health systems to meet the needs of people. WHO will provide global leadership for attainment of *Health for All* and will promote international collective action. More information on healthy people can be found in Chapter 7, "The Nurse as Health Promoter and Care Provider."

SUMMARY

Changes in the delivery of health care have resulted in changes in the practice of nursing. Two influences on these changes are cost-containment measures mandated by third-party payers and the commitment to providing care that is accessible to people in their communities. Cost containment has resulted in more focus on resource management and created the need for nurses to become skillful in the utilization of scarce resources, the development of critical pathways that provide accountability for outcomes, and the use of unlicensed assistive personnel. Focus of care has expanded from acute inpatient care to include primary and preventive care that is community-focused.

The changes in nursing require a new perspective on health as more than the absence of illness or disease, also involving a high level of wellness or the fulfillment of one's maximum potential for physical, psychosocial, and spiritual functioning. Wellness is an active, five-dimensional process of becoming aware of and making choices toward a higher level of well-being. The five dimensions of wellness are the physical, social, emotional, intellectual, and spiritual dimensions. Well-being is considered a subjective perception of balance, harmony, and vitality. It is a state rather than a process. Illness is usually associated with disease but may occur independently of it. Illness is a highly personal state in which the person feels unhealthy or ill. Disease alters body functions and results in a reduction of capacities or a shortened life span.

Because notions of health are highly individual, the nurse must determine each client's perception of health to provide meaningful assistance. This involves well-developed communication skills. Nurses also need to be aware of their own personal definitions of health. Many people describe health as freedom from symptoms of disease, the ability to be active, and a state of being in good spirits. Various models have been developed to explain health. They include the agent-host-environment mode, the high-level wellness grid, and the health belief model.

A person's decision to implement health behaviors or to take action to improve health depends on a number of factors. Such factors include the importance of health to the person, perceived threat of a particular disease or severity of the health care problems, perceived benefits of preventive or therapeutic actions, inconvenience and unpleasantness involved, degree of lifestyle change necessary, cultural ramifications, and cost.

The movement toward health and wellness has an international impetus through the work of the World Health Organization. *Health for All* is promoted through international collaboration to meet global health targets set by the organization.

Bookshelf

Anders, G. 1996. *Health against wealth.* **New York: Houghton Mifflin Company.**
This book discusses the background of the rise of HMOs and the breakdown of medical trust. It addresses ways to build a better system.
O'Brien, L. J. 1999. *Bad medicine: How the American medical establishment is ruining our healthcare system.* **Amherst, N.Y.: Prometheus Books.**
This book analyzes the decline of health care services in the United States from the perspective of medicine and proposes approaches to change.

SELECTED REFERENCES

American Nurses Association. 1980. *Nursing: A social policy statement.* Kansas City, Mo.: ANA.

American Nurses Association. 1991. *Nursing's agenda for health care reform.* Washington, D.C.: ANA.

American Organization of Nurse Executives. 1992. Eight premises for a reformed American health-care system. *Nursing Management* **23**: 42, 44.

Anderson, E. T., and McFarlane, J. 2000. *Community as*

partner: Theory and practice in nursing. Philadelphia: J. B. Lippincott.

Anspaugh, D. J., Hamrick, M. H., and Rosata, F. D. 2000. *Wellness: Concepts and applications,* 4th ed. St. Louis: Mosby-Year Book.

Becker, M. H., ed. 1974. *The health belief model and personal health behavior.* Thorofare, N.J.: Charles B. Slack.

Becker, M. H., Haefner, D. P., and Kasi, S. V. 1977. Selected psychosocial models and correlates of individual health-related behaviors. *Medical Care* **15:** 27–46.

Donatelle, R. J., and Davis, L. G. 2000. *Access to health,* 6th ed. Boston: Allyn and Bacon.

Dubos, R. 1978. Health and creative adaptation. *Human nature* **74**(1).

Dubos, R. 1968. *So human the animal.* New York: Scribners.

Dunn, H. L. 1959a, June. High-level wellness in man and society. *American Journal of Public Health* **49:** 786.

Dunn, H. L. 1959b, Nov. What high-level wellness means. *Canadian Journal of Public Health* **50:** 447.

Dunn, H. L. 1973. *High-level wellness.* Arlington, Va.: Beatty.

Glick, D. F. 1999. Advanced practice community health nursing in community nursing centers: A holistic approach to the community as client. *Holistic Nursing Practice* **13**(4): 19–27.

Leavell, H. R., and Clark, E. G. 1965. *Preventive medicine for the doctor in his community,* 3d ed. New York: McGraw-Hill.

Leddy, S., and Pepper, J. M. 1998. *Conceptual bases of professional nursing,* 4th ed. Philadelphia: J. B. Lippincott.

Lewis, F. M. 1982, March/April. Experienced personal control and quality of life in late-stage cancer patients. *Nursing Research* **31:** 113–118.

McAllister, G., and Farquhar, M. 1992, Dec. Health beliefs: A cultural division? *Journal of Advanced Nursing* **17:** 1447–1454.

Milstead, J. A. 1999. *Health policy and politics: A nurse's guide.* Gaithersburg, Md.: Aspen Publishers.

Murray, R. B., and Zentner, J. P. 1989. *Nursing concepts for health promotion,* 4th ed. Norwalk, Conn.: Appleton & Lange.

Nightingale, F. 1969. *Notes on nursing: What it is and what it is not.* New York: Dover Books (original work published in 1860).

Parsons, T. 1972. Definitions of health and illness in the light of American values and social structure. In E. G. Jaco, ed., *Patients, physicians, and illness,* 2d ed. New York: Free Press.

Pender, N. J. 1987. *Health promotion in nursing practice,* 2d ed. Norwalk, Conn.: Appleton & Lange.

President's Commission on Health Needs of the Nation. 1953. *Building Americans' Health.* Vol. 2 Washington, D.C.: U.S. Government Printing Office.

Price, S. A., Koch, M. W., and Bassett, S. 1998. *Health care resource management: Present and future challenges.* St. Louis: Mosby.

Rosenstock, I. M. 1974. Historical origins of the health belief model. In M. H. Becker, ed., *The health belief model and personal health behavior.* Thorofare, N.J.: Charles B. Slack.

Salmond, S. W. 1999. Delivery-of-care systems using clinical nursing assistants: Making it work. In S. O. Turner, *Essential readings in nursing managed care.* Gaithersburg, Md.: Aspen Publications, pp. 215–224.

Travis, J. W., and Ryan, R. S. 1988. *Wellness workbook,* 2d ed. Berkeley, Calif.: Ten Speed Press.

World Health Organization. 1947. *Constitution of the World Health Organization: Chronicle of the World Health Organization I.* Geneva: WHO.

World Health Organization. 1998. *The world health report 1998: Life in the 21st century—a vision for all.* Geneva: WHO.

World Health Organization. 2000. *Health for all in the twenty-first century.* Geneva: WHO.

CHAPTER 18

Health Care Economics

Outline

Objectives

- Identify selected issues related to nursing and health care economics.
- Define common terms used in the discussion of health care financing.
- Discuss cost-containment strategies implemented in health care.
- Examine the economics of providing health care services.
- Apply economics to nursing.
- Describe approaches to financial management in health care.

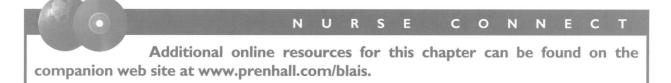

NURSE CONNECT

Additional online resources for this chapter can be found on the companion web site at www.prenhall.com/blais.

The decade of the 1990s focused on health care reform, accompanied by considerable debate regarding the resulting changes in financing. There was general recognition of the need for fundamental changes in health care delivery but no consensus about what these changes should be. There are basically three types of reform proposals: (1) complete governmental control with national health insurance and universal coverage with a single payer; (2) incremental changes to the current system of private-provider fee-for-service by means of malpractice reform, expansion of coverage for the poor, and the use of vouchers; (3) requiring employers to offer health insurance to all employees, along with increasing coverage for the poor.

Two central questions are raised by health care reform. Who should control the health care system? Who should pay for health care? A number of issues need to be addressed. People in the United States are paying more for health care and getting less in return. The cost of health care is implicated in the decline of the United States in the global economy. The cost of long-term care is a major concern with a growing percentage of the population aging and a smaller workforce bearing the burden of providing service. Curbing the costs of prescription drugs and other medical technologies was an issue in the 2000 presidential campaign for both major-party candidates.

CHALLENGES AND OPPORTUNITIES

The economic changes in health care have made it necessary for nurses to find new ways of delivering needed services within new structures of payment. An era of cost cutting arising from changes in financing has resulted in reductions in nursing staff, higher nurse-patient ratios, and higher productivity expectations as values seemingly moved from quality of care to cost effectiveness and profits.

The necessity of lowering the cost of health care has created many opportunities for nursing to expand practice and create new roles. Advanced-practice nursing has flourished in the era of health care reform. Nursing has an opportunity to exert its influence in new directions for policy and delivery of care.

ISSUES

Demand versus Supply of Health Care

During the 1980s, the cost of medical care was increasing faster than the gross national product. Coupled with the increased expense of care was the consumer's expectation that any and all services should be available and paid for by third-party payers regardless of cost. The demand for expensive care was outstripping the ability of payers to pay and spiraling out of control as consumers demanded a total continuum of care and unlimited access.

Further imbalance in supply and demand is created by the resulting increased cost of insurance coverage in the private sector. Many employers believe they cannot afford to provide coverage to employees at the levels previously provided. Individuals who must provide their own insurance because their employers do not offer that benefit can no longer afford premiums to maintain coverage.

These increases in costs have resulted in a diminished ability of consumers to afford care, yet they continue to expect care on demand. Health care economics cannot supply health care at a level demanded by the public (Milstead, 1999; Feldstein, 1999).

When there is an imbalance of supply and demand, an outcome may be rationing of health care. No country can afford to provide unlimited amounts of medical services to everyone, and each must decide upon a mechanism to ration, or limit access to, medical services. This can happen in two ways; the first is by having the government set limits. In this approach, the cost of services is kept low and people wait for availability. This type of rationing has been used in Great Britain. Scarce services are kept at a reasonable cost, but they are allocated according to particular criteria, such as age or a waiting list. In the United States, only Oregon has suggested such an approach. The Oregon legislature enacted a program to limit access to expensive procedures such as transplants and then increase Medicaid eligibility to a larger number of low-income people. The second rationing approach is to ration by ability to pay. This limits demand for more expensive procedures by offering them only to those who are willing to pay out of pocket or who have sufficient health insurance coverage (Feldstein, 1999).

There are important differences between these rationing methods. One is the freedom of the individual to choose the amount and type of health care used and to select who should deliver it. This has been a traditional value of health care consumers in the United States. Under a method using ability to pay, a consumer can spend as much as he or she can afford. For those who cannot afford it, that service is not an option. Under a system of government rationing, a patient will not be able to purchase a service unless it has been made available to everyone by the government. In order to decide the rationing technique to use, decisions must be made regarding how much health care will be provided to whom and at what cost.

Paying for Health Care

The United States is the only industrialized nation without a national health policy. Although the specific

Table 18–1 Comparison of Health Care Values Between the United States and Other Developed Countries

United States	Other Countries
Pluralism and choice	Universality
Individual accountability	Equity
Ambivalence toward government	Acceptance of the role of government
Progress, innovation, and new technology	Skepticism about markets and competition
Volunteerism and communitarianism	Global budgets
Paranoia about monopoly	Rationing
Competition	Technology assessment and innovation control

Source: Based on I. Morrison, *Health Care in the New Millennium: Vision, Values, and Leadership,* San Francisco: Jossey-Bass, 2000, pp. 2–5.

details of coverage and the availability of certain services vary by country, governments provide financing (Powell and Wesson 1999). Table 18–1 compares the U.S. and other developed countries in terms of values underlying health care.

In the past, private insurers, for the most part, have paid for U.S. health care. In 1965 the federal government entered into health care financing with the passage of Medicare, followed by Medicaid. These programs have grown and expanded until nearly half of the cost of health care is covered by at least one of them. The dilemma in health care reform is whether the federal programs should continue to expand until there is a national health care payment structure or whether private insurance should continue. The debate about national health care versus private insurance has been vigorous, with significant support on each side of the issue (Feldstein, 1999).

Separate Billing for Nursing Services

Bills submitted to third-party payers and consumers from health care organizations such as hospitals continue to bundle nursing services with flat daily charges, such as the cost of the room and housekeeping. The specific cost of nursing has neither been separated out nor given a dollar value. This has hindered the ability of nurses to receive payment from third-party payers. Many leaders think that for nursing to be a profession, nursing services must be accounted for separately from flat room fees to the health care institution.

Several developments within nursing have provided ways of quantifying nursing care (Peters, 2000;

Kerr, 2000). Some of the better-known projects have resulted in nursing diagnoses that can be used to categorize nursing interventions (NANDA), nursing intervention classification (NIC), and nursing outcome classification (NOC).

COST-CONTAINMENT STRATEGIES

Efforts have been made for many years to control health care costs, yet they continue to rise. Some of the main cost-containment strategies are competition, price controls, alternative insurance delivery systems, managed care, health promotion and illness prevention, and alternative care providers.

Competition

In the 1970s in the United States, regulations were changed to permit competition among the agencies that deliver health care and provide insurance. Currently, there appears to be little reduction in costs that can be attributed to competition. Competition has, however, led to the establishment of walk-in clinics, urgent-care clinics, and alternative health care providers, such as advanced registered nurse practitioners, for example, which offer additional care choices for clients.

Price Controls

Price controls for health care services have been established in various ways. Freezes on physicians' fees have been imposed at various times for short periods, and many states limit reimbursement to physicians and hospitals for services provided to Medicaid clients.

Group self-insurance plans are another means to reduce costs. These plans involve a designated group, such as employees in a large company, a group of companies, or a union, for example. The designated group assumes all or part of the costs of health care for its members. They can often provide coverage at a lower cost than insurance companies because they are exempt from certain taxes and fees.

The passage of the Tax Equity and Fiscal Responsibility Act (TEFRA) in 1982 brought about a dramatic restructuring of health care delivery in the United States. Through this act, the federal government changed the payment method for Medicare from a retrospective system to a **prospective payment system.** This legislation limits the amount paid to hospitals that are reimbursed by Medicare. Reimbursement is made according to a classification system known as **diagnostic-related groups** (DRGs). The system establishes pretreatment diagnosis billing categories and a payment schedule.

Using DRGs, a hospital is paid a predetermined amount for clients with a specific diagnosis. For example, a hospital that admits a client with a diagnosis of myocardial infarction is reimbursed with a specific dollar amount, regardless of the cost of services, the length of stay, or the acuity or complexity of the client's illness. Prior to the DRG system, hospitals billed retrospectively, that is, after services were rendered. In contrast, prospective payment or billing is determined *before* the client is ever admitted to the hospital. DRG rates are set in advance of the year during which they apply and are considered fixed unless major, uncontrollable events occur. The Health Care Financing Administration (HCFA) is authorized to administer and enforce this system.

This legislation has had a tremendous impact on health care delivery in the United States because hospitals and providers, rather than Medicare or other third-party payers, run the risk of monetary losses. If a hospital's costs exceed the fixed amount, the hospital loses money. Thus, this type of prospective payment system offers financial incentives for withholding unnecessary tests or procedures and avoiding prolonged hospital stays and excessive expenditures.

Notable effects of prospective payment systems include the earlier discharge of clients, a decline in admissions, a rise in the number and type of outpatient services, and an increased focus on the costs of care. One result of the decline in admissions is that most of those clients who are admitted to acute-care hospitals are seriously ill and have complex health care needs. The earlier discharge of clients has led to an expansion of home care services and an increased use of technology and specialists.

To protect clients from DRG abuses, Medicare introduced state **peer review organizations** (PROs). Made up of physicians, nurses, and other health care professionals, PROs are intended to monitor the hospitals and ensure high-quality care under DRGs. PROs have developed screening guidelines that determine whether admissions should occur or procedures should be performed. PROs also review health care records, render payment decisions, and handle related problems, such as admission criteria.

The cost-containment strategies have resulted in new trends in health care delivery. These are shown in the box on page 295.

Alternative Delivery Systems

With the advent of increased costs, alternative delivery systems were created. Private insurers created new programs, such as the health maintenance organization (HMO) and the preferred provider organization (PPO), as strategies to control costs. Insurers also encouraged outpatient diagnostic testing and surgery, required second opinions for surgery, and implemented a variety of other cost-cutting initiatives.

Health maintenance organizations are group health care agencies that provide basic and supplemental health maintenance and treatment services to voluntary enrollees. The enrollees or their employers prepay a fixed periodic fee that is set without regard to the amount or kind of services provided. To receive federal funds, an HMO must offer physician services, hospital and outpatient services, emergency services, short-term mental health services, treatment and referral for drug and alcohol problems, laboratory and radiologic services, and preventive health services. By encouraging preventive and wellness services and by offering ambulatory services, HMOs have reduced the cost of health insurance to the consumer.

The **preferred provider organization** emerged as another alternative health care delivery system. It consists of a group of physicians or a hospital that provides companies with health services at a discounted rate. Hospitals, physicians, and insurance companies are major sponsors of PPOs. Physicians can belong to one or more PPO, and the client chooses a primary care provider among the physicians who belong to a particular PPO.

Physician/hospital organizations (PHOs) are joint ventures between a group of private practice physicians and a hospital. PHOs combine both resources and personnel to provide managed care alternatives and medical services. PHOs work with a variety of in-

Trends in Health Care Delivery

FROM		TO
Illness emphasis	→	Preventive emphasis
Acute care	→	Preventive, home care
Hospital/institution-based	→	Noninstitution-based (clinic/home)
Fee-for-service (cost-based)	→	Prospective payment and managed care
Physician-directed	→	Diverse decision-makers and managed care
If it helps (at all), use it (regardless of cost)	→	Outcomes measurement and cost-effectiveness
Independent decisions (practice variation)	→	Protocols/guidelines (best practice)
Local perspective (practice variation, standards/benchmarking)	→	Global perspective (protocols/guidelines/practice)
Introduce new technologies (regardless of cost)	→	Outcomes measurement and cost-effectiveness
Paper records, medical charts	→	Information systems, computer records

CHANGE IN

Orientation

Illness, crisis	→	Prevention
Specific, specialist	→	Holistic
Quantity of care	→	Quality of care

Location of Service

Inpatient	→	Outpatient, clinic, home

Payment Mode

Retrospective	→	Prospective
Fee-for-service	→	Managed care

Outlook

Just do it	→	Outcomes measurement
Just do it	→	Quality of care; quality of life

Source: Used by permission of B. Cherry and S. R. Jacob, *Contemporary Nursing: Issues, Trends, and Management,* St. Louis: Mosby, 1999, p. 162.

surers to provide services. A typical PHO will include primary care providers and specialists.

Managed Care

Managed care describes a health care system whose goals are to provide cost-effective, quality care that focuses on improved outcomes for groups of clients. In managed care, health care providers and agencies collaborate so as to render the most appropriate, fiscally responsible care possible. Managed care denotes an emphasis on cost controls, customer satisfaction, health promotion, and preventive services. Health maintenance organizations and preferred provider organizations are examples of provider systems committed to managed care.

Hospitals and other health care agencies have adopted many of the principles of managed care. Hospitals have developed strategies to reduce costs and ensure quality outcomes for groups of clients. They have adopted practice innovations, including case management, critical pathways, and patient-focused care. These models require nurses, physicians, and ancillary providers to collaborate as they develop and implement health care.

Case management describes a model of integrating health care services for individuals or groups. Various case management models exist that strive to provide cost-effective care and ensure quality outcomes. Generally, case management involves nurse-physician teams that assume collaborative responsibility for assessing needs, and planning, coordinating, implementing, and evaluating care for groups of clients from preadmission to discharge or transfer and recuperation. Case managers, however, may be a social worker or other appropriate professional.

Case managers generally coordinate care for a specific client population, such as clients with AIDS, in a particular setting. A critical component of their role is collaboration with other health care professionals and the client to achieve established outcomes. Key responsibilities for case managers are shown in the accompanying box.

Vertically Integrated Health Services Organizations

Prior to the 1970s, the typical delivery system for medical and surgical care was the single, not-for-profit hospital and its medical staff or small group practices. Very little care was provided in the home. In the current health care environment, new organizations have emerged, with new relationships between hospitals and physicians. The scope of responsibility has widened to wellness, ambulatory care, outpatient surgery, and home health services. Many physicians' practices are owned and managed by this new organization.

Two trends have contributed to this organizational change. The first—and probably the most important—is the change in payment structures, and the other is medical technology. Prior to the health care reform movement, hospitals and physicians were reimbursed separately on a fee-for-service basis regardless of how high the costs rose, as long as the patient had insurance coverage. Hospitals invested in services and facilities regardless of whether there was duplication in the community.

As insurers became more concerned about the rising costs of health care in the 1970s, hospitals began horizontal integration by forming multihospital systems. Thus, hospitals could band together to offer services within the community rather than duplicate them. The disadvantage was a loss of autonomy; as the system grew larger there was less control of operating budgets and decision making.

As a result of the changes in Medicare's payment under fixed-priced diagnostic related groups, the move to vertical integration began. Hospitals were then affected by physicians' hospital practices and began to monitor discharge practices and lengths of stay. It became more cost effective to discharge some patients to another suitable setting such as a nursing home or the patient's home, and it became advantageous for hospitals to own or contract with agencies, such as home health, providing this type of care. This vertical integration allowed hospitals to reduce inpatient costs and receive additional Medicare revenues.

Advances in medical technology contributed to this move from a traditional hospital to an outpatient setting. Many surgeries, such as cholecystectomies, hernia repairs, and some orthopedic surgeries that had necessitated several days in the hospital at one time, can now be done on an outpatient basis. These outpatient services are less costly.

Another stimulus to vertical integration came with provider capitation payments. The move to paying for the full range of health care per person, rather than a per-diem amount for the stay, changed hospitals from profit centers to cost centers. In other words, it became more costly to the hospital to keep people in the hospital than treat them in other less costly settings.

Within the integrated system, there has been a goal to create a "seamless" system of patient care, where movement from service to service is coordinated and well organized. Such a plan could improve quality of care and outcomes while increasing patient satisfaction. It provides better control of costs by more efficient use of resources. If it is efficient, it can decrease transaction costs and allows greater accountability.

A disadvantage of a vertically integrated organization is that the financial incentives need to be aligned among all the different providers within that organi-

Key Responsibilities of Case Managers

Assessing clients and their homes and communities
Coordinating and planning client care
Collaborating with other health professionals

Monitoring clients' progress
Evaluating client outcomes

zation. Medical groups must be well integrated both philosophically and in decision making regarding care.

HEALTH CARE ECONOMICS

Because health care is an exceedingly expensive entity in contemporary society, many approaches have been developed to finance it and, at the same time, maintain quality.

Billing Methods

There are three main types of billing for health care services: fee-for-service, capitation, and fee-for-diagnosis.

Fee-for-Service

In the fee-for-service method, clients pay the practitioner for each health service they receive rather than the professional receiving a fixed amount of compensation. Ideally, clients choose the service they need and each pays for this service. In reality, not all clients are willing or able to choose the service they require and not all health care providers are willing to relinquish their prescriptive power or work for a fixed amount. Therefore, collaboration is required to select mutually acceptable health services in the fee-for-service billing.

Capitation

Under **capitation,** health care providers are paid a fixed dollar amount per person for providing an agreed-upon set of health services to a defined population for a specific period of time. If the costs of providing service are lower than the fixed amount, the provider organization makes a profit. If costs exceed payment, however, then the provider organization takes a financial loss.

Health maintenance organizations, preferred provider organizations, and physician/hospital organizations discussed earlier are managed-care systems and thus subject to capitation. In other words, payers negotiate health care costs, and the providers take both the potential financial risks and benefits.

Fee-for-Diagnosis

Fee-for-diagnosis is a type of prospective payment system (PPS). Agencies are provided with a fixed dollar amount for the care of a client based on the client's main and secondary diagnoses, demographic information (e.g., age and sex), and the usual treatment provided for the health problems. The diagnosis-related group system is an example of a fee-for-diagnosis system.

Because a diagnosis is needed to establish a fee for the health care provider, the fee-for-diagnosis system does not provide incentives for reducing costs by providing preventive care.

Payment Sources

United States

In the United States, there are three main sources of payment: government health plans, private insurance, and personal payment.

Government Health Plans

The federal government, through Social Security, has in place a number of health care programs, including Medicare and Medicaid.

- ■ **MEDICARE** Medicare is designed to provide health care to people 65 years and older. Medicare clients pay a deductible and coinsurance. **Coinsurance** is the 20% share of a payment that is paid by the client; the other 80% is paid by the government.

  Medicare is divided into two parts: Part A is available to the disabled and to people 65 years and over. It provides insurance toward hospitalization, home care, and hospice care. Part B is voluntary and provides partial coverage of physician services to people eligible for Part A. Clients pay a monthly premium for this coverage.

  Medicare does not cover dental care, dentures, eyeglasses, hearing aids, or examinations to prescribe and fit hearing aids. Most preventive care, including routine physical examinations and associated diagnostic tests, is not included.

- ■ **MEDICAID** Medicaid is a public assistance program paid out of general taxes for people who require financial assistance (i.e., low-income groups). Medicaid is paid by federal and state governments. Each state program is distinct. Some states provide very limited coverage, whereas others pay for dental care, eyeglasses, and prescription drugs.

Private Insurance

In the United States, numerous commercial health insurance carriers offer a wide range of coverage plans. There are two types of private health insurance: not-for-profit (e.g., Blue Cross–Blue Shield) and for-profit (e.g., commercial companies such as Metropolitan Life, Travelers, and Aetna). Private health insurance pays either the entire bill or, more often, 80% of the costs.

With these plans, insurance may be purchased either as an individual plan or as part of a group plan through a person's employer, union, student association, or similar organization. The individual usually pays a monthly premium to obtain this protection. Group plans offer premiums at lower costs. Some employers share the costs of the premiums, and this benefit is often a major item in labor contracts.

Personal Payment

Direct personal payment is the payment of money for services not covered by insurance. The percentage of health care costs paid personally by an individual is higher in the United States than that paid by people in England, Germany, or Canada, for example.

The International Perspective

Health care systems worldwide have had to respond to challenging conditions regarding economic, political, and social circumstances. In Great Britain, massive changes referred to as *internal market reforms* were a response to the need for greater efficiency and value to community needs. The Swedish health care system has progressively decentralized in order for local governments to find innovative ways to meet local desires within the goals of the national health care framework. In Canada, budgetary and economic restrictions have stimulated the provinces to enact management reforms for cost containment and develop programs for primary care. Germany has had to respond to budgetary problems resulting from the costs of national reunification by adopting a more centralized management of health insurance (Powell and Wesson, 1999).

Each of these countries has dealt with the problem of medical cost inflation more or less successfully. In Great Britain and Germany, reform has taken place through the national governments. In Canada and Sweden, the changes have taken place at the regional level of government. Whether the response was regional or national, these countries have responded to economic difficulties while maintaining universal coverage. This is likely due to their commitments to equitable access to services for their populations.

Germany

Germany was the first country to institute national insurance-based social and health programs by adopting the Health Insurance Act in 1883, the Accident Insurance Law in 1884, and the Old Age and Invalidity Act in 1889 (Powell and Wesson, 1999, p. 49). Germany's health care system is based on private-practice physicians and on community, church, and municipality af-

filiated hospitals using a large number of nonprofit and for-profit insurers and autonomous sickness funds. The cost of sickness funds is paid by an income-adjusted fee; half of this fee is paid by the worker and half is paid by the employer. Individuals and their families are obligated to become members of a sickness fund if they fall below certain income levels or are in certain occupations. It is a pluralistic, private system that ensures universal coverage and contains costs. In 1977, the need for more effective cost-containment efforts led to the creation of an advisory group called Concerted Action in Health Care, with the very specific duty of maintaining stability in the contribution rates to the sickness funds by placing expenditure controls on the funds. This required changes in provider-payment methods.

Canada

The Canadian national health insurance program was developed over a period of time to make access to care more equitable. The Hospital Insurance and Diagnostic Services Act in 1957 and the Medical Care Act in 1966 are the cornerstones. The national program was fully adopted in Canada in 1971 (Powell and Wesson, 1999, p. 115). Each province funds and administers its own health insurance plan that covers hospital and medical services. The federal government contributes financially on the condition that provinces meet national standards for eligibility and coverage. Most of the resources are in the private sector, and the system is often described as publicly funded and privately delivered. The basic tenets are (1) universal health insurance for all citizens of the province, (2) government funding from general tax revenues, (3) no point-of-service charges, (4) no private insurance for universal medical benefits, (5) central control of budget levels but discretion for institutions to spend within the budget, and (6) central control of dissemination of technology.

Enacted in 1984, the Canada Health Act (CHA) penalizes provinces that permit extra billing of clients and creates incentives for home care, community health clinics, and health-promotion services. In addition, many provincial initiatives are currently under way to improve quality and efficiency and decrease health care costs. As in the United States, hospital beds are decreasing and community resources are increasing. However, there are serious concerns about increasing health care costs.

Australia

Australia's Medicare system provides health care for all who are legally permanent residents of Australia or are visitors from countries with which Australia has a health care agreement. The Medicare system consists of two parts: (1) free or subsidized treatment by a general practitioner, medical specialist, dentist or optometrist; and (2) free treatment as public patients in a public hospital. Clients may choose their own general practitioner; however, treatment by a specialist requires referral by a general practitioner.

The Medicare system is funded through the Australian tax system and pays 85% of the schedule fee, which is set by the government. If a client or client family spends in excess of the government-set amount on health care costs within a given year (A$302.30 in 2001), the Medicare system will pay 100% of schedule fees for the remainder of that year through the Medicare Safety Net. This entitlement is designed to protect individuals and families from high medical expenses.

Australia's public hospital system is funded jointly by the commonwealth, state, and territory governments and is administered by the state/territory health departments. Medicare does not pay for private accommodation in either a public or private hospital, so individuals who choose to be treated as private patients must pay the difference between the amount Medicare subsidizes and the cost of service. Medicare pays 75% of the schedule fee for private physician services. Private patient services can also be paid for through private insurance.

Sweden

The Swedish health care system developed through politics of compromise forged by executive-induced conciliation. It represents the extreme of government financing and delivery of health care. The Swedish government introduced national health insurance and controls on doctor's fees and put doctors on full-time salary; it restricted the private practice of physicians, converting the system to a national health service (Immergut, 1992).

Great Britain

Britain's National Health Service provides remarkably comprehensive service to the entire population. It is tax-financed and free at the point of delivery, with relatively low administrative costs. Although the quality of care is usually high, the environments are often dreary, and there are often long waits for service. Britain's system of primary health care contributes to the success of the system. Every member of the population is registered with a general practitioner (GP); each person makes an average of four visits per year to the GP (Day and Klein,

1991). The GP is the gatekeeper to the more expensive services in the hospital sector or to specialty care.

The previous examples from other countries illustrate systems used to provide a national health care policy that provides equity in access to services. All these systems face continuous challenges to cost containment that require adjustments and change. However, the commitment to providing quality care for all the population has allowed them to survive and evolve.

NURSING ECONOMICS

Few efforts have been made to determine the actual costs of nursing care. Traditionally, the cost of nursing services has been included in the average hospital bill within the general category of "room rate." Often, the number of patients determined the number of nurses needed. However, when the prospective payment system was introduced, it became necessary for hospitals to determine their staffing needs more efficiently. In the early 1960s, a *patient classification system* (PCS) was developed at Johns Hopkins Hospital that identified the needs for nursing care in quantitative terms. Since that time, various PCSs have been developed that assess the acuity of illness and the corresponding complexity and amount of nursing care required.

Quality care and cost trade-offs in hospitals dominate the literature of the past decade. Both consumers and health care professionals are expressing concerns about diminished quality of care resulting from cost constraints, early discharge, nursing shortages, and the increased use of unlicensed assistive personnel (UAPs). Determining the precise cost of nursing services is a major challenge for nursing. What are the exact costs of high-quality nursing care? How many nursing care hours are required for each DRG? What is the best *skill mix*—that is, ratio of registered nurses to licensed practical nurses and nursing assistants—on each hospital unit? Since 1983, many studies have been undertaken to determine the actual costs of nursing care and the cost-effectiveness of nursing care. Researchers have investigated such topics as the impact of nurse-physician collaboration; new cost-effective interventions; cost benefits of primary nursing, nurse practitioners, and nurse midwives; cost-effectiveness of home care; and so on. The quality of the nursing care of the future will rely on ongoing research.

Consider . . .

■ whether cost-containment programs implemented in your agency have influenced nursing care.

- measures that have been implemented in your agency to relieve nurses of nonnursing tasks.
- the role nurses play in maintaining quality nursing care in your agency.
- what cost-effective care nurses could provide that may substitute for physicians' services in your community.
- who should reimburse the nurse for services.

The Nursing Shortages

Since the 1940s, there have been periods of concern over a national shortage of nurses. The shortages have been cyclic in their occurrence; there have been periods in which the shortage has seemed to be acute, followed by a period of time where the problem seems to have been resolved, only to have it emerge again. The measure commonly used to indicate a shortage of nurses is the nursing **vacancy rate,** or the percent of unfilled positions for which an organization is recruiting. When the national nursing vacancy rate is high, commissions and committees study the problem and make recommendations. The federal government has spent billions of dollars in nursing education through the Nurse Training Act that was passed in 1964 (Feldstein, 1999).

In theory, the reason for a nursing shortage is that organizations cannot hire enough nurses at the wage offered. If the demand for nurses exceeds the supply, then organizations will compete to employ them and wages will increase. As the wages increase, nurses who are not employed in nursing or who are working part time either seek employment or increase their work time. As the organizations are able to fill the positions, they no longer need to compete with higher wages until employment falls off and another shortage begins.

In part, this theory explains the cycles, but trends of the past 15 years in health care have added to the complexity of the problem. When length of stay decreased, patients were sent home "sicker and quicker." The acuity level within inpatient settings increased and care shifted to the home, outpatient settings, and skilled-nursing facilities. Cost-containment companies began hiring nurses to do utilization review and case management. For a period of time, hospitals were downsizing nursing departments as a cost-cutting measure and adding unlicensed assistive personnel. Some nurses experienced disillusion with health care and left the profession, feeling that they could no longer provide quality care.

Ending the cycle of nursing shortages will require some adjustment to the approaches used by employers and nurses. New opportunities and new roles for nurses may attract more people into the profession. To the extent that RNs are able to perform more highly valued functions, their presence will be more valuable to administrators in health care organizations.

FINANCIAL MANAGEMENT

Profit versus Not-for-Profit Organizations

Hospitals in the United States have three forms of ownership: public, private for-profit, and private nonprofit (Baker et al., 2000). Federal, state, or local government agencies govern public nonprofit hospitals, which provide care regardless of the client's ability to pay. Private for-profit hospitals are owned by private investors to make profits, and they primarily serve paying clients. They provide limited charitable care. Private not-for-profit hospitals are owned by a voluntary board of trustees to provide care for both paying clients and those who require charitable care.

Health care in the United States has been and continues to be mostly a nonprofit enterprise. The for-profit sector has accounted for about 15% of hospital beds over the past 20 years (Morrison, 2000). For-profit organizations have shareholders who invest money and expect a return on the investment. Not-for-profit organizations operate according to mission statements that usually refer to community service. The not-for-profit organizations are often referred to as the public sector; they receive tax exemptions based on their benefits to the community. The for-profit organizations are often referred to as the private sector and are taxed by the government.

During the health care reform movement of the 1980s, the shift of hospitals and physician groups to the private sector was referred to as the *corporatization* of health care. The emphasis placed upon profits for shareholders led to the criticism that quality of care was no longer important; rather, the focus was on cost cutting and revenue production.

Increased attention has been paid to the for-profit sector due to its visibility in acquiring struggling hospitals and HMOs and creating corporate chains. The pattern has been for these chains to undergo turmoil as a result of low profits or even losses, with the divesting of struggling organizations and the buyout of other institutions. According to Morrison (2000, p. 64), "It is likely that when the accounting is all done, the net amount of capital brought into health care from shareholders exceeds the amount of capital that has gone out of the system in the form of profits." In other words, the for-profit organizations have not been profitable.

The not-for-profit organizations operate in much

the same way as the private sector in that their leaders use the language of business and they pay attention to financial margins. They are also under pressure to show evidence of community benefit, as required by their tax-exempt status. Because much of the cost cutting was generated by changes in health care financing by third-party payers rather than by a profit motive, public institutions have suffered the same impact of tightened financial resources.

Costs and Budgeting

It is extremely important for nurses to understand the business of health care. Financial considerations and accounting drive many management decisions, and familiarity with the basic concepts can empower nurses.

Cost accounting is used by hospitals and other organizations; it is a method of accounting for total costs of the business and tracking and allocating those costs to the specific service. For instance, the cost of providing a service is calculated and then used to determine the charge for the service. In the mid-1980s this was applied to DRGs. This method is used when the organization negotiates capitated rates.

Total costs of care are a sum of fixed costs and variable costs. Fixed costs are those that do not fluctuate with census or volume. Examples are salaries of managers and salaries of the minimum number of nurses needed to staff a unit. Variable costs are a function of census or volume and are over and above the fixed costs. An example is medical supplies for a particular patient. The total costs are used to calculate the cost per unit of service, which in many hospitals is the cost per patient day.

Full costing includes direct and indirect costs. Direct costing compares a department's actual outflow with its inflow from the services it delivers. Indirect costs are necessary but not directly related to delivery of service; examples are administrative salaries or bed linens. Productivity measures also figure in determining costs. These measure how efficiently resources are utilized in providing the service. For nursing, productivity is often measured in hours per patient day and compares actual staffing with projected hours under some patient acuity classification system.

Costing and productivity measures are used to develop a budget for the unit of service. The budget is an educated guess or estimate of the expenses to be encountered in the next year. It operationalizes management functions of planning, ongoing activities, and spending control. There are different budgeting methods that may be used. The simplest method is the flat percentage increase that develops a budget based on

year-to-date expenses and multiplies it by the inflation rate. Management by objective supports programs and services that assist the organization to reach its predetermined goals and usually requires cost-benefit analysis. Zero-based budgeting requires analysis of services on three levels: minimum, current, and improvement levels. It requires ranking by priorities.

Marketing concepts are applied to health care in order to maximize the potential utilization and satisfaction with a service. Four variables are involved in marketing:

1. Product—the service to be provided

Research Box

Baker, C. M., Messmer, P. L., Gyurko, C. C., Domagala, S. E., Conly, F. M., Eads, T. S., Harshman, K. S., and Layne, M. K. 2000. Hospital ownership, performance, and outcomes: Assessing the state-of-the-science. *Journal of Nursing Administration* 30 (5): 227–244.

An analysis of the research literature from 1985 to 1999 was done to achieve three objectives related to hospital ownership, performance, and outcomes: (1) identify research evidence, (2) assess the state of the science in acute-care hospitals, and (3) identify measurable components of performance and outcomes. Examination and synthesis of the published research indicated that hospital ownership has an impact on hospital performance in relation to costs, prices, financial management issues, and personnel issues. For-profit hospitals offer fewer unprofitable services, but regardless of ownership, market share influences the availability of services and pricing. The for-profit hospitals also employ fewer employees and fewer full-time-equivalent employees, and they offer lower salaries, except in competitive markets. Hospital ownership has an impact on type and degree of community benefits. The association with patient outcomes varies with the dimension measured; the evidence is mixed or inconclusive regarding access to care, morbidity, and mortality.

Assessment of the state of the science was determined to be in its infancy. The evidence is described as fragmented. There is a need for better-defined and more consistent outcome measurements for performance and outcomes.

2. Place—the agency where the service is to be provided
3. Promotion—advertising and publicity
4. Price—the charge for the service

The goals of marketing are to maximize marketplace consumption of a service and to maximize customer satisfaction to create more demand. Marketing of nursing's product or services may emphasize the quality of nursing provided in the organization compared to others. Many public relations campaigns emphasize care that is more family-centered, for example, so that the potential customer will want to receive care at that

agency. Some marketing strategies may focus more on one variable than others, but health care marketing tends to focus more on the product or quality of a particular service (Turner, 1999).

Consider . . .

- how your organization fits into the vertical integration of health care.
- how nursing can work toward achieving a seamless health care–delivery system.
- marketing strategies that could be used to promote nursing.

SUMMARY

The demand for controlling the spiraling costs of health care resulted in changes in health care financing. Cost containment became the goal of many changes in the way health care is delivered and paid for. Billing, which was once retrospective payment for services rendered, is now done through capitation or costs allowed for particular diagnoses.

As health care reform progresses, controversy regarding universal health care arises. There is little agreement on who should pay. Third-party payers in the form of insurance companies and benefits provided by the federal government (Medicare and Medicaid) provide the vast majority of financing, with self-pay by consumers accounting for a very small percentage.

Nursing is attempting to meet the challenge of payment for nursing care by developing its business savvy. One of these attempts is the development of ways of documenting the costs of nursing by using outcomes and measurements that allow it to be separated from the indirect and direct costs of the health care institution. Hospitals and health care organizations, whether they are for-profit or not-for-profit, are being managed in a business-oriented manner, and nurses need to be familiar with costing, budgeting, and marketing. Changes in health care delivery and financing

are challenging the traditional practice of nursing. The challenges produced by changes in health care economics have provided opportunities for the nursing profession to take a leadership role in shaping the future of health care.

Bookshelf

Armstrong, H., Armstrong, P., and Fegan, C. 1998. *Universal healthcare: What the United States can learn from the Canadian experience.* **New York: New Press: Distributed by W.W. Norton.**
The book compares the U.S. and Canadian systems and examines the mechanisms of care that are universal, accessible, comprehensive, portable, and publicly administered.

Andrews, C. 1995. *Profit fever: The drive to corporatize health care and how to stop it.* **Monroe, Maine: Common Courage Press.**
The author is an advocate of single-payer health care coverage. From this perspective, the history of health insurance in the United States is provided.

SELECTED REFERENCES

About Medicare (Australia). 2001. www.hic@gov.au/yourhealth/our_services/am.htm.

Aiken, L. H., Clarke, S. P., and Sloane, D. M. 2000. Hospital restructuring: Does it adversely affect care and outcomes? *Journal of Nursing Administration* **30**(10): 457–465.

American Nurses Association. 1985. *Code for nurses with interpretive statements.* Kansas City, Mo.: ANA.

American Nurses Association. 1991. *Nursing's agenda for health care reform.* Washington, D.C.: ANA.

American Nurses Association. 2000. *Achieving access for all Americans: A proposal from the American Nurses Associ-*

ation for Health Coverage 2000. www.nursingworld.org/readroom/rwjpaper.htm.

American Nurses Association. 2000. *Nursing's values challenged by managed care: Executive summary.* www.nursingworld.org/products/nti0198.htm.

Baker, C. M., Messmer, P. L., Gyurko, C. C., Domagala, S. E., Conly, F. M., Eads, T. S., Harshman, K. S., and Layne, M. K. 2000. Hospital ownership, performance, and outcomes: Assessing the state of the science. *Journal of Nursing Administration* **30**(5): 227–245.

Cherry, B., and Jacob, S. R. 1999. *Contemporary nursing: Issues, trends, and management.* St. Louis: Mosby.

Day, P., and Klein, R. 1991. The British health care experiment. *Health Affairs* **10**(3): 39–59.

Feldstein, P. J. 1999. *Health policy issues: An economic perspective on health reform,* 2d ed. Chicago: Health Administration Press.

Haugh, R. 2000. New directions in managed care. *Hospitals and Health Networks.* www.hhnmag.com.

Immergut, E. 1992. *Health politics. Interests and institutions in Western Europe.* Cambridge, U.K.: Cambridge University Press.

Kerr, P. 2000. Comparing two nursing outcome reporting initiatives. *Outcomes Management for Nursing Practice* **4**(3): 144

Mark, B. A., Salyer, J., and Wan, T. T. H. 2000. Market, hospital, and nursing unit characteristics as predictors of nursing unit skill mix: A contextual analysis. *Journal of Nursing Administration* **30**(11): 552–560.

Milstead, J. A. 1999. *Health policy and politics: A nurse's guide.* Gaithersburg, Md.: Aspen Publications.

Morrison, I. 2000. *Health care in the new millennium: Vision, values, and leadership.* San Francisco: Jossey-Bass.

Peters, R. M. 2000. Using NOC outcome of risk control in prevention, early detection, and control of hypertension. *Outcomes Management for Nursing Practice* **4**(1):39–45.

Powell, F. D., and Wessen, A. F., eds. 1999. *Health care systems in transition: An international perspective.* Thousand Oaks, Calif.: Sage.

Rambur, B. 1998. Ethics, economics, and the erosion of physician authority: A leadership role for nurses. *Advances in Nursing Science* **20**(4): 62–71.

Turner, S. O. 1999. *The nurse's guide to managed care.* Gaithersburg, Md.: Aspen.

Providing Care in the Home and Community

Objectives

- Describe the roles of the home health and community health nurse.
- Compare differences in applying the nursing process in the home setting versus the hospital setting.
- Describe characteristics of a healthy community.
- Discuss various elements and settings for community-based nursing practice.
- Apply the nursing process to the community as client.
- Discuss the interrelationship between the home health and community health nurse.

NURSE CONNECT

Additional online resources for this chapter can be found on the companion web site at www.prenhall.com/blais.

In the past decade there has been an observable increase in the delivery of nursing services in home and community settings. A number of factors have contributed to this trend, among them rising health care costs, an aging population, and a growing emphasis on managing chronic illness and stress, preventing illness, and enhancing the quality of life. Important concepts related to providing nursing care in the home and community include the following:

- The goals of home and community nursing practice are health promotion, disease prevention, health maintenance, and health restoration.
- Increasing access to preventive health services is a goal of *Healthy People 2010*. This goal can best be achieved by delivering services where people live, work, play, or attend school, in their homes and communities.
- For the home- and community-based nurse, nursing care generally focuses on the individual client and the persons who provide support for that client.
- Community-based nursing focuses on local, state, federal, and international health initiatives. For the community health nurse, there are three general types of clients: individuals, families, and groups. Groups may be communities, at-risk aggregates, or persons with similar problems and needs.
- Home health nursing practice and community-based nursing practice differ from nursing in acute-care settings in many ways. For example, home- and community-based nurses assume a higher degree of autonomy and independence.

CHALLENGES AND OPPORTUNITIES

One of the greatest challenges of the 21st century will be for nurses to continue to work within the health care system to provide safe and effective nursing care. Nurses will need to join community leaders in advocating for those in need. Anderson and McFarlane (2000, p. 6) describe the challenges as follows:

> If current trends are any indication, the peoples and nations of the 21st century will continue to face many of the same health-related problems that we struggle with today: poverty, hunger, unemployment, homelessness, illiteracy, racism, sexism, ageism, environmental deterioration, militarism, and human rights violations.

The opportunities for addressing these health problems will increase. Technology will provide opportunities for instant communication in the most remote areas of the world. New and effective partnerships with communities will be developed. Nurses will have the responsibility to be on the forefront of planning for the nation's health care future.

HOME HEALTH NURSING

Historically, nurses who provided direct services in the home were strong generalists who focused on long-term preventive, educational, remedial, and rehabilitative outcomes. Today, **home health** services center on individualized, episodic care with curative, short-term outcomes. Many home health care nurses are generalists or specialists possessing high-technology skills that were formerly used only in acute-care settings. For example, nurses provide a variety of intravenous therapies in the home setting and monitor clients who are dependent on technologically complex medical equipment, such as ventilators and central lines. These nurses collaborate with physicians and other health care professionals in providing care; usually, third-party payers pay for their services.

Home nursing care is one of the fastest growing sectors of the health care system. More than six million Americans currently receive care at home (Stackhouse, 1998). Several factors have contributed to the growth of home health care. These factors include (1) the increase in the older population, who are frequent recipients of home care; (2) third-party payers who favor home care to control costs; (3) the ability of agencies and institutions to successfully deliver high-technology services in the home; and (4) consumers who prefer to receive care in the home rather than an institution (Stulginsky, 1993a, p. 402).

By the year 2020, the growth rate of the population over 65 years of age will increase by 73% and will be more than twice the growth rate of the general population (Stackhouse, 1998).

Definitions of Home Nursing

The delivery of nursing services in the home has been called by a variety of terms, including home health nursing, home care nursing, and visiting nursing. Spradley and Allender (1996, p. 484) define home health care as "all the services and products provided to clients in their homes to maintain, restore, or promote their physical, mental, and emotional health." Stanhope and Lancaster (1996, p. 806) add that "home health care cannot simply be defined as 'care at home' but includes an arrangement of disease prevention, health promotion, and episodic illness–related services provided to people in their places of residence." This suggests that home health nursing services might be provided in long-term care facilities, residential hospices, residential shelters for abused women and children and the homeless, and adult congregate living facilities (ACLFs). According to the American Nurses Association (1992), home health nursing is a "synthesis of community health nursing and selected technical skills from other nursing specialties," including medical-surgical nursing, psychiatric-mental health nursing, gerontologic nursing, parent-child nursing, and community health nursing. The Department of Health and Human Services presented a more comprehensive definition of home health care in 1980 (Warhola, 1980). The USDHHS states that:

> home health care is that component of a continuum of comprehensive health care whereby health services are provided to individuals and families in their places of residence for the purposes of promoting, maintaining or restoring health, or of maximizing the level of independence while minimizing the effects of disability and illness, including terminal illness. Services appropriate to the needs of the individual patient and family are planned, coordinated, and made available by providers organized for the delivery of home care through the use of employed staff, contractual arrangements, or a combination of the two patterns.

Today, home health nurses work primarily with ill clients. However, home health nurses must also incorporate their knowledge of social, economic, and environmental influences on health when planning care. Although the primary focus is on the individual, the family must be considered. Home health nurses apply community health principles to the ill population. The American Nurses Association supports the view that home health is a subspecialty of community health nursing (Clark, 1999).

Perspectives of Home Health Nursing

Stulginsky (1993a, p. 404) interviewed home health care nurses who identified their practice as "meeting the acute and chronic care needs of patients and their families in the home environment." These nurses maintained that care centers on the client and that their role is to advocate for the client despite possible conflict in the opinions and needs of various care providers. Because the home is the family's territory, power and control issues in delivering nursing care differ from those in the institution. For example, entry into a home is granted, not assumed; the nurse must therefore establish trust and rapport with the client and family. Families also may feel more free to question advice, to ignore directions, to do things differently, and to set their own priorities and schedules.

Home health care nurses have identified significant advantages in caring for individuals and families in the home. The home setting is intimate; this intimacy fosters familiarity, sharing, connections, and caring between clients, families, and their nurse. Behaviors are more natural, cultural beliefs and practices are more visible, and multigenerational interactions tend to be displayed. Home health care nurses become realistic about what they can remedy and learn how to provide various supports and use creative interventions for what they cannot remedy (Stulginsky, 1993b, pp. 477–480).

Home health care nurses have also identified issues that negatively impact care in the home. More than any other care providers, these nurses have firsthand knowledge and experience about the burden of caregiving. In the interest of cutting health care costs, policy makers, third-party payers, and medical providers are placing increasingly complex responsibilities on clients' families and significant other(s). Caregiving demands may go on for months or years, placing the caregivers themselves (many of whom are older adults) at risk for physiologic and psychosocial problems. Additionally, nurses enter homes where the living conditions and support systems may be inadequate. When additional support or improved caregiving cannot be obtained for the client, home health care nurses face difficult decisions (Stulginsky, 1993a, p. 406).

Because home health care nurses must function independently in a variety of home settings and situations, employers generally prefer that the nurse be prepared at the baccalaureate level or above. In 1995, the American Nurses Credentialing Center approved a certification for clinical specialist in home health nursing. This certification requires a master's degree in nursing and recognizes the need for home health clinical specialists who can provide direct care, manage client care, and engage in consulting, education, administrative, and research activities ("ANCC approves," 1995, p. 11). As employment opportunities for registered nurses decrease in acute-care institutions, the growth of home health care is providing nurses with additional career choices and career opportunities.

Hospice nursing is often considered a subspecialty of home health nursing as hospice services are frequently delivered to terminally ill clients in their residence. See the box on page 308 for an interview of a hospice nurse.

The majority of reimbursement payments for home health services are from Medicare. This federally funded insurance covers services for those over age 65 and the disabled. Medicare eligibility criteria for home care services require the need for skilled nursing or physical, occupational, or speech therapy. The client

Hospice Nurse

Jace Martinson, RN, BSN, MSN

Why did you choose this practice setting? I worked in an intensive care unit in Alaska and found that I was very comfortable and effective in dealing with families before and after their loved one died. I also liked the flexible schedule and autonomy that hospice nursing offers.

What qualities do you think are necessary to be a nurse in this setting? The most important quality is compassion. Additionally, it is important to be truly empathetic and sympathetic but also therapeutic during interactions with families.

What has been your most gratifying moment as a nurse in this setting? Hospice nursing is the only job I ever had where I entered the client's home as a stranger and two hours later emerged as part of the family. I watched families come together, become prepared, and know what to expect before and after their family member's death.

What encouragement would you give a nurse considering practice in your setting? I would encourage nurses to be well aware of their feelings about death and their own mortality. I would tell them that the job is very satisfying, and that the client and family really do benefit from the service.

---

must be homebound and receive restorative care on an intermittent basis. In the past, agencies were reimbursed for each visit. Currently, reimbursement is changing to prospective pay, similar to acute-care reimbursement. This type of reimbursement may severely limit the number of visits a client receives for each diagnosis. Medicare also provides reimbursement for hospice care.

Medicaid is the largest source of reimbursement for home care services. This state-funded insurance is provided for medically indigent clients of all ages. Medicaid also provides for clients with chronic conditions needing custodial care. Through Medicaid, many frail, elderly clients can remain in their own homes with the services of a home health aide.

Private insurance, managed-care plans, worker's compensation insurance, and private pay are other methods of home care reimbursement. Free or sliding-scale fees are often provided by home care agencies such as the Visiting Nurse Association. (Stackhouse, 1998).

Applying the Nursing Process in the Home

The application of the nursing process is focused on the needs of individual clients and their caregivers. According to the American Nurses Credentialing Center (2000, p. 20), "the framework of home health practice is care management, which includes: the use of the nursing process to assess, diagnose, plan, and evaluate care; performing nursing interventions, including teaching; coordinating and using referrals and resources; providing and monitoring all levels of technical care; collaborating with other disciplines and providers; identifying clinical problems and using research knowledge; supervising ancillary personnel; and advocating for the client's right to self-determination."

ASSESSING Nurses must assess the health care needs of the client and family in the context of the home and community environment. The home health nurse obtains a health history from the client, reviews documents from the referral agency, examines the client, observes the client and caregiver relationship, and assesses the home and community environment. Parameters of assessment of the home environment include client and caregiver mobility, client ability to perform self-care, the cleanliness of the environment, the availability of caregiver support, safety, food preparation, financial supports, and emotional status of the client and caregiver.

DIAGNOSING In addition to nursing diagnoses specific to the client's health needs, nursing diagnoses related to the home environment may be identified. An example of a nursing diagnosis appropriate for home care is **impaired home maintenance management,** which is defined by Carpenito (1999) as the "state in which an individual or family experiences or is at risk to experience a difficulty in maintaining self or family in a home environment." Impaired home maintenance management may be related to a physical disability such as arthritis or neuromuscular degeneration, loss of support systems because of the death of a spouse, insufficient finances, impaired cognition, or fatigue.

PLANNING AND INTERVENTION Planning and intervention, done in collaboration with the client and caregivers, focuses on establishing a realistic plan for home health management, teaching the client and family the techniques of home care, and identifying appropriate resources to assist the client and family in maintaining self-sufficiency.

EVALUATING Evaluation can be done by the nurse on subsequent home visits by observing the same parameters assessed on the initial home visit. The nurse can also teach caregivers parameters of evaluation so that they can obtain professional intervention if needed.

Differences Between Home Health Nursing and Hospital Nursing

The role of the home care nurse is different than the role of the nurse in acute care. Stackhouse (1998) has identified some of the major considerations in home health nursing:

- The nurse works within the client's environment. The nurse is a guest in the client's home. In the hospital, there is often the feeling that the nurses and doctors own the hospital and the client is a guest.
- The need for clear and complete communication is essential as other health team members are usually not present with the nurse.
- Knowledge of reimbursement systems is essential. Clients must know what services are available, because most people do not pay directly for services.

- The home health nurse works alone. The hospital nurse is surrounded by other colleagues, whereas the home health nurse has only a telephone.
- The nurse in the hospital setting has a large variety of supplies and equipment. The home health nurse often must create or adapt equipment to fit the home.
- Knowledge of community resources is important. Community resources can often bring a great deal of improvement to the client's quality of life. Home health nurses should have a resource file to share with the client and the client's family.

Consider . . .

- the differences in professional autonomy between the home health care nurse and the hospital nurse. What are the legal and ethical implications of the independence experienced by the home health care nurse?
- the different roles of the professional nurse. What differences might there be in the practice of the nurse's professional roles between the home health care nurse and the hospital nurse?
- how the availability of computer technology assists the home health care nurse in providing and documenting better nursing care.

COMMUNITY-BASED NURSING

The goal of many public and private efforts is to develop and maintain healthy communities. Characteristics of a healthy community are described in the accompanying box. Nursing, as a caring profession,

---

Ten Characteristics of a Healthy Community

A HEALTHY COMMUNITY:

- Is one in which members have a high degree of awareness that "we are a community."
- Uses its natural resources while taking steps to conserve them for future generations.
- Openly recognizes the existence of subgroups and welcomes their participation in community affairs.
- Is prepared to meet crises.
- Is a problem-solving community; it identifies, analyzes, and organizes to meet its own needs.

- Possesses open channels of communication that allow information to flow among all subgroups of citizens in all directions.
- Seeks to make each of its systems' resources available to all members.
- Has legitimate and effective ways to settle disputes that arise within the community.
- Encourages maximum citizen participation in decision making.
- Promotes a high level of wellness among all its members.

Source: Adapted from *Community Health Nursing: Concepts and Practice,* 4th ed. by B. W. Spradley and J. A. Allender, Philadelphia: Lippincott, 1996, p. 206.

exists because individuals, families, and groups (and, therefore, communities) are not always healthy or self-sufficient. The focus in community nursing is the *community*: it is a practice that is comprehensive and continuous, takes place in a wide variety of settings, is directed toward all age groups, and commands the utilization of all professional nursing roles. Although definitions of community health nursing by the American Nurses Association; the American Public Health Association Public Health Nursing Section; and the 1990 Task Force on Community Health Nursing Education, Association of Community Health Nursing Educators define community health differently, they all agree that community health nurses focus on nursing service to the population as a whole. Through providing care for individuals, families, and groups, the health of the community is enhanced (Hitchcock, Schubert, and Thomas, 1999).

The **community health nurse specialist** is prepared in graduate nursing programs at universities and colleges. These programs usually prepare the nurse for leadership and coordinating functions in the community. The many roles of the community health nurse can include care provider, client advocate, consultant, coordinator, manager, educator, collaborator, and researcher. See the accompanying interview box for a community health nurse specialist's description of her practice.

Definitions of Community and Community-Based Nursing

To understand community-based nursing one must first define the word community and other terms associated with community health. A **community** is a collection of people who share some attribute of their lives. It may be that they live in the same locale, attend a specific church, or even share a particular interest, such as painting. Groups that constitute a community because of common member interests are often referred to as a *community of interest* (e.g., religious and ethnic groups). A community can also be defined as a *social system* in which the members interact formally or informally and form networks that operate for the benefit of all people in the community. Five of the functions of the community are described in the box on page 311. In community health, the community may be viewed as having a common health problem, for example, populations where there is a high incidence of infant mortality or communicable disease, such as tuberculosis or HIV infection.

Community-based nursing is the "synthesis of nursing and public health practice. Community health nurses use the knowledge and skills of professional nursing and the philosophy, content, and methods of public health when delivering services in the commu-

Community Health Nurse

Mary Jorda, ARNP, BSN, MPH

Why did you choose this practice setting? After a year of working in a poor public hospital in Honduras (when I was in the Peace Corps), I noticed that the same patients were returning frequently with the same problems. I began to think that a more effective solution would be to provide education and health promotion in the community.

What qualities do you think are necessary to be a nurse in this setting? Working in the community requires patience, persistence, understanding, and flexibility. The clients set the agenda and priorities; we as health care workers are "guests" in assisting communities to realize their goals in improving health.

What has been your most gratifying moment as a nurse in this setting? While I was working in a refugee camp in Honduras, we transported a young girl who was very ill to a makeshift hospital. She was diagnosed with typhoid fever and started on IV antibiotics. The next morning I found her back in her hut. Her brother reported that "spirits" had entered her body through the IV. I realized that she had been delirious, but her family would not return her to the hospital. I conferred with the family and neighbors and we developed a plan to care for the girl in the camp. I administered antibiotics and bathed her, and her family gave her fluids. Some neighbors prayed; others boiled water. I also provided continuing education in the camp on the transmission of the disease. She survived. It was gratifying to see her well again and to realize the important role the family and community played in recovery.

What encouragement would you give a nurse considering practice in your setting? If you believe in preventing health problems before they arise, then community health nursing is the place to be.

Five Functions of a Community

1. *Production, distribution, and consumption of goods and services.* These are the means by which the community provides for the economic needs of its members. This function includes not only the supplying of food and clothing but also the provision of water, electricity, police and fire protection, and the disposal of refuse.

2. *Socialization.* Socialization refers to the process of transmitting values, knowledge, culture, and skills to others. Communities usually contain a number of established institutions for socialization: families, churches, schools, media, voluntary and social organizations, and so on.

3. *Social control.* **Social control** refers to the way in which order is maintained in a community. Laws are enforced by the police; public health regulations are implemented to protect people from certain diseases. Social control is also exerted through the family, church, and schools.

4. *Social interparticipation.* **Social interparticipation** refers to community activities that are designed to meet people's needs for companionship. Families and churches have traditionally met this need; however, many public and private organizations also serve this function.

5. *Mutual support.* **Mutual support** refers to the ability to provide resources at a time of illness or disaster. Although the family is usually relied on to fulfill this function, health and social services may be necessary to augment the family's assistance if help is required over an extended period.

nity" (Clemen-Stone, McGuire, and Eigsti, 1998, p. 32). The major goal of the community health nurse is to provide primary health care as defined by the World Health Organization. Zotti, Brown, and Stotts (1996, p. 212) describe the four major assumptions of this philosophy as follows:

■ Health is a political and social right. Equity is fundamental and universal coverage is the norm, with care provided according to need.

■ The community as a whole, rather than the individual, is the client, and the community determines its greatest priority and resources allocation in health care. Thus the overall public good is promoted, but needs of individuals may go unmet.

■ Because conditions in many sectors of communities affect health, multisectoral cooperation is necessary to promote, maintain, or improve the health of the community.

■ The philosophy of primary health care can be applied to any country or community.

The U.S. Department of Health and Human Services has identified *Healthy People 2010* as the prevention agenda for the nation. This statement of national health objectives is designed to identify significant preventable threats to health and the establishment of goals to reduce these threats. Nurses in the home and community will have increasing responsibilities in assisting individuals, families, and groups in meeting these goals. See the accompanying box for the leading health indicators for *Healthy People 2010*.

Leading Health Indicators for *Healthy People 2010*

- Physical activity
- Overweight or obese
- Tobacco use
- Substance abuse
- Responsible sexual behavior
- Mental health
- Injury and violence
- Environmental quality
- Immunization
- Access to health care

Keller et al. (1998) identified 17 interventions taken by public health nurses on behalf of communities, systems, individuals, or families in an effort to improve or protect their health status. See the accompanying box.

Elements of Community-Based Nursing Practice

There are six basic elements of community-based practice: (1) promotion of healthful living, (2) prevention of health problems, (3) remedial care for health problems, (4) rehabilitation, (5) evaluation, and (6) research (Spradley and Allender, 1996, p. 13).

Promotion of Healthful Living

The promotion of the health of individuals and groups has long been recognized as an important aspect of community health nursing. Health-promotion programs are provided to raise the levels of wellness of individuals, families, groups, and the entire community.

At the individual level, programs may include smoking cessation, reduction of alcohol and drug abuse, exercise and fitness, and stress management. At the family level, preventive health services such as family planning, pregnancy and infant care, immunizations, and information about sexually transmitted diseases may be offered. At the group level, occupational safety and health and accidental injury may be considered. At the community level, toxic agent control, fluoridation of water supplies, and infectious agent control are of significance.

Prevention of Health Problems

Health-protection activities are highly varied. They may include the prevention of nutritional deficiency, accidents at work and at home, communicable diseases, cardiovascular disease, lung cancer, child abuse, poisoning, pollution, and so on. Three levels of prevention were first discussed by Leavell and Clark in the 1950s. Their concept was based on public health concepts.

Public Health Interventions

- *Surveillance* is the ongoing and systematic collection, analysis, and interpretation of health data for the purpose of planning, implementation, and evaluation.
- *Disease investigation* is the process of gathering and analyzing data regarding threats to the health of populations.
- *Outreach* is the process of locating populations of interest or at risk in order to provide information.
- *Screening* is the process of identifying individuals with unrecognized or asymptomatic health conditions.
- *Case-finding* locates individuals and families with identified risk factors.
- *Referral and follow-up* assist individuals, families, and groups to obtain resources.
- *Case management* is the process of coordinating services for optimal use.
- *Delegated functions* are those direct-care tasks that the RN carries out or delegates under the nurse practice act.
- *Health teaching* is the communication of facts, ideas, and skills in order to change knowledge, behavior, attitudes, values, and practices of others.

- *Counseling* is the engaging of the family, individual, or group at an emotional level in order to establish an interpersonal relationship.
- *Consultation* is interactive problem solving through the community system, family, or individual.
- *Collaboration* is two or more persons working together to achieve a goal.
- *Coalition building* is the process of promoting and developing alliances and linkages with organizations and constituencies to solve problems or provide for a common goal.
- *Community organizing* is the working together of groups to identify and solve common problems.
- *Advocacy* is acting on behalf of oneself or another to plead a cause.
- *Social marketing* uses marketing principles and technology to influence the behaviors, attitudes, knowledge, values, and practices of a population.
- *Policy development* is the placement of issues on a decision-maker's agenda.

Source: L. O. Keller, S. Stohschein, B. Kia-Hoagberg, and M. Schaffer. "Population-based Public Health Nursing Interventions: A Model from Practice." *Public Health Nursing* **115**(3): 207–215, 1998.

Primary prevention is action taken prior to the occurrence of health problems. Teaching clients to select a well-balanced diet or develop a stress-management program are examples of primary prevention. **Secondary prevention** focuses on the early identification and treatment of existing health problems. Yearly mammograms or glaucoma testing are examples of secondary prevention programs. The goal of **tertiary prevention** is to return the client to optimal level of health while preventing further deterioration. Assisting the diabetic client by teaching proper nutrition and foot care is an example of tertiary prevention (Clark, 1999).

Remedial Care for Health Problems

Community health care nurses provide direct and indirect services to individuals with chronic health problems. A variety of health care services provide **direct services,** such as home visits for the assessment and monitoring of health problems, dietary planning, administration of injections, personal care, homemaking services, and information about equipment resources (e.g., bath seats, wheelchairs, canes, walkers, syringes, dressing materials, and so on). **Indirect services** focus on assisting people with health problems to obtain treatment. For example, a community health nurse may assist a person to get a physician's appointment after eliciting data about an elevated blood pressure, a persistent cough, or vaginal bleeding. In other instances, the nurse may refer an individual or family to other agencies that provide information and/or therapy such as (1) a family therapy and counseling program, (2) a self-help group or association, or (3) a chemical dependency counseling and treatment center.

On a community level, individual community members and health workers may lobby for the development of programs to remedy unhealthy situations or to initiate services that are lacking. Examples of unhealthy situations are an inadequate school lunch program, inhumane conditions in a nursing home, and excessive pollution of water supplies from industrial wastes. Examples of new initiatives are increased shelters for abused women, low-cost housing for the elderly, the establishment of nursing services on the streets, and provision of health care to the homeless.

Rehabilitation

Rehabilitation services that focus on reducing disability and/or restoring function are provided at the individual, family, and community level. At the individual level, a community health nurse in conjunction with other health professionals (e.g., physical and occupational therapists) may assist physically disabled persons (e.g., those with cerebrovascular accidents, heart conditions, amputations, or paralysis) regain some degree of lost function, prevent further disability, and develop new skills that enable them to assume an appropriate vocation or degree of independence. Many rehabilitative community groups are available to assist families and individuals with chronic health problems. Examples are colostomy clubs, postmastectomy groups, halfway houses for the discharged mentally ill, and Alcoholics Anonymous. The community health nurse can be instrumental in informing clients of available services.

Evaluation

Ongoing evaluation of health and health care services at the individual, national, and international levels is an essential component of community health practices. Its aim is to (1) determine the effectiveness of current activities, (2) determine needs, and (3) develop improved services. For example, evaluation of services available for rape victims may reveal a need for more comprehensive counseling programs.

Research

Research, a critical component of community health care practice, provides the means to identify problems and examine improved methods of providing health services. Research occurs at all levels—from federal agencies such as the U.S. Public Health Service to state and municipal groups. Researchers may investigate (1) patterns of illness and health, (2) possible causes and means of preventing specific problems such as child abuse, suicide, homicide, trauma, and substance abuse, (3) deficiencies in services such as day-care centers or services for the elderly, (4) the effectiveness of treatment programs such as weight reduction, stress management, or substance abuse programs, (5) the effect of societal and environmental changes on existing services, and (6) utilization of existing health services.

Settings for Community-Based Nursing Practice

Community-based nursing is practiced in diverse settings, including community centers, schools, and the workplace, among others.

Community Centers

Community-based nurses utilize a variety of community sites for practice. In community centers, the client is usually a group of individuals with common needs or interests. Nurses may provide health-related education and influenza immunizations for older adults in an adult day-care center, offer blood pressure screenings and nutritional counseling at a community health fair, lead a discussion in stress management at a local church, and teach cardiopulmonary resuscitation (CPR) in a school. Community-based nurses also staff stationary or mobile clinics that provide primary care and health screening services for the medically indigent or disadvantaged. Using clinics increases nurse efficiency and decreases nurse travel time. Community health nurses may also collaborate with other community professionals, such as environmental health professionals who regulate day-care facilities. This collaboration provides opportunities for the nurse to educate day-care staff on managing ill children, identifying children who are neglected or abused, preventing injuries, and promoting normal growth and development (Stanhope and Lancaster, 1996, p. 614).

Schools

Community schools reflect the society they are part of. Today, school systems are encountering increasingly complex health-related morbidities in children, such as substance abuse and pregnancies; dealing with major environmental risks, such as violence and poverty; and accommodating children with significant physical and psychosocial impairments. The core components of a **school health** program are health services, health education, and a healthy environment (Stanhope and Lancaster, 1996, p. 884). Nursing services are an integral part of the school health program. School nurses provide direct care in school clinics, manage immunization programs, provide health education in classrooms, offer health-related expertise during student conferences, coordinate student health services, promote safety, and advocate for student health programs at the local and state level. Although the health needs of today's children have increased, many school systems have cut support for school health programs in order to cut costs. Other school systems recognize that providing health services today is an investment in children's future, and they directly or indirectly support health services at school sites by, for example, maintaining primary care clinics. Nurses who wish to pursue a specialty and certification in school nursing will find a variety of graduate programs that provide advanced degrees in this field. See the interview box on page 315, in which a school nurse describes her role.

Research Box

Kelly, C. S., Morrow, A. L., Shults, J., Nakas, N., Strope, G. L., and Adelman, R. D. 2000. Outcomes evaluation of a comprehensive intervention program for asthmatic children enrolled in Medicaid. *Pediatrics* 105(5): 1029–1035.

The purpose of this study was to evaluate health care and financial outcomes in a population of Medicaid-insured asthmatic children after a comprehensive asthma intervention program. The subjects were eight children 2 to 16 years old with a history of frequent use of emergent health care services for asthma in a pediatric allergy clinic. Children in the intervention group received asthma education and medical treatment in the setting of a tertiary care pediatric allergy clinic. An asthma outreach nurse maintained monthly contact with the families enrolled in the intervention group. Baseline demographics did not differ significantly between the two groups. In the year before the study there were no significant differences between intervention and control children in emergency department visits (mean = 3.5 per patient), hospitalizations (mean = 0.6 per patient), or health care charges (mean = $2969 per patient). During the study year, emergency department visits decreased to a mean of 1.7 per patient in the intervention group and 2.4 in the control group, whereas hospitalizations decreased to a mean of 0.2 per patient in the intervention group and 0.5 in the control group. Asthma health care charges decreased by a mean of $721 per child per year in the intervention group and by a mean of $178 per child per year in the control group.

The conclusion is that a comprehensive asthma intervention program for Medicaid-insured asthmatic children can significantly improve health outcomes while reducing health care costs, decreasing emergency department visits, and decreasing hospitalizations.

Faith Communities

Parish nursing is practiced in faith communities, such as churches, synagogues, temples, and other places of worship. According to Stanhope and Lancaster (1996), parish nursing began in the United States in

School Nurse

Nancy Humbert, ARNP, MSN

Why did you choose this practice setting? I chose school health in order to participate in holistic, family-centered, and multidisciplinary nursing practice.

What qualities do you think are necessary to be a nurse in this setting? To function effectively in a school health setting, a nurse must have clinical expertise in public health and pediatrics. The school health nurse must be flexible, patient, creative, and culturally competent.

What has been your most gratifying moment as a nurse in

this setting? My most gratifying moment as a school health nurse was when I helped empower an adolescent to overcome a severe case of bulimia.

What encouragement would you give a nurse considering practice in your setting? I would encourage any nurse to consider the school health practice setting after first developing strong basic nursing skills. School health is by far the most rewarding and challenging setting I've ever encountered. One must love change, challenge, and children.

---

the late 1960s when churches used nurses to provide health care to their congregations. Parish nurses are defined by the American Nurses Association (1998, p. 7) as registered nurses "who serve as members of the ministry staff of a faith community to promote health as wholeness of the faith community, its family and individual members, and the community it serves." The International Parish Nurse Resource Center (2001) describes the role of the parish nurse as one that balances "knowledge and skill, the sciences, theology, and humanities; service and worship; and nursing care with pastoral care functions." Ryan (1997, p. 4) states that the "intent of parish nursing is to create the environment within which the parish nurse, patient, family, and congregation can interact, understand, and care for one another in light of their relationships to God, themselves, each other, the congregation, and the community around them." Parish nursing is nondenominational and includes nurses of all religious faiths. Parish nurses are found in nations around the world, including Canada and Jamaica.

Occupational Health

Occupational health nurses consider an organization's needs as well as workers' needs (Stanhope and Lancaster, 1996, p. 908). The primary functions of the occupational nurse are to provide emergency treatment and promote worker health and safety; however, rapid changes in technology, the health care system, and societal expectations have expanded the nurse's role and made it increasingly complex. Occupational health nurses may now develop and carry out health promotion, health maintenance, and risk-management programs and consult with their employers in reducing health-related costs. They may offer direct care to employees, manage program evaluation, and analyze work-related injuries and illnesses. In companies where management positions have been pared, the occupational health nurse may assume expanded responsibilities in job analysis, safety, and benefits management. Specialization in the field is often a requirement for additional responsibilities. Nurses who wish to pursue specialization and certification in occupational health will find a number of graduate programs that offer advanced education in this field. See the interview box on page 316, in which an occupational health nurse describes her practice.

Consider . . .

- organizations within your community where health care is currently delivered or where health and nursing services could be delivered. What are the advantages to delivering health care in these various settings?
- whether nursing and health services are better provided to the traditionally underserved (e.g., the poor, older adults, minorities) by providing that care in the community and in the home.
- which nursing services can be effectively delivered in the home and community. Are there any nursing services that can be delivered only in the hospital? If yes, which services and why? Are there nursing services that are more effectively delivered in the home or community? If yes, which services and why?

Occupational Health Nurse

Ethel Oatman, RN, BSN, MS

Why did you choose this practice setting? I found that I enjoyed working with adults in an ambulatory setting. There is so much to offer in the field of occupational health. The workplace is a natural environment for building a rapport with employees. Even though there is treatment of injuries and illnesses, much more can be done through employee health education, especially in the areas of health promotion and disease and injury prevention.

What qualities do you think are necessary to be a nurse in this setting? It is helpful to have medical-surgical and emergency nursing skills and be able to work independently. To be credible and effective, occupational health nurses must possess skills and knowledge in the areas of workers' compensation, health education, counseling,

and human relations. Good verbal and written skills are also required.

What has been your most gratifying moment as a nurse in this setting? The focus of many of our clinics is on prevention and early detection of disease. I was coordinating a skin cancer clinic and three malignant melanomas were found. Since all of the melanomas were in the early, treatable stage, I feel I saved three lives that day.

What encouragement would you give a nurse considering practice in your setting? In order to stay in business, companies must address health cost containment, usually through managed care. Occupational health nurses have opportunities to assume leadership roles in ensuring high-quality, appropriate health care while remaining a client advocate.

APPLYING THE NURSING PROCESS IN THE COMMUNITY

Assessing

Nurses assess community health by using epidemiologic studies and by using an established community assessment framework or tool.

Epidemiologic Studies

"**Epidemiology** is the study of the distribution of states of health and of the causes of deviations from health in populations and the application of this study to control the health problems" (Stanhope and Lancaster, 1996, p. 1090). Epidemiologic studies provide health professionals with information about the health and illness patterns of a specified population, the people involved, and any causal factors. Most health problems are currently thought to be the result of multiple causes. That is, a multiplicity of factors interact to result in coronary heart disease or teenage pregnancy, for example.

Epidemiologists use three types of studies: analytic, descriptive, and experimental. In *analytic studies,* the epidemiologist uses prospective (forward-looking) and retrospective (backward-looking) and/or experimental studies to test hypotheses about health and illness. In a *prospective study,* the epidemiologist determines the variables and the investigation method and

establishes possible hypotheses. Data are then collected to see whether the hypothesis is supported. For example, a nurse may establish a hypothesis about the relation of dietary habits to weight, then follow a group of people, collecting data regarding their diet. In a *retrospective study* the investigator goes back over existing records to collect data that may or may not support a hypothesis. For example, when studying weight loss patterns among a group of people, a nurse might refer to records about the activity and diet of these people.

Descriptive studies rely primarily on existing data. The epidemiologist describes the people most likely to be affected by a disease, the geographic region in which it will occur, when it will occur, and its overall effect.

Experimental studies are often conducted to determine the effectiveness of a particular therapeutic modality. Subjects are assigned to one of two groups: the experimental group or the control group. People in the experimental group are, for example, exposed to a condition thought to improve health, to prevent disease, or to influence a person's health status in some manner, such as walking for a half hour each day. The members of the matched control group are not exposed to the experimental condition. Any subsequent differences in the health patterns between the two groups are then attributed to the manipulated factor.

Two types of rates are commonly used when describing health patterns in a population: the incidence rate and the prevalence rate. The **incidence rate** reflects the number of people with a particular health problem or characteristic over a given unit of time, such as a year.

The **prevalence rate** describes a situation at a given point in time. For example, if 63 students in a school have chickenpox, the number of students who have the disease is divided by the number of students in the school.

Community Assessment Framework

There are many sources for obtaining data for community assessment (see the accompanying box). Stewart (1985) proposes a general systems theory as a framework for community assessment. She identifies nine subsystems of the community for analysis: health, communication, economy, education, law, politics, recreation, religion, and social life. See Table 19–1 for details about assessment data for these subsystems.

Assessment of the **health subsystem** of a community includes collecting data about population size, rate of growth, density, and composition; life expectancy; overall health status of individuals; health care facilities and services and accessibility to the facilities; and quantity and types of caseloads of health professionals. The **communication subsystem** is an important part of the health of a community since a community relies on the abilities of individuals and groups to exchange ideas and feelings and work toward common goals. The **economic subsystem** or economic status of the community significantly affects the physical and emotional health of its citizens. Successful industries and high income and employment levels provide financial support for health, education, and recreational services. The **education subsystem** promotes intellectual development and socialization of the community's youth. Communities that expend a great deal of energy on educational, social, and cultural activities achieve a higher level of development than those whose energies are directed toward law enforcement and economic concerns (Hanchett, 1979). The **law subsystem** ensures social order and the safety of a community and thus preserves the emotional and physical security of its members. In regard to the **political subsystem,** "political jurisdictions identify the formal boundaries of many of a community's subsystems such as school, health, and police districts" (Stewart, 1985, p. 371). Local and other governments carry specific responsibilities for all community subsystem services that directly and indirectly affect the health of a community. The **recreational subsystem** provides facilities and activities that are essential for the physical, emotional, and social health of individuals and families. The **subsystem of religion** functions to promote the spiritual health of citizens. It is often a pervading force in providing support to individuals and families

Sources of Community Assessment Data

- City maps to locate community boundaries, roads, churches, schools, parks, hospitals, and so on.
- State or provincial census data for population composition and characteristics.
- Chamber of Commerce for employment statistics, major industries, and primary occupations.
- Municipal, state, or provincial health departments for location of health facilities, occupational health programs, numbers of health professionals, numbers of welfare recipients, and so on.
- City or regional health planning boards for health needs and practices.
- Telephone book for location of social, recreational, and health organizations, committees, and facilities.
- Public and university libraries for district social and cultural research reports.

- Health facility administrators for information about employee caseloads, prevalent types of problems, and dominant needs.
- Recreational directors for programs provided and participation levels.
- Police department for incidence of crime, vandalism, and drug addiction.
- Teachers and school nurses for incidence of children's health problems and information on facilities and services to maintain and promote health.
- Local newspapers for community activities related to health and wellness, such as health lectures or health fairs.
- Online computer services that may provide access to public documents related to community health.

Table 19–1 Systems Framework for Community Assessment

System	Assessment Data	Rationale
Health	Size	Size influences the number and size of health care agencies.
	Rate of growth or decline	Rapid growth may place excessive demands on health care services.
	Density	Density affects the availability of health care services.
	Composition	Composition may identify the types of health care needs.
	Life expectancy	Life expectancy indicates the need for services for the aged or the physically and mentally incapacitated.
	Health status, including nutritional status	This reflects the overall physical, emotional, and social health of the members of the community.
	Health care facilities and services, including resource allocation and utilization, health programs, and age groups served	These indicate the degree to which the health needs of the community are being met.
	Geographic, economic, and cultural accessibility to health care services	Accessibility to health care services is considered a basic right by many people regardless of economic status, ethnic origin, or geographic location.
	Consumer participation in health care programs	Consumer participation reflects people's interest in and values about health maintenance and promotion.
	Number, type, and routine caseloads of health professionals (e.g., community health nurses, nutritionists, dental hygienists, family physicians and specialists, public health inspectors)	Caseload numbers and types indicate physical and emotional health problems prevalent in the community.
	Sources of health knowledge	This identifies information about agencies and available services for consumers.
	Levels of immunization among children	This information reflects the citizens' knowledge and values about disease prevention.
	Ambulance services	The availability of emergency services indicates the ability of the community to respond to life-threatening situations.
	Sanitation services	Quality sanitation services prevent disease.
	Opinions about community health services	Satisfaction with current services and proposed improvements can be determined.
	Environmental conditions of air, water, and soil	The state of the environment can affect physical and emotional health.
Communication	Existence and frequency of public forums	Public forums enable inputs or feedback to the system, thus enhancing satisfaction with and survival of the system.

Table 19–1 Systems Framework for Community Assessment (Cont.)

System	Assessment Data	Rationale
	Telephone services	Telephones promote communication among members and ability to contact health services.
	Newspapers and television	Newspapers and television provide an ongoing flow of information about community activities and health care.
	Transportation and road networks	Transportation influences access to health care facilities and programs, as well as to recreational and educational facilities that indirectly affect health.
Economy	Industries and occupations	A strong industrial base in a community provides financial support for health, education, and recreational facilities.
	Number or percentage of population employed or attending school	Social health problems such as stress, depression, drug abuse, and crime are frequently widespread where there are economic problems such as high unemployment.
	Income levels and quality and types of housing (private dwellings, apartments, mobile homes, and so on)	Overcrowded and poor-quality dwellings may affect the health of residents.
	Occupational health programs	The presence of occupational health programs can help workers maintain health and prevent accidents.
Education/schools	School health facilities, services, and personnel	Quality health facilities and services can provide information and assistance to maintain and promote health.
	Existence of nutritious lunch programs, extracurricular sports activities, libraries, and counseling services	These services contribute to children's physical, emotional, and social health.
	Number and types of health problems handled by the school nurse	The number and types of problems reflect individual and family health problems in the community.
	Adjunctive services (e.g., resource teachers, community volunteers) for individuals with physical and mental disabilities	Available services and resources for the disabled indicate the attitudes of the community toward these citizens.
	Type of continuing education or evening extension classes provided	Continuing education programs can affect the development of a community, the literacy of its adults, and its overall health values.
	Parent-teacher associations and the extent of parental involvement in the schools	Maximum parental involvement in the schools can indicate minimal individual and family health problems such as school dropouts, teenage pregnancies, drug abuse, vandalism, etc.
Law	Caseloads of police force and lawyers	These caseloads identify the social problems of a community (e.g., child abuse, vandalism, drug addiction, alcoholism, juvenile crime, etc.). Such problems reflect the social order of the community, the safety of the citizens, and the need for special programs such as youth recreation, arts and crafts for older adults, and child abuse programs.

Table 19–1 Systems Framework for Community Assessment (Cont.)

System	Assessment Data	Rationale
Politics	Responsibilities of local and other governments and community councils for all community subsystem services (e.g., health and welfare councils, housing authorities, transportation authorities, sanitation authorities)	Formal political channels and authority to direct use of the health care dollar are reflected in government responsibilities.
	Political leaders or other influential people in community affairs	This helps the nurse determine and recognize the power framework and perhaps leaders' issues of concern.
	Election issues and average election turnout	Election turnouts can indicate the degree of citizen involvement, community cohesiveness, and desire to influence change.
Recreation	Location of *inexpensive* recreational services for all age groups, including use of schools and other vacant buildings	Recreational activities provide physical and emotional outlets and intellectual stimulation that promote and maintain health.
	Number of playgrounds, pools, sports fields, and parks and utilization of them	Existence and use of recreational facilities indicates the community system's goals and values about them.
	Participation levels in fitness programs	Low participation levels may indicate the need to provide inexpensive programs for certain age groups, such as senior citizens.
	Number of family-centered programs	Family-centered programs assist in the maintenance of family health and cohesiveness.
	Persons responsible for developing and maintaining playgrounds and parks	Knowledge of those responsible for playgrounds and parks helps the citizens provide direct input about any problems.
Religion	Number and types of churches and religious programs	Church members provide support to individuals and families, particularly in times of crisis.
	Level of participation in various church programs	Church programs help people grow spiritually and morally, both of which are important influencing factors in the development and maintenance of a healthy self-concept.
Social life	Predominant social classes, racial and ethnic makeup, language, values, and childrearing practices	The community's classes, cultures, and values affect its health and its ability to make use of input from the environment.
	Number and type of social committees, organizations, and clubs, and kinds of services offered	These groups promote cohesiveness of the system's citizens. Such groups, whether formal government agencies or informal friendship groups, often provide financial assistance, emotional support, counseling, and rehabilitation services to the handicapped and to senior citizens.
	Number of persons who belong to social groups and participate in volunteer activities	The level of participation and numbers of volunteers are indicators of community health.

Source: Modified from "Community and Aggregates: Systematic Community Health Assessment" by M. Stewart, J. Innes, S. Searl, and C. Smillie, *Community Health Nursing in Canada,* Toronto, Ontario: Gage Educational Publishing, 1985, pp. 363–377.

in times of crisis. **Social life** as a subsystem consists of all the social, economic, and ethnic classes of people in the community and the social clubs and organizations that function to promote cohesiveness of all members of the community.

Diagnosing

After assessing, validating, and summarizing data, the nurse identifies nursing diagnoses for the community. NANDA diagnoses have largely focused on individual and family responses. McCloskey and Bulechek (1996, p. 704) identify three community-focused NANDA nursing diagnoses:

- **Ineffective community coping:** a pattern of community activities for adaptation and problem solving that is unsatisfactory for meeting the demands or needs of the community (p. 618).
- **Potential for enhanced community coping:** a pattern of community activities for adaptation and problem solving that is satisfactory for meeting the demands or needs of the community but can be improved for management of current and future problems/stressors (p. 619).
- **Ineffective community management of therapeutic regimen:** a pattern of regulating and integrating into the community processes programs for treatment of illness and the sequelae of illness that are unsatisfactory for meeting health-related goals (p. 619).

Planning and Implementing

Planning community health may be oriented toward improved crisis management, disease prevention, health maintenance, or health promotion. The responsibility for planning at the community level is usually broadly based. The exact resources and skills of members of the community will often depend on the size of the community. A broadly based planning group is most likely to create a plan that is acceptable to members of the community. Also, people who are involved in planning become educated about the problems, the resources, and the interrelationships within the system relative to health and problems.

When setting priorities, health planners must work with consumers, interest groups, or other involved persons to prioritize health problems. The priority areas established in *Healthy People 2010* can be used as a guide in this stage (USDHHS, 2000). It is important to take into consideration the values and interests of community members, the severity of the problems, and the resources available in order to identify and act on the problems. Because any plan will

probably result in change, members of the planning group should be cognizant of and employ planned change theory. (See Chapter 14, "Change Process.")

Establishing goals also requires consumer participation. The goals should reflect a desirable state—for example, to reduce infant mortality by 15%. National statistics and/or *Healthy People 2010* goals may be helpful in keeping goals realistic. Among the many other factors that must be considered are the traditions of people in the community, vested interests, current organizations, and resources, all of which may be barriers to change. An example of a goal of a community would be to reduce the incidence of infectious disease in a school.

Outcome criteria or objectives are specific, measurable targets. An example of such an objective is an increase in immunization levels by 20%, to be achieved by September 2003.

Implementing nursing strategies in community health is generally a collaborative action. Nurses are also frequently catalysts and facilitators in implementation of plans. The primary goal in community health nursing is to help people help themselves.

McCloskey and Bulechek (1996), through the Nursing Intervention Classification (NIC) Project, describe three specific interventions appropriate to the management of community health problems: **environmental management, community health policy monitoring,** and **health education.** In implementing health education (NIC 5510) as an intervention, the nurse "develops and provides instruction and learning experiences to facilitate voluntary adaptation of behavior conducive to health in individuals, families, groups, or communities." See Chapter 8, "The Nurse as Learner and Teacher," for more information about the nurse as a health educator. In promoting community environmental management (NIC 6486), the nurse "monitors and influences the physical, social, cultural, economic, and political conditions that affect the health of groups and communities" through the following activities (McCloskey and Bulechek, 1996, p. 258):

- Initiating screening for health risks from the environment
- Participating in multidisciplinary teams to identify threats to safety in the community
- Monitoring the status of known health risks
- Participating in community programs to deal with known risks
- Collaborating in the development of community action programs
- Promoting governmental policy to reduce specified risks

- Encouraging neighborhoods to become active participants in community safety
- Coordinating services to at-risk groups and communities
- Conducting educational programs for targeted risk groups
- Working with environmental groups to secure appropriate governmental regulations

McCloskey and Bulechek also describe the nurse's role in political advocacy in the nursing intervention health policy monitoring (NIC 7970), which is defined as the "surveillance and influence of government and organization regulations, rules, and standards that affect nursing systems and practices to ensure quality care of patients." The nurse does this by carrying out the following activities (McCloskey and Bulechek, 1996, p. 310):

- Reviewing proposed policies and standards in organizational, professional, and governmental literature, and in the popular media
- Assessing implications and requirements of proposed policies and standards for quality client care
- Comparing requirements of policies and standards with current practices
- Assessing negative and positive effects of health policies and standards on nursing practice, client, and cost outcomes
- Identifying and resolving discrepancies between health policies and standards and current nursing practice
- Acquainting policy makers with implications of current and proposed policies and standards for client welfare
- Lobbying policy makers to make changes in health policies and standards to benefit clients
- Testifying in organizational, professional, and public forums to influence the formulation of health policies and standards that benefit clients
- Assisting consumers of health care to be informed of current and proposed changes in health policies and standards and the implications for health outcomes

Evaluating

In community health, evaluation determines whether the planned interventions have led to the achievement of the established goals and objectives; for example, was the immunization rate of preschool children improved. Because community health is usually a collaborative process between health providers, including nurses, community leaders, politicians, and consumers, all may be involved in the evaluation process. Often the community health nurse is the agent of evaluation in collecting evaluation data that determines the effectiveness of implemented programs. Evaluation data may include community statistics related to changes in disease incidence rates, mortality and morbidity rates, the costs to provide programs and the availability of required financial and other resources, and citizen program utilization and satisfaction rates. Leaders must decide whether the benefits of a program merit the costs in money, time, and other resources. Based on such evaluation, effective programs may be continued, ineffective programs may be discontinued, existing programs may be modified, or new programs might be implemented.

Consider . . .

- the responsibility and role of the hospital-based nurse in promoting community health. What activities can all nurses pursue to promote community health?
- the value of collaboration among various health professionals in promoting community health. How can health professionals influence legislators and policy makers, who have little or no knowledge and experience related to health care, to make wise and effective decisions regarding community health?

INTEGRATION OF HOME AND COMMUNITY NURSING

"Home care has been an organized system of care in the United States for approximately 100 years. Home care was developed in response to (1) the needs and preferences of families to care for ill and infirm members at home and (2) limitations and costs of institutional care" (Barkauskas, 1990, p. 394). The focus of home nursing has always been on the individual client and his or her family. Community nursing has an equally prestigious history as nurses focused on the health needs of the community as a whole. In many ways the roles and practice settings of the home health care nurse and the community health nurse are separate and distinct. For example, the home health care nurse works exclusively in the client's residence. Community nurses may work in the home but are more frequently found in clinics, immigrant and refugee centers, public health centers, community nursing centers, and other community-based providers of care outside the home or hospital. The home health care nurse is usually providing care to a client who is recovering from illness or injury; the community health nurse is usually working in areas of health promotion and illness prevention.

The home health care nurse is the care provider,

teacher, and advocate for the client and their family. The nurse may intervene to mobilize the resources of the community or the hospital to meet the client's identified needs, but the focus remains the client and family. The community nurse may work with the individual client and their family but often must subjugate the needs of the individual to the needs of the community. For example, a client with a highly communicable disease may have his or her freedom of movement restricted in order to protect the community, or a client diagnosed with a sexually transmitted disease may have to defer their right of confidentiality for the identification and treatment of their contacts.

Some consider home health nursing an aspect of community nursing as the client's residence is within his or her community and the strengths and weaknesses of the community impact the client's ability to stay well or recover from illness in the home. While the issue of whether home health nursing is community nursing may be debated, it is more important that nurses recognize the wide range of professional opportunities for nurses to influence the health of individuals, and families, in their homes and communities.

Consider . . .

- what academic and experiential qualifications a nurse should have to practice in the home or community setting. What are the differences in knowledge and skill required to become certified as a home care nurse or a community health nurse?

- the differences in autonomy in decision making and practice between the hospital nurse, the home care nurse, and the community nurse. Does one type of nurse have greater autonomy than another, or are there simply differences in the types of independent decision making and practice?

SUMMARY

Because of changing demographics and a need for health care cost containment, the focus of health care has shifted from hospital-based illness treatment to community-based health promotion and disease prevention in home and community settings. While not new nursing practice settings, this shift in focus has created new opportunities for nurses to impact the health of individuals, families, and communities.

Home health care nursing is a rapidly growing industry providing a wide range of nursing services to clients in their places of residence. It may include the administration of physician prescribed treatments, independent nursing interventions, and high-tech therapies, including chemotherapy and dialysis. The home health care nurse assesses the care needs of clients in their home; plans, implements, and supervises that care; teaches clients and their families self-care; and mobilizes the resources of hospitals, physicians, and community agencies in meeting the needs of the clients and their families.

Community health nurses may provide nursing services in the home, but are more frequently found in clinics, schools, and other community-based settings. Community health nurses focus on the health needs of the community as a whole, providing health education, illness prevention through immunization programs, and communicable disease follow-up.

Both home health care nurses and community health nurses are essential components of a health care delivery system that ensures access to quality health care at an affordable cost.

Bookshelf

Friedman, M. 1998. *Family nursing: Research, theory, and practice.* **New York: Prentice Hall.**
This text presents a holistic approach to the nursing care of families. A family-assessment tool is provided for nurses to use in practice.

Friedemann, M. 1995. *The framework of systemic organization: A conceptual approach to families and nursing.* **Thousand Oaks, Calif.: Sage Publications.**
The author provides a theoretical framework for assisting families within the context of their various communities—social, environmental, cultural, and economic. The author guides the reader through the application of family theory to practice and research as the practitioner seeks to advocate and support health and well-being in individuals and families.

SELECTED REFERENCES

American Nurses Association. 1992. *A statement on the scope of home health nursing practice.* Washington, D.C.: ANA.

American Nurses Association. 1998. *Scope and standards of parish nursing practice.* Washington, D.C.: ANA.

American Nurses Credentialing Center. 2000. *Certification catalog.* Washington, D.C.: ANA. http//www.ana.org/ancc/cert/catalogs/2000.

ANCC approves new certification program for clinical specialist in home health nursing. 1995, July 4. *Vital signs: The pulse of Florida's health care opportunities,* p. 11.

Anderson, E., and McFarlane, J. 2000. *Community as partner,* 3d ed. Philadelphia: Lippincott.

Barkauskas, V. H. 1990. Home health care: Responding to need, growth, and cost containment. In N. L. Chaska, ed., *The nursing profession: Turning points.* St. Louis: Mosby, pp. 394–405.

Carpenito, L. J. 1999. *Nursing diagnosis: Application to clinical practice,* 8th ed. Philadelphia: Lippincott.

Clark, M. J. 1999. *Nursing in the community,* 3d ed. Norwalk, Conn.: Appleton & Lange.

Clemen-Stone, S., McGuire, S. L., and Eigsti, D. G. 1998. *Comprehensive community health nursing: Family, aggregate, and community practice,* 5th ed. St. Louis: Mosby.

Hanchett, E. 1979. *Community health assessment: A conceptual tool kit.* New York: John Wiley & Sons.

Hitchcock, J., Schubert, P., and Thomas, S.. 1999. *Community health nursing.* New York: Delmar.

International Parish Nurse Resource Center. 2001. *What is parish nursing?* www.advocatehealth.com/about/faith/parishn/index.

Keller, L. O., Stohschein, S., Kia-Hoagberg, B., and Schaffer, M. 1998. Population-based public health nursing interventions: A model from practice. *Public Health Nursing* **115**(3): 207–215.

Leavell, H. R., and Clark, E. G. 1965. *Preventive medicine for the doctor in his community,* 3d ed. New York: McGraw-Hill.

McCloskey, J. C., and G. M. Bulechek. 1996. *Iowa Intervention Project: Nursing interventions classification (NIC),* 2d ed. St. Louis: Mosby.

Ryan, J. 1997. Assuring the future quality of parish nursing practice. *Perspectives in Parish Nursing Practice* **5**(3): 4.

Spradley, J. W., and Allender, J. A. 1996. *Community health nursing: Concepts and practice,* 4th ed. Philadelphia: Lippincott.

Stackhouse, J. 1998. *Into the community.* Philadelphia: Lippincott.

Stanhope, M., and Lancaster, J. 1996. *Community health nursing: Promoting health of aggregates, families, and individuals,* 4th ed. St. Louis: Mosby.

Stewart, M. 1985. Community and aggregates: Systematic community health assessment. In M. Stewart, J. Innes, S. Searl, and C. Smillie, eds., *Community health nursing in Canada.* Toronto, Ontario: Gage Educational Publishing, pp 363–377.

Stulginsky, M. M. 1993a, Oct. Nurses' home health experience. Part 1: The practice setting. *Nursing & Health Care* **14**(8): 402–407.

Stulginsky, M. M. 1993b, Nov. Nurses' home health experience. Part 2: The unique demands of home visits. *Nursing & Health Care* **14**(9): 476–485.

U.S. Department of Health and Human Services. 2000. *Healthy people 2010 national health promotion and disease prevention objectives.* http://www.health.gov/healthypeople.

Warhola, C. 1980, Aug. *Planning for home health services: A resource handbook.* (Pub No. HRA 80-14017). Washington, D.C.: USDHHS, Public Health Service.

Zotti, M., Brown, P., and Stotts, C. 1996. Community-based nursing versus community health nursing. What does it all mean? *Nursing Outlook* **44**(5): 211–217.

Nursing in a Culture of Violence

Outline

Objectives

- Define domestic violence and abuse.
- Recognize the incidence of violence within the family, in the community, and in the workplace.
- Discuss theoretical perspectives of violence.
- Identify essential aspects of assessing the effects of violence and abuse.
- Explain the nurse's role in assisting victims of abuse and violence.
- Discuss methods of violence prevention.

N U R S E   C O N N E C T

Additional online resources for this chapter can be found on the companion web site at www.prenhall.com/blais.

Violence and abusive behavior have become major health problems in North America, and they are the source of injury and both physical and mental morbidity in people of all ages. The context of the violence and abuse may be the family, the community, or the workplace.

- Approximately 1000 workers are murdered and 1.5 million workers are assaulted in the workplace each year in the United States (Occupational Safety and Health Administration, 1999).
- Approximately 25% of women and 8% of men report being raped and/or physically assaulted by a current

or former spouse, cohabiting partner, or date at some time in their life (Tjaden and Thoennes, 1998).

■ A survey of public school principals estimates approximately 4000 rapes or sexual batteries occur on school grounds or at school-sponsored events, along with 7000 robberies, 11,000 physical attacks or fights with a weapon, and 188,000 attacks or fights without a weapon (U.S. Department of Education, 1997).

■ The National Committee for the Prevention of Child Abuse reports that 1,054,000 children were confirmed by child protective agencies as victims of child maltreatment in 1997 (Wang and Daro, 1998).

CHALLENGES AND OPPORTUNITIES

The high incidence of violence in society affects large segments of the population with direct impact on health care. Nurses are challenged in their practice to identify and intervene when providing care for a victim of violence. Because the victims often attempt to hide the fact that they have been attacked, it requires high levels of skill in communication and in assessment on the part of the nurse.

In meeting the challenge of providing care for victims of violence, the nurse has an opportunity to have a positive impact on the client outcomes. Nurses are strategically placed to have a role in primary and secondary prevention programs. The focus on the community that is embraced by professional organizations, such as the ANA agenda for health care reform, places nurses in roles and settings that enable them to have influence on reducing the effects of violence within the community and within families.

VIOLENCE AND ABUSE

Traditionally the term *domestic abuse* has been thought of as violence against a woman by a spouse or boyfriend. More recently, the term has expanded to include other forms of violence, such as child abuse, elder abuse, abuse of male partners, and violence between same-sex partners. The CDC now uses the term **intimate partner violence,** which is defined as "the intentional emotional and/or physical abuse by a spouse, ex-spouse, boyfriend/girl-friend, ex-boyfriend/ex-girlfriend, or date" (CDC, 2000).

Domestic Violence

Family violence includes intimate partner abuse, child abuse, and elder abuse ranging from verbal abuse to light slaps to severe beatings to homicide. It occurs in all strata of society; it crosses all racial, religious, ethnic, socioeconomic, and educational boundaries, and it is not con-

fined to any particular age group or occupation. It is a myth that domestic violence occurs only in poor minority families.

Emotional abuse is equally damaging (Fontaine, 1996, p. 565). Words can hit as hard as a fist, and the damage to self-esteem can last a lifetime. Emotional abuse involves one person shaming, embarrassing, ridiculing, or insulting a loved one. It may include the destruction of personal property or the killing of pets in an effort to frighten or control the victim. Emotional abuse may also include statements that are devastating to the victim's self-esteem, such as, "You can't do anything right," "You're ugly and stupid—no one else would want you," "I wish you had never been born" (Fontaine, 1996).

Abusive individuals come from all walks of life but have certain traits or characteristics in common:

■ Overpossessiveness: viewing family members in terms of ownership and property
■ Excessive jealousy
■ Desire to control and dominate
■ Poor control of impulses
■ Low tolerance for frustration
■ Belief that physical measures are necessary to control children
■ Dependence on an elder for financial support and accommodation
■ Drug or alcohol abuse
■ History of poor mental health or a personality disorder
■ History of abuse as a child by own parents

Intimate Partner Abuse

Most intimate partner abuse is perpetrated by men against women; however, abuse is also perpetrated by women against men and between partners of the same gender. Women are more vulnerable, generally speaking, to this violence because of their disadvantage in size and strength and their social and economic dependence on men. However, men who are victimized in this way have fewer resources available, such as 24-hour toll-free-assistance numbers or shelters. Abused men may be less likely to seek help because of the stigma.

Societal acceptance regarding violence against women by husbands has existed historically; it was considered a private domestic matter. Before 1700, laws allowed a husband to chastise his wife with any reasonable instrument, such as a rod not thicker than the husband's thumb (the origin of the phrase "rule of thumb") (Henderson, 1992, p. 27).

Abuse can be categorized as physical abuse, sexual abuse, psychosocial abuse, and property violence. *Physical abuse* involves any physical harm or nonconsensual touching. It may involve pushing and shoving, dragging

Research Box

Yarn, M. 2000. Seen but not heard: Battered women's perceptions of the ED experience. *Journal of Emergency Nursing* **26 (5): 464–470.**

This qualitative study described battered women's perceptions of their experience in the emergency department. A phenomenological approach was used to interview women recruited from shelters for battered women. Participants in the study had been treated at a hospital emergency department for abuse-related injuries within the past 12 months. In-depth interviews and a demographic data sheet were used to collect the data. Data analysis used Colaizzi's procedural steps.

Several categories emerged from the data. Feelings experienced during the ED visit were fear of their partner, concern for the children, and loneliness. The women's perceptions were that nurses in the ED do not understand abuse. They were satisfied with the treatment of the injuries but dissatisfied with how the issue of abuse was managed. They indicated that they had difficulty disclosing the abuse due to fear, embarrassment, and a lack of resources. They wanted health care professionals to be compassionate, provide referrals, and offer options.

or pulling; kicking, hitting, or beating with fists or objects; locking a person out of the home or in a room or closet or abandoning him or her in a dangerous place; or biting, choking, physically restraining, or threatening with a weapon. *Sexual abuse* involves any forced or nonconsensual sex. It includes sexually criticizing the person, hurting during sex, and/or treating that person as property or a sex object. *Psychosocial abuse* can involve threats of harm, abuse of pets, constant criticism and downgrading in front of others, insulting family or friends, keeping the person from talking to or seeing friends and family, and threats to kidnap the children. It may involve keeping the person from working or going to school, censoring mail, taking away car keys or money, accusations of having affairs, or forbidding use of the telephone. *Property violence* is threatened or actual destruction of material possessions.

It is especially difficult for many victims to leave an abusive relationship. Women who do leave an abusive relationship attempt an average of three to five separa-

tions before finally ending the relationship. Some women are threatened with loss of children or with death if they do not return home. Social and cultural beliefs also play a role. Women have been socialized to be self-sacrificing for the good of others and feel responsible for keeping the family together at almost any cost, and cultural beliefs about loyalty and duty may reinforce the role of victim. In addition, many women are financially dependent on their abusive partners; if they have outside employment, they are unlikely to earn as much as their male counterparts. If there are children, the woman may desperately need child support, and many fathers do not honor this obligation and default on the payments. The burdens of child care have traditionally fallen entirely on the mother. Thus, lack of affordable and adequate child care facilities has become a major problem for the single mother seeking employment.

Many people believe that abused spouses can end the violence by divorcing their abuser or that the victim can learn to stop doing those things that provoke violence. These beliefs are myths and not supported by facts. According to the United States Department of Justice, about 75% of all spousal attacks occur between people who are separated or divorced. In many cases, the separation process brings on an increased level of harassment and violence. In a battering relationship, moreover, the abuser needs no provocation to become violent. Violence is the abuser's pattern of behavior, and the victim can't learn how to control it. Even so, many victims blame themselves for the abuse, feeling guilty—even responsible—for doing or saying something that triggers the abuser's behavior. Friends, family, and service providers reinforce this attitude by laying the blame and the need to change on the shoulders of the victim. Many people who do try to disclose their situation are met with disbelief or denial; this discourages them from persevering.

Effects of Domestic Violence on Children

Children experience domestic violence as victims and as witnesses, affecting not only their physical health and safety but also their psychological adjustment, social relations, and academic achievement. The experience affects their perception of the world, self-concept, ideas about the purpose of life, future expectations, and moral development (Margolin and Gordis, 2000). Domestic violence violates a child's safe haven, and the immediate reaction is likely to be helplessness, fear, anger, and high arousal, which can disrupt the child's efforts in age-appropriate academic and social pursuits.

Children of any age, race, religion, or socioeconomic status can be victims of abuse and neglect. Perpetrators may be parents, siblings, a boyfriend or girlfriend, or a baby-sitter, and the form of the abuse may be physical battering, physical neglect, sexual abuse, or emotional abuse and neglect. Laws mandate the reporting of suspected child abuse to child-protection authorities, and these laws also protect health care professionals from any liability that might result from their reporting, in good faith, suspected cases of child maltreatment.

Physical abuse is nonaccidental injury of a child and is relatively easy to recognize and treat. The most common types of physical abuse are burns, bruises, fractures, abdominal injuries, and head or spinal injuries. The location and pattern of injuries help determine the likelihood of abuse. For example, accidental scalds usually occur on the front of the body; scald burns on the back and feet are suspicious. Bruises over bony surfaces such as the shin, forehead, knees, forearms, and chin are common occurrences among active children; bruises on the cheek, abdomen, back, buttocks, and thighs raise suspicion of abuse.

Whiplash-shaking can lead to severe injury in infants. Cerebral damage, neurologic defects, blindness, and mental retardation can result. These findings are often seen without external evidence of head injury. Nurses should suspect **shaken baby syndrome (SBS)** in infants less than one year of age who present with apnea, seizures, lethargy or drowsiness, bradycardia, respiratory difficulty, coma, or death. Subdural and retinal hemorrhages accompanied by the absence of external signs of trauma are hallmarks of the syndrome.

Another common, but often unrecognized, form of family violence occurs between siblings (Fontaine, 1996, p. 522). Many people assume that it is natural, and even appropriate, for children to use physical force with one another: "It is a good chance for him to learn how to de-fend himself," "She had a right to hit him; he was teasing her," or "Kids will be kids." These attitudes teach children that physical force is an appropriate method of resolving conflicts. Sibling violence is highest in the early years and decreases with age. In all age groups, girls are less violent toward their siblings than are boys.

Physical neglect is failure to meet the basic needs of children by those persons responsible for doing so. Basic needs include adequate nourishment, clothing, housing, supervision, and medical care. Nurses must exercise caution, however, "not to define as willful neglect a case in which an impoverished or uneducated family is providing . . . the best care possible within their means" (Srnec, 1991, p. 476).

Sexual abuse is the occurrence of any sexual activity between an adult and child. It includes either *assaultive* abuse, which produces physical injury and severe emotional trauma, or *nonassaultive* abuse, which produces minimal or no physical trauma. Nonassaultive abuse is often chronic and severely disruptive of the child's sexual development. Children who have been sexually abused may demonstrate the following clinical signs: perineal rashes, genital-rectal irritation or tissue trauma, frequent urinary tract infections, evidence of vaginal or anal penetration by a foreign body, presence of sexually transmitted disease, and an unusually mature knowledge of sexual terminology and slang. Some children may become involved in promiscuous sexual activities and juvenile prostitution or pornography. Because child sexual abuse often involves the parent of the child, this form of abuse is the least reported.

Emotional abuse and neglect is failure to provide an environment in which the child can thrive, learn, and develop. Obviously, this type of abuse is more difficult to identify and manage than physical abuse.

Abused children manifest various characteristics (see the accompanying box). Childhood abuse may have

Behavioral Characteristics of Abused Children

The child may

- Be unusually aggressive, withdrawn, overly compliant, or attention seeking.
- Appear afraid of a parent or wary of physical contact with an adult.
- Be inappropriately clothed during winter.
- Manifest developmental delay and failure to thrive.

- Express violence toward pets.
- Run away from home.
- Demonstrate changes in school performance.
- Be habitually late for school or avoid spending time at home by arriving early and staying late.
- Verbalize fault for injuries: "I deserved it."
- Attempt suicide or abuse alcohol or drugs.

far-reaching consequences for the victim's health. Empirical data link child maltreatment and exposure to domestic violence with numerous outcomes, including aggression and violent behavior problems with peers, delinquency, depression, delayed cognitive functioning, poor academic performance, and symptoms of post-traumatic stress disorder (Margolin and Gordis, 2000).

Elder Abuse

Older adults who can no longer live independently may be vulnerable to mistreatment in the forms of physical abuse, psychological or emotional abuse, sexual abuse, financial manipulation, or neglect. The most likely perpetrators are persons in continual contact with the dependent elder and could be family or nonfamily caregivers such as spouses, children, or professional caregivers (Marshall, Benton, and Brazier, 2000). Federal definitions of elder abuse, neglect, and exploitation first appeared in the Amendments to the Older Americans Act in 1987 and appeared as guidelines for identifying problems, not for law-enforcement purposes (National Center on Elder Abuse, 2000). Currently, elder abuse is defined by state laws, and definitions vary somewhat by state.

According to the National Center on Elder Abuse (2000), there are three categories of elder abuse: (1) domestic elder abuse, (2) institutional elder abuse, and (3) self-neglect. Domestic abuse refers to any of several forms of maltreatment of an older person by someone who has a special relationship with the elder. Institutional abuse refers to abuse occurring in residential facilities such as nursing homes. Self-neglect is characterized as the behavior of the elderly person that threatens health and safety; it is usually a failure to provide sufficiently for himself or herself.

The types of abuse that can occur are physical abuse, which includes not only striking, but also inappropriate use of drugs, physical restraints, and force-feeding. Sexual abuse is nonconsensual sexual contact of any kind, even if the elder is not capable of giving consent. Emotional or psychological abuse is defined as the infliction of anguish, pain, or distress through verbal or nonverbal acts. Neglect is the refusal or failure to fulfill any part of a person's obligations or duties to an elder, and abandonment is the desertion by an individual who has assumed responsibility for providing care for the elder. Financial exploitation is the illegal or improper use of an elder's funds, property, or assets, such as cashing checks or forging the signature, or improper use of power of attorney.

Elder abuse is complex, but some of the reasons researchers have found to be associated with it are caregiver stress, impairment of the dependent elder, continuation of a cycle of violence (because the tendency for violent responses is perpetuated in some families), and personal problems of the abusers. Typically, the abusers are adult children. The incidence is probably underreported because of the dependent status of the abused and their embarrassment at disclosing abuse or fear of retribution (Beers and Berkow, 2000). The accompanying box describes clinical situations suggestive of elder abuse. Although the incidence is difficult to determine, it is estimated that there are about 1 million known cases annually in the United States and that

---

Clinical Situations Suggestive of Elder Abuse

- When there is a delay between the injury or illness and the seeking of medical attention
- When the accounts of the patient and caregiver do not agree
- When the severity of the injury does not fit the explanation given by the caregiver
- When the explanation of the patient or caregiver is implausible or vague
- When visits to the emergency department for chronic disease exacerbations are frequent despite an appropriate care plan and adequate resources
- When a functionally impaired patient presents to the physician without a designated caregiver in attendance
- When laboratory findings are inconsistent with the history
- When the caregiver is reluctant to accept home health care (e.g., a visiting nurse) or to leave the elderly person alone with a health care practitioner

Source: Used by permission of M. H. Beers and R. Berkow, eds. *The Merck Manual of Geriatrics,* 3rd ed. Whitehouse, N.J.: Merck Research Laboratories, 2000, p. 152.

reported numbers in Canada and Western Europe are comparable (Beers and Berkow 2000; Marshall, Benton, and Brazier 2000).

Consider . . .

■ how a nurse's previous abusive relationships might affect his or her practice with victims of domestic violence.

■ the available resources for victims of abuse in your area of practice. What additional resources might be needed?

Violence in the Community

Violence in the community has ripple effects. People who are not directly victimized may observe violent acts or at the least may hear about them repeatedly from the news media. Data suggest that in inner-city neighborhoods, one-third or more of children have been directly victimized, and almost all children have been exposed to community violence (Margolin and Gordis, 2000). Children are particularly vulnerable because violence can result in a disruption to the normal developmental trajectory. Anxiety, depression, and post-traumatic stress syndrome symptoms are results that can disrupt the child's developing socialization, social interactions, and concentration in school. In Western culture, the home and the neighborhood are considered safe havens for children, but they lose those protective and comforting qualities in the aftermath of violence in the community. Exposure to community violence has been linked to the development of aggressive and antisocial behavior on the part of the child (Miller et al., 1999).

Although exposure to violence clearly puts children at risk for developing psychological problems, these negative outcomes are not inevitable. It is important for nurses to identify those factors that mediate or moderate the effects and use them to help children who experience violence in the community. Mediating factors identified in research fall into three categories: (1) child characteristics, (2) factors related to the frequency, severity, and chronicity of the violence, and (3) quality of family and social relations, along with the level of disruption and chaos in the child's life (Hughes, 1997).

The elderly are particularly vulnerable to violence in the community. They are often easy victims of crimes such as mugging, theft, and robbery. In addition, the threat of violence in the community may keep them from leaving the perceived safety of their homes to go out alone. This contributes to isolation, loneliness, fear, and depression.

The causes of violence have been investigated extensively by many disciplines in the social sciences. According to a review by Gilligan (2000), the experience of shame and humiliation is at the root of violent behavior, along with a lack of guilt or remorse. When individuals experience shame and humiliation without the ability to feel guilt or remorse, they may be prone to violence as a way of striking out without self-control. Worldwide, the most powerful predictor of the murder rate is the size of the gap between the income of the rich and the poor. The primary prevention suggested is to ensure that people have access to the means by which they can achieve feelings of self-worth, such as education and employment and equitable levels of income, wealth, and power.

Nurses need to be involved in creating safer communities through social policies. This may be approached with political advocacy, as discussed in Chapter 11, "The Nurse as Advocate."

School Violence

School shootings have raised concern about the risk of violence by children and youths. Risk factors have been investigated so that violence potential can be identified and preventive measures can be implemented. The Seattle Social Development Project conducted a prospective study of a panel of youths and studied potential risk factors for violence at age 18. They sampled the risk factors at ages 10, 14, and 16 years. The parent rating of hyperactivity, low academic performance, peer delinquency, and availability of drugs in the neighborhood predicted violence at all three ages. Multiple risk factors increased the likelihood of later violence. The recommendation from the project was that prevention efforts must be comprehensive and developmentally sensitive, responding to populations exposed to multiple risks (Herrenkohl et al., 2000).

Other research has identified the victimization by peers as a risk factor. Violent acts committed at school are often associated with bullying and ostracizing of the perpetrators (Hanish and Guerra, 2000). The National School Safety Center has made recommendations for school personnel to help create a safe school environment (Miller et al., 2000). School nurses may be directly involved in prevention measures.

Violence in the Workplace

Workplace violence is defined as "any act against an employee that creates a hostile work environment and which negatively affects the employee, either physically or psychologically" including physical or verbal assaults, threats, coercion, intimidation, or harassment"

(Lenius, 1999). The costs of workplace violence include loss of productivity, work disruptions, employee turnover, litigation and legal costs, and other incident-related costs.

According to the Department of Justice's National Crime Victimization Survey (Warchol, 1998), assaults and threats of violence against Americans at work number almost 2 million per year. The most common type of workplace violent crime is simple assault, followed by aggravated assault, rape and sexual assault, robbery, and homicide. Retail sales workers were most frequently the victims of violence, followed by police officers (Warchol, 1998).

Workplace homicides are the second leading cause of job-related deaths. Robbery is the primary motive of job-related homicide, accounting for 85% of the fatalities. Disputes among coworkers and with customers or clients accounted for about 10% of fatalities (Bureau of Labor Statistics, 1998).

The National Institute for Occupational Safety and Health (NIOSH, 1996) has identified risk factors for workplace assault:

- Contact with the public
- Exchange of money
- Delivery of passengers, goods, or services
- Having a mobile workplace, such as taxi or police cruiser
- Working with unstable or volatile persons in health care, social services, or criminal justice settings
- Working alone or in small numbers
- Working late at night or during early morning hours
- Working in high-crime areas
- Guarding valuable property or possessions
- Working in a community-based setting

The Occupational Safety and Health Administration (OSHA) does not have a specific standard for workplace violence. They encourage employers to develop workplace violence-prevention programs through recommended guidelines related to creation of barriers and administrative controls. Preemployment selection procedures, 24-hour hotlines for reporting concerns, and restricted or monitored building entry are measures employers have initiated to reduce the occurrence of violence.

ASSESSING THE EFFECTS OF VIOLENCE AND ABUSE

Often the nurse is the first one outside a person's family to discover that the person is being abused. Some victims may not disclose the abuse, or they may minimize its impact. However, it is the nurse's responsibility to assess for and be alert to signs of abuse and not deny the violence.

During the assessment interview, the nurse must ensure privacy. The victim must feel safe from the perpetrator. It may be difficult for the client to admit to the reality of family violence until a trusting nurse-client relationship evolves. The nurse should assure the client of genuine desire to help the entire family system. The nurse should also approach this topic as if it were any other health risk. In addition, the nurse can offer the option of answering questions about incidents of abuse with "sometimes" instead of "yes" or "no"; this may encourage the client to make a first step to acknowledge the abuse.

Victims of violence enter the health care system for a variety of conditions associated with abuse. For example, common physical complaints include chronic pelvic pain, headache, irritable bowel syndrome, arthritis, pelvic inflammatory disease, and neurologic damage. Psychiatric illness (e.g., alcoholism) may also be the result of a history of sexual or physical abuse. Depression is also common.

Research Box

Nabb, D. 2000. Visitor's violence: The serious effects of aggression on nurses and others. *Nursing Standard* 14(23): 36–38.

One hundred British nurses in acute medical, rehabilitation, and long-term care units caring for older people completed a questionnaire and a personal interview. A majority (59%) reported they had experienced verbal abuse from patient's visitors within the past 12 months and 72% of those incidents had been repeated from two to five times. Twenty percent of the nurses reported experiencing some sort of physical violence within that same period of time; for these nurses, it occurred from one to five times. The type of physical violence included being pushed, grabbed, and being struck. Eighty-four percent of the nurses believed that violence from visitors is increasing.

Analysis of the interview data identified effects of the violence on the nurses. They reported (1) increased incidence of illness, (2) not wanting to come to work, (3) thinking about leaving, and (4) feeling vulnerable.

Nursing History

Because domestic violence is so prevalent, many health care professionals now believe that questions concerning abuse should be part of any health history. To detect the presence of abuse, various assessment tools may be used.

The Canadian Nurses Association (1992, p. 9) proposes that the nurse assess the frequency of family conflict and aggression by asking such questions as these:

> "Many times, families don't handle problems in the way that they would like to. How does your family handle problems?"

> "Has anyone ever used physical force? Who? When?"

The nurse must clarify vague or evasive answers and further explore any such areas by asking, for example, "What happens when you and your partner get angry?" or "Has anything happened to you that might have caused these symptoms?"

When assessing a child, the nurse may ask, "Moms and dads try to help their children learn how to behave well. What happens to you when you do something wrong?" or "Can you tell me more about this?"

If the responses to initial questions indicate possible abuse, the nurse needs to conduct a detailed assessment. Some agencies supply nursing history tools for this purpose.

Physical Examination

Victims of physical abuse may suffer a variety of injuries. During a head-to-toe assessment, the nurse observes for indications of abuse, such as the following:

- *Head:* Bald patches on the scalp where hair has been pulled out; evidence of trauma from blows to the head, such as hematoma, facial bruises, facial fractures, bruised or swollen eyes, hemorrhages into the eyes; petechiae around the eyes from attempted strangulation.
- *Skin:* Swelling or tenderness, bruises, burns, or scars of past injuries on the skin, genitals, and rectal areas.
- *Musculoskeletal system:* Fractures or evidence of previous fractures, particularly of the face, arms/legs and ribs; dislocated joints, especially in the shoulder when the victim is grabbed or pulled by the arm.
- *Abdomen:* Bruises, wounds, or intra-abdominal injuries, especially if the person is pregnant.
- *Neurologic system:* Hyperactive reflexes due to neurologic damage; paresthesias, numbness, or pain from old injuries.

If the nursing assessment reveals possible domestic violence, a team assessment needs to take place.

The victim's medical condition and emotional state must be assessed. The severity and potential fatality of the situation must be considered, as well as the needs of dependent children and the legal ramifications.

The American Academy of Pediatrics (AAP, 1999) has published guidelines for the evaluation of sexual abuse of children. These were developed by the committee on child abuse and neglect and are available from the AAP.

Consider . . .

- nursing and medical assessment instruments used in your practice setting. Are there areas or questions that specifically assess for abuse or violence? Do self-report instruments ask questions that would elicit a history of abuse?
- the possibility that abuse is underreported in practice settings whose staff are not attuned to the signs and symptoms of violence. How might the ignorance of health care providers exacerbate the problem of abuse?
- the responsibility of the nurse if evidence of abuse is detected during assessment.

PLANNING/IMPLEMENTING INTERVENTIONS FOR THE ABUSED

The goals of treating abuse are (a) to empower the client to take control, (b) to support the client, and (c) to maximize the client's safety (CNA, 1992, p. 10).

Most people involved in intrafamily violence are disturbed by this behavior and would like it to end. Even though they want help to stop the abuse, they may not know how to seek the assistance they need. It is extremely important for nurses to be nonjudgmental in their interactions with all family members. The abusers may be distrustful of the motives of the nurse. Initially, the victims may be unwilling to trust because of family shame and fear of being blamed for remaining in the violent situation. The nurse should convey a nonjudgmental manner; in other words, the nurse should avoid blaming the victim or the abuser or looking for pathological elements in anyone's behavior. It is vital not to impose personal values on the family by offering quick and easy solutions to intrafamily violence (Fontaine, 1996).

Short-Term Interventions

Because the nurse may have the only contact with the client, it is essential that the nurse (1) determine the immediacy of danger, (2) convey that the person is not to blame and has the right to be safe, (3) explore options for help, and (4) provide information regarding available services.

It is important that the nurse avoid a judgmental attitude and support the person's choice about whether to leave the unsafe situation or return to the abusive relationship. Because severely battered women are at risk for homicide, the nurse needs to inform the client about associated risk factors and determine the immediacy of danger.

Many agencies now provide protocols for health care professionals to follow. These offer specific guidelines for the identification, treatment, and referral of battered women seeking emergency care. A simple mnemonic tool developed by Holtz and Furniss (Furniss, 1993) provides guidelines for essential interventions during this early contact with the client (see the accompanying box).

A collaborative team of nurse administrators and clinical nurses at Harris County Health Department in Houston, Texas, developed a screening and intervention triage tool for abuse. The triage structure facilitates appropriate intervention according to screening data. Each of the triage levels includes related interventions and essential documentation. See Table 20–1.

Abused children need to be encouraged to talk, but they must also be protected from having to provide multiple reports. Nurses need to tell an abused child that they believe the story, and they must reassure the child that he or she has done nothing wrong. The nurse should also avoid making negative comments about the abuser and to follow established protocols for mandatory reporting, documentation, and use of available support services (e.g., the police department, social service agencies, and child welfare agency).

Interventions for abused older adults include developing a positive relationship with both the victim and the abuser, exploring ways for the older person to maximize independence, and exploring the need for additional home care services or alternative living arrangements.

Nurses must familiarize themselves with agency protocols and resources available for victims of domestic violence. Most municipalities have crisis helplines and hotlines to provide assistance to victims of abuse. The nurse should also keep a record of telephone numbers for transition houses and rape crisis centers, alcohol and drug abuse information, support groups, religious organizations, and legal services. There are also several national organizations that offer toll-free contacts, such as the National Organization

---

The Holtz and Furniss Mnemonic Tool to Guide Immediate Treatment of Abused Women

A. Reassure the woman that she is not *alone* and that assistance and support are available from caregivers who can help.

B. Express *belief* that violence is not acceptable, no matter what she has been told by the batterer. Tell her that she should never be physically hurt.

C. Ensure *confidentiality*. Let the person know that her disclosure is private but will be documented on her medical record in case it is needed for legal purposes at a future date.

D. *Document* clear descriptions of all physical and psychologic symptoms; a history of at least the first, worst, and most recent incidents of abuse; what was said, done, and observed; date, time, and direct quotes of the client. Notes may be needed for legal purposes.

E. *Educate* the woman about (a) the cycle of violence and likely escalation of abuse and (b) assistance available for shelter or housing, jobs, legal issues, social services, medical care, crisis counseling, support groups (for victims and abusers), and other local agencies.

F. Ensure the woman's *safety*. Provide telephone numbers for a local shelter, the police, and telephone help lines. Discuss a safety plan for quick escape. Hide or place a suitcase containing personal belongings with a neighbor or friends. The suitcase should contain a change of clothes for the client and each child, a small amount of money, essential telephone numbers, a toy for each child, and copies of essential documents, such as marriage license, children's birth certificates, medical insurance number or plan, and, if possible, last income tax return. Explore all legal options, such as orders of protection or restraining orders.

Source: Adapted from "Screening for Abuse in the Clinical Setting" by K. K. Furniss, *AWHONN's Clinical Issues* 4(3): 404, 1993.

Table 20–1 Screening and Intervention Triage for Abuse

Steps	TRIAGE		
	Level I	Level II	Level III
SCREEN	No history or present threat of abuse.	Recent or present abuse.	Client presents with injuries.
INTERVENE	Group or individual education about domestic violence; give handouts and pamphlets of community resources to client.	Crisis intervention; individual counseling; assist client with escape plan; identify shelter and other emergency resources; assist client in contacting shelter.	Crisis intervention; notify police; refer client to hospital for treatment (call ambulance); notify shelter; transport patient to shelter.
DOCUMENT	Statement of no abuse or threat of abuse; give handouts/education materials to client.	Statement of present or recent abuse; counsel client; give numbers to shelter and police; plan escape route; note if client declines shelter assistance at this time, or if shelter should be contacted per client's request.	Give statement of medical care given; notify emergency services; note where client was transported and in what condition.

Source: "Establishing a Screening Program for Abused Women" by M. V. Lazzaro and J. McFarlane, *Journal of Nursing Administration* 21: 10, October 1991. Reprinted with permission.

for Victim Assistance, the National Coalition Against Domestic Violence (in the United States), and the National Clearinghouse on Family Violence (in Canada).

Long-Term Interventions

Goals for ongoing counseling and care may include (1) helping the client continue to choose to be safe from violence, (2) helping the client explore options for self-development, and (3) helping the client improve quality of life through increasing self-esteem (CNA, 1992, p. 14).

Usually, the best way to treat violent families is a multidisciplinary approach involving nurses, physicians, social workers, police, protective services personnel, and, often, lawyers. Most families are more open to accepting help during a time of crisis than at other times. They will most likely be willing to develop new behavior patterns for up to 4 to 6 weeks following a crisis. If they are not helped during that time, they will most likely return to previous behavior patterns, including violence.

Nurses should know the laws associated with reporting physical abuse. In the United States and Canada, nurses are required to report any suspected child abuse. The courts and child protective agencies make decisions in the child's interest. They may allow a child to remain in the home but under court supervision; they may remove the child from the home; and,

in some instances, they may terminate parental rights if the abuse was severe.

State and provincial laws about reporting adult and elder abuse vary. Domestic violence is considered a violent crime; the victim has a right to be protected, and the perpetrator of the violence can be prosecuted.

PREVENTION OF VIOLENCE AND ABUSE

Nurses in all areas of practice (e.g., maternal/child health; school; community and occupational health; mental health; primary and acute care; and academic settings) need to take a proactive role to prevent family violence. Early screening of vulnerable people and efforts to promote a change in attitudes and beliefs about family violence are essential.

If they are to assist victims effectively, nurses must be aware of their own feelings about family violence. Nurses who are unclear about their own feelings about family violence may deny its existence, blame the victim in crisis, or minimize the effects of the violence (CNA, 1992, p. 8).

Nurses can also be instrumental as advocates in developing policies and programs, and providing inservice training and education to health care professionals and the public.

Table 20–2 *Healthy People 2010* Objectives for Violence and Abuse Prevention

Objective	Target	Baseline
Reduce homicides	3.0 per 100,000 population	6.5 per 100,000 population in 1998
Reduce maltreatment of children	10.3 per 1000 children under 18 years	12.9 per 1000 in 1998
Reduce child maltreatment fatalities	1.4 per 100,000 children under 18 years	1.6 per 100,000 in 1998
Reduce the rate of physical assault by current or former intimate partners	3.3 per 1000 persons aged 12 years and older	4.4 per 1000 persons aged 12 years and older in 1998
Reduce the annual rate of rape or attempted rape	0.7 per 1000 persons	0.8 per 1000 persons aged 12 years and older in 1998
Reduce sexual assault other than rape	0.4 per 1000 persons aged 12 years and older	0.6 per 1000 persons aged 12 years and older in 1998
Reduce physical assaults	13.6 per 1000 persons aged 12 years and older	31.1 per 1000 persons aged 12 years and older in 1998
Reduce physical fighting among adolescents	32%	35% in grade 9 through 12 within a year in 1999
Reduce weapon carrying by adolescents on school property	4.9%	6.9% of students in grades 9 through 12 during a 30-day period in 1999

Comprehensive violence prevention programs require a variety of different disciplines and organizations working together, such as state or provincial and local health care agencies, criminal justice agencies, and social service agencies.

Many of these programs are generated by *Healthy People 2010,* a national health-promotion and disease-prevention initiative to increase health for all. The objectives for violence and abuse prevention are shown in Table 20–2 (USDHHS, 2000, pp. 45–60).

SUMMARY

The prevalence of violence and abusive behavior in North America is alarming. National health care organizations now view violence as a major health problem and are directing attention to its recognition, prevention, and treatment. Nurses need to know how to identify victims of violence, to appreciate potential risk factors for future injury, and to understand some of the unique considerations regarding care of victims of abuse. Acts of violence often escalate in frequency and severity and may ultimately result in homicide.

Family violence includes intimate partner abuse, child abuse and neglect, and elder abuse, neglect, or mistreatment. It occurs in all strata of society. Abusive individuals have certain traits in common, such as overpossessiveness, desire to dominate, poor control of impulses, and a history of drug or alcohol use. Vic-

tims of domestic violence most often are women, many of whom have difficulty leaving the abusive relationship largely because of fear, shame, guilt, and economic dependence. Laws mandate the reporting of suspected child abuse. Elder abuse can involve not only physical, sexual, or emotional abuse but also active or passive neglect, violation of human or civil rights, and financial abuse. Those most vulnerable to elder abuse are females over 75 years of age, physically or mentally impaired, and dependent for care on the abuser.

Often the nurse is the first one outside the family to discover that a person is being abused. Appropriate assessment, intervention, and documentation are essential to prevent the abuse from continuing. The nurse needs to empower the client to take control, pro-

Bookshelf

Victor, B. 1996. *Getting away with murder: Weapons for the war against domestic violence.* **New York: Simon and Schuster.**
This text gives interviews with victims and abusers as well as police, social workers, district attorneys, and judges about the violent crimes committed against women by intimate partners. Suggestions are given from each of these sources regarding how to stop the attacks.

Levy, B. 1998. *In love and in danger: A teen's guide to breaking free of abusive relationships.* **Seattle: Seal Press.**
The book examines abusive relationships among teenagers. It is appropriate for grades 9 and up.

Rodriguez, S. 1999. *Time to stop pretending: A mother's story of domestic violence, homelessness, poverty, and escape.* **Middlebury, Vt.: P.S. Eriksson.**
This book is one woman's story of her life of domestic violence, poverty, and homelessness with her eight children in New York City.

Plain, B. 1994. *Whispers.* **New York: Dell Publishing.**
This novel is the story of a contemporary family and the story beneath the surface of their perfect lives. A woman struggles to free herself from the cycle of violence–contrition–more violence and finally emerges in triumph.

vide support, and maximize the client's safety. Treatment of violent families requires a multidisciplinary approach among nurses, social workers, physicians, family therapists, vocational trainers, police, protective services personnel, and lawyers.

If they are to assist victims effectively, nurses need to be aware of their own feelings about family violence. They also need to take a proactive role in preventing family violence. Nurses can advocate in developing programs and policies and provide in-service training and education to other health care professionals and the public.

SELECTED REFERENCES

American Academy of Pediatrics. 1999. Guidelines for the evaluation of sexual abuse in children: Subject review. *Pediatrics* **103**(1): 186.

American Nurses Association. 1991. *Position statement on physical violence against women.* Washington, D.C.: ANA.

Beers, M. H., and Berkow, R. 2000. *The Merck manual of geriatrics,* 3rd ed. White House Station, N.J.: Merck Research Laboratories.

Boychuk-Duchscher, J. E. 1994, June. Acting on violence against women. *Canadian Nurse* **91:** 20–25.

Brown, L. 1992a, Jan./Feb. Family violence. Part I. Hidden secrets: Elder abuse. *Nursing BC* **24:** 18–20.

Brown, L. 1992b, March/April. Family violence. Part II. Hidden secrets: Child abuse and wife abuse. *Nursing BC* **24:** 10–15.

Bureau of Labor Statistics. 1998. National census of fatal occupational injuries, 1997. www.bls.gov/opub/.

Campbell, J. C. 1993. Woman abuse and public policy: Potential for nursing action. *AWHONN's Clinical Issues* **4**(3): 503–512.

Canadian Nurses' Association. 1992. *Family violence: Clinical guidelines for nurses.* Ottawa: CNA.

Centers for Disease Control. 2000. *What is domestic violence?* www.cdc.gov/ncipc/dvp/fivpt/spotlite/home.htm.

Chez, N. 1994, July. Helping the victim of domestic violence. *American Journal of Nursing* **94:** 33–37.

Chiocca, E. M. 1995, Jan./Feb. Shaken baby syndrome: A nursing perspective. *Pediatric Nursing* **21:** 33–38.

Devlin, B. K., and Reynolds, E. 1994, March. Child

abuse: How to recognize it, how to intervene. *American Journal of Nursing* **94**: 26–32.

Fontaine, K. L. 1996. Rape and intrafamily abuse and violence. In H. S. Wilson and C. R. Kneisl, *Psychiatric Nursing*, 5th ed, pp. 555–584. Menlo Park, Calif.: Addison-Wesley Nursing.

Frost, M. H., and Willette, K. 1994, Aug. Risk for abuse/neglect: Documentation of assessment data and diagnoses. *Journal of Gerontological Nursing* **20**: 37–45.

Furniss, K. K. 1993. Screening for abuse in the clinical setting. *AWHONN's Clinical Issues* **4**(3): 402–406.

Gilligan, J. 2000. Violence in public health and preventive medicine. *Lancet* **355**: 1802–1804.

Greene, B. 1991. *The war against women. Report of the Standing Committee on Health and Welfare, Social Affairs, Seniors and the Status of Women.* Issue No. 31. Ottawa: Canada Communications Group, Publishing, Supply and Services.

Grunfeld, A. F., Ritmiller, S., Mackay, K., Cowan, L., and Hotch, D. 1994, Aug. Detecting domestic violence against women in the emergency department: A nursing triage model. *Journal of Emergency Nursing* **20**(4): 271–274.

Hall, L. A., Sachs, B., Rayens, M. K., and Lutenbacher, M. 1993, Winter. Childhood physical and sexual abuse: Their relationship with depressive symptoms in adulthood. *Image: Journal of Nursing Scholarship* **25**(4): 317–323.

Hanish, L. D., and Guerra, N. G. 2000. The roles of ethnicity and school context in predicting children's victimization by peers. *American Journal of Community Psychology* **28**(2): 201–223.

Henderson, A. 1992, Feb. Critical care nurses need to know about abused women. *Critical Care Nurses* **12**(2): 27–30.

Herrenkohl, T. I., Maguin, E., Hill, K. G., Hawkins, J. D., Abbott, R. D., and Catalano, R. F. 2000. Developmental risk factors for youth violence. *Journal of Adolescent Health* **26**(3): 176–186.

Hoag-Apel, C. 1994, Sept. Protocol for domestic violence intervention. *Nursing Management* **25**: 81–83.

Horsham, P. 1992, Sept. Child sexual abuse: What parents need to know. *Canadian Nurse* **88**: 32–35.

Hughes, H. M. 1997. Research concerning children of battered women: Clinical implications. In *Violence and sexual abuse at home: Current issues in spousal battering and child maltreatment*, R. Geffner, S. B. Sorenson, and P. K. Lundberg-Love, eds., pp. 225–244. New York: Haworth.

Jezierski, M. 1994, Oct. Abuse of women by male partners: Basic knowledge for emergency nurses. *Journal of Emergency Nursing* **20**(5): 361–372.

Johnson, T. 1991. *Elder mistreatment: Deciding who is at risk.* Westport, Conn.: Greenwood Press.

Kennedy, L. 1994, June. Women in crisis. *Canadian Nurse* **91**: 26–32.

Lazzaro, M. V., and McFarlane, J. 1991, Oct. Establishing a screening program for abused women. *Journal of Nursing Administration* **21**: 24–29.

Lenius, P. 1999, Oct. Workplace violence is a growing concern. *Contractor*.

Limandri, B. J., and Tilden, V. P. 1993. Domestic violence: Ethical issues in the health care system. *AWHONN's Clinical Issues* **4**(3): 493–502.

Margolin, G., and Gordis, E. B. 2000. The effects of family and community violence on children. *Annual Review of Psychology* **51**: 445–479.

Marshall, C. E., Benton, D., and Brazier, J. M. 2000. Elder abuse: Using clinical tools to identify clues of mistreatment. *Geriatrics* **55**: 42–53.

McFarlane, J., Parker, B., Soeken, K., and Bullock, L. 1992, June 17. Assessing for abuse during pregnancy: Severity and frequency of injuries and associated entry into prenatal care. *Journal of the American Medical Association* **267**: 3176–3178.

Miller, L. S., Wasserman, G. A., Neugebauer, R., Gorman-Smith, D., and Kamboukos, D. 1999. Witnessed community violence and antisocial behavior in high-risk urban boys. *Journal of Clinical Child Psychology* **28**: 2–11.

Miller, T. W., Clayton, R., Miller, J. M., Bilyeu, J., Hunter, J, and Kraus, R. F. 2000. Violence in the schools: Clinical issues and case analysis for high-risk children. *Child Psychiatry and Human Development* **30**(4): 255–272.

Mondor, E. E., and Wray, M. R. 1994, April. What's the matter with Johnny? *Canadian Nurse* **90**: 35–38.

Nabb, D. 2000. Visitor's violence: The serious effects of aggression on nurses and others. *Nursing Standard* **14**(3): 36–38.

National Center on Elder Abuse. 2000. *What is elder abuse?* http://www.elderabusecenter.org/basic/indes.html.

National Institute for Occupational Safety and Health. 1996. Violence in the workplace: Risk factors and prevention strategies. *NIOSH Current Intelligence Bulletin* **57**.

Occupational Safety and Health Administration. 1999. *Workplace violence.* www.osha.gov/oshinfo/priorities/violence.html.

Ozmar, B. 1994, Sept. Encountering victims of interpersonal violence: Implications for critical care nursing. *Critical Care Clinics of North America* **6**(3): 515–523.

Parker, B., McFarlane, J., Soeken, K., Torres, S., and Campbell, D. 1993, May/June. Physical and emotional abuse in pregnancy: A comparison of adult and teenage women. *Nursing Research* **42**(3): 173–178.

Patterson, R. J., Brown, G. W., Salassi-Scotter, M., and Middaugh, D. 1992, Aug. Head injury in the unconscious child. *American Journal of Nursing* **92**: 22–30.

Ross, M. M., and Hoff, L. A. 1994, June. Teaching nurses about abuse. *Canadian Nurse* **90**: 33–36.

Saveman, B. I., Hallberg, I. R., and Norberg, A. 1993, Sept. Identifying and defining abuse of elderly people, as seen by witnesses. *Journal of Advanced Nursing* **18**: 1393–1400.

Sheridan, D. J., and Taylor, W. K. 1993. Developing hospital-based domestic violence programs, protocols, policies, and procedures. *AWHONN's Clinical Issues* **4**(3): 471–482.

Simon, M. L. 1992. *An exploratory study of adult protective services programs' repeat elder abuse clients.* Washington, D.C.: American Association of Retired Persons.

Srnec, P. 1991, Sept. Children, violence, and intentional injuries. *Critical Care Nursing Clinics of North America* **3**: 471–478.

Tjaden, P., and Thoennes, N. 1998. Prevalence, incidence, and consequences of violence against women: Findings from the National Violence Against Survey. Institute of Justice, Research in Brief, November, 1998.

United States Department of Education. 1997. Principal/school disciplinarian survey on school violence. *Fast Response Survey System* **63**. Washington, D.C.: National Center for Educational Statistics. http://nces.ed.gov/pubs98/violence/98030003.html.

United States Department of Health and Human Services. Public Health Service, Health Resources and Services Administration. 1986. *Surgeon General's workshop on violence and public health.* DHHS Pub. no. HRS-D-MC 86-1. Washington, D.C.: Government Printing Office.

United States Department of Health and Human Services. 1989. Education about adult domestic violence in U.S. and Canadian medical schools, 1987–88. *Morbidity and Mortality Weekly Report* **38**(2): 17–19.

United States Department of Health and Human Services. 1990, Sept. *Healthy people 2000: National health promotion and disease prevention objectives.* DHHS Publ. No. (PHS) 91-50212. Washington, D.C.: Government Printing Office.

United States Department of Health and Human Services. 2000. *Healthy people 2010 injury and violence prevention objectives,* pp. 15.3–15.60. Washington, D.C.: U.S. Government Printing Office.

United States Department of Justice, Federal Bureau of Investigation. 1986. U.S. Department of Justice Crime Reports: *Crime in the U.S. 1985.* Washington, D.C.: U.S. Department of Justice.

Wang, C.T., and Daro, D. 1998. Current trends in child abuse reporting and fatalities: The results of the 1997 annual fifty-state survey. Chicago: National Committee on the Prevention of Child Abuse.

Warchol, G. 1998. Workplace violence, 1992–1996. *National Crime Victimization Survey.* Report No. NCJ-168634.

Yarn, M. 2000. Seen but not heard: Battered women's perceptions of the ED experience. *Journal of Emergency Nursing* **26**(5): 464–470.

CHAPTER 21

Nursing in a Culturally and Spiritually Diverse World

Objectives

■ Analyze concepts related to cultural diversity in nursing.

■ Discuss components of culture pertinent to nursing care.

■ Analyze concepts related to spirituality in nursing.

■ Describe the components of Leininger's Sunrise Model.

■ Differentiate among spirituality, religion, and faith.

■ Discuss the influence of spiritual beliefs on health and healing.

■ Describe barriers to cultural and spiritual sensitivity.

■ Assess clients from a cultural perspective and plan culturally competent care.

■ Assess clients from a spiritual perspective and plan spiritually competent care.

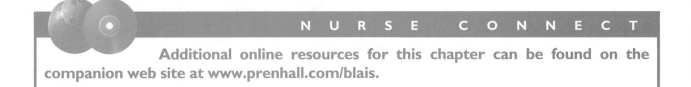

N U R S E   C O N N E C T

Additional online resources for this chapter can be found on the companion web site at www.prenhall.com/blais.

Nurses need to become informed about and sensitive to culturally and spiritually diverse subjective meanings of health, illness, caring, and healing practices. A transcultural perspective is considered essential for nurses and other health care professionals to deliver quality health care to all clients.

North America is a continent of many cultural and spiritual groups. See Tables 21–1 and 21–2. In addition to the indegenous peoples (Native Americans and Aboriginals), there is much diversity in immigrant groups in North America. The term *cultural mosaic* is used to describe the way in which many people of different cultures maintain the cultural values, beliefs, traditions, and practices of their homelands for many generations. The same term can be applied to the diverse spiritual beliefs and practices that influence health care decision making.

Nurses must understand how their own cultural and spiritual beliefs and biases relate to people whose beliefs are different. Health care professionals are not expected to know and understand all cultures and religions of the world; it is possible, however, for health care professionals to develop an awareness of those cultural and spiritual belief systems that are prevalent in the region where they practice.

Nurses must be aware that although people from a given ethnic group share certain beliefs, values, and experiences, often there is also widespread intra-ethnic diversity. Major differences within ethnic groups may be related to age, sex, level of education, socioeconomic status, religious affiliation, and area of origin in the home country (rural or urban). These factors influence the client's beliefs about health and illness, health and illness practices, health-seeking behaviors, and expectations of health professionals.

In 1991 the American Nurses Association stated that "culture is one of the organizing concepts upon which nursing is based and defined" (ANA, 1991, p. 1). Nurses need to understand how cultural groups understand life processes, how cultural groups define health and illness, what cultural groups do to maintain wellness, what cultural groups believe to be the causes of illness, how healers cure and care for members of cultural groups, and how the cultural background of a nurse influences the way in which the nurse provides care. Because a nurse is expected to provide individualized care based on an assessment of the client's physiologic, psychologic, and developmental status, the nurse must understand how the client's cultural beliefs and practices can affect the client's health and illness (ANA, 1991).

Table 21–1 United States Population Diversity 1990–1999

	1990	1995	1999
White	83.9%	83.0%	82.4%
Black	12.3%	12.6%	12.8%
Asian/Pacific Islander	3.0%	3.6%	4.0%
American Indian, Eskimo/Aleut	0.8%	0.9%	0.9%
Hispanic	9.0%	8.7%	11.5%
Foreign Born	8.0%	8.7%	9.5%

Source: United States Census Bureau. *USA Statistics in Brief—Population and Vital Statistics,* 2001. www.census.gov/statab/www/part1.html.

Table 21–2 United States Religious Diversity 1997

Protestant	58%
Catholic	26%
Jewish	2%
Other*	6%
None**	8%

*Includes Muslim, Hindu, and other specified religions not included in other categories.
**Includes those who specified atheist and those who did not designate their religious preference.
Source: Statistical Abstracts of the United States, 1998. www.census.gov/prod/religions.html.

Nurses also need to understand how individuals' spiritual beliefs influence their health decision making, how their spiritual beliefs provide strength during illness and times of adversity, and how their faith communities can provide support for health, healing, and, at the end of life, dying.

CHALLENGES AND OPPORTUNITIES

The challenges of working in a culturally diverse environment require nurses to be open to differences in beliefs about health and illness, different types of cultural healers and healing behaviors, and the use of traditional healing practices that may be considered untested to modern health practitioners. Establishing trust with people whose beliefs are different depends on a nurse's willingness to accept difference and to work with the client's different beliefs to effect a healing relationship. Spiritual beliefs also influence clients' health beliefs. Is illness the result of God's will? Is it punishment for doing evil? Can prayer heal? Can faith prevent illness? It is important for nurses to respect clients' spiritual beliefs and integrate them into the healing relationship.

Working with clients of different cultures and spiritual beliefs provides nurses with the opportunity to enrich their own lives through an understanding of the differences of others. Traditional remedies such as acupuncture, massage, meditation, and some herbs increasingly are being shown to have healing properties. Researchers are examining the effects of prayer and faith on health and healing. New knowledge derived from traditional beliefs and practices can provide new ways of healing and helping.

CONCEPTS RELATED TO CULTURE

All groups of people face similar issues in adapting to their environment: providing nutrition and shelter, caring for and educating children, division of labor, social organization, controlling disease, and maintaining health. Humans adapt to varying environments by developing cultural solutions to meet these needs. An understanding of the cultural dimension of people is the focus of the field of anthropology. Cultural anthropologists attempt to understand culture by studying both similarities and differences among human groups. Nurses use the cultural information gained by cultural anthropologists to understand and help clients (individuals, their families, or groups) to achieve optimum health.

Culture is a universal experience, but no two cultures are exactly alike. Two important terms identify the differences and similarities among peoples of different cultures. **Culture-universals** are the commonalities of values, norms of behavior, and life patterns that are similar among different cultures. **Culture-specifics** are those values, beliefs, and patterns of behavior that tend to be unique to a designated culture and do not tend to be shared with members of other cultures. For example, most cultures have ceremonies to celebrate the passage from childhood to adulthood; this practice is a culture-universal. However, different cultural groups celebrate this important life event in very different ways. In Latin or Hispanic cultures, the "quince" or "quinceañero" party, which celebrates a girl's fifteenth birthday, signifies that the young girl has now become a woman. In the Jewish tradition, the bar mitzvah (for boys) and the bat mitzvah (for girls) are celebrations of the passage to adulthood.

Anthropologists have also traditionally divided culture into material and nonmaterial culture. **Material culture** refers to objects (such as dress, art, religious artifacts, or eating utensils) and ways these are used. **Nonmaterial culture** refers to beliefs, customs, languages, and social institutions.

The terms *culture, diversity, ethnicity,* and *race* are often used interchangeably, but they are not synonymous. **Culture** is defined as "the learned, shared, and transmitted values, beliefs, norms, and lifeway practices of a particular group that guide thinking, decisions, and actions in patterned ways" (Leininger, 1988, p. 158).

Because cultural patterns are learned, it is important for nurses to note that members of a particular group may not share identical cultural experiences. Thus, each member of a cultural group will be somewhat different from his or her own cultural counterparts. For example, third-generation Japanese Americans, or Sansei, will differ in cultural understandings from first-generation Japanese Americans, or Issei. The same is also true for spiritual patterns; for example, white Roman Catholics will have cultural patterns and beliefs different from those of white Seventh Day Adventists.

Large cultural groups often have cultural subgroups or subsystems. A subculture is usually composed of people who have a distinct identity and yet are also related to a larger cultural group. A subcultural group generally shares ethnic origin, occupation, or physical characteristics with the larger cultural group. Examples of cultural subgroups include occupational groups (e.g., nurses), societal groups (e.g., feminists), and ethnic groups (e.g., Cajuns, who are descendants of French Acadians).

Bicultural refers to the integration of two cultures within the individual. In the 2000 U.S. census, individuals could identify themselves as multiracial for the first time. For an immigrant, biculturalism may be the integration of the culture of the native country, or homeland, with the culture of the new country. Children whose parents are from two different cultures may grow up in an environment that practices and respects both cultures. The values, beliefs, rituals, and traditions of both cultures may be practiced. For example, a young man whose father is Native American and whose mother is European American may maintain his traditional Native American heritage while also being influenced by his mother's cultural values.

Diversity refers "to differences in race, ethnicity, national origin, religion, age, gender, sexual orientation, ability/disability, social and economic status or class, education, and related attributes of groups of people in society" (Andrews and Boyle, 1999, p. 5). Diversity therefore occurs not only between cultural groups, but also within cultural groups.

The term *ethnic* refers to a group of people who share a common and distinctive culture and who are members of a specific group. An ethnic group is a subgroup of a larger social system whose members "have common ancestral, racial, physical or national characteristics and who share cultural symbols such as language, lifestyle, religion, and other characteristics that are not fully understood or shared by outsiders" (Andrews and Boyle, 1999, p. 10). The characteristics of the group give an individual a sense of cultural identity. Ethnicity has been defined by Sprott (1993, p. 190) as " a consciousness of belonging to a group that is differentiated from others by symbolic markers (culture, biology, territory). It is rooted in bonds of a shared past and perceived ethnic interest." Other factors that help to define ethnicity are religion and geographic background of the family.

Race is the classification of people according to shared biologic characteristics, genetic markers, or features. They have common characteristics such as skin color, bone structure, facial features, hair texture, and blood type. Different ethnic groups can belong to the same race, and different cultures can be found within the same ethnic group. For example, the term *Caucasian* and *European American* describe the race of people whose origins are in Europe. Whereas British Americans are a subgroup of European Americans, Scottish Americans (an ethnic subgroup of British Americans) may share different cultural practices than other British Americans. It is important to understand that not all people of the same race have the same culture. Culture should not be confused with either race or ethnic group.

Acculturation is the process of "becoming a competent participant in the dominant culture" (Spector, 2000, p. 76). Acculturation, also referred to as assimilation, is the integration of the cultural patterns of the dominant or host culture into the person's way of life. Spector suggests that it takes three generations for a family to become fully assimilated into the American culture.

The cultural beliefs and practices regarding the health and illness of North America's many different ethnic and cultural groups are important considerations for nurses in planning nursing care. Nursing ethnoscientists study the health beliefs of cultures so that nurses can provide culturally competent care to clients of different cultures. Madeleine Leininger, a nurse anthropologist, described **transcultural nursing** as the study of different cultures and subcultures with respect to nursing and health illness caring practices, beliefs, and values (1978, p. 493). The goal of transcultural nursing is to provide culture-specific and culture-universal nursing care. Cultural awareness and cultural sensitivity are prerequisite to the provision of culturally competent nursing care. **Cultural awareness** is the conscious and informed recognition of the differences and similarities between different cultural or ethnic groups. Cultural awareness is not knowledge derived solely from myths and stereotypes. **Cultural sensitivity** is the respect and appreciation for cultural behaviors based on an understanding of the other person's perspective. Cultural competence is "having the knowledge, understanding and skills regarding a diverse culture that allows one to provide acceptable, congruent care" (Purnell and Paulanka, 1998, p. 481). The culturally competent nurse, therefore, works within the cultural belief system of the client to resolve health problems. To provide culturally competent care, nurses need data about the client's personal and cultural views regarding health and illness. To make valid assessments, nurses need to try to see and hear the world as their clients do. When developing care plans, nurses need to consider the client's world and daily experiences. Although a client's needs and behaviors can be better understood when particular cultural health norms are identified, nurses must take care to avoid stereotyping clients by culture norms. This allows for individualized care.

Culture shock can occur when members of one culture are abruptly moved to another culture or setting. **Culture shock** is the state of being disoriented or unable to respond to a different cultural environment because of its sudden strangeness, unfamiliarity, and incompatibility to the stranger's perceptions and expectations (Leininger, 1978, p. 490). For example, when immigrants first enter the United States or Canada, language and behavior differences may initially cause them difficulty in carrying out normal activities. People can also experience culture shock when they are abruptly thrust into the health care subculture. Nursing students, for example, may experience culture shock when they enter nursing school and must learn medical terminology (a new language) and provide care for clients in clinical environments with which they are unfamiliar. Expressions of culture shock can range from silence and immobility to agitation.

Consider . . .

- the various cultural and ethnic groups in your community. Is cultural difference valued? If cultural and ethnic difference is valued, in what ways is this value manifested in your community, the nation, and the world? In what ways are negative responses to cultural difference manifested in your community, the nation, the world?

Characteristics of Culture

Culture exhibits several characteristics.
- *Culture is learned.* It is neither instinctive nor innate. It is learned through life experiences from birth.
- *Culture is taught.* It is transmitted from parents to children over successive generations. All animals can learn, but only humans can pass along culture. Verbal and nonverbal communication patterns are the transmitters of culture.
- *Culture is social.* It originates and develops through the interactions of people: families, groups, and communities.

- *Culture is adaptive.* Customs. beliefs, and practices change as people adapt to the social environment and as biologic and psychologic needs of people change. Some traditional norms in a culture may cease to provide satisfaction and are eliminated. For example, in many cultures it is customary for family members of different generations to live together (extended family); however, education and employment considerations may require children to leave their parents and move to other parts of the country. In such cases, the extended family norm may change.
- *Culture is satisfying.* Cultural habits persist only as long as they satisfy people's needs. Gratification strengthens habits and beliefs. Once they no longer bring gratification, they may disappear.
- *Culture is difficult to articulate.* Members of a specific cultural group often find it difficult to articulate their own culture. Many of the values and behaviors are habitual and are carried out subconsciously.
- *Culture exists at many levels.* Culture is most easily identified at the material level. For example, art, tools, and clothes usually reveal aspects of a culture relatively readily. More abstract concepts, such as values, beliefs, and traditions, are often more difficult to find out about. Nurses may need to ask culture-sensitive questions of the client or support persons to obtain this information.

Components of Culture

Cultures are very complex. They consist of facets that relate to all aspects of life: language, art, music, values systems (beliefs, morals, rules), religion, philosophy, family interaction, patterns of behavior, childrearing practices, rituals or ceremonies, recreation and leisure activities, festivals and holidays, nutrition, food preferences, and health practices. Many facets of culture (e.g., health and illness practices, attitudes about touch, territory and privacy, childbirth, and death and dying practices) have an impact on nursing practice.

Religious values are part of the cultural values of groups that have one dominant religion. For example, the roles of men and women in Islamic cultures are clearly defined by the Koran. The tenets of Roman Catholicism dictate the value for life and family and influence both laws and customs in many Roman Catholic cultures around the world. Culture and religion are deeply intertwined among many Jews, most notably in the nation of Israel, which is founded on Jewish beliefs and traditions.

Religious values associated with any culture influence many facets of life, including dietary restrictions, family planning, use of blood transfusions, and death-related practices, such as autopsy, organ donation, cremation, and prolonging life.

Consider . . .

■ your own cultural values, beliefs, and practices. How do you describe yourself culturally? What meaning does your cultural identification have for you? How do you celebrate your cultural identification?

CULTURE AND HEALTH CARE

Two transcultural health care systems generally exist side by side with limited awareness by practitioners of both systems: an indigenous health care system and a professional health care system (Leininger, 1993, p. 36). The *indigenous health care system* refers to traditional folk health care methods, such as folk medicines and other home treatments. The modern *professional health care system* refers to a structured system maintained by individuals who have engaged in a formal program of study. The indigenous system is the older system and has often provided health care long before a professional system enters the culture. According to Leininger, few professional health care workers are knowledgeable about the indigenous health care system or its practitioners. Some professionals regard the indigenous system as unscientific, "primitive," or even as "quackery." Leininger emphasizes that the goal of health care should be to use the best of both systems and that health professionals need to consider ways to interface with the two systems for the benefit of the people served. "Every culture has health, caring, and curing processes, techniques, and practices viewed as important to the people" (p. 38).

Currently there is much interest in and inquiry into the efficacy of folk healing methods and herbal remedies. These healing practices are considered complementary or alternative to Western or scientific medicine. In 1998 the National Center for Complementary and Alternative Medicine (NCCAM) was established at the National Institutes of Health to stimulate, develop, and support research on the benefits of complementary and alternative medicines to the public (NCCAM, 2001).

Leininger's Sunrise Model

Leininger produced the Sunrise Model to depict her theory of cultural care diversity and universality (Figure 21–1). This model emphasizes that health and care are influenced by elements of the social structure, such as technology, religious and philosophical factors, kinship and social systems, cultural values, political and legal factors, economic factors, and educational factors. These social factors are addressed within environmental contexts, language expressions, and ethnohistory. Each of these systems is part of the social structure of any society; health care expressions, patterns, and practices are also integral parts of these aspects of social structure (Leininger, 1993).

Technologic factors, such as the availability of technical and electrical equipment, greatly determine what health equipment will be used. For example, many European Americans regard resuscitative equipment as essential. The *economic* system determines the quality of health care within a culture, for example, the availability of funds for health care services materially affects the health of the culture's infants and aged. The *political* system is a major determinant of what health programs will be available and which health practitioners may provide health services. *Legal* aspects govern the roles, functions, and standards of health professionals within cultures. *Kinship and the social system* often influence who will or will not receive health care and how promptly it will be provided. For example, in some cultures a person of high status (e.g., tribal leader, CEO, or king) may receive prompt care; a person of lower status (e.g., a peasant, housewife, or child) may experience a considerable waiting period for care. Because of male dominance in many cultures, men may receive care before a wife or female child. *Cultural, educational, religious,* and *philosophical* factors are closely related. They influence the type, quality, and quantity of health care considered desirable, appropriate, or acceptable to the culture. *Environmental* and *demographic* factors relate to the health needs of the culture and which strategies of care can be used in the setting.

Since the development of Leininger's Sunrise Model, several other transcultural nursing models have been developed. These include Murdock's Outline of Cultural Material, appropriate for community cultural assessment (Murdock, 1971); Bloch's Assessment Guide for Ethnic/Cultural Variation (Orque, Bloch, and Monrroy, 1983); Giger and Davidhizar's (1995) Model of Cultural Assessment; The Felder Cultural Diversity Practice Model (Felder, 1995); Purnell's Conceptual Model for Cultural Competence (Purnell and Paulanka, 1998); and the Model for Developing Cultural Sensitivity (Baldwin et al., 1996). All models are useful for assessing the belief systems and health practices of individuals and groups of different cultures and religions.

CULTURALLY SENSITIVE CARE

Kittler and Sucher (1990) suggest a four-step process to improve cultural sensitivity:

Figure 22–1

Leininger's Sunrise Model

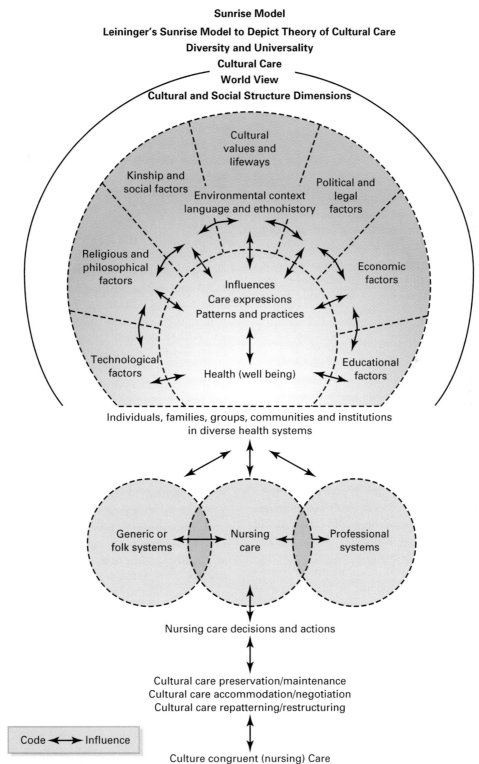

Sunrise Model

Leininger's Sunrise Model to Depict Theory of Cultural Care Diversity and Universality

Cultural Care

World View

Cultural and Social Structure Dimensions

Cultural values and lifeways

Kinship and social factors

Environmental context language and ethnohistory

Political and legal factors

Religious and philosophical factors

Economic factors

Influences
Care expressions
Patterns and practices

Technological factors

Health (well being)

Educational factors

Individuals, families, groups, communities and institutions in diverse health systems

Generic or folk systems

Nursing care

Professional systems

Nursing care decisions and actions

Cultural care preservation/maintenance
Cultural care accommodation/negotiation
Cultural care repatterning/restructuring

Culture congruent (nursing) Care

Code ◄—► Influence

Source: Culture Care Diversity and Universality: A Theory of Nursing by M. Leininger, New York: National League for Nursing Pub. No. 15-2402, 1991, p. 43. Reprinted with permission.

1. *Become aware of one's own cultural heritage.* Nurses should identify their own cultural values and beliefs. For example, does the nurse value stoic behavior in relation to pain? Are the rights of the individual valued over and above the rights of the family? Only by knowing one's own culture (values, practices, and beliefs) can a person be ready to learn about another's.

2. *Become aware of the client's culture as described by the client.* It is important to avoid assuming that all people of the same ethnic background have the same culture. When the nurse has a knowledge of the client's culture, mutual respect between client and nurse is more likely to develop.

3. *Become aware from the client of adaptations made to live in a North American culture.* During this interview, a nurse can also identify the client's preferences in health practices, diet, hygiene, and so on.

4. *Form a nursing care plan with the client that incorporates his or her culture.* In this way, cultural values, practices, and beliefs can be incorporated with care and judgment.

Barriers to Cultural Sensitivity

Many factors can be barriers to providing culturally sensitive or culturally congruent care to clients and their support persons. These factors can also affect communication and working relationships with other health care personnel. Ethnocentrism, stereotyping, prejudice, and discrimination are some of these factors.

Ethnocentrism refers to an individual's belief that his or her culture's beliefs and values are superior to those of other cultures. In the health care area, ethnocentrism means that the only valid health care beliefs and practices are those held by the health care culture. Nurses who take a transcultural view, however, value their own beliefs and practices while respecting the beliefs and practices of others. It is important for nurses to realize that although many people of differing racial and religious backgrounds have combined their traditional health practices with Western health practices, other people may be unable to do so.

Most people are gradually exposed to their cultural beliefs, values, and practices over a period of years starting at birth. Ethnocentricism is thought to result from lack of exposure or knowledge of cultures other than one's own. **Ethnorelativity** is the ability to appreciate and respect other viewpoints different from one's own.

Stereotyping is assuming that all members of a culture or ethnic group are alike. For example, a nurse may assume that all Italians express pain verbally or

that all Chinese people like rice. Stereotyping may be based on generalizations founded in research, or it may be unrelated to reality. For example, research indicates that Italians are likely to express pain verbally; however, an Italian client may not verbalize pain. Stereotyping that is unrelated to reality may be either positive or negative and is frequently an outcome of racism or discrimination.

It is important for nurses to realize that not all people of a specific group will have the same health beliefs, practices, and values. It is therefore essential to identify a specific client's beliefs, needs, and values rather than assuming they are the same as those attributable to the larger group.

Prejudice is strongly held opinion about some topic or group of people. A prejudice may be positive or negative. A positive prejudice often stems from a strong sense of ethnocentrism (Eliason, 1993, p. 226), that is, beliefs that one's cultural group holds are vastly superior to the beliefs held by others. One example is that American nursing education is superior to European nursing education. Prejudice may also derive from ignorance, misinformation, past experience, or fear. Other types of negative prejudice are ageism, which includes negative attitudes toward older adults; sexism, meaning negative attitudes toward women; and homophobia, which is negativism toward lesbians and gay men.

Discrimination is the differential treatment of one person or group over another based on race, ethnicity, gender, age, social class, disability, sexual preference, or other distinguishing characteristic. For example, a nurse takes a child who is waiting in an emergency department ahead of another child. The child taken first appears clean, is neatly dressed, and is smiling; the other child appears dirty, is wearing worn clothes, and is angry. **Racism** is a form of discrimination related to ethnocentrism where a person believes that race is the primary determinant of human traits and capacities and that racial differences produce an inherent superiority of a particular race.

Conveying Cultural Sensitivity

It is important for nurses to be culturally sensitive and to convey this sensitivity to clients, support persons, and other health care personnel. Some of the ways to do so follow.

- Always address clients by their last names (e.g., Mrs. Aylia, Dr. Rush) until they give you permission to use other names. In some cultures, the more formal style of address is a sign of respect, whereas the informal use of first names may be considered disrespect. It is important to ask clients how they wish to be addressed.

- When meeting a person for the first time, introduce yourself by name, and, when appropriate, explain your position. This helps establish a relationship and provides an opportunity for both clients and nurses to clarify pronunciation of one another's names, and so on.
- Be authentic with people, and share your lack of knowledge about their culture.
- Use language that is culturally sensitive; for example, say gay, lesbian, or bisexual rather than homosexual; do not use man or mankind when referring to a woman; African American and Latino are currently preferred over black or Hispanic. Asian is more acceptable than Oriental (Eliason, 1993, p. 228). However, nurses need to keep up with language changes.
- Find out what the client knows about his or her health problems, illness, and treatments. Assess whether this information is congruent with the dominant health care culture. If the beliefs and practices are incongruent, establish whether this will have a negative effect on the client's health.
- Do not make any assumptions about the client, and always ask about anything you don't understand.
- Respect the client's values, beliefs, and practices, even if they differ from your own or from those of the dominant culture. If you don't agree with them, it is important to respect the client's right to hold these beliefs.
- Show respect for the client's support people. In some cultures males in the family make decisions affecting the client, while in other cultures females make the decisions.
- Make a concerted effort to obtain the client's trust, but do not be surprised if it develops slowly or not at all.

CONCEPTS RELATED TO SPIRITUALITY

Religious and spiritual beliefs are an integral part of a person's cultural beliefs and can influence a client's beliefs about the cause of illness, healing practices, and the choice of healer or health care provider. Spiritual and religious beliefs can be a source of strength and comfort for clients experiencing illness or crisis or approaching death.

Spirituality, Religion, and Faith

Spirituality, religion, and faith, although often used interchangeably, are different. The nurse must be aware of the differences to understand the depth of feeling that clients have about their beliefs. The word *spiritual* derives from the Latin word *spiritus,* which means "to blow" or "to breathe" (the same word origin for inspire

and respiration), and has come to mean that which gives life or essence to the soul. According to O'Brien (1999, p. 6), spirituality includes "love, compassion, caring, transcendence, relationship with God, and the connection of body, mind, and spirit." **Spirituality** is the belief in or relationship with a higher power, creative force, divine being, or infinite source of energy. For example, a person may believe in God, Jehovah, Allah, the Creator, or a Higher Power. Burkhardt (1993, p. 12) describes the following aspects of spirituality:

- Dealing with the unknown or uncertainties in life
- Finding meaning and purpose in life
- Being aware of and able to draw upon inner resources and strength
- Having a feeling of connectedness with oneself and with God or a Higher Being

"The spiritual dimension tries to be in harmony with the universe, strives for answers about the infinite, and especially comes into focus or sustaining power when the person faces emotional stress, physical illness, or death. It goes outside a person's own power" (Murray and Zentner, 2001, p. 116). Characteristics of spirituality are listed in the box on page 348.

Religion is defined by Dossey, Keegan, and Guzzetta (2000, p. 92) as "an organized system of beliefs shared by a group of people and the practices, including worship, related to that system." It provides a way of spiritual expression that guides people in responding to life's questions and crises. According to Vardey (1995, p. xv), the organized religions offer (1) a sense of community bound by common beliefs, (2) the collective study of scripture (the Bible, Torah, Koran, or others), (3) the performance of ritual, (4) the use of disciplines and practices, commandments, and sacraments, and (5) ways of taking care of the person's soul (such as fasting, prayer, and meditation). Many traditional religious practices and rituals are related to life events such as birth, transition from childhood to adulthood, marriage, illness, and death. Religious rules of conduct, like cultural beliefs, may also apply to matters of daily life such as dress, food, social interaction, and sexual relationships. Religious development of an individual refers to the acceptance of specific beliefs, values, rules of conduct, and rituals. Religious development may or may not parallel spiritual development. For example, a person may follow certain religious practices yet not internalize the symbolic meaning behind the practices. **Faith** is "deeper and more personal than organized religion. . . . [It relates] to one's transcendent values and relationship with a higher power, or God" (O'Brien, 1999, p. 58).

Characteristics of Spirituality

RELATIONSHIP WITH SELF

Inner strength/self-reliance

- Self-knowledge (who one is, what one can do)
- Attitudes (trust in self, trust in life and the future, peace of mind, harmony with self)

RELATIONSHIP WITH NATURE

Harmony

- Knowing about plants, trees, wildlife, weather
- Communing with nature (gardening, walking, being outside); preserving nature

RELATIONSHIP WITH OTHERS

- Sharing time, knowledge, and resources; reciprocating
- Caring for children, elderly, sick
- Reaffirming the living and the dead (visiting, photos, cemetery meetings)

RELATIONSHIP WITH DEITY

Religious or nonreligious

- Prayer-meditation
- Religious articles
- Being in nature
- Church participation

Source: M. Burkhardt, "Characteristics of Spirituality in the Lives of Women in a Rural Appalachian Community." *Journal of Transcultural Nursing,* 4: 12–18, Winter, 1993. Used with permission.

Prayer and Meditation

Prayer is a communication or petition to God in word or thought. Meditation is an internal reflection or contemplation. Prayer or meditation are part of most religions. Depending on the specific religion, prayer is a communication with God, Jehovah, Allah, or some Higher Power. In some religions, prayers may be channeled through another; for example, Catholics may pray to God through a saint or the Virgin Mary. Prayers may be a petition or request (e.g., cure from illness or relief from pain), a thanksgiving (e.g., for healing), or a spiritual communion (e.g., to find peace or acceptance). Dossey (1993) identifies seven forms of prayer that may be used when someone is ill (see the accompanying box). Some religions have formal prayers that are printed in a prayer book, such as the Anglican or Episcopal Book of Common Prayer or the Catholic Missal. Some religious prayers are attributed to the source of faith; for example, the Lord's Prayer is at-

Types of Prayer

Petition	Asking something for oneself
Intercession	Asking something for another
Confession	Repentance of wrongdoing and asking forgiveness
Thanksgiving	Offering gratitude
Adoration	Giving honor and praise
Invocation	Summoning the presence of the Almighty
Lamentation	Crying in distress and asking for vindication

Source: Adapted from L. Dossey, *Healing Words: The Power of Prayer and the Practice of Medicine.* New York: Harper San Francisco, 1993, p. 5.

tributed to Jesus, and the first sutra for Muslims is attributed to Mohammed.

Daily prayers are prescribed by some religions. For example, Muslims perform the five daily prayers, or Salat, while facing toward Mecca, at dawn, noon, midafternoon, sunset, and evening. Jews may say the daily Kaddish. People who are ill may want to continue their prayer practices. Moschella et al. (1997) report that patients may even increase their prayer practices in response to illness (see the accompanying box). People may memorize prayers during childhood, and their repetition becomes a source of comfort during illness or adversity. Clients may need uninterrupted quiet time or want to have their prayer books, rosaries, prayer beads, or other sacred symbols available to them. Some clients may want their minister, priest, rabbi, mullah, or other spiritual advisor with them when they pray.

Consider . . .

- your own spiritual and religious beliefs. How do they affect your beliefs about health and illness? How important would it be for you to be able to practice your spiritual and religious traditions if you were ill?
- the various spiritual and religious groups in your community. Is religious difference valued? Where could you go to learn more about the religious groups

---

Research Box

Moschella, V. D., Pressman, K. R., Pressman, P., and Weissman, D. E. Spring 1997. The problem of theodicy and religious response to cancer. *Journal of Religion and Health* **36**(1): 17–20.

The researchers studied the religious response to cancer in a group of 45 hematology/oncology-clinic patients. Of the 45 patients 67% ($n = 30$) increased their amount of prayer, 51% ($n = 23$) gained faith, and 16% ($n = 7$) increased the frequency of church attendance in response to their illness. The majority of patients across all levels of religious belief endorse a belief that God is good and omnipotent in the face of evil and suffering and that God has a reason for their suffering, but this reason cannot be explained or understood. The authors conclude that "religious cancer patients intensify their religious belief and practice in response to their illness. Despite the elusiveness of an explanation for their suffering in religious terms, patients remain confident in their faith."

Nurses must understand the importance of a client's spiritual beliefs as they relate to the client's potential for healing or acceptance of their illness or injury. With this understanding, nurses can better support clients in their spiritual practices.

Research Box

McSherry, W. M. 1998. Nurses' perceptions of spirituality and spiritual care. *Nursing Standard* **13**(4): 36–40.

A descriptive survey was used to discover and discuss perceptions of spirituality and spiritual care of 1029 nurses employed in a large national health service trust in Yorkshire, U.K. A questionnaire consisting of five parts (demographics, work issues, spirituality and spiritual care rating scale [SSCRS], provision of spiritual care, religious affiliation, and comments) was mailed to participants; 559 (55.3%) were returned. The SSCRS consisted of items rated on a five-point Likert scale. Factor analysis was used to analyze the SSCRS statements. Frequencies and qualitative analysis were used on the remainder of the questionnaire.

Findings of the study indicate that nurses do not perceive spirituality as a concept that embraces only religious beliefs and formal religious worship. It is perceived as a universal concept experienced by and relevant to all. Findings of the factor analysis indicate that the nurses are aware of the existential, universal, and individual nature of spirituality. Nurses perceive that they are able to identify patients experiencing spiritual needs but report they are not totally comfortable addressing such needs. Lack of education and training were identified as concerns about providing spiritual care; they called for the formal integration of the spiritual dimension into the nursing curricula. The provision of spiritual care was seen as a part of the nurse's role, but nurses believe that a team approach is needed. Little evidence was found to support the idea that nurses who practice a formal religion are more effective. Findings suggest that nurses strive to be nonjudgmental in providing spiritual care.

in your community? In what ways could you as a professional nurse support the spiritual and religious practices of your clients?

SELECTED CULTURAL AND SPIRITUAL PARAMETERS INFLUENCING NURSING CARE

This section outlines selected cultural, ethnic, and spiritual phenomena of significance to nursing.

Health Beliefs and Practices

Andrews and Boyle (1995, pp. 22–29) describe three health belief views: magico-religious, scientific, and holistic. In the **magico-religious health belief view,** health and illness are controlled by supernatural forces. The client may believe that illness is the result of "being bad" or opposing God's will. Getting well is also viewed as dependent on God's will. The client may make statements such as, "If it is God's will, I will recover," or "What did I do wrong to be punished with cancer?" Some cultures believe that magic can cause illness. A sorcerer or witch may put a spell or hex on the client. Some people view illness as possession by an evil spirit. Although these beliefs are not supported by empirical evidence, clients who believe that such things can cause illness may, in fact, become ill as a result. Such illnesses may require magical treatments in addition to scientific treatments. For example, a man who experiences gastric distress, headaches, and hypertension after being told that a spell has been placed on him may recover only if the spell is removed by the culture's healer.

The scientific, or **biomedical health belief view** is based on the belief that life and life processes are controlled by physical and biochemical processes that can be manipulated by humans (Andrews and Boyle, 1995, p. 23). The client with this view will believe that illness is caused by germs, viruses, bacteria, or a breakdown of the human machine, the body. This client will expect a pill, or treatment, or a surgery to cure health problems.

The **holistic health belief view** holds that the forces of nature must be maintained in balance or harmony. Human life is one aspect of nature that must be in harmony with the rest of nature. When the natural balance or harmony is disturbed, illness results. The Medicine Wheel is an ancient symbol used by Native Americans of North and South America to express many concepts. Related to health and wellness, the Medicine Wheel teaches the four aspects of the individual's nature: the physical, the mental, the emotional, and the spiritual. Each of the dimensions must be in balance to be healthy. The Medicine Wheel can also be used to express the individual's relationship with the environment as a dimension of wellness. The concept of yin and yang in the Chinese culture and the hot/cold theory of illness in many Spanish cultures are examples of holistic health beliefs. When the client has a yin illness, or a "cold" illness, the treatment will need to include a yang, or "hot," food. For example, a Chinese client who has been diagnosed with cancer, a yin disease, will want to eat cultural foods that have yang properties. What is considered as hot or cold varies considerably across cultures. In many cultures, the mother who has just delivered a baby should be offered warm or hot foods and kept warm with blankets, because childbirth is seen as a cold condition. Conventional scientific thought recommends cooling the body to reduce a fever. The physician may order liquids for the client and cool compresses to be applied to the forehead, the axillae, or the groin. Galanti (1991, p. 97) states that many cultures believe that the best way to treat a fever is to "sweat it out." Clients from these cultures may want to cover up with several blankets, take hot baths, and drink hot beverages. Giger and Davidhizar (1995, p. 84) state that the nurse must keep in mind that a treatment strategy that is consistent with the client's beliefs may have a better chance of being successful. For example, the Mexican-American client who avoids "hot" foods when he has a stomach disturbance such as an ulcer may be eating foods consistent with the bland diet that is normally prescribed by physicians for clients with ulcers.

Sociocultural forces, such as politics, economics, geography, religion, and the predominant health care system, can influence the client's health status and health care behavior. For example, people who have limited access to scientific health care may turn to folk medicine or folk healing. **Folk medicine** is defined as those beliefs and practices relating to illness prevention and healing which derive from cultural traditions rather than from modern medicine's scientific base. The nurse may recall special teas or "cures" that were used by older family members to prevent or treat colds, fevers, indigestion, and other common health problems. For example, many people continue to use chicken soup as a treatment for flu.

Why do individuals use these nontraditional folk healing methods? Folk medicine, in contrast to biomedical health care, is thought to be more humanistic. The consultation and treatment takes place in the community of the recipient, frequently in the home of the healer. It is less expensive than scientific or biomedical care, because the health problem is identified primarily through conversation with the client and the family. The healer often prepares the treatments, for example, teas to be ingested, poultices to be applied, or charms or amulets to be worn. A frequent component of treatment is some ritual practice on the part of the healer or the client to cause healing to occur. Because folk healing is more culturally based, it is often more comfortable and less frightening for the client.

It is important for the nurse to obtain information about folk or family healing practices that may have been used prior to the client's seeking Western medical treatment. Often clients are reluctant to share home remedies with health care professionals for fear of being laughed at or rebuked. The nurse should remember that treatments once considered to be folk treatments, including acupuncture, therapeutic touch, and massage are now being investigated for their therapeutic effect.

Consider . . .

■ nursing situations in your experience that reflect each of the health belief views as described by Andrews and Boyle: the magico-religious health belief view, the biomedical health belief view, and the holistic health belief view. Describe culturally competent nursing interventions that would be appropriate to each of your nursing situations.

Family Patterns

The family is the basic unit of society. Cultural and religious values can determine communication within the family group, the norm for family size, and the roles of specific family members. In some families the man is usually the provider and decision maker. The woman may need to consult her husband prior to making decisions about her medical treatment or the treatment of her children (Galanti, 1991). Some families are matriarchal; that is, the mother or grandmother is viewed as the leader of the family and is usually the decision maker. The nurse needs to identify who has the "authority" to make decisions in a client's family. If the decision maker is someone other than the client, the nurse needs to include that person in health care discussions.

The value placed on children and elderly within a society is culturally derived. In some cultures, children are not disciplined by spanking or other forms of physical punishment. Rather, children are allowed to interact with their environment and to learn from their environment while caregivers provide subtle direction to prevent harm or injury. In other cultures, the elderly are considered the holders of the culture's wisdom and are therefore highly respected. Responsibility for caring for older relatives is determined by cultural practices. In many cultures, older relatives who cannot live independently often live with a married daughter and her family.

Culture and religious norms about sex-role behavior may also affect nurse-client interaction. In some countries, the male dominates and women have little status. The male client from these countries may not accept instruction from a female nurse or physician but be receptive to the same instruction given by a male physician or nurse (Galanti, 1991). In some cultures, there is a prevailing concept of machismo, or male superiority. The positive aspects of machismo require that the adult male provide for and protect his family, including extended family members. The woman is expected to maintain the home and raise the children.

Cultural family values may also dictate the extent of the family's involvement in the hospitalized client's care. In some cultures, the nuclear and the extended family will want to visit for long periods of time and participate in care. In other cultures, the entire clan may want to visit and participate in the client's care (Galanti, 1991). This can cause concern on nursing units with strict visiting policies. The nurse should evaluate the positive benefits of family participation in the client's care and modify visiting policies as appropriate.

Cultures that value the needs of the extended family as much as those of the individual may hold the belief that personal and family information must stay within the family. Some cultural groups are very reluctant to disclose family information to outsiders, including health care professionals. This attitude can present difficulties for health care professionals who require knowledge of family interaction patterns to help clients with emotional problems.

In many cultures naming systems differ from those in North America. In some cultures (e.g., Japanese and Vietnamese) the family name comes first and the given name, second. One or two names may or may not be added between the family and given names. Other nomenclature may be used to delineate sexual, child, or adult status. For example, in traditional Japanese culture, adults address other adults by their surname followed by *san*, meaning *Mr., Mrs.,* or *Miss.* An example is Murakami san. The children are referred to by their first names followed by *kun* for boys and *chan* for girls. Sikhs and Hindus traditionally have three names. Hindus have a personal name, a complimentary name, and then a family name. Sikhs have a personal name, then the title *Singh* for men and *Kaur* for women, and lastly the family name. Names by marriage also vary. In Central America, a woman who marries retains her father's name and takes her husband's. For example, if Louisa Viccario marries Carlos Gonzales she becomes Louisa Viccario de Gonzales. The connecting *de* means "belonging to." A male child will be Pedro Gonzales Viccario. Nurses need to become familiar with appropriate ways to address clients. In many cultures, using a client's first name is considered patronizing.

Communication Style

Communication style and culture are closely interconnected. Through communication, the culture is transmitted from one generation to the next, and knowledge about the culture is transmitted within the group and to those outside the group. Communicating with clients of various ethnic and cultural backgrounds is critical to providing culturally competent nursing care. Luckmann (2000, p. 15) identifies the following influencing factors for implementing transcultural communication:

1. The increase in ethnic, racial, and cultural diversity in the United States

2. The increase in cultural, ethnic, and disenfranchised populations who seek health care

3. Multicultural and multinational settings for health care delivery

4. The commitment of health care professions to provide high-quality, culturally appropriate care.

Verbal Communication

The most obvious cultural difference is in verbal communication: vocabulary, grammatical structure, voice qualities, intonation, rhythm, speed, pronunciation, and silence (Giger and Davidhizar, 1995, p. 23). In North America, the dominant language is English; however, immigrant groups who speak English still encounter language differences, because English words can have different meanings in different English-speaking cultures. For example, in the United States a boot is a type of footwear that comes to the ankle or higher; in England, a boot can also be the trunk of a car. Spanish is spoken by people in several regions of the world: Spain, South America, Central America, Mexico, the Caribbean, and the Philippines. It is the second most commonly spoken language in the United States. Nevertheless, each cultural group that speaks Spanish may use different vocabulary, apply rules of grammar differently, and use different pronunciation, so that often two people of different

Latino cultures, speaking Spanish together, may not completely understand each other.

Initiating verbal communication may be influenced by cultural values. The busy nurse may want to complete nursing admission assessments quickly. The client, however, may be offended when the nurse immediately asks personal questions. In some cultures, it is believed that social courtesies should be established before business or personal topics are discussed. Discussing general topics can convey that the nurse is interested in the client and has time for the client. This enables the nurse to develop a rapport with the client before progressing to more personal discussion.

Verbal communication becomes even more difficult when an interaction involves people who speak different languages. Both clients and health professionals experience frustration when they are unable to communicate verbally with each other. For clients who have limited knowledge of English, the nurse should avoid slang words, medical terminology, and abbreviations. Augmenting spoken conversation with gestures or pictures can increase the client's understanding. The nurse should speak slowly, in a respectful manner and at a normal volume. Speaking loudly does not help the client understand and may be offensive. The nurse must also frequently validate the client's understanding of what is being communicated. The nurse must be wary of interpreting a client's broad smiling and head nodding to mean that the client understands; the client may only be trying to please the nurse and not understand what is being said.

For the client who speaks a different language, a translator may be necessary. Luckmann (2000) suggests that it is best to use a professional medical interpreter who can facilitate communication between people speaking different languages in a health care setting. Guidelines for using an interpreter are shown in the box on page 353.

Translators should be objective individuals who can provide accurate translation of the client's information and of the health professional's questions, information, and instruction. Many institutions that are located in culturally diverse communities have translators available on staff or maintain a list of employees who are fluent in other languages. Embassies, consulates, ethnic churches (e.g., Russian Orthodox, Greek Orthodox), ethnic clubs (e.g., Polish-American Club, Italian-American Club) or telephone communication companies may also be able to provide translating services. Nursing and other health personnel can use pictures and gestures to augment verbal communication. Some schools of nursing and health care in-

Using an Interpreter

- Avoid asking a member of the client's family, especially a child or spouse, to act as interpreter. The client, not wishing family members to know about his or her problem, may not provide complete or accurate information.
- Be aware of gender and age differences; it is preferable to use an interpreter of the same sex as the client to avoid embarrassment and faulty translation of sexual matters.
- Avoid an interpreter who is politically or socially incompatible with the client. For example, a Bosnian

Serb may not be the best interpreter for a Muslim, even if he speaks the language.
- Address the questions to the client, *not* to the interpreter.
- Ask the interpreter to translate as closely as possible to the words used by the nurse.
- Speak slowly and distinctly. Do *not* use metaphors, for example, "Does it swell like a grapefruit?" or "Is the pain stabbing like a knife?"
- Observe the facial expressions and body language that the client assumes when listening and talking to the interpreter.

stitutions do not permit nursing students to translate for a procedure consent because a lack of knowledge about the procedure may lead the student to give inaccurate information. The student should check the institution's policy prior to agreeing to translate for institutional staff and physicians.

Nurses and other health care providers must remember that clients for whom English is a second language may lose command of their English when they are in stressful situations. It is not uncommon for clients who have used English comfortably for years in social and business communication to forget and revert back to their primary language when they are ill or distressed. It is important for the nurse to assure the client that this is normal and to promote behaviors to facilitate verbal communication.

Nonverbal Communication

To communicate effectively with culturally diverse clients, the nurse needs to be aware of two aspects of nonverbal communication behaviors: what nonverbal behaviors mean to the client and what specific nonverbal behaviors mean in the client's culture. It is not required that the nurse be knowledgeable about the nonverbal behavior patterns of all cultures; however, before the nurse assigns meaning to nonverbal behavior, the nurse must consider the possibility that the behavior may have a different meaning for the client and the family. Furthermore, to provide safe and effective care, nurses who work with specific cultural groups should learn more about cultural behavior and communication patterns within those cultures.

Nonverbal communication can include the use of

silence, touch, eye movement, facial expressions, and body posture. Some cultures are quite comfortable with long periods of silence, whereas others consider it appropriate to speak before the other person has finished talking. Many persons value silence and view it as essential to understanding a person's needs or use silence to preserve privacy. Some cultures view silence as a sign of respect, whereas to other persons silence may indicate agreement (Giger and Davidhizar, 1995, p. 28).

Touch and touching is a learned behavior that can have both positive and negative meanings. In the American culture, a firm handshake is a recognized form of greeting that conveys character and strength (Giger and Davidhizar, 1995, p. 28). In some European cultures, greetings may include a kiss on one or both cheeks along with the handshake. In some societies, touch is considered magical and because of the belief that the soul can leave the body on physical contact, casual touching is forbidden. In the Hmong culture, only certain elders are permitted to touch the head of others, and children are never patted on the head. Nurses should therefore touch a client's head only with permission (Rairdan and Higgs, 1992, p. 55). The sex of the person touching and being touched often has cultural significance. Purnell and Paulanka (1998, p. 18) describe how among Egyptian-Americans, touch between men and women is accepted "in private and only between husband and wife, parents and children, and adult brothers and sisters."

Cultures also dictate what forms of touch are appropriate for individuals of the same sex and opposite sex. In many cultures, for example, a kiss is not appropriate for a public greeting between persons of the opposite sex, even those who are family members; however, a kiss on the cheek is acceptable as a greeting among individuals of the same sex. The nurse should watch interaction among clients and families for cues to the appropriate degree of touch in that culture. The nurse can also assess the client's response to touch when providing nursing care, for example, by noting the client's reaction to the physical examination or the bath.

Facial expression can also vary between cultures. Giger and Davidhizar (1995, p. 13) state that Italian, Jewish, African-American, and Spanish-speaking persons are more likely to smile readily and use facial expression to communicate feelings, whereas Irish, English, and northern European persons tend to have less facial expression and are less open in their response, especially to strangers. Facial expression can also convey the opposite meaning of what is felt or understood. For example, clients who have difficulty understanding English may smile and nod their heads as though they understood what is being said, when, in fact, they do not understand at all, but do not want to displease the caregiver.

Eye movement during communication has cultural foundations. In Western cultures, direct eye contact is regarded as important and generally shows that the other is attentive and listening. It conveys self-confidence, openness, interest, and honesty. Lack of eye contact may be interpreted as secretiveness, shyness, guilt, lack of interest, or even a sign of mental illness. Other cultures may view eye contact as impolite or an invasion of privacy. In the Hmong culture, continuous direct eye contact is considered rude, but intermittent eye contact is acceptable (Rairdan and Higgs, 1992, p. 53). The nurse should not misinterpret the character of the client who avoids eye contact.

Body posture and gesture are also culturally learned. Finger pointing, the "V" sign with the index and middle fingers, and the "thumbs up" sign may have different meanings. For example, the "V" sign means victory in some cultures, whereas it may be an offensive gesture in other cultures (Galanti, 1991, p. 22). In the Hmong culture, bowing the head slightly when entering the room where an elder is present or using both hands to give something to someone are considered signs of respect (Rairdan and Higgs, 1993, p. 52).

Communication is an essential part of establishing a relationship with a client and their family. It is also important for developing effective working relationships with health care colleagues. To enhance their practice, nurses can observe the communication patterns of clients and colleagues and be aware of their own communication behaviors. The accompanying box provides strategies for communicating with clients

Strategies for Communicating with Clients from Different Cultures

- Consider the cultural component of communication, and integrate it into the relationship.

- Encourage the client to communicate cultural interpretations of health, illness, treatments, and planned care. Incorporate this into the plan of care so that it is congruent with the client's lifestyle and needs as the client views them.

- Understand that respect for clients and their communicated needs is crucial to the effective helping relationship.

- Use an open and attentive approach so that the client knows you are really listening.

- Relate to the client in an unhurried manner that considers the social and cultural amenities. Give the client time to answer. Engage in appropriate social conversation prior to discussing more intimate or personal details.

- Use validation techniques while communicating to check that the client understands. Note that big smiles and frequent head nodding may indicate merely that the client is trying to please you, not necessarily that the client understands you.

- Sexual concerns may be difficult for clients to discuss. Try to have a nurse of the same sex as the client discuss sexual matters.

- Use alternative methods of communication for clients who do not speak English: foreign language dictionaries or phrase books, interpreter, gestures, pictures, facial expressions, tone of voice.

- Learn key phrases in languages that are commonly spoken in the community. For example, medical phrase books are available in Spanish and French.

from different cultures. The same strategies can be used in communication with professional colleagues.

Consider . . .

■ your own values, beliefs, and practices related to verbal and nonverbal communication. How might your values, beliefs, and practices related to communication conflict with those of people from the different cultural groups in your community?

Space Orientation

Space is a relative concept that includes the individual, the body, the surrounding environment, and objects within that environment. The relationship between the individual's own body and objects and persons within space is learned and is influenced by culture. For example, in nomadic societies space is not owned; it is occupied temporarily until the tribe moves on. In Western societies people tend to be more territorial, as reflected in phrases such as "This is my space" or "Get out of my space." In Western cultures, spatial distances are defined as the intimate zone, the personal zone, the social and the public zones. The intimate zone is the smallest area of space around the individual, the public zone the largest area. The size of these areas may vary with the specific culture. Nurses move through all four zones as they provide care for clients. The nurse needs to be aware of the client's response to movement toward the client. The client may physically withdraw or back away if the nurse is perceived as being too close. The nurse will need to explain to the client why there is a need to be close to the client. To assess the lungs with a stethoscope, for example, the nurse needs to move into the client's intimate space. The nurse should first explain the procedure and await permission to continue.

Clients who reside in long-term care facilities, or are hospitalized for an extended time, may want to personalize their space. They may want to arrange their space differently and control the placement of objects on their bedside cabinet or over-bed table. The nurse should be responsive to clients' needs to have some control over their space. When there are no medical contraindications, clients should be permitted and encouraged to wear their own clothing and have objects of personal significance. Wearing cultural dress or having personal, cultural, and spiritual items in one's environment can increase self-esteem by promoting not only one's individuality but also one's cultural and spiritual identity. Of course, the nurse should caution the client about responsibility for loss of personal items.

Time Orientation

Time orientation refers to an individual's focus on the past, the present, or the future. Most cultures combine all three time orientations, but one orientation is more likely to dominate. The European-American focus on time tends to be directed to the future, emphasizing time and schedules (Purnell and Paulanka, 1998). Nursing students know what times they "must" be in class or clinical. They know what courses they will take in future semesters. European Americans often plan for next week, their vacation, or their retirement. Other cultures may have a different concept of time. Leininger (1978, pp. 256, 262) describes the Navajo emphasis as "on the flow of life within the natural environment without specific time boundaries." For example, a Navajo mother may not be concerned about when her child achieves developmental milestones, such as walking or toileting.

The culture of nursing and health care values time. Appointments are scheduled and treatments are prescribed with time parameters (e.g., changing a dressing once a day). Medication orders include how often the medicine is to be taken and when (e.g., digoxin 0.25 mg, once a day, in the morning). Nurses need to be aware of the meaning of time for clients. Giger and Davidhizar (1995, p. 109) state that when caring for clients who are "present-oriented," it is important to avoid fixed schedules. The nurse can offer a time range for activities and treatments. For example, instead of telling the client to take digoxin every day at 10:00 A.M., the nurse might tell the client to take it every day in the morning, or every day after getting out of bed.

Nutritional Patterns

Most cultures have staple foods, that is, foods that are plentiful or readily accessible in the environment. For example, the staple food of Asians is rice; of Italians, pasta; and of Eastern Europeans, wheat. Even clients who have been in the United States or Canada for several generations often continue to eat the foods of their cultural homeland.

The way food is prepared and served is also related to cultural practices. For example, in the United States, a traditional food served for the Thanksgiving holiday is stuffed turkey; however, in different regions of the country the contents of the stuffing may vary. In Southern states, the stuffing may be made of cornbread; in New England, of seasoned bread and chestnuts.

The ways in which staple foods are prepared also varies. For example, some Asian cultures prefer steamed rice; others prefer boiled rice. Southern Asians from India prepare unleavened bread from wheat flour rather than the leavened bread of Anglo-Americans.

Food-related cultural behaviors can include whether to breast feed or bottle feed infants, and when to introduce solid foods to them. Food can also be considered part of the remedy for illness. Foods classified as "hot" foods or foods that are hot in temperature may be used to treat illnesses that are classified as "cold" illnesses. For example, corn meal (a "hot" food) may be used to treat arthritis (a "cold" illness). Each cultural group defines what it considers to be hot and cold entities.

Religious practice associated with specific cultures also affects diet. Some Roman Catholics avoid meat on certain days, such as Ash Wednesday and Good Friday, and some Protestant faiths prohibit meat, tea, coffee, or alcohol. Both Orthodox Judaism and Islam prohibit the ingestion of pork or pork products. Orthodox Jews observe kosher customs, eating certain foods only if they are inspected by a rabbi and prepared according to dietary laws. For example, the eating of milk products and meat products at the same meal is prohibited. Some Buddhists, Hindus, and Sikhs are strict vegetarians. The nurse must understand the importance of religious dietary practices.

Consider . . .

- the nutritional content of the foods of various cultures. Identify the food preferences of cultural groups in your community. How do these diets fulfill nutritional requirements? What nutritional deficiencies exist in these diets?

Pain Responses

It has been demonstrated that beliefs about and responses to pain vary among ethnic/racial groups. Cultural and spiritual response to pain must be viewed in relation both to the actual perception of pain and to the meaning or significance of pain to the client and family. In some cultures, pain may be considered a punishment for bad deeds; the individual is, therefore, to tolerate pain without complaint in order to atone for sins. In other cultures, self-infliction of pain is a sign of mourning or grief. In other groups, pain may be anticipated as a part of the ritualistic practices of passage ceremonies, and therefore tolerance of pain signifies strength and endurance. In yet other cultures, the expression of pain elicits attention and sympathy, while in other cultures, boys especially are taught "to take pain like a man" and "big boys don't cry."

Cavillo and Flaskerud (1991, p. 16) found that nurses and clients assess pain differently. In a study of Mexican-American clients with pain, they found that nurses and physicians tend to underestimate and undertreat their client's pain in relation to the client's expression of pain. Client responses to pain should be assessed within the context of their culture. If the client does not complain of pain, it should not be assumed that the client is not experiencing pain. The nurse must be aware of what conditions are likely to cause pain and offer clients pain relief as appropriate.

Treatment for pain may also vary with culture. In European-American cultures, medication is typically used for pain relief. In other cultures, heat, cold, relaxation, meditation, or other techniques and treatments may be used.

Death and Dying

Death is a universal experience, and people want to die with dignity. Various cultural and religious traditions and practices associated with death, dying, and the grieving process help people cope with these experiences. Nurses are often present through the dying process and at the moment of death, especially when it occurs in a health care facility. Knowledge of the client's religious and cultural heritage helps nurses provide individualized care to clients and their families, even though they may not participate in the rituals associated with death.

Dying in solitude is generally unacceptable in most cultures. In many cultures, people prefer a peaceful death at home rather than in the hospital. Some ethnic groups may request that health professionals not reveal the prognosis to dying clients. They believe the person's last days should be free of worry and pain. People in other cultures prefer that a family member (preferably a male in some cultures) be told the diagnosis so that the client can be tactfully informed by a family member in gradual stages or not be told at all. Nurses also need to determine whom to call, and when, as the impending death draws near.

Beliefs and attitudes about death, its cause, and the soul also vary among cultures. Unnatural deaths, or "bad deaths," are sometimes distinguished from "good deaths." The death of a person who has behaved well in life is considered less threatening because that person will be reincarnated into a good life next time.

Beliefs about preparation of the body, autopsy, organ donation, cremation, and prolonging life are closely allied to the person's religion. *Autopsy,* for example, may be prohibited, opposed, or discouraged by Eastern Orthodox religions, Muslims, Jehovah's Witnesses, and Orthodox Jews. Some religions prohibit the removal of body parts and dictate that all body parts be given appropriate burial. *Organ donation* is prohibited by Jehovah's Witnesses and Muslims, whereas Buddhists in America consider it an act of mercy and encourage it. *Cremation* is discouraged, opposed, or prohibited by the Mormon, Eastern Orthodox, Islamic, and Jewish faiths. Hindus, in contrast, prefer cremation and cast the ashes in a holy river. *Prolongation of life* is generally encouraged; however, some religions, such as Christian Science, are unlikely to use medical means to prolong life, and the Jewish faith generally opposes prolonging life after irreversible brain damage. In hopeless illness, Buddhists may permit euthanasia.

Nurses also need to be knowledgeable about the client's death-related rituals, such as last rites and administration of Holy Communion, chanting at the bedside, and other rituals, such as special procedures for washing, dressing, positioning, and shrouding the dead. For example, certain immigrants may wish to retain their native customs, in which family members of the same sex wash and prepare the body for burial and cremation. Muslims also customarily turn the body toward Mecca. Nurses need to ask family members about their preference and verify who will carry out these activities. Burial clothes and other cultural or religious items are often important symbols for the funeral. For example, faithful Mormons are often dressed in their "temple clothes." Some Native Americans may be dressed in elaborate apparel and jewelry and wrapped in new blankets with money. The nurse must ensure that any ritual items present in the health care agency be given to the family or to the funeral home.

Consider...

■ cultural beliefs and practices related to death and dying among people of the different cultural groups in your community. How can the nurse support the client and family in the performance of death and dying practices?

Childbirth and Perinatal Care
Prenatal Care

In North America, emphasis is placed on regular prenatal medical visits, dental care, prenatal classes for both parents, and avoidance of communicable disease. These practices are accepted in varying degrees by people of other cultures. To some for example, regular medical checkups are often avoided because they are equated with problems or abnormalities. Traditionally, these women will see a physician only if there is a problem. Many immigrants may also prefer not to attend prenatal classes for a variety of reasons. Some of these relate to language problems or discomfort and embarrassment about doing exercises in front of others, discussing sexual matters, or seeing movies about childbirth.

Because in many cultures pregnancy and childbirth are considered the exclusive realm of women, some women prefer to have a female friend or relative attend prenatal classes and the birth rather than the husband. Nurses need to respect this choice. However, some new immigrant husbands, in the absence of a mother, mother-in-law or other female, may indicate interest in attending prenatal classes and the birth, if only to act as interpreters for their wives.

Research Box

Carolan, M. 2000. Menopause: Irish women's voices. *Journal of Obstetric, Gynecologic, and Neonatal Nursing* 29(4): 397–404.

This phenomenological study focused on understanding the cultural meanings of menopause for Irish women. It was Colaizzi's method to analyze the stories of Irish women. Six Irish women were interviewed 1 to 6 years after menopause; they were each the mother of five or more surviving children. Women who wished for more children were excluded. They lived in small villages in rural southern Ireland and were interviewed in their homes.

Three themes were predominant in the stories of the women. One was a sense of relief, principally relief from continued childbearing. The second theme was acceptance as a natural event; they expressed that life was as full as ever, and menopause had not significantly impacted their lives. The third theme was a sense of satisfaction at having successfully raised their families; they looked forward to a quieter life invested in grandparenting.

These results were interpreted in the sociocultural context of predominantly Catholic religion with high values on family. Family sizes tend to be large and spacing options for births are limited. The women have very busy lives with homemaking, child care, and farmwork. Rural Irish women experience menopause as a normal process of aging and do not associate it with illness. This supports the view that menopause is a complex phenomenon experienced within a sociocultural context.

Prenatal practices vary in regard to safeguarding the health of the fetus and mother. People in several cultures (e.g., Mexican Americans, Asians, Chinese) emphasize the equilibrium model of health—that is, balancing yin and yang or hot and cold—during pregnancy. Pregnant women therefore avoid too much "hot" or "cold" food as determined by their culture. Some women believe that hot foods during the first trimester of pregnancy can cause miscarriage or a premature delivery; as a result, they emphasize the ingestion of cool foods, such as some fruit, coconut, buttermilk, and yogurt, and the avoidance of hot foods, such as meat, nuts, and eggs, during this period.

Labor and Delivery

In some cultures, pregnant women traditionally return to their parents' home for the delivery of the first child and, sometimes, subsequent births. Births in the home are usually managed by a midwife, with the assistance of the woman's mother, mother-in-law, or married sister. Traditionally, the husband is not present. In other cultures, childbirth takes place in homes, hospitals, and clinics and is attended by physicians and certified midwives.

Positions used for delivery vary from the standard lithotomy position of North Americans. For example, squatting, kneeling, sitting, or standing may be preferred.

Responses to labor pain vary. Some women of certain cultures tolerate considerable pain and stoically accept pain for many reasons. They may, for example, want to avoid showing weakness or calling undue attention to themselves for fear of shaming themselves and their families, or they may act accordingly simply because it is expected behavior within their culture. In other cultures, women express pain and anguish more freely. For example, screaming and sobbing are acceptable and expected responses. It is important for the nurse to know that the absence of crying and moaning does not necessarily mean that pain is absent, nor does the presence of crying and moaning necessarily mean that pain relief is desired at that moment. With clients from some cultures, nurses may use touching and the support of others (husband, female relative, or friend) to decrease pain during labor. Various other cultures may or may not value the same comfort measures. Pain-relief medications may also be used, but some clients are hesitant to request them.

Postpartum Care

Most cultures emphasize certain postpartal routines or rituals for mother and baby. These are frequently de-

signed to restore harmony or the hot-cold balance of the body. In many cultures, the mother's health status is classified as cold due to stress and the loss of blood. Thus, people take care to warm the body and to avoid cold after birth. This prohibition includes cold air and wind, as well as designated foods and fluids. Showers, tub baths, and shampoos are restricted, often until the lochia stops or longer, to avoid chilling. Sponge baths may be taken using warm water and/or special products that have medicinal properties. Foods considered "hot" by the specific culture are provided, whereas foods considered "cold" are avoided. Some women may wear binders around the abdomen and perineum not only to protect the body from cold but also to aid the uterus to return to its normal size. Mexican Americans may also cover the head, body, and feet to avoid cold air, infection, and other problems, such as sterility.

Confinement periods also vary and in many cultures are considerably longer than that of the health care system of North America. For example, traditional Chinese practice a "sitting in" period for one month to avoid cold winds. This confinement also applies to the newborn. New Mexican American mothers may remain in bed for three days following delivery, begin to walk inside the home after one week and may go outside after two weeks.

For most cultures, the extended family frequently plays an essential role during the postnatal period. A grandmother, mother, mother-in-law, aunt, or married sister may be the primary helper for the mother and newborn. This gives the new mother time to rest as well as access to someone who can help with problems and concerns as they arise.

The Newborn

Breast-feeding is the traditional feeding method in most cultures. However, bottle feeding is becoming more common among women who are employed. The current emphasis in North America on breast-feeding is confusing to some new immigrants because effective advertising campaigns have convinced women of the superiority of bottle feeding; they believe babies grow faster on the formulas. Nurses need to provide additional encouragement and clear explanations for these women.

In some cultures, newborn babies may have a coin placed on the umbilicus or their waist tied with a belly band to prevent a protruding umbilicus or hernia. Islamic practice requires a family member to pray in the newborn's ear as soon as possible after birth. Circumcision is mandatory according to some religious doctrines and cultural practices. However, in many cultures, circumcision is not performed.

It is important to remember that younger members of a specific cultural group may have been acculturated to the dominant culture and no longer follow traditional practices. In other instances, they follow some practices but not others. Sensitive nurses can work toward a blending of old and new behaviors to meet the goals of all concerned.

PROVIDING CULTURALLY AND SPIRITUALLY COMPETENT CARE

All phases of the nursing process are affected by the client's and the nurse's cultural and spiritual values, beliefs, and behaviors. As the client and the nurse come together in the nurse-client relationship, a unique cultural and spiritual environment is created that can improve or impair the client's outcome. Self-awareness of personal biases can enable nurses to modify behaviors or (if they are unable to modify behaviors) to remove themselves from situations where care might be compromised. Nurses can become more aware of their own cultural and spiritual values through values-clarification activities. Nurses must also consider the cultural values of the health care setting because they, too, may influence a client's outcome.

To obtain cultural- and spiritual-assessment data, nurses use broad statements and open-ended questions that encourage clients to express themselves fully. The important principle to remember when conducting an assessment is that "the client is the teacher and expert regarding his or her culture, and the nurse is the learner" (Rosenbaum, 1995, p. 188). At this stage nurses make no conclusions but obtain information from clients.

There are several cultural- and spiritual-assessment tools available. Nurses need to use tools that are appropriate to the situation and adapt them as required. For example, a nurse in an emergency department of an urban hospital may need a different format than a nurse working in a home care setting. It is unnecessary to complete a total cultural or spiritual assessment for every client. Instead, nurses need to collect enough basic data to identify patterns of behavior that may either facilitate or interfere with a nursing strategy or treatment plan.

Anderson et al. (1990, pp. 256–262) emphasize the following points relevant to cultural assessment.

- A cultural assessment takes time and usually needs to extend over several time periods.
- Recognition of one's own ethnicity and social

background is essential. Even when the nurse and client share the same ethnic background, the nurse should expect differences in beliefs and values.
- The *process* of assessment is important. How and when questions are asked requires sensitivity and clinical judgment.
- The timing and phrasing of questions needs to be adapted to the individual. Timing is important in introducing questions. Sensitivity is needed in phrasing questions.
- Trust needs to be established before clients can be expected to volunteer and share sensitive information. The nurse therefore needs to spend time with the clients, introduce some social conversation, and convey a genuine desire to understand their values and beliefs.

Before a cultural assessment begins, the nurse determines what language the client speaks and the client's degree of fluency in the English language. The nurse can also learn about the client's communication patterns and space orientation by observing both verbal and nonverbal communication. For example, does the client speak for himself or herself or defer to another? What nonverbal communication behaviors does the client exhibit (e.g., touching, eye contact)? What significance do these behaviors have for the nurse-client interaction? What is the client's proximity to other people and objects within the environment? How does the client react to the nurse's movement toward the client? What cultural or spiritual objects within the environment have importance for health promotion/ health maintenance?

For the initial cultural assessment, regardless of the approach used, nurses should ask themselves the following questions (Grant, 1994, pp. 180–181):

- What does the client think about the nature of the illness? What does the client believe to be its cause? How does the client usually deal with the problem? How can others help?
- What support systems are available to the client? Is support from family, religious, community, or ethnic groups available to the client during and after treatment? Does the client need assistance contacting these individuals?
- What treatments is the client using to maintain health and fight illness? Are nontraditional healers involved? What remedies or treatments are ongoing or under consideration? What assistance will be needed from the health care institution or staff to accommodate a combined approach to the problem?
- What biologic and social factors should the nurse consider when planning client care? What health care risks and individual needs characterize the client's culture? What communication problems might occur?

■   What does the client want from traditional medicine? What problems are foreseeable? What decisions can be anticipated? How might any legal or ethical problems be addressed?

As the client answers these questions, the sensitive nurse will identify other concerns and issues that can be queried. Examples of open-ended questions to elicit cultural data are shown in the accompanying box.

Information about spiritual and religious beliefs and practices may be elicited during a cultural assessment. However, nurses also need to be cognizant of statements, behaviors, relationships, and objects in the client's environment that may indicate spiritual or religious beliefs and needs. The box on page 361 provides parameters for assessing spiritual needs of culturally diverse clients.

To provide *culturally congruent care* that benefits, satisfies, and is meaningful to the people nurses serve, Leininger (1991, pp. 41–42) conceptualizes three major modes to guide nursing judgments, decisions, and actions:

1. *Cultural care preservation and/or maintenance.* The nurse accepts and complies with the client's cultural beliefs. For example, the nurse provides herbal tea to ease a "nervous stomach," a practice the client says has worked well in the past.

2. *Cultural care accommodation and/or negotiation.* The nurse plans, negotiates, and accommodates the client's culturally specific food preferences, religious practices, kinship needs, child care practices, and treatment practices.

3. *Cultural care repatterning or restructuring.* The nurse is knowledgeable about cultural care and develops ways to repattern or restructure nursing care.

Examples of Open-Ended Questions for a Cultural Assessment

CULTURAL AFFILIATION

I am interested in learning about your cultural heritage. Can you tell me about your cultural group, where you were born, and how long you have lived in this country?

BELIEFS ABOUT CURRENT ILLNESS

What do you call your problem? What name do you give it? What do you think has caused it? Why did it start when it did? What does your sickness do to your body? How severe is it? What do you fear most about your sickness? What are the chief problems your sickness has caused for you personally, for your family, and at work?

HEALTH CARE PRACTICES

What kinds of things do you do to maintain health? For example, what types of food do you eat to maintain health? What foods do you eat during illness, and how is food prepared? What other activities do you or your family do to keep people healthy (e.g., wearing amulets, religious or spiritual practices)? How do you know when you are healthy?

ILLNESS BELIEFS AND CARE PRACTICES

What kind of things do you do to treat illnesses? Do you use traditional healers (shaman, curandero, priest, spiritualist, minister, monk)? Who determines when a person is sick? How would you describe your past experiences with cultural healers and Western health professionals? What special remedies are generally used for the illness you have? What remedies are you currently using (e.g., herbal remedies, potions, massage, wearing of talismans, copper bracelets, or charms)? What remedies have you used in the past, and which did you find helpful? What remedies or treatments are you considering now, and how can we help?

FAMILY LIFE AND SUPPORT SYSTEM

I would like to learn about your family. Who are the members of your family? What family duties do women and men usually perform in your culture? Whom do you consult when making health care decisions (e.g., other family member, cultural or religious leader)? Who will be able to help you during and after treatment? Do you need help to contact these people?

Sources: Transcultural Concepts in Nursing Care, 2d ed., by M. M. Andrews and J. S. Boyle, Philadelphia: Lippincott, 1995, pp. 439–444; *Cross Cultural Caring: A Handbook for Health Professionals in Western Canada* by N. Waxler-Morrison, J. Anderson, and E. Richardson, eds., Vancouver, B.C.: UBC Press, 1990, pp. 245–267; "A Cultural Assessment Guide: Learning Cultural Sensitivity" by J. N. Rosenbaum, *Canadian Nurse* **88**: 32–33, April 1991; and "Culture, Illness and Care" by A. Kleinman, L. Eisenberg, and B. Good, *Annals of Internal Medicine* **88**: 251–258, 1978.

Assessing Spiritual Needs in Culturally Diverse Clients

ENVIRONMENT:

- Does the client have religious objects, such as a bible, prayer book, devotional literature, religious medals, rosary or other type of beads, photographs of historic religious persons or contemporary church leaders (e.g., pope, church president), paintings of religious events or persons, religious sculptures, crucifixes, objects of religious significance at entrances to rooms (e.g., holy water founts, a *mezuzah*, or small parchment scroll inscribed with an excerpt from the Bible), candles of religious significance (e.g., Pascal candle, menorah), shrine, or other?

- Does the client wear clothing that has religious significance (e.g., head covering, undergarment, uniform)?

- Are get-well greeting cards religious in nature or from a representative of the client's church?

- Does the client receive flowers or bulletins from his or her church?

BEHAVIOR:

- Does the client appear to pray at certain times of the day or before meals?

- Does the client make special dietary requests (e.g., kosher diet, vegetarian diet, or diet free from caffeine, pork, shellfish, or other specific food items)?

- Does the client read religious magazines or books?

VERBALIZATION:

- Does the client mention God (Allah, Buddha, Yahweh), prayer, faith, church, or religious topics?

- Does the client ask for a visit by a clergy member or other religious representative?

- Does the client express anxiety or fear about pain, suffering, or death?

INTERPERSONAL RELATIONSHIPS:

- Who visits? How does the client respond to visitors?

- Does a priest, rabbi, minister, elder, or other church representative visit?

- How does the client relate to the nursing staff? To his or her roommate(s)?

- Does the client prefer to interact with others or to remain alone?

Source: Spiritual Care: The Nurse's Role, 3d ed., by Judith Allen Shelly and Sharon Fish. © 1988 by InterVarsity Press, Christian Fellowship of the USA. Used by permission of InterVarsity Press, P.O. Box 1400, Downers Grove, IL 60515.

Cultural care preservation may involve, for example, encouraging the use of cultural health care practices, such as ingesting herbal tea, chicken soup, or "hot foods" to the ill client. Accommodating the client's viewpoint and negotiating appropriate care require expert communication skills, such as responding empathetically, validating information, and effectively summarizing content. Negotiation is a collaborative process. It acknowledges that the nurse-client relationship is reciprocal and that differences exist between the nurse and client about notions of health, illness, and treatment. The nurse attempts to bridge the gap between the nurse's (scientific) and the client's (cultural and spiritual) perspectives. During the negotiation process, the nurse first elicits the client's views and acknowledges these views and then, if appropriate, provides relevant scientific information. If the client's views reveal that certain behaviors would not affect the client's condition adversely, then the nurse incorporates these views in planning care. If the client's views

can lead to harmful behaviors, then the nurse attempts to shift the client's perspectives to the scientific view. Negotiation therefore occurs when cultural treatment practices or spiritual practices conflict with those of the health care system and when the cultural or spiritual practices are considered harmful to the client's well-being. The nurse must determine precisely how the client is managing the illness, what practices could be harmful, and which practices can be safely combined with Western medicine. For example, reducing dosages of an antihypertensive medication or replacing insulin therapy with herbal measures may be detrimental. In situations where harm may occur, the nurse needs to inform the client about possible outcomes. When a client chooses to follow only cultural or spiritual practices and refuses all prescribed medical or nursing interventions, the nurse needs to adjust the client's goals. Anderson et al. (1990, p. 264) point out that monitoring the client's condition to identify changes in health state and to recognize impending crises before they become irreversible may be all that is realistically achievable. At a time of crisis, the nurse may then have the opportunity to renegotiate the original care approach.

Transcultural nursing care is challenging. It requires discovery of the meaning of the client's behavior, flexibility, creativity, and knowledge to adapt nursing interventions. For example, a culturally sensitive nurse knows that a Chinese woman who has just given birth and refuses to eat fruit and vegetables, refuses to drink the cold water at her bedside, stays in bed, and refuses to take sitz baths, baths, or showers needs to increase the return of yang forces. The nurse will make plans to adapt nursing interventions accordingly.

Nurses also need to identify community resources that are available to assist clients of different cultures or spiritual or religious beliefs. Nurses should try to learn from each transcultural nursing situation they encounter to improve the delivery of culture-specific care to future clients. The accompanying box offers suggestions for providing culturally competent nursing care.

Bookshelf

Books that describe the African American experience:

Angelou, M. 1997. *I know why the caged bird sings.* **New York: Bantam Books.**

Ellison, R. 1947. *Invisible man.* **New York: Vintage.**

Walker, A. 1982. *The color purple.* **New York: Washington Square Press.**

Books that describe the Asian experience:

Tan, A. 1989. *The joy luck club.* **New York: Vintage.**

Books that describe the Hispanic experience:

Marquez, G. G. 1985. *Love in the time of cholera.* **New York: Penguin Books.**

Santiago, E., and M. Asher. 1994. *When I was Puerto Rican.* **Cambridge, Mass.: Perseus Publishing.**

Books that describe the Irish American experience:

McCourt, F. 1999. *Angela's ashes.* **New York: Simon & Schuster.**

Consider . . .

■ resources (e.g., churches, synagogues, or mosques; civic groups; embassies or consulates; and so on) available in your community that will assist health care providers in delivering culturally competent care.

■ the value of learning the language of culturally different clients in your community. What resources are available in your community for nurses to learn different languages or phrases related to health care?

Providing Culturally Competent Care to Families

- Learn the rituals, customs, and practices of the major cultural groups with whom you come into contact. Learn to appreciate the richness of diversity as an asset rather than a hindrance in your practice.

- Identify personal biases, attitudes, prejudices, and stereotypes.

- Incorporate culture practices into care. Recognize that cultural symbols and practices can often bring a client comfort.

- Include cultural assessment of the client and family as part of overall assessment.

- Recognize that it is the client's (or family's) right to make their own health care choices.

- Provide the services of an interpreter if one is needed.

- Convey respect and cooperate with traditional healers and caregivers.

SUMMARY

North Americans come from a variety of ethnic, cultural, spiritual, and religious backgrounds, and many North Americans retain at least some of their traditional values, beliefs, and practices. Many groups in North America are bicultural; i.e., they embrace two cultures: their original ethnic culture and a North

American culture. An individual's ethnic, cultural, spiritual, and religious background can influence values, beliefs, and practices. Through acculturation, most ethnic and cultural groups in North America modify some of their traditional cultural characteristics.

Nurses must be aware of their own cultural, spiritual, and religious beliefs because they may impact the care they give.

Health beliefs and practices, family patterns, communication style, space and time orientation, nutritional patterns, pain response, death and dying practices, childbirth and perinatal care, and ethnic-related problems influence the relationship between a nurse and a client who have different cultural and spiritual backgrounds.

When assessing a client, a nurse considers the client's cultural and spiritual values, beliefs, and practices related to health and health care. It is the responsibility of nurses not only to be aware of cultural difference, but also to be culturally sensitive and to provide culturally competent nursing care.

SELECTED REFERENCES

American Nurses Association. 1991. *Position statement on cultural diversity in nursing practice.* Washington, D.C.: ANA.

Anderson, J. M., Waxler-Morrison, N., Richardson, E., Herbert, C., and Murphy, M. 1990. Delivering culturally-sensitive health care. In N. Waxler-Morrison, J. Anderson, and E. Richardson, *Cross cultural caring: A handbook for health professionals in Western Canada,* pp. 245–267. Vancouver, B.C.: UBC Press.

Andrews, M. M., and Boyle, J. S. 1995. *Transcultural concepts in nursing,* 2d ed. Philadelphia: Lippincott.

Andrews, M. M., and Boyle, J. C. 1999. *Transcultural concepts in nursing care.* Philadelphia: Lippincott.

Baldwin, D., Cotanch, P., Johnson, P., and Williams, J. 1996. *An Afrocentric approach to breast and cervical cancer early detection and screening.* Washington, D.C.: ANA.

Barnum, B. S. 1996. *Spirituality in nursing: From traditional to new age.* New York: Springer Publishing Company.

Burkhardt, M. 1993. Characteristics of spirituality in the lives of women in a rural Appalachian community. *Journal of Transcultural Nursing* **4:** 12–18.

Calvillo, E. R., and Flaskerud, J. H. 1991, Winter. Review of literature on culture and pain of adults with focus on Mexican Americans. *Journal of Transcultural Nursing* **2:** 16–23.

Carolan, M. 2000. Menopause: Irish women's voices. *Journal of Obstetric, Gynecologic, and Neonatal Nursing* **29**(4): 397–404.

Dossey, B. M., Keegan, L., and Guzzetta, C. E. 2000. *Holistic nursing: A handbook for practice,* 3d ed. Gaithersburg, Md.: Aspen.

Dossey, L. 1993. *Healing words: The power of prayer and the practice of medicine.* New York: Harper San Francisco.

Eliason, M. J. 1993, Sept./Oct. Ethics and transcultural nursing care. *Nursing Outlook* **41:** 225–228.

Felder, E. 1995. Integrating culturally diverse theoretical concepts into the education preparation of the advanced practice nurse: The cultural diversity practice model. *Journal of Cultural Diversity* **2:** 88–92.

Galanti, G. 1991. *Caring for patients from different cultures.* Philadelphia: University of Pennsylvania Press.

Giger, J. N., and Davidhizar, R. 1995. *Transcultural nursing: Assessment and interventions,* 2d ed. St. Louis: Mosby-Year Book.

Grant, A. B. 1994. *The professional nurse: Issues and actions.* Springhouse, Pa.: Springhouse.

Kavanaugh, K. H., and Kennedy, P. H. 1992. *Promoting cultural diversity.* Newbury Park, Calif.: Sage Publications.

Kittler, P. G., and Sucher, K. P. 1990, March/April. Diet counseling in a multicultural society. *Diabetes Educator* **16:** 127–134.

Kleinman, A., Eisenberg, L., and Good, B. 1978. Culture, illness and care. *Annals of Internal Medicine* **88:** 251–258.

Lea, A. 1994, Aug. Nursing in today's multicultural society: A transcultural perspective. *Journal of Advanced Nursing* **20:** 307–313.

Leininger, M. M. 1978. *Transcultural nursing: Concepts, theories, and practices.* New York: Wiley.

Leininger, M. M. 1988, Nov. Leininger's theory of nursing: Cultural care diversity and universality. *Nursing Science Quarterly* **14:** 152–160.

Leininger, M. M. ed. 1991. *Culture care diversity and universality: A theory of nursing.* New York: National League for Nursing Press. Pub. No. 15-2402.

Leininger, M. M. 1993, Winter. Towards conceptualization of transcultural health care systems: Concepts and a model. *Journal of Transcultural Nursing* **4:** 32–40.

Luckmann, J. 2000. *Transcultural communication in health care.* Albany, N.Y.: Delmar.

McSherry, W. M. 1998. Nurses' perceptions of spirituality and spiritual care. *Nursing Standard* **13**(4): 36–40.

Moschella, V. D., Pressman, K. R., Pressman, P., and Weissman, D. E. Spring, 1997. The problem of theodicy and religious response to cancer. *Journal of Religion and Health* **36**(1): 17–20.

Murdock, G. 1971. *Outline of cultural materials,* 4th ed. New Haven, Conn.: Human Relations Area Files.

Murray, R. B., and Zentner, J. P. 2001. *Health promotion strategies through the life span.* Upper Saddle River, N.J.: Prentice Hall.

National Center for Complementary and Alternative Medicine. 2001. http://nccam.nih.gov.

O'Brien, M. E. 1999. *Spirituality in nursing: Standing on holy ground.* Boston: Jones and Bartlett.

Orque, M. S., Bloch, B., and Monrroy, L. S. A. 1983. *Ethnic nursing care: A multicultural approach.* St. Louis: Mosby.

Purnell, P. D., and Paulanka, B. J. 1998. *Transcultural health care: A culturally competent approach.* Philadelphia: F. A. Davis.

Rairdan, B., and Higgs, Z. R. 1992, March. When your patient is a Hmong refugee. *American Journal of Nursing* **92**: 52–55.

Rosenbaum, J. N. 1991, April. A cultural assessment guide: Learning cultural sensitivity. *Canadian Nurse* **88**: 32–33.

Rosenbaum, J. N. 1995, April. Teaching cultural sensitivity. *Journal of Nursing Education* **34**: 188–189.

Shelly, J. A., and Fish, S. 1988. *Spiritual care: The nurse's role,* 3rd ed. Downers Grove, Ill.: InterVarsity Press.

Spector, R. E. 2000. *Cultural diversity in health and illness.* Upper Saddle River, N.J.: Prentice Hall Health.

Sprott, J. 1993. The black box in family assessments: Cultural diversity. In S. Feetham, S. Meister, J. Bell, and C. Gilliss, eds., *The nursing of families: Theory, research, education, practice,* pp. 189–199. Beverly Hills, Calif.: Sage Publications.

Statistical Abstracts of the United States. 1998. www.census.gov/prod/religions.html.

Tripp-Reimer, T., Brink, P. J., and Saunders, J. M. 1984, March/April. Cultural assessment: Content and process. *Nursing Outlook* **32**: 78–82.

United States Census Bureau. 2001. *USA statistics in brief—Population and vital statistics.* www.census.gov/statab/www/part1.html.

Vardy, L. 1995. *God in all worlds.* Toronto: Vintage Canada.

Waxler-Morrison, N., Anderson, J., and Richardson, E., eds. 1990. *Cross cultural caring: A handbook for health professionals in Western Canada.* Vancouver, B.C.: UBC Press.

Wenger, A.F.Z. 1993, Jan. Cultural meaning of symptoms. *Holistic Nursing Practice* **7**: 22–23.

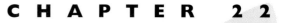

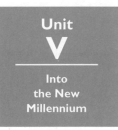

Unit

V

Into
the New
Millennium

C H A P T E R   2 2

Advanced Nursing Education and Practice

Objectives

■ Discuss education for advanced nursing roles.

■ Differentiate among functional advanced nursing roles, including clinical nurse specialist, nurse practitioner, nurse-educator, and nurse administrator.

■ Describe the historical development of advanced-practice nursing.

■ Discuss certification and regulation of advanced-practice roles.

■ Compare graduate education programs in advanced-practice nursing.

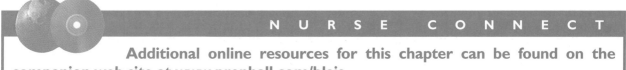

N U R S E   C O N N E C T

Additional online resources for this chapter can be found on the companion web site at www.prenhall.com/blais.

Graduate education provides specialized knowledge and skill to enable nurses to assume advanced roles in education, administration, research, and practice. It also prepares nurses for advanced practice in a variety of specialized roles in primary, secondary, and tertiary settings. Graduate programs prepare clinical nurse specialists, nurse practitioners, nurse-midwives, and nurse-anesthetists.

■ Choosing a graduate nursing program involves identifying one's personal career goals and then selecting the best program to enable one to meet those goals.

■ Nurses with graduate education can influence the health care system from within by assuming positions of leadership in administration, education, and practice. They can also influence the political system to effect needed change through the research process.

- The growth of advanced-practice nursing occurs through education, professional role advancement, and legislation.
- Nurses prepared to assume advanced nursing roles bring new ideas, insights, and enlightenment to the total health care system. Their creativity, competence, commitment, and courage will influence the quality of care in a changing health system.

CHALLENGES AND OPPORTUNITIES

Advanced-practice nursing has proliferated in response to managed care. As a result of health care reform, societal changes, an increasing international perspective, and demographic population changes, new advanced-practice roles and changes in old ones have evolved. This has challenged the traditional ways of educating nurses and of practicing nursing. The changes in health care delivery continue, and the development of advanced-practice roles must also continue to meet new demands.

The opportunities for nursing to redefine its role and practice in response to demands for change are tremendous. The evolution of advanced-practice nursing to more autonomous roles needs to be driven by the nursing profession's vision as opposed to being reactive to outside pressures. Nursing education and advanced-practice roles will need to develop in tandem if nursing is to be effective in preserving the best of what nursing has been and to take the profession into the future of health care.

ADVANCED NURSING EDUCATION

Historically, basic education in nursing prepared the graduate to be a nurse generalist. Nurses obtained education for specialization after completing the basic program, usually through hospital-based postgraduate courses designed to provide knowledge and skill in a specialized area. This type of specialized preparation in the early part of the twentieth century generally focused on obstetric nursing and private-duty nursing. As nurses acquired a greater body of knowledge in the sciences of anatomy, physiology, microbiology, chemistry, pathophysiology, and pharmacology, they became better able to make assessments about the nature of clients' problems. Nurses' increasing skills enabled them to assume a more active role in the care of their clients. Knowledge and skill that had previously been the physician's domain gradually crossed over into nursing practice. For example, nurses acquired the skills to conduct in-depth physical assessments, venipuncture, suturing, ordering basic diagnostic studies, and administering life-saving medications under protocols.

As the nurse's role expanded, nurses became more specialized, and standards of practice required greater consistency in what nurses were permitted to do and could be expected to do. As the settings for practice became more specialized, postbasic specialty courses proliferated to include oncology nursing, critical care nursing, recovery room nursing, operating room nursing, rehabilitation nursing, and so on. These developments created a need for more formalized programs of study to ensure consistency of education and skill training.

Preparation for Advanced Clinical Practice

Specialty education provided in universities and colleges at the master's degree level evolved during the 1940s and 1950s. The idea was greatly facilitated by the return of nurses from military service during World War II. These nurses often had GI benefits to return to school for advanced education. Passage of the National Mental Health Act in 1946 provided additional funds for education of nurses in the area of psychiatric/mental health nursing. During a 1952 conference sponsored by the National League for Nursing (NLN), it was agreed that the purpose of baccalaureate education was to prepare nurse generalists, whereas master's education was devoted to the preparation of nurse specialists. Master's level education was envisioned as the appropriate foundation for the preparation of nurses for specialty practice. Early graduate degrees in nursing focused on the functional roles of educator and administrator; for example, the degree offered at Columbia University's Teacher College focused on the preparation of nurse educators. The first clinical master's program was developed in 1954 by Hildegard Peplau at Rutgers University to prepare advanced-practice nurses in psychiatric/mental health nursing. At this time, nurses prepared with graduate degrees in clinical specialties were referred to as **nurse clinicians** or **clinical nurse specialists.** The primary purpose of the clinical nurse specialist (CNS) was to improve client care and nursing practice by functioning as an expert nurse in the practice setting. The clinical nurse specialist was considered to be an expert in a specialized area of nursing practice, usually in the acute care setting, and served as an expert care provider, a resource to novice nurses or general staff nurses for education and development, a consultant to the physician and other health professionals, and an active participant in research related to the specialized area of practice. Some believed that the clinical nurse specialist should not be used as a direct care provider, but rather as a clinical educator, consultant, or researcher. There was also concern that the role of the clinical nurse specialist was not clearly defined because nurses performed different roles and functions (educator, researcher, consultant, direct care provider, administrator) in different settings (Hamric, Spross, and Hanson, 2000).

During the 1960s, the United States experienced a health care personnel shortage as a result of the Vietnam War. Also during this time, a maldistribution of primary care physicians exacerbated the problem. In response to this problem, Dr. Loretta Ford and Dr. Henry Silver (a physician) developed in 1965 the first nurse practitioner program at the University of Colorado focusing on the care of children. Within nine years, there were 65 nurse practitioner programs in pediatrics; additional programs were developed that focused on women's health or family health. Nurses moved into other advanced-practice roles of nurse-midwives and nurse-anesthetists (Wilson, 1994, p. 28).

Because of society's need to meet its health care needs and the lack of graduate-level clinical nursing programs, short-term certificate programs were created to prepare nurse practitioners to meet health care demands. There was no consistency in the educational prerequisites, the length of the program, and the goals and content of the program in these early nurse practitioner programs. Some programs required the nurse to have a baccalaureate degree for admission, while others simply required registered nurse licensure and varying numbers of years of nursing experience. Program lengths ranged from a few months to two years. Some programs were taught only by physicians; others were taught by both physicians and nurses. Today, most advanced-practice education takes place at the graduate level, and American Nurses Association (ANA) certification at the advanced-practice levels of clinical specialist and nurse practitioner require the master's degree.

There remains controversy related to the role of the clinical nurse specialist (CNS) and its differences from and similarities to the advanced nurse practitioner (ANP). The different titles and the various perceptions about these advanced-practice roles cause confusion among health care consumers as well as health care professionals. In 1994, the American Association of Colleges of Nursing (AACN) held a conference on role differentiation of the nurse practitioner and the clinical nurse specialist. At consensus-building work groups, the participants identified the characteristics of the two advanced-practice roles, their strengths, and the outcomes that might be expected if the two roles merged or remained separate (see accompanying box). The

Clinical Nurse Specialist

Characteristics

Expertise in specific populations

Research projects—team member and evaluator

Case management

Staff development and teaching

Use of systems approach to problem solving

Strengths

Specialized knowledge and skills, in-depth knowledge, expertise

Systems skilled

Role flexibility—time and practice

Nurse Practitioner

Characteristics

Primary care, health-promotion focus

Client-centered focus

Diagnosing and prescribing

Case management

Teacher

Strengths

Autonomy of practice

Cost-effective and reimbursable

Popular with consumers and legislators

Diagnostician

Holistic approach (prevention and wellness)

Source: Adapted from L. R. Cronenwett, *Role differentiation of the nurse practitioner and clinical nurse specialist: Reaching toward consensus.* Proceedings of the Master's Education Conference, American Association of Colleges of Nursing, December 1994, San Antonio, Texas, pp. 69–70.

reasons cited for merging the CNS and ANP roles included (1) less confusion to the public, (2) clarification of competencies and titles, (3) greater professional and political power, (4) greater marketability of the advanced-practice nurse designation, (5) guarantees that preparation of advanced-practice nurses would occur at the graduate level, and, perhaps most important, (6) increased benefits to clients resulting from the more comprehensive preparation of their nurses. In a vote taken following the work groups, 68% of the participants voted to merge the ANP and CNS roles (AACN, 1994, p. 71). Nursing schools are beginning to merge their existing clinical nurse specialist programs with nurse practitioner programs, providing all graduates with the knowledge and skills to achieve national certification and to be eligible for state licensure at the advanced-practice level. (Regulation of advanced practice is discussed later in the chapter.)

Consider . . .

- what knowledge and skills are shared by nurses and physicians. Which specific skills fall in the domain of basic nursing practice, which fall into advanced nursing practice, and which are specific to the practice of medicine?
- how the role of the primary care advanced practice nurse differs from the role of the primary care physician. How does the focus of care differ?
- the societal benefits of having advanced-practice nurses provide primary care.

Master's Degree in Nursing

According to the position statement of the American Association of Colleges of Nursing, advanced-practice nursing requires preparation at the master's degree level and may include preparation as a clinical nurse specialist, nurse-anesthetist, nurse-midwife, or nurse practitioner (AACN, 2001a). Most of these advanced-practice nurses must have both a graduate degree and certification in the specialty area.

The number of programs offering master's preparation for advanced-practice nursing, particularly nurse practitioners, has increased dramatically in the past decade in response to the demand for cost-effective primary care. However, schools of nursing continue to offer specialization in indirect care roles such as management, administration, education, and informatics. These roles will continue to be important as nurses are prepared to be leaders in systems of care (AACN, 2001b).

Regardless of the advanced practice or functional role, the curricula should have a core that is common to all graduate programs. Priorities for the core curriculum include the following:

- Critical thinking and clinical judgment
- Primary health care, patient education, health promotion, rehabilitation, self-care, and alternative methods of healing
- Practice across multiple settings, including nontraditional settings
- Case management, health care policy and economics, research methods, quality indicators, outcome measures, financial management, legislative advocacy, and management of data and technology (AACN, 2001c)

Key topics for teaching these requirements include health care policy, organization of the health care delivery system, health care economics and finance, ethical issues in health care, professional role development, theoretical foundations of nursing practice, human diversity and social issues, and health promotion and disease prevention (Robinson and Kish, 2001).

Doctoral Programs in Nursing

The majority of doctoral programs in nursing emphasize clinically relevant research that builds the science for nursing practice and also prepares faculty for academic roles in colleges and universities that offer nursing programs. These doctoral programs must prepare faculty for the future by providing frameworks and tools for moving to new ways of educating for new roles and ways of practice (AACN, 2001c).

Graduates of doctoral programs in nursing are prepared for research, education, and practice and may assume careers as advanced clinicians, administrators, researchers, or public policy makers. The degree granted may be a doctor of philosophy (Ph.D.) in nursing, doctor of nursing science (D.N.S.), or nursing doctorate (N.D.). The differences among these degrees may be minimal in reality but generally reflect a greater emphasis on research (Ph.D.), greater emphasis on the development of nursing science (D.N.S.), or greater emphasis on nursing practice (N.D.). Nurses interested in enrolling in a doctoral program in nursing should review the curriculum plan and philosophy of the selected program to select a match for their professional goals.

ADVANCED NURSING PRACTICE

Almost 140,000 advanced-practice nurses are delivering health care in the United States, and the numbers are increasing (ANA, 1997). They are delivering cost-effective and high-quality health care to chronically underserved populations in particular. The advanced-practice nurse (APN) is an umbrella term for the registered nurse who has met advanced education and clinical practice requirements. This umbrella covers four principal types of APNs: certified nurse-midwives (CNM), clinical nurse specialists (CNS), certified registered nurse-anesthetists (CRNA), and nurse practitioners (NP). Table 22–1 gives examples of the role and scope of each of these four APN roles.

Much of the primary and preventive care provided traditionally by physicians can be provided by APNs at a lower cost. These nurses work collaboratively with physicians and other health professionals to coordinate health services for the benefit of the client. Each of the 50 states provides regulatory oversight through its board of nursing, which sets competency standards and continuing education requirements. Restrictions on the scope of practice have resulted from the lack of prescriptive authority and eligibility for reimbursement from third-party payers.

In Canada, advanced practice in nursing has developed in three categories: the clinical nurse specialist, the nurse practitioner, and a variety of new roles that are often developed by health care facilities to meet specific needs (CNA, 1997). Advanced nursing practice refers to the role of a nurse working within a specialty area where superior skills are developed through a combination of education and experience. Advanced nursing synthesizes research-based theory and expert nursing in a clinical area and combines the roles of practitioner, teacher, consultant, and researcher.

The advanced-practice role with the most consistency in Canada is the clinical nurse specialist, a nurse with a master's degree or doctoral degree in nursing with expertise in a specialty area. There are five interrelated components to this CNS role; they are practitioner, educator, consultant, researcher, and leader (CNA, 1996). In the other advanced-practice roles, there is not a firm position on the educational preparation. Certificate programs may prepare nurse practitioners. Certification in specialty areas is offered through the Canadian Nurses Association, but eligibility is based on experience in the clinical area or on a combination of experience and post-basic education (CNA, 1997).

Table 22–1 Examples of the Role and Scope of Advanced-Practice Nurses

Advanced-Practice Nurses	Application of Advanced Knowledge and Skills	Patient Population Served	Practice Settings
Certified Nurse-Midwives	Well-women health care, management of pregnancy, childbirth, antepartum and postpartum care. Health promotion.	Childbearing women	Homes Hospitals Birthing centers Ambulatory care
Clinical Nurse Specialists	Management of complex patient health care problems in various clinical speciality areas through direct care, consultation, research, education, and administrative roles.	Individuals with physical or psychiatric disability, maternal and child health problems gerontologic problems	Tertiary care Ambulatory care Community care Home health care Rehabilitation
Nurse-Anesthetists	Preoperative assessment, administration of anesthesia; and management of postanesthesia recovery.	Individuals in all age groups undergoing surgical procedures	Hospital operating rooms Ambulatory care Surgical settings
Nurse Practitioners	Management of a wide range of health problems through physical examination, diagnosis, treatment, and patient/family education and counseling. Primary care and health promotion.	Individuals and families: Women Infants and children Elderly Adults and others	Primary care Long-term care Ambulatory and community care Tertiary care

Source: American Association of Colleges of Nursing, *Certification and Regulation of Advanced Practice Nurses.* Washington, D.C.: AACN, 2001.

Types of Advanced Practice

Advanced-practice nursing has evolved into four main types of advanced practitioners: clinical nurse specialist, nurse practitioner, nurse-midwife, and nurse-anesthetist. As health care–delivery systems continue to change and develop, other roles may emerge to meet future needs. Each advanced role has a distinguishable scope of practice, but knowledge and skills still overlap.

Clinical Nurse Specialist (CNS)

The American Nurses Association describes the role of CNS as "an expert clinician and client advocate in a particular specialty or subspecialty of nursing practice" (ANA, 1996, p. 3). According to Hamric, Spross, and Hanson (1996), the role is implemented in direct or indirect patient care as the CSN integrates the subroles of expert nurse clinician, consultant, educator, and researcher. These subroles require skill in collaboration, role modeling, patient advocacy, clinical leadership, and being a change agent. The CNS may also assume administrative and management roles, but there is controversy about whether that is appropriate to a role dependent upon expertise in clinical practice. The scope of practice can be described as fluid as the subroles are implemented and as the CNS interacts with other health care professionals.

The education and expertise should be such that the clinical nurse specialist is eligible for certification in a specialty area. Eligibility requirements vary somewhat from specialty to specialty, and applications are reviewed individually to determine eligibility for certification. The American Nurses Credentialing Center provides national certification of clinical nurse specialists in a number of areas; the certification is valid for a period of five years, and renewal requires either a minimum number of continuing education hours or retaking a certification exam.

Nurse Practitioner (NP)

The NP, according the the American Nurses Association, is "a skilled health care provider who utilizes critical judgment in the performance of comprehensive health assessments, differential diagnosis, and the prescribing of pharmacologic and nonpharmacologic treatments in the direct management of acute and chronic illness and disease" (1996, p. 4). Health promotion and illness and injury prevention are important focuses. The NP works in a variety of settings, both autonomously and in interdisciplinary groups, providing care for individuals, families, and communities.

Certification of NPs is available from the American Nurses Credentialing Center in the areas of acute-care nurse practitioner, adult nurse practitioner, family nurse practitioner, gerontological nurse practitioner, and pediatric nurse practitioner. Other specialty areas where nurse practitioners work are women's health, occupational health, mental health, and emergency and acute care (American Academy of Nurse Practitioners, 1998a).

The **acute-care nurse practitioner** is a registered nurse with a graduate degree in nursing who is prepared for advanced practice using a collaborative model to provide direct services to adult patients who are acutely or critically ill in a variety of settings. They use diagnostic reasoning and advanced therapeutic interventions, and their practice includes independent and interdependent decision making and direct accountability for clinical judgment. The **adult nurse practitioner** is prepared for advanced practice in adult health across the health continuum. The role includes case management, consultation, leadership, education, research, and health policy development. The **family nurse practitioner** is prepared for advanced practice with individuals and families throughout the life span and across the health continuum. The **gerontological nurse practitioner** provides primary care to older adults in a variety of settings and practices, both collaboratively and independently. In this role the NP works to maximize functional abilities; promotes, maintains, and restores health; prevents or minimizes disabilities; and promotes death with dignity. The **pediatric nurse practitioner** provides primary and specialty care for children from birth through 21 years of age. These services are provided within family and developmental contexts to children who are essentially well or who have acute illness, chronic illness, or disabilities. Prior to December 31, 2000, certification was also offered to school nurse practitioners, but the exam is no longer offered. Previously certified school nurse practitioners can be recertified through continuing education (ANCC, 2000). The accompanying interview boxes provide further information about these roles.

Certified Nurse-Midwife (CNM)

A **certified nurse-midwife (CNM)** is a registered nurse who has advanced educational preparation in midwifery, which includes theory and extensive supervised clinical experiences in prenatal care, management of labor and delivery, postpartum care of the mother and infant, family planning, and gynecological care for well women. The focus of education is on normal obstetrics

Adult Nurse Practitioner

Bonnie Hammack, MSN, ARNP

What was your area of practice before you became an advanced-practice nurse? "I practiced in medical-surgical nursing for about four years."

Why did you decide to become an advanced-practice nurse? "I was working for some doctors and found I was performing some advanced practice skills. They encouraged me to become a nurse practitioner. I liked the independent practice, the ability to have more control over patient outcomes. I could give holistic care from a nursing perspective, not just medical treatment."

Where do you practice? "I work in the clinic and long-term care unit at the Veterans Administration (VA) Hospital. I also teach nursing in an associate degree program and an RN-BSN program. As a U.S. Air Force Reserve nurse, I used my advanced practice skills when I was activated during Desert Storm to work in a military hospital emergency room."

What do you do in your area of practice? "I kind of fill in the blanks. When I'm working on the long-term care unit I provide follow-up care for patients with chronic health problems and deliver episodic care for acute problems. When I'm assigned to the outpatient clinic, I provide follow-up treatment and counseling. I practice autonomously and independently, but we're a team; the physician is available as a resource."

Describe your best experience as an advanced-practice nurse. "I really like taking care of the elderly—it's like taking care of my grandparents. (I don't have any.) It's good to be able to answer their questions to put their mind at ease, to tell them that some things are a normal part of aging and some things can be treated. They don't always have to live with their discomforts; many of the discomforts can be treated."

What encouragement would you give a nurse considering becoming an advanced-practice nurse? "The sky's the limit! They can do as much or as little as they want; however, the advanced-practice nurse must learn some business and consumer skills. They have to be the best and deliver quality care to clients, but they must also seek just compensation for their work."

Pediatric Nurse Practitioner

Sandra Levin, MSN, ARNP

What was your area of practice before you became a pediatric nurse practitioner? "I have been a nurse for 24 years, during which time I have worked as a pediatric staff nurse in the hospital setting and a classroom and clinical educator."

Why did you decide to become a pediatric nurse practitioner? "I always wanted to be a nurse practitioner, but there were very few programs available. I wanted a more autonomous role caring for children and educating their families about effective parenting."

Where do you practice? "I practice in an ambulatory pediatric setting in an urban community with a group of pediatricians. There is one other nurse practitioner and two physicians. We see children and families from across the socioeconomic continuum."

What do you do in your area of practice? "I perform many of the same things as a physician in relation to diagnosis and treatment of minor illnesses, but from a nursing view of health promotion, wellness, and holism. I prefer to work with well children assessing their achievement of developmental milestones. I then provide anticipatory guidance to parents about their child's development and related needs, such as safety, nutrition, immunizations, etc."

Describe your best experience as a pediatric nurse practitioner. "I like identifying subtle changes in a child that may indicate a larger health problem. I like working with parents helping them to recognize their child's potential and assisting them with their parenting skills. I especially like working with families who have a child with attention deficit/hyperactivity disorder. I like helping them plan behavioral interventions to help their child realize his/her full potential."

What encouragement would you give to a nurse considering becoming a pediatric nurse practitioner? "Go for it!" Especially in pediatrics there is a need for education of parents, helping them to have family harmony and have a child achieve his/her full potential."

and newborn care. Most nurses who choose to become nurse-midwives have extensive prior nursing experience in maternity and public health nursing. The majority of nurse-midwifery programs in the United States offer the master's degree, and all are accredited by the American College of Nurse-Midwives (ACNM). The ACNM is also the credentialing organization that sets the standards by which nurse-midwifery is practiced in the United States. Certified nurse-midwives practice in all 50 states in the United States delivering babies in hospitals, in birthing centers, and in the home. Although most nurse-midwives practice independently providing care for women and children, all maintain an affiliation with a physician specialist in obstetrics and gynecology for consultation and referral of clients with complications.

Nurse-midwives also practice in Great Britain, Canada, Australia, Europe, Africa, and many of the island nations in the Caribbean. The education, regulation, and extent of practice of nurse-midwives vary around the world. See the accompanying interview box for a description of a nurse-midwife's role and practice setting.

Nurse-Midwife

Terry DeFilippo, MSN, CNM

What was your area of practice before you became a nurse-midwife? "I was a labor and delivery nurse and a childbirth educator for about 10 years. I was also a hospital inservice educator prior to becoming a nurse-midwife. I started once to become a midwife, but the program didn't start as planned, so I went back to labor and delivery nursing and then returned to graduate school when the midwifery program became available."

Why did you decide to become a nurse-midwife? "After my experience working in labor and delivery, I wanted to extend my role and provide more total patient care. Midwifery was an extension of what I was doing. I didn't become a midwife to get out of what I was doing as a nurse but rather to go forward and provide more care to patients during the childbirth experience."

Where do you practice? "I work for a group practice which contracts to a large public hospital. We provide prenatal and postpartum care and family planning education in the clinic. We provide intrapartum and immediate postpartum care in the labor and delivery suite. We also provide care in a school setting for pregnant teenagers and for teenage mothers while they are finishing high school.

"My practice is somewhat different from the typical midwife. I previously worked in a private practice where we provided care for healthy women throughout life. My patients were primarily women who wanted a female practitioner or physician. Many were women who wanted a female practitioner for their daughters for their first pelvic exam."

What do you do in your area of practice? "I provide antepartum, intrapartum, and postpartum care for healthy women and their newborns. I also provide some gynecologic care for healthy women, mostly family planning. I care for high-risk patients or patients with obstetric complications under detailed protocols with obstetrician/gynecologists. Most of my care is independent; some of my patients are co-managed with the physician who provides various levels of assistance depending on the patient's need. Sometimes the physician is simply reviewing the case and providing feedback.

"Studies have shown that nurse-midwives are especially effective in prevention of preterm labor in teenagers because of personal support they provide and because they take time and show an interest in the patient. I think these patients identify more with the nurse-midwife."

Describe your best experience as a nurse-midwife. "I'm privileged to be present at a birth. I feel like I'm participating in a miracle every time I'm there."

What encouragement would you give to a nurse considering becoming a nurse-midwife? "A nurse-midwife has to be realistic about the personal commitment she is making. You have to be willing to put in the time/hours. You're not on a fixed schedule—you have to take calls and be there when you're expected. This is especially so if you are in private practice; there may be no one else to cover you.

"You also have a great deal of autonomy and have a tremendous opportunity to have an impact on your patient, but with it comes a great deal of responsibility. The nurse-midwife has the ability to empower women, which is very important. We need to give each other the respect we deserve. I assist patients in achieving what they want; they have choices, and they can make decisions about their care."

Bookshelf

Breckinridge, M. 1981. *Wide neighborhoods: The story of the frontier nursing service.* **Lexington, Ky.: University Press of Kentucky.**

The author describes the story of the beginning of the frontier nursing service and of providing nursing and health care to an underserved area of Appalachia. She founded the Frontier Nursing Service by gathering dedicated nurses willing to serve in an isolated area where little health care was available.

Wells, R., and McCarty, P. 1998. *Mary on horseback: Three mountain stories.* **New York: Dial Books for Young Readers.**

This is a book to recommend to younger readers, grades 2–5. It tells the stories of three families who were helped by Mary Breckinridge, the first nurse to go into the Appalachian Mountains and provide medical care.

Certified Registered Nurse-Anesthetist (CRNA)

The nurse-anesthetist was one of the earliest advanced practice roles in the United States: Nurses started administering anesthesia as early as 1889. A **certified registered nurse-anesthetist (CRNA)** is a registered nurse who has advanced educational preparation, including classroom and laboratory instruction and supervised clinical practice, in the delivery of anesthesia to clients in a variety of practice settings, including hospitals, ambulatory surgical centers, birthing centers, and clinics. The American Association of Nurse Anesthetists, founded in 1931, established a certification program for nurse-anesthetists in 1945 and an accreditation program for educational programs for nurse anesthesia in 1952. Nurse-anesthetists working with physician-anesthesiologists administer approximately 65% of the anesthesia given to clients in the United States. In some settings, such as birthing centers and ambulatory surgical centers, nurse-anesthetists may deliver anesthesia independently to clients with uncomplicated vaginal deliveries or minor surgeries.

A CRNA takes care of a patient's anesthesia needs before, during, and after surgery. The tasks they assume in performing the role include:

- Performing physical assessment
- Participating in preoperative teaching
- Preparing for anesthetic management
- Administering anesthesia to keep the patient free of pain
- Maintaining anesthesia intraoperatively
- Overseeing recovery from anesthesia
- Following the patient's postoperative course from recovery room to patient care unit

CRNAs practice in traditional operating rooms, ambulatory surgery centers, pain clinics, and physicians offices. Many practice on a solo basis and have independent contracting arrangements with physicians and hospitals (AANA, 2001). Nurse-anesthetists maintain an affiliation with a physician-anesthesiologist for consultation prior to or during the delivery of anesthesia to a client (AANA, 2001). See the interview box on page 374 for a description of a nurse-anesthetist's role and practice setting.

Consider . . .

- the various roles and specialty practice areas of advanced nurse practitioners, especially the differences between the clinical nurse specialist and the nurse practitioner. What are the differences? What are the similarities?
- the practice of various advanced-practice nurses whom you know. How does their practice conform to the roles and functions described in this chapter? What are their relationships with physician specialists in their practice area?
- client satisfaction with the advanced-practice nurse. What client needs does the advanced-practice nurse meet that the physician may not meet? What client needs does the physician meet that the advanced-practice nurse may not meet?

Regulation of Advanced Practice

The regulation of advanced-practice nursing in the United States varies from state to state. Each state has the jurisdiction to determine the requirements for licensure of the advanced-practice nurse, including the use of a particular title and the definition of the scope of practice. The majority of state boards of nursing use certification examinations for the regulation of advanced-practice nurses and provide coverage under their registered nurse license. Only three states (California, Florida, and New York) provide either dual licenses or separate certification for advanced-practice nurses (Hickey, Ouimette, and Venegoni, 2000).

Various legal titles are conferred by the states to designate the advanced-practice nurse, including nurse practitioner, advanced-practice registered nurse, advanced-practice nurse, and advanced registered

Certified Registered Nurse-Anesthetist

William Maybury, MS, CRNA

What was your area of practice before you became a nurse-anesthetist? "I worked in an intensive care unit for two years."

Why did you decide to become a nurse-anesthetist? "I wanted to advance my skills beyond that of a floor nurse. Also, as a male nurse and knowing that someday I would be the main financial supporter of a family, I needed a job in nursing where I could earn enough to support a family possibly without having my wife work and be away from our children when they were young and in need of her."

Where do you practice? "I have been a CRNA for the past 28 years. I work for a group of anesthesiologists who contract to provide anesthesia services for a number of large and small public and private hospitals."

What do you do in your area of practice? "I administer anesthesia—general, regional, and local—and monitor anesthesia care. I do preoperative evaluations on patients to determine their most appropriate anesthesia needs during surgery. I give anesthesia to pediatric, neuro, ob-

stetric, trauma, as well as other types of general surgery patients."

Describe your best experience as a nurse-anesthetist. "My best experience is working one on one with patients as I give anesthesia. This means you use knowledge of all the specialties in medicine. You must know internal medicine, cardiology, respiratory, as well as other medical fields in order to administer anesthesia. As for myself, I enjoy pediatrics the most."

What encouragement would you give to a nurse considering becoming a nurse-anesthetist? "As in any job or profession, you should advance in your knowledge and skills as far as you can. As you become an advanced-practice nurse, you will have more knowledge and skills in that specific area. The job market for the future will be more open to an advanced-practice nurse than a routine nurse, and the financial benefits are greater than those of a regular nurse."

nurse practitioner. In addition, certification titles such as certified nurse-midwife, clinical nurse specialist, and certified registered nurse-anesthetist cause confusion in the public's mind about who advanced-practice nurses are and what they do. The state boards of nursing as well as the professional nursing organizations are currently considering this issue of advanced-practice nurse titling.

Certification is a voluntary process by which an agency or an association grants recognition to a person who has met specified qualifications. Certification is intended to protect the public by enabling the identification of competent people. It signifies the attainment of specific criteria and knowledge, skills, and abilities in a specific specialty field (ANCC, 2001). Many advanced-practice nurses are certified by national professional organizations that have developed educational and experiential criteria for specialty certification. For example, the National Certification Board of Pediatric Nurse Practitioners and Nurses (NCBPNP/N) provides pediatric nurses certification opportunities as certified pediatric nurse practitioners (CPNP) and certified pediatric nurses (CPN). It is the largest certification organization for this specialty and has granted more than 85% of the national pediatric nursing certifications

(NCBPNP/N, 2000). Most states require certification by a recognized national certification body before a nurse can function at the advanced practice level. Table 22–2 shows specialties and the resulting credential for advanced practice nurses in the United States.

Advanced-practice nurses, with the assistance of national professional organizations, have fought hard to obtain legal authority to practice, to be directly reimbursed for their service, and to prescribe medications. Whereas most states recognize the nurse-anesthetist, the nurse-midwife, and the nurse practitioner roles, many states do not recognize the clinical nurse specialist as an advanced-practice role. Most states require the completion of a master's degree in nursing with an advanced-practice specialty for licensure as an advanced-practice nurse.

Advanced-practice nurses have sought to receive direct reimbursement for their services from private insurers, Medicaid, Medicare, and other governmental funders of health care services. Whereas many states provide for some level of direct reimbursement from governmental sources, usually at a percentage of what a physician will receive for providing the same service, a few states provide full reimbursement for advanced-practice nursing services. Some states authorize a per-

Table 22–2 Certified Advanced-Practice Nurses in the United States

Specialty	Credential	# Certified	Certifying Organization	Year: 1st Exam
Clinical Specialists				
Community Health	RN,CS	437	American Nurses Credentialing Center (ANCC)	1990
Gerontology	RN, CS	878	ANCC	1989
Home Health	RN, CS	67	ANCC	1996
Medical/Surgical	RN, CS	2268	ANCC	1976
Psychiatric—Mental Health: Adult	RN, CS	6916	ANCC	1977
Psychiatric—Mental Health: Child/ Adolescent	RN, CS	909	ANCC	1977
Oncology	AOCN	431	Oncology Nursing Certification Corp.	1995
Critical Care	CCNS		American Association of Critical-Care Nurses (AACN) Certification Corporation	1999
Other				
Anesthetist	CRNA	21,966	Council on Certification of Nurse Anesthetists	1945
Midwife	CNM	6000	American College of Nurse Midwives	1971
Nurse Practitioners				
Acute Care	RN, CS	1051	ANCC and AACN Certification Corporation	1995
Adult	RN, CS	10,224	ANCC	1976
Adult	NP-C	—*	American Academy of Nurse Practitioners (AANP)	1994
Family	RN, CS	17,900	ANCC	1976
Family	NP-C		AANP	1994
Gerontology	RN, CS	2938	ANCC	1979
Neonatal	RN, C	41,193**	National Certification Corporation for the Obstetric, Gynecologic and Neonatal Nursing Specialties (NCC)	
Pediatric	RN, CS	2890	ANCC	1974
Pediatric	CPNP	6000	National Certification Board of Pediatric Nurse Practitioners and Nurses	1974
School	RN, CS	240	ANCC	1979
Women's Health	RN, C	41,193	NCC	1979

*Unable to obtain number of certified nurses from AANP.
**NCC statistics do not differentiate between neonatal and women's health nurses.
Source: Hickey, J. V., R. N. Ouimette, and S. L. Venegoni. *Advanced Practice Nursing: Changing Roles and Clinical Applications.* Philadelphia: Lippincott, 2000, p. 77.

centage of reimbursement (usually around 80%) when the nurse bills directly but will reimburse at 100% if the nurse bills indirectly through a physician/nurse collaboration.

The right to prescribe medications and other therapies is a third area requiring legal authority. The majority of states allow advanced-practice nurses to prescribe, but many require that such prescriptions follow physician protocols and be cosigned by a physician or include the physician's name and drug number on the prescription form. Some states require pharmacist approval. Many states limit the advanced-practice nurse's prescriptive authority to certain classifications of drugs, often prohibiting the nurse from prescribing controlled drugs. Some states have developed a formulary of drugs from which nurses can prescribe. Some states grant prescriptive privileges only to nurses who are working in public health clinics, rural health facilities, or other underserved settings. In those states where advanced-practice nurses have some level of prescriptive authority, they may be required to have a course in advanced pharmacology, some specified period of supervised clinical practice, or a master's degree in nursing. Some states mandate continuing education in pharmacology to maintain prescriptive privileges.

In Canada, a CNS is a registered nurse who holds a master's or doctoral degree in nursing with expertise in a clinical nursing specialty. The nurse practitioner has been defined by the Ontario Ministry of Health as "a registered nurse with additional nursing education to provide services within the scope of nursing, in all five areas of comprehensive health services (promotion, prevention, cure, rehabilitation, and support) and at all levels in the health care system" (CNA, 1997, p. 2). The nurse practitioner role can be acquired by obtaining a master's degree or by attending a certificate program.

The Canadian Nurses Association offers a certification program that provides a clinical credential in a number of clinical specialties. Eligibility for certification is based on experience in the specialty or a combination of experience and postbasic education. Nursing legislation across Canada is built on professional responsibility and accountability, and nurses must not act beyond their individual level of competence and preparation. Recent developments in two provinces have added special registration. The College of Nurses in Ontario proposed an extended class of registration for the nurse practitioner role. This would allow them to perform additional controlled acts. The Alberta Association of Registered Nurses is establishing an extended-practice roster for nurses who (1) have a baccalaureate in nursing, (2) have three to five years of experience, (3) attend an approved program preparing them to provide extended health services, (4) demonstrate expertise in their area of practice, and (5) have personal qualities congruent with the responsibilities (CNA, 1997).

In Nordic countries, the CNS role is similar to that in the United States. The nurse practitioner role has not developed because there is not a doctor shortage creating problems with access to care. The pattern suggests that hospitals are employing nurses with graduate education as clinicians. They are expected to promote research, scholarship, and the development of advanced-practice nurses to become expert caregivers to patients and families (Lorenson, Jones, and Hamilton 1998).

In Australia, there are two levels of nurses: the registered nurse and the enrolled nurse. The registered nurse is a first-level nurse, educated in preregistration degree-level courses in universities. The enrolled nurse is a second-level nurse who provides nursing care within the limits specified by education. They are educated primarily through advanced-certificate or associate-diploma-level courses in colleges of technical and fur-

Research Box

Chang, E., Daly, J., Hawkins, A., McGirr, J., Fielding, D., Hemmings, L., O'Donoghue, A., and Dennis, M. 1999. An evaluation of the nurse practitioner role in a major rural emergency department. *Journal of Advanced Nursing* 30(1): 260–268.

The purpose of this study was to test the hypothesis that there would be no significant difference in the quality of care or level of patient satisfaction provided by medical officers and nurse practitioners. A randomized trial design was used to collect both qualitative and quantitative data. The 232 participants were randomly assigned to have care provided by nurse practitioners or medical officers in a rural area of New South Wales, Australia. Telephone interviews were done to evaluate client satisfaction. Information was collected on demographics, health service use, clinical assessment, clinical management plan, and clinical care plan. Client records were reviewed by the directory of emergency services and clinical nurse consultant according to a protocol to evaluate care. Client satisfaction was measured on a five-item Likert scale. Multivariate and chi-square statistics were used to analyze differences between the two groups. There were no significant differences between groups on any area of care. Very positive outcomes of treatment were consistent across both groups. The study concluded that there is strong support for the role of nurse practitioner in the rural emergency setting.

ther education. The Australian Nursing Council, Inc., establishes competency standards for both levels, and these standards assist in establishing the scope of practice. State and territory nurse regulatory authorities establish and maintain standards and processes for the regulation of nursing. The standards cover clinical practice, management of care, counseling, health promotion, client advocacy, facilitation of change, clinical teaching, supervising, mentoring, and research. Nurses in Australia work in a variety of settings, and nurse practitioner roles are currently being introduced in a number of states (Australian Nursing Council, Inc., 2000, 2001).

The Future of Advanced-Practice Nursing

Advanced-practice nurses fill a need for quality primary care services at an affordable cost to clients in both rural and urban settings. Access to affordable care has been one of the driving forces in the increased number of APNs in recent years. That societal need is likely to continue to influence the delivery of health care. Nursing is strategically positioned to be a major player in policy development for the future.

Registered nurses, advanced-practice nurses, and professional nursing organizations will need to educate not only the public, but also the politicians and legislators about the proper role of the advanced-practice nurse. The advanced-practice nurse has a major role in preventing illness and promoting health for individuals, families, and communities. As APNs expand their roles and become more autonomous, role conflict with primary care physicians develops. In order for the advanced-practice roles to fulfill their potential, there must be a cooperative and collaborative relationship established with other health care providers, particularly with physicians. The need for further expansion of the scope of practice to include prescriptive privileges and other procedures traditionally performed by physicians will continue into the future.

Professional nursing organizations will need to ensure a high standard for those who aspire to advanced-practice certification. Educational institutions will need to collaborate and cooperate with professional nursing organizations and employers of advanced-practice nurses to ensure that the classroom and clinical instructional experiences prepare graduates to assume the advanced-practice nurse role effectively. Recently there has been much discussion about merging the role of the advanced nurse practitioner with the clinical specialist to decrease professional and public con-

fusion. Many educational institutions are already changing their curricula to integrate the two roles in graduate education.

Consider . . .

- the future of advanced practice in your community, state (province, territory), and nation. How do you see advanced-practice nurses solving some of the problems in today's health care system?
- whether advanced practice is a professional career choice for you. Do you have the assertiveness required to perform in an independent role?
- the role differences between the registered nurse and the advanced-practice nurse. Consider which nurses may not be appropriate for advanced-practice roles. What will be the relationship between registered nurses and advanced-practice nurses?

SELECTING A GRADUATE PROGRAM

Choosing a graduate program is an important decision for a nurse who is committed to lifelong work in nursing. Several factors must be considered, including professional career goals, personal and family factors, and characteristics of the proposed program (see the box on page 378).

Professional Career Goals

The nurse must first identify personal career goals. Graduate education is preparation for specialized practice. Not all graduate programs will provide the course work to meet the requirements for all advanced nursing roles and all clinical practice settings. Some graduate schools of nursing focus on nurse practitioner roles; other focus on the roles of nurse educator and administrator. Some schools are highly specialized and may provide only a single program, for example, in nurse anesthesia. Some schools of nursing have become innovative and offer highly specialized graduate programs of study, such as nursing informatics, aerospace nursing, or forensic nursing. Some graduate schools of nursing integrate advanced clinical practice roles with functional roles of education or administration but still require that the nurse choose an area of clinical specialization, such as adult health or child health, women's health, gerontology, physiologic health, or psychiatric/mental health. Graduate study may include shared core or common courses that all students take (e.g., nursing theory, nursing research); however, the student must be assured that the program provides the course work and clinical experiences that

Criteria for Considering a Graduate Program

- Professional career goals
- Personal and family factors
- Program characteristics
    1. Type of graduate programs offered
    2. School's philosophy of nursing and education
    3. Accreditation status
    4. National standing

5. Admission requirements
6. Faculty qualifications
7. Institutional climate
8. Resources
9. Clinical facilities
10. Assistantships and other financial support
11. Program graduation requirements

Source: Adapted from "Graduate Education: Making the Right Choice" by G. W. Poteet, L. C. Hodges, and S. Tate, in *Current Issues in Nursing,* 4th ed., by J. McCloskey and H. K. Grace (Eds.), St. Louis: Mosby, 1994, pp. 182–187.

the student will need to achieve personal goals. For example, the nurse who wants to become a teacher in a school of nursing should take courses in teaching methods and clinical evaluation of students; the nurse who wants to become a child health nurse practitioner must have clinical experience in pediatrics with appropriate faculty and preceptors.

The nurse must also decide whether to pursue a graduate degree in nursing or a graduate degree in another field. For example, some nurses who want to become administrators in health care organizations may choose a graduate degree in business or health care administration. Nurses in psychiatric/mental health nursing may choose a graduate degree in mental health counseling. Before selecting a nonnursing graduate degree, the nurse should investigate the requirements for nursing licensure and certification in the desired field and consider possible future requirements. Currently, some national certification programs require the graduate degree in nursing (e.g., American Nurses Credentialing Center [ANCC] clinical nurse specialist in medical-surgical nursing or gerontologic nursing), whereas others do not (e.g., Association of Operating Room Nurses [AORN] nurse anesthesia). Many professional nursing organizations are developing or planning changes in certification requirements that will mandate the graduate degree in nursing. Many state boards of nursing are also developing rules that will mandate the graduate degree in nursing to practice in an advanced nursing role. Further, the nurse who wants to teach nursing will need to consider employment requirements. Accreditation criteria for schools and colleges of nursing specify that graduate preparation be in the content area being

taught. In other words, someone teaching nursing must have an advanced degree in nursing rather than education, psychology, or another discipline.

Clearly defining professional goals enables the nurse to identify those graduate programs that provide the education and experiences to meet those goals. The nurse then considers personal and family factors and program characteristics to determine which program is most appropriate.

Personal and Family Factors

Several personal and family factors may affect a nurse's choice of a graduate nursing program. Is the nurse able to travel or relocate to another city or state to pursue graduate education? If there is a long commute to school, should the nurse relocate to be closer to school and its resources, such as the library or computer laboratories? Must the nurse support self or family while going to school? If so, the availability of employment opportunities are important. If the nurse is working while going to graduate school, the nurse may desire flexible school or work schedules to facilitate balancing study and work time. It may be best for the nurse to select a program that allows part-time study if work and family demands are heavy.

The nurse who is married needs the support of spouse and other family members while going to school. Working and going to school may limit the nurse's ability to fulfill spousal and parenting responsibilities. At the same time, children who see their parent continuing professional education have a role model for lifelong learning. The nurse who is returning to school needs to strategize with family members about how to meet family responsibilities.

Program Characteristics

Poteet, Hodges, and Tate (1994, p. 184) identify the following essential elements for assessing a graduate program: accreditation status, national standing, admission requirements, faculty qualifications, institutional climate, resources, clinical facilities, assistantships and other financial support, and program requirements. In addition, they recommend that the nurse should obtain information about what specific programs of study are offered and the school's philosophy of nursing and education. This information may be obtained from the institution's catalog or website, a telephone or in-person interview, or through discussion with a current student or graduate.

1. *Programs of study offered.* Does the school offer the specific program of study to enable the nurse to achieve professional goals? Are programs offered on campus only or through distance learning techniques such as video conferencing, community-based learning, Internet courses, or correspondence?

2. *School's philosophy of nursing and education.* Does the school subscribe to the philosophy of one nursing theorist, or do they have an eclectic model, that is, an integration of several theorists? Knowing the school's philosophy helps the prospective student understand the foundational beliefs of the school, its faculty, and the curriculum. Is the school's philosophy of nursing and education consistent with the nurse's philosophy? Inconsistency between the nurse's philosophy and the program's philosophy may interfere with success in the program.

3. *Accreditation status.* Accreditation may be conferred by a state government; by a regional accreditation association, such as the Southern Association of Colleges and Schools (SACS); or by a professional organization, such as the National League for Nursing Accreditation Commission (NLNAC) or American Association of Colleges of Nursing (AACN). Specialty nursing organizations may also accredit specific programs; for example, the American College of Nurse Midwifery accredits graduate programs in midwifery. Graduation from an accredited program may be important for the graduate to meet national certification requirements and to obtain licensure for advanced practice.

4. *National standing.* Programs may have a national reputation for excellence in certain fields of study. This reputation is usually based on the achievements of the faculty, the facilities for learning, and the achievements of its graduates. Attending a program with a national reputation for excellence may enhance the graduate's opportunities for employment.

5. *Admission requirements.* Admission requirements may include a minimum grade-point average (GPA) for undergraduate work, a minimum score on a national entrance examination such as the Graduate Record Examination (GRE) or the Miller Analogy Test (MAT), and successful completion of specific prerequisite courses such as physical assessment, statistics, or computer science. Most graduate nursing programs require completion of a baccalaureate degree in nursing. Some graduate programs allow nurses with a baccalaureate degree in another field to enter the graduate nursing program but require that the student complete any undergraduate nursing courses that were not previously taken (McGriff, 1996, p. 9). Because admission to graduate nursing programs is competitive, students need to be aware of specific admission requirements so that they can take action to meet or exceed the requirements; if they fail to meet the requirements, they may be denied admission. The student who is denied admission should question whether there are any admission waivers under which they might still qualify, such as a minority waiver or conditional admission.

6. *Faculty qualifications.* All faculty who teach at the graduate level should have a doctoral degree and a history of scholarly productivity. Students should expect to be taught by faculty who are expert in their fields. Students should seek a program where there are faculty who have expertise in the area of their interest.

7. *Institutional climate.* Prospective students may want to question students currently in the program about the climate of the school of nursing and the university/college. Do the university and school of nursing provide an environment of diversity where students can experience the value and strength of human difference? Is there an open climate in the school of nursing and the university community that allows scholarly inquiry without fear of retribution? Are relationships among faculty, students, administration, and other staff open and conducive to learning? Do faculty members have a reputation of being "student friendly"; that is, are they readily available for student consultation, or are they difficult to contact outside scheduled class times? Do faculty members challenge students to achieve their fullest potential in an atmosphere of academic rigor? Do faculty members teach most of the courses, or do teaching assistants or adjunct faculty teach a high percentage of classes?

8. *Resources.* What resources are available to support and enhance student learning? Are library materials adequate, including books and journals to support the student's field of study, computer services, and statistical consultation to facilitate student research? Are study areas, lounges, and dining facilities adequate? Students should also inquire about hours of operation, especially evening, weekend and holiday hours, to determine whether resources are available when the student needs them. Is there on-campus housing available for the student who must relocate for graduate study?

9. *Clinical facilities.* Are adequate clinical sites and preceptors available to support students, especially those who are in programs preparing the advanced nurse practitioner? Clinical facilities should include primary, secondary, and tertiary settings that provide diverse practice opportunities. Preceptors should be available who are experts in the desired specialty and who like working with students. If this is a nurse practitioner program, is most of the teaching and clinical precepting done by qualified nurse practitioner faculty or is there a heavy reliance on physician preceptors? Clinical practice settings should provide opportunities for graduate students to demonstrate critical thinking in the delivery of care to diverse clients with complex problems. Some graduate programs may provide clinical opportunities that are international in scope, for example, clinical experience study programs to provide primary care in underdeveloped nations.

10. *Assistantships and other financial support.* What is the availability of financial assistance? Many graduate programs provide teaching or research assistantships, in which the student receives tuition assistance in exchange for providing either teaching or research support to faculty. For the student whose professional goals involve teaching or research, assistantships provide an opportunity to gain experience in the role while completing formal graduate education. Many professional nursing organizations provide scholarship assistance for graduate nursing students. Other financial assistance may be available, especially for the student pursuing a graduate degree as an advanced nurse practitioner. Students should inquire about opportunities for financial assistance from their professional organizations, the school of nursing, and the university financial aid office.

11. *Program requirements.* What are the requirements for degree completion? Specifically, how many credit hours, what type of course work, and how many classroom and clinical hours are required? A requirement of nurse practitioner certification, in most clinical areas, is a specified minimal number of hours in clinical practice. Will graduates of the program be eligible to take the national certification exam?

Some graduate programs may be offered in cooperation with another academic discipline; for example, some programs in nursing administration are offered jointly with schools of business. These may result in dual degrees in each discipline; they are typically lengthy because of the need to meet requirements for each discipline. Other programs grant only a nursing degree but cooperate with other schools in offering course content. A joint position statement on nursing administration education by the American Organization of Nurse Executives (AONE) and AACN states that the educational preparation should take place in schools of nursing and include interdisciplinary education in business, economics, and/or health service administration (AACN, 2001d).

SUMMARY

Advanced-practice nursing has evolved from the early 1900s to become a well-defined area of practice that provides services related to disease prevention, health promotion, health restoration, and rehabilitation. Advanced nursing practitioners include clinical nurse specialists, nurse practitioners, nurse-midwives, nurse-anesthetists, and clinical nurse specialists. Advanced-practice nurses work in a variety of practice settings across the health care continuum but are most suited to the delivery of primary care to rural and urban populations, especially underserved populations, such as the poor and the elderly.

In some countries, the CNS role is well established, but the nurse practitioner role is not as widespread. Certification and regulation of advanced practice has been developed by professional nursing organizations and state boards of nursing to ensure safe practice by qualified practitioners. Increasingly, nurses are required to obtain education for advanced practice in graduate programs to be eligible for certification and/or state licensure.

The future of advanced practice includes redesign of graduate nursing curricula to incorporate the clinical specialist role with the nurse practitioner role. Continued legislative activity by advanced-practice nurses will be needed to ensure equitable compensation and a broader scope of practice. The advanced-practice nurse will be a major contributor to the delivery of quality health care at an affordable cost to clients in a changing health care environment.

Nurses planning to pursue graduate study must determine their professional goals before choosing a program. After identifying specific programs that will enable the nurse to meet desired goals, the nurse needs to evaluate the programs based on personal and family needs and program characteristics. Graduate programs in nursing may focus on nursing education, nursing administration, or advanced-practice nursing.

SELECTED REFERENCES

American Academy of Nurse Practitioners. 1998a. *Nurse practitioner as an advanced practice nurse role-position statement.* www.aanp.org.

American Academy of Nurse Practitioners. 1998b. *Scope of practice for nurse practitioners.* www.aanp.org.

American Association of Colleges of Nursing. 1994. *Role differentiation of the nurse practitioner and clinical nurse specialist: Reaching toward consensus.* Proceedings of the Master's Educational Conference. December, 1994. San Antonio, Texas: AACN.

American Association of Colleges of Nursing. 2001a. *Certification and regulation of advanced practice nurses.* Washington, D.C.: AACN.

American Association of Colleges of Nursing. 2001b. *Nursing education's agenda for the 21st century.* Washington, D.C.: AANC.

American Association of Colleges of Nursing. 2001c. *A vision of baccalaureate and graduate nursing education: The next decade.* Washington, D.C.: AACN.

American Association of Colleges of Nursing. 2001d. *Joint position statement on nursing administration education.* Washington, D.C.: AACN.

American Association of Nurse Anesthetists. 2001. *Questions and answers about a career in nurse anesthesia.* www.aana.com/information.

American College of Nurse Midwives. 1999. *The CNM profession.* www.acnm.org/educ.

American Nurses Association. 1997. Advanced practice nursing: A new age in health care. *Nursing Facts.* Washington, D.C.: ANA.

American Nurses Association. 1996. *Scope and standards of advanced practice registered nursing.* Washington, D.C.: ANA.

American Nurses Credentialing Center. 2000. *Nurse practitioner certification.* www.nursingworld.org/ancc/certify/catalogs/2000/cbt/nursprac.htm.

American Nurses Credentialing Center. 2001. *Fre-quently asked questions.* www.nursingworld.org/ancc/faqs.htm.

Australian Nursing Council, Inc. 2000. *ANCI national competency standards for the registered nurse and the enrolled nurse.* www.anci.org.au/competencystandards.htm.

Australian Nursing Council, Inc. 2001. *Nursing in Australia.* www.anci.org.au/nursing.htm.

Canadian Nurses Association. 1996. *Policy statement on clinical nurse specialist.* http://206.191.29.104/pages/policies/clinical_nurse.

Canadian Nurses Association. 1997. Out in front—advanced nursing practice, *Nursing Now* **2.**

Chang, E., Daly, J., Hawkins, A., McGirr, J., Fielding, K., Hemmings, L., O'Donoghue, A., and Dennis, M. 1999. An evaluation of the nurse practitioner role in a major emergency department. *Journal of Advanced Nursing* **30**(1): 260–268.

Cronenwett, L. R. 1994. Molding the future for advanced practice nurses: Education, regulation, and practice. *Role differentiation of the nurse practitioner and clinical nurse specialist: Reaching toward consensus.* Proceedings of the Master's Education Conference. American Association of Colleges of Nursing. December 8–10, 1994, San Antonio, Texas, pp. 1–20.

Hamric, A., Spross, J., and Hanson, C. 1996. *Advanced nursing practice: An integrative approach.* Philadelphia: W.B. Saunders.

Hamric, A., Spross, J., and Hanson, C. 2000. *Advanced nursing practice: An integrative approach,* 2d ed. Philadelphia: W. B. Saunders.

Hickey, J. V., Ouimette, R. M., and Venegoni, S. L. 2000. *Advanced practice nursing: Changing roles and applications,* 2d ed. Philadelphia: Lippincott.

Lorenson, M., Jones, D., and Hamilton, G. 1998. Advanced practice nursing in the Nordic countries. *Journal of Clinical Nursing* **7**(3): 257–264.

McGriff, E. P. 1996, Jan. Graduate education in nursing. *NSNA/Imprint,* pp. 9–11.

National Certification Board of Pediatric Nurse Practitioners and Nurses. 2000. *About NCBPNP/N.* www.pnpcert.org.

Poteet, G. W., Hodges, L. C., and Tate, S. 1994. Graduate education: Making the right choice. In J. McCloskey and H. K. Grace, eds., *Current issues in nursing,* 4th ed. St. Louis: Mosby.

Robinson, D., and Kish, C. P. 2001. *Core concepts in advanced practice nursing.* St. Louis: Mosby.

Sheehy, C. M., and McCarthy, M. C. 1998. *Advanced practice nursing: Emphasizing common roles.* Philadelphia: F.A. Davis.

Wilson, D. 1994, Dec. Nurse practitioners: The early years (1965–1974). *Nurse Practitioner* **19**(12): 26, 28, 31.

CHAPTER 23

Visions for the Future

Objectives

■ Identify past events that have shaped and molded nursing.

■ Discuss projections of future events that will affect nursing.

■ Identify anticipated changes in health care and nursing in the future.

N U R S E   C O N N E C T

Additional online resources for this chapter can be found on the companion web site at www.prenhall.com/blais.

The approach of the year 2000, marking a new millennium, saw many articles published on changes in nursing and predictions about the future. One future role in nursing was described as gatekeeper for complementary alternative medicine (Jones, 1998). As nurses move into greater roles in case management, they will need to understand which therapies are appropriate for each client, and when nontraditional therapies are appropriate, nurses will assist clients in making decisions regarding alternative treatments.

Patricia Benner predicted that in the new millennium nurses will be doing more in the community but will also continue to be even more integral to the provision of intensive care that will increasingly comprise hospital care. She advocates that a major task should be to recover the "Nightingale vision of attending to the real world of embodiment, and social, emotional, and physical environments that support well-being and promote health"(Benner, 2000, p. 35). She expresses the hope that caring practices will be recognized as good in themselves regardless of more objective and measurable outcomes.

Heller, Oros, and Durney-Crowley (2000) identify ten trends that will affect the future of nursing education. They are driven by socioeconomic factors, developments in health care delivery, and professional issues unique to nursing:

1. Changing population demographics and increasing ethnic and cultural diversity of nursing students
2. The technological explosion, particularly information technology
3. Globalization of the world's economy and society
4. The era of the educated consumer, alternative therapies and genomics, and palliative care
5. The shift to population-based care and the increasing complexity of patient care
6. The cost of health care and the challenge of managed care
7. The impact of health policy and regulation
8. The growing need for interdisciplinary education for collaborative practice
9. The current nursing shortage and opportunities for lifelong learning and workforce development
10. Significant advances in nursing science and research

Transformations are already taking place in nursing and nursing education based upon these trends, and change is expected to continue.

Nursing is described as being at a crossroads with a chance to grow and develop its vision for practice and education (Jenkins, 1997). The signposts at this crossroad are identified as cultural diversity, reorganization, interdisciplinary functions, managed care, creation and dissemination of nursing research knowledge, and the information superhighway. In the past, patients had to adapt to the culture of health care and, particularly, of hospitals. Now nursing has the opportunity to adapt health care to the culture of the people for whom nurses care.

The rapid changes in health care delivery and changing population demographics have affected supply and demand of nurses. The future will require effective identification and planning for personnel needs. Further, national trends indicate an overall decrease in enrollment in baccalaureate and master's degree nursing programs. The demand for nurse practitioners will likely continue in the role of primary-care providers, especially in managed-care settings. Nursing administrators will need to ensure adequate staffing of skilled and qualified nurses while maintaining a cost-effective staffing mix (Mailer et al., 2000).

CHALLENGES AND OPPORTUNITIES

In today's health care environment, there are many challenges facing the nursing profession and nurses as individuals. Nursing roles are expanding and developing at a rapidly increasing pace. Old roles and skills are no longer adequate, and education must make adjustments in order to keep pace and provide leadership. The challenge for nurses is to take control of these changes and become proactive in meeting society's needs for health care now and in the future.

Today's challenges provide opportunities to actualize the ANA vision: Every patient deserves a nurse. Professional organizations provide an opportunity for nurses to unite in vision and growth for nursing practice and education. There are many opportunities for growth of nurses both professionally and personally. With the vast resources of information technology and of distance education, continuing development of knowledge, skills, and experiences provide an avenue to advancing nursing in the future.

PAST EVENTS THAT HAVE AFFECTED NURSING

Events That Promoted Nursing's Growth and Development

Many events of the past spurred the growth and development of nursing as a profession; many events and public policy changes that were never intended to help or harm nursing's development nevertheless changed nursing. Social movements and technologic advancements also have propelled nursing into both favorable and hazardous positions.

A discussion about nursing's growth must include the impact of World War II on the quantity and quality of nurses in many countries. World War II and the period following were times of major change, both for health care and for women. Major medical and surgical advances were discovered (some by intent, others by accident), and new techniques for care were developed. Women played a major role in the military and performed valiantly in front-line medical units; some served as volunteers in the American and International Red Cross, whereas others entered the workforce in areas they had never before encountered. With most men at war, women were drawn into a work life that was new to them.

Nursing both advanced during this period and suffered. In answering the call to patriotic duty, many women chose nontraditional roles, particularly because the salaries available to "war workers" were higher. The changing work opportunities for women had a negative effect on nursing: The challenge of doing "men's work" attracted many women who might have otherwise pursued nursing. This shift in work choice caused a shortage of nurses in America, even after the war was over. In response to the shortage and in line with the desire of professional nursing organizations in the United States to advance nursing's professional standing, a two-year associate degree nursing program was developed for the junior/community colleges.

Although before World War II nurses were educated primarily in hospitals, the first university baccalaureate degree program in nursing (BSN) in the United States had been in existence since 1909. However, the number of BSN programs has not increased at the same rate as ADN programs. These changes in the education of nurses have significant implications for the future of professional nursing, which is discussed later in this chapter.

Another event that has affected nursing's growth and development is the position paper issued by the American Nurses Association in 1965, which suggested that all education for nurses take place in institutions of higher learning. Although both ADN and BSN programs existed throughout the United States at that time, most nurses were prepared in hospital-based diploma programs, and the position paper met with much resistance and even anger. By 1978, the ANA issued another recommendation, one that was even stronger. The ANA recommended there be two levels of nurses prepared in universities or colleges: ADN and BSN nurses. In 1985, ANA went even further, suggesting different titles for the two levels of nurses. By then, several nursing organizations, including the NLN, had joined the movement. However, it was not long before the NLN withdrew its support in an attempt to avoid an intraprofessional fight. In 1995, the ANA reaffirmed its position and encouraged ways to move on the recommendation while preserving the integrity of the profession. As professional nursing moved toward the goal of requiring the baccalaureate degree as the minimum credential for professional practice, RN/BSN transition programs were developed to enable the ADN nurse to move upward. RN/MSN programs have also been developed to enhance career mobility. Although these developments have advanced nursing, the continued inability to reach consensus on the "entry to practice" preparation has resulted in divisiveness among nurses with different educational preparation.

In Canada, two-year programs and four-year degree nursing programs developed to augment the hospital training schools. In Australia and Great Britain, baccalaureate nursing programs emerged as those nations moved toward the goal of educating nurses in institutions of higher learning. It is interesting to note that individual nurses in the United States, Great Britain, Australia, Canada, and other British Commonwealth nations elected to advance their own professional development by obtaining baccalaureate and master's degrees in other disciplines, most notably education, social work, and health service administration.

Another historical event that has affected nursing, especially in the United States, is the development of the role of the advanced nurse practitioner. This role evolved from two sources: the nurse practitioners and the clinic nurse specialist (CNS). In 1965, Dean Loretta Ford, in collaboration with Dr. Steven Silver (a physician) initiated a new kind of nurse preparation as a solution for the physician shortage in Colorado. Registered nurses were given 6 weeks of continuing education in which they learned assessment skills and then functioned as physician extenders. Almost immediately that education was increased, and currently most nurse practitioners hold master's degrees and are certified. The CNS role developed within acute-care settings and was found within higher education from the outset. The development of advanced practice is another example of nursing responding to a societal need; and a resulting change in the practice of some nurses. This historical event has been an advancement and a problem: Nursing now struggles for legislation that will enable advanced nurse practitioners to receive third-party reimbursement and prescriptive authority.

In the United States in the mid-1990s, President Clinton's attempts at national health care reform and increases in the number of for-profit health care corporations also affected nursing. In an effort to avoid national regulation and the perceived problems associated with 'socialized health care' in other countries, insurance companies, physicians, and hospitals moved toward a system of managed care. This resulted in redesign of hospital-based client care delivery and consequent downsizing of both professional and support staff. To reduce costs, hospitals have instituted shorter length of stays, integrated systems, case management, and the use of unlicensed assistive personnel (UAPs). Other countries have implemented similar changes in order to provide their citizens with affordable health care.

A shift from curing illness to promoting health and preventing illness has, however, provided new opportunities for nurses. This shift in health care from the hospital to the community has increased the need for primary practitioners; more opportunities exist for advanced nurse practitioners and other advanced-practice nurses, such as nurse-midwives, nurse-anesthetists, and clinical nurse specialists. This trend to involve more nurses in the care of the public outside the hospital setting has major implications for nursing education and for the future utilization of nurses (Bower, 1997).

Events That Have Indirectly Affected Nursing

Medical advances (e.g., new surgical procedures, the proliferation of diagnostic and monitoring instrumentation, and new pharmacologic preparations) have changed not only the physician's practice but also nursing practice. In the past, the nurse's hands, eyes, and ears were the principal tools for assessing clients; today, the nurse augments these tools with data from monitoring equipment that can provide more subtle and accurate information. Some of these advances have made the nurse's job easier; others, such as the development of new and more powerful drugs, have broadened the nurse's responsibilities. Knowing the drug's expected action, adverse effects, and compatibility with other drugs is a complicated responsibility. Nurses have significantly more responsibility and accountability today than they had in the past.

Cost-containment measures instituted by hospitals in many countries have also changed nursing practice. Changes that began as downsizing, or a reduction in staff to save money, quickly became a redesign of the entire hospital delivery system. Cross-training, focusing on the client, streamlining processes using continuous quality improvement (CQI), and the increased use of unlicensed assistive personnel (UAPs) or minimally trained support staff are only a few of the outcomes of the redesign. In some cases, the result was a redesign of the nurse's role; in other instances, an elimination of RN positions. RN and LPN/LVN ratios were shifted, and more management and delegation skills were required of the RN. Some RN activities were delegated to other, "cross-trained," health care workers (paramedics, respiratory therapists, phlebotomists, EKG technicians), and the RN was educated to assume additional responsibilities. Some RNs, for example, have returned to school to become respiratory therapists so that they might be able to provide total care to clients who have respiratory disorders or are ventilator dependent.

Managed care in the United States has been another cost-containment method that has affected the nurse's role. Managed care refers to a system in which hospitals (with subsidiary clinics, home care, skilled nursing facilities, and so on) and physician groups provide comprehensive care for groups of people who purchase their insurance and agree to use the program for health services. It is expected that free-market competition will provide the system with the lowest cost for care. And because the price for that care is based on the total number of members, the cost of caring for those who need care will be balanced by those members who are well and don't require services. Keeping members well so that they do not need the system is how costs are contained.

Case managers are needed as "gatekeepers" of the system so that only care that is deemed essential is provided. Cost for the care is determined proactively, so the system must be careful not to spend more than it is paid by capitation (numbers of those insured). Thus, in the new managed care environment nurses must have case management, coordination, assessment, health promotion, illness prevention, and cost-containment skills. The goal of keeping people focused on staying well and out of the hospital constitutes an entirely new paradigm of care. The way the goal is met and funded impacts the role expectations and responsibilities of the nurse.

Public policy has changed everyone's lives. Informed consent laws have increased the public's knowledge about and participation in decisions about their health care. The Self-Determination Act of 1991 has allowed people to make decisions in advance about their future health care, before they are unable to make such decisions. People have more choice about how and when health care will be delivered. These laws have also affected the role of the nurse. Monitoring the procedures for gaining consent and implementing procedures to ensure that the client's living will or durable power of attorney for health care is understood and documented are now a part of the nurse's responsibility. Issues such as the "right to die," assisted suicide, and other ethical dilemmas are of daily concern to the nurse in all practice settings. These and other added duties change the nurse's role, both in scope and accountability (Bower, 1997).

Social Movements and Technological Initiatives That Have Affected Nursing

The women's movement that began in the 1960s has made a major impact on nursing. Predominantly a women's profession (about 10% of nurses are men), nursing has benefited from the recognition of women as a force for social change. As a result of the gains made by the feminist movement, nurses have gained better salaries, better working conditions, access to higher education, and access to opportunities as middle managers and executives in many occupations as well as nursing. Nurses have recently seized the opportunity to become entrepreneurs. Many nurses would have been unlikely to rise to such challenges if the women's movement had not opened the door to opportunity.

No discussion of the changes in nursing would be complete without indicating the impact of the information age and the way that computers have changed daily life. Computer technology is impacting health care by improving storage of and access to health care information. Nurses will be able to access and input client information at bedside computers or in the client's home through portable laptop computers. Computers will improve the accuracy and efficiency of documentation. By touching the computer screen, nurses record client information and make it available to the physician, the pharmacy, and any other service who is online.

Clients can carry a card that contains information about their insurance coverage, status, medical history, medications, and demographic information. Insertion of this card into a computer sends that information to all who need to know; as a result, traditional health and medical records and files may soon become unnecessary. Instead of spending hours on manual recording, the nurse can spend that time with the client. Because the computer is often in the hospital room, at the clinic, or even in the home, the client can also share and participate in the development of the record.

Computers have also affected nursing education. Computer technology has facilitated supervision of students at a distance. Hand-sized computers provide information to students visiting clients in the home and act as vehicles for distributing client data to the college or clinic. Computerized instruction allows faculty to focus on the student's ability to think critically rather than on the ability to accumulate facts. A major advantage of computer technology is that it enables students to interact with information, classmates, faculty, and other nurses online at home, in the computer laboratory or library, in the classroom, or in the clinical setting. Thus, computerized instruction expands the instructional environment so that learning is portable, accessible, and always available. There are no constraints of time, person, or place. These advances

in computer technology and their application to nursing and health care require that nurses broaden their knowledge still further, so that they become computer literate.

Through technology and travel, the world has become a smaller place. Immigrants and refugees readily cross national borders to seek opportunity in new lands. Nurses are more able to move rapidly to assist with the delivery of care to victims of natural and manmade health disasters. The shrinking of the worldwide community requires that nurses become more knowledgeable about and accepting of cultural difference. Nurses need to be aware of different beliefs about health and illness and different cultural healing practices. The nurses of tomorrow need to be more than culturally aware—they need to strive for cultural competence in providing nursing care.

This overview of changes that have affected nursing and nursing practice is not meant to be comprehensive; there are many more good examples of events that have directly or indirectly changed nursing. Rather, this overview was intended to show that any changes in nursing in the past were usually linked to professional or societal change. As one considers the future, it is important to keep this point in mind (Bower, 1997).

Consider . . .

- how the changes in health care financing have changed the practice of nursing where you work. What has nursing gained from these changes? What might have been lost from health care?
- how the information technology advances have impacted nursing practice. Do some nurses have a more difficult time adapting to these changes? What might be some helpful strategies for nurses?
- the societal changes in population demographics as they relate to health care. How has nursing adapted to these changes? What related needs might have gone unmet or been undermet?

FUTURE EVENTS THAT WILL AFFECT NURSING

During the past century, there have been tremendous advances in health care, such as immunizations and antibiotics, and these have contributed to a greatly increased life expectancy. The 2000 census, for the first time, had a three-digit space for age. In the 1900s, when pneumonia and tuberculosis were the leading causes of death, no one could have forecast the advances that would be developed to manage these diseases as well as other health problems. Neither could they have predicted health hazards that were to come, such as motor vehicle–related injuries and AIDS. The future will no doubt present anticipated challenges based upon what society is experiencing at the present as well as unanticipated ones.

Computer Technology and Its Effect on Health and Nursing Care

The computer systems of tomorrow will require that all health care providers be knowledgeable and practiced in the use of computers. It will take more than being computer literate to function in the computer world of tomorrow. Knowledge of word processing using several software packages, the ability to use spreadsheets, and the ability to adapt to ever-changing computer systems will be necessary. For awhile, health care facilities will need to train their personnel, but eventually all workers will be expected to have computer skills when hired. This means that schools of nursing and other departments of colleges and universities will need to ensure that all graduates of their programs are able to access computers and obtain the information needed.

Some of the projections can be provocative, particularly those that relate to innovative technology. The use of virtual computerization in the learning environment is one of those. Much of that technology has been applied to games, but not to education.

> Imagine wearing a headset with two small screens located in front of your eyes, used to project computer graphic images, and earphones to receive computer-generated sound. On your hands you wear data gloves, which contain position sensors. These sensors tell the computer exact positions, especially of your body and arms. The computer responds to the movement of your head, eyes, hands, and arms. It might even have voice recognition and respond to your commands (Justice, 1999, p. 14).

Any number of clinical scenarios could be displayed in this virtual world, allowing students and nurses to learn skills and refresh previously learned ones. A trainer may be involved for guidance and may even control the progression of the scenario to assess the ability to respond to changes and crises and fit the experience to the learner's level of expected performance. The computer can be programmed to score the performance, providing new avenues for testing skills and perhaps even testing for licensure.

The 3-D images can be made even more lifelike by the use of head-mounted displays, allowing total visual immersion, and of auditory feedback in response to the viewer's movements and contact with virtual objects. Pilot training has used flight simulators for some time, but the use of this technology has been fairly limited in other contexts. This advancement is likely to impact education and perhaps even the practice of nursing in the future, particularly if the technology were to be applied to client education.

More applications for online services will be implemented in the future. Patient information sources will be used to an even greater degree, creating a more educated health care consumer. Nurses can be developers of these information services as well as referral agents. Online continuing education and formal education will probably continue as a trend in the near future, creating new opportunities for nurses to update their own knowledge base and advance their careers. Programs using digital interactive television that offers two-way communication are being piloted and have tremendous opportunity for creative applications in health care.

Physician and nonphysician offices should soon be able to access the hospital system so that they do not need a paper trail or their own electronic system. With managed care, the system should expand to connect the hospital, the insurance company (or payer), and the physician and nonphysician care providers. Soon, with a tap of the finger, a client's record can be accessed from any of those entities.

It will not be long before nurses will carry pocket computers on their uniform belts to record data and make assessments at the site of the client (whether in hospital, home, school, or job). These data will simultaneously be entered in the client's personal record and be available to any department in the hospital as long as the client is there. This capacity for simultaneous entry and distribution is already possible in restaurants, where the server enters the order in the computer at table side, records it, and notifies the kitchen without ever going near the kitchen until the order is ready. That same entry creates a bill that is ready for customers when they leave.

Similar activities will soon be part of every health care facility to ensure smooth, quick care and accurate accounting. The capacity is there; all that is necessary is to find ways to fund the systems and to put them in place so they "talk" to one another.

Robotics is another area of advanced technology that could affect the practice of nursing. There have been applications of early robotic technology to the use of programmable machines for the delivery of supplies and even trays within hospitals, but thus far, uses have been fairly limited. Speculation about future applications can conjure up images of robotic nurses in the image of R2D2 and C3P0 from the Star Wars movies, but other possibilities may be closer to implementation. Some medical and surgical procedures could be robotically assisted. Robotic devices are likely to become more integrated into rehabilitation and prosthetics.

Technologies have changed the practice of nursing in the recent past, and that trend is expected to continue. More and more sophisticated devices for monitoring and administering care have made the delivery of care very different in recent decades. With the shortage of highly skilled nurses that are needed for the high-tech environments, aggressive recruitment and retention strategies are being implemented. The unique body of knowledge needed for these roles is not acquired in undergraduate nursing programs as they are now taught. This has led to a new model of offering speciality education in some Canadian schools. A partnership among Queen Elizabeth Hospital II, the Health Science Center, and Dalhousie University School of Nursing will provide a strategy for specialty education at three educational levels in acute-care nursing. The areas offered are emergency, critical care, and perioperative nursing (Robertson, 2000). Nursing education will need to adapt to prepare nurses for practice in the future, and new templates will emerge.

Responses to demographic and societal changes within the changing paradigms of health care delivery create challenges to the public's health, both now and in the future. Leaders at the Centers for Disease Control and Prevention have identified at least ten future health challenges. These challenges encompass not only the changes in health care delivery and the aging of society, but also such things as risks imposed by lifestyles, the environment, and new scientific frontiers, such as the brain and human behavior and genome mapping (Koplan and Fleming 2000). These challenges for the future include:

1. Instituting a rational health care system that balances equity, cost, and quality
2. Eliminating health disparities by improving access to health care using innovative community-based strategies tailored to a diverse population
3. Focusing on children's emotional and intellectual development, as well as physical health, to permit them to achieve full potential

4. Achieving a longer "health span" so that people are not merely living longer
5. Integrating physical activity and healthy eating into daily lives to counteract the trend toward obesity and its consequences for health
6. Cleaning up and protecting the environment, which is likely to be increasingly challenged
7. Preparing to respond to emerging infectious diseases resulting from microbial adaptation and antibiotic resistance
8. Recognizing and addressing the contributions of mental health to overall health and well-being
9. Reducing the toll of violence in society
10. Using new scientific knowledge and technological advances wisely by applying them equitably, ethically, and responsibly

Some of these challenges have strategies that can easily be identified and evolved from earlier attempts to improve health and health care. Others need an approach that is less clear and may create controversy or even divisiveness in the planning. Nevertheless, there are valuable opportunities to make a difference in future health.

Many factors will affect nursing in the future. What nurses do, how they are educated, and where they practice will undoubtedly change. Nurses need to embrace the changes and be a part of shaping the future.

Consider . . .

■ the rapid changes in technology that have come about since you have been a nurse. Were these changes embraced by everyone when they were new? Has practice improved because of them?

■ the changes in the nurse-client relationship that has been associated with new nursing roles and the use of technological advances. How does the nurse maintain a therapeutic relationship with the client when machines take over some of the nursing functions?

■ the skills you believe will be important in the future. How should they be taught?

Health Care System Changes

As the health care system struggles to provide care for all people at a reasonable cost, it will undergo many changes. Although managed health care is only the latest attempt to reverse the escalating costs of care, time and the outcomes will determine its impact. However, while managed care is available, there will be fewer professional nurses in hospitals and more multiskilled workers supervised by professional nurses. The term *multiskilled worker* refers to a person who is prepared to provide basic care under supervision but who is not licensed. Basic care will also change as technology takes over the measuring of vital signs and other parameters of assessment. The client's history, which is already on their personal computer card, will need revising only as new events occur and information is added to the computer record.

Because the length of stay for a hospitalized person will become shorter, the care provided will address the very acute phase of the illness episode and will be directed toward pain management, respiratory facilitation, cardiac support, and neurologic monitoring. Preparing the client for recovery at home will be a major aspect of the nurse's role. In order to plan and implement effective care, nurses will need to maintain and increase their knowledge of physiologic and psychologic functioning, technologic monitoring systems, client care, and computer systems.

Seriously ill clients confined to a hospital bed will require intensive care administered by professionals who will administer medications using equipment that is computer driven. There will be less worry about turning clients because the hospital beds of tomorrow will be designed to rotate the occupant periodically so that skin integrity is preserved. The professional nurse will assign dressing changes and other treatments to the multiskilled workers, so the cost of care will be contained by the number and level of the workers assigned to the units. Self-directed work teams made up of cross-trained professionals and multiskilled workers will direct, provide, and evaluate the care.

One of the most exciting possibilities for what might occur in the United States is described by Jeffrey Bauer, who proposes that the health care system be changed by breaking the monopoly held by physicians over the delivery of health care to American citizens. Bauer proposes that health care costs will not decrease until citizens are allowed to select the provider they want. He proposes that health care be placed on the free market so that maximum choice and quality competition are available. He believes we must "take the shackles off America's many competent non-physician providers and allow the American consumer free access to their services" (Bauer, 1994, p. 19).

If Bauer's plan were to come into being—and there are good reasons to believe that it will—then advanced nurse practitioners, certified nurse-midwives, dentists, pharmacists, certified nurse-anesthetists, physical therapists, occupational therapists, and respiratory therapists, to name only a few, would be able to respond directly to the public's needs. The consumer would be free to choose from an expanded menu of qualified providers, a development that would bring the cost of care down while providing quality care for all. Nurses will be needed in increasing numbers in ambulatory surgical centers, diagnostic centers, home care, nursing homes, and skilled nursing facilities as hospitals become smaller and health care moves to the community. Those nurses with baccalaureate and master's degrees will have first choice as nonphysician providers because they are the best prepared for the role required of the nurse in the community. The nurse's role will include direct and indirect care; nurses will care for and manage others who provide care. In rural areas, advanced nurse practitioners will act as primary care providers as they assess, treat, and follow up on common, ordinary health care problems. Problems that require surgery or specialty consultation will be referred to physicians and other nonphysician providers. Physicians, nurses, and other health care providers will work together as interdisciplinary teams providing the consumer with the expertise of many care providers. Collaborative efforts will be necessary as the world of health care becomes more complex and technology continues to improve and change. The anticipated changes in the health care delivery system of the future require that everyone, health professional and consumer alike, must change his or her expectations and behaviors. The changing health care system requires more personal health responsibility on the part of the consumer and greater responsiveness on the part of health care providers.

Regulatory Changes

In the future there will probably be some major changes in the regulation of physicians and nonphysician health care providers. The National Council of State Boards of Nursing (which is composed of representatives from each state's board) has proposed that there be national standards for licensing entry-level nurses and measuring the competency of nurses over time. The PEW Health Professions Commission (1995) went even further, proposing that the regulation of all physician and nonphysician health care providers be carried out at the national level and that the approach be an interdisciplinary one.

What would this mean? It could mean that regulations would be competency based, broad enough to allow for change, and yet definitive enough to assure the public that the provider, regardless of title, is qualified to offer the service. It could mean that quality control would be the key ingredient in determining universal standards for all health care providers, no matter where they practice or what title they hold. The state could provide the entry exam, and the professions could be held legally and financially responsible for the conduct of their members under state and federal guidelines based on general norms set across all health care disciplines. Would this work? Several professional organizations believe so, and there is enough pressure from legislators to indicate that kind of modification could occur.

The value of this kind of approach to regulation is that competency standards, not titles, would drive decisions; as a result, nonphysician providers would be considered equal partners in health care delivery. Having the state control entry to practice based on national standards and the profession control certification based on their own specific practice expectations for general and advanced practice results in more meaningful recertification of providers with the least amount of government intrusion. These radical changes are becoming necessary to the removal of traditional practice barriers between physicians, nurses, and other health care providers. Advanced nurse practitioners have demonstrated that they are excellent primary caregivers, but most state regulations, which generally are influenced by physician lobbyists, have kept legislators from making the changes needed for the legitimate use of advanced nurse practitioners. The argument of cost could be used to make the case for national, standardized regulation, but the argument that advanced nurse practitioners are adequately prepared and have demonstrated their value as primary care providers is a better one.

Continued Medical, Surgical, and Pharmacological Advances

The list of advancements in medicine is a long one. For example, it is possible to clone people (although whether to do so is an ethical controversy); treat highly infectious diseases with potent chemicals; keep people alive with machines that breathe for them and keep the heart pumping; and remove, sterilize, and replace a person's bone marrow to cure disease. It is possible to perform surgery while the client's blood is cycled through an artificial heart and lungs, transplant organs from human and animal donors, and replace old worn-out joints with new artificial ones. It is possible to save the life of a 26-week premature infant through mechanical breathing, intravenous feedings, and highly potent drugs. It is possible to replace amputated limbs with artificial ones and to provide computer and mechanical support that can enable a paralyzed person to pursue a career and be self-supporting.

The development of medications that produce desired physiologic effects and change psychologic moods has prolonged life, made it more comfortable, and enhanced people's ability to enjoy it. Drugs can be a vital part of healthy living for those with chronic physiologic or psychologic illnesses. Some drugs, however, have also caused dependence, making people less able to cope or function without them.

Medical treatment of chronic conditions and acute phases of infection and much after-trauma care often centers around pharmacologic therapy. Furthermore, the number of nonprescription medications has increased in number as the Food and Drug Administration (FDA) releases many prescription drugs for over-the-counter purchase. The consumer now has even more choices than before. A trip to the drugstore or local supermarket or discount store allows the consumer access to a vast variety of remedies for a stuffy nose, sore throat, respiratory congestion, bowel problems, joint aches, heartburn, urinary discomfort, worry, or whatever else is causing distress. It is very easy to acquire drugs, and the public uses many drugs; in fact, polypharmacy has become a major problem in America because many people combine prescription drugs and nonprescription drugs in a haphazard manner.

Pharmacological advancements have also had a significant impact on nursing. Nurses have had to expand their knowledge base of pharmacology and their skills in caring for clients who have had surgery or who are undergoing medical treatment. Keeping informed about the newest drugs means the nurse must consult the *National Drug Formulary* or other drug references more often. Moreover, it is becoming even more urgent for nurses to face the inevitable ethical dilemmas. The need for more information and more discussion about ethical issues will continue and escalate as health care in hospitals becomes more acute, as arguments rage over the distribution of financial resources for expensive "experimental treatment" (e.g., complex organ transplants) versus less expensive preventive care (childhood immunizations), and as more nonphysician providers deliver care in homes, malls, the office or place of work, the school, the church, clinics, ambulatory centers, and nursing homes.

In the past, nurses have responded to the events that confront them; no doubt they will again. In the 21st century, however, nurses' responses will need to be quicker and more flexible. This means nurses will need more education and a greater understanding of the community and aggregate care. Nurses will also have to see themselves as "knowledge workers" and facilitators of care rather than individual caregivers. This is a major paradigm shift.

Teaching, preparing educational materials, and

teaching others how to teach will consume more of a nurse's time. Interactive video, distance learning, and using computers and other audio-visual equipment for learning will expand the market for instructional materials and good teachers. Because people will learn in their homes and at work, instructional materials will need to be portable and self-contained. Group learning will become as common as individual learning, and the use of the "information highway" will be a key mode of delivery. With satellites available and cables throughout the United States, North America, and the world, disseminating information will not be difficult.

Surgical procedures, medical treatment, and pharmacological therapies will continue to advance. In fact, there is every reason to believe the advancements will develop even more rapidly, so that only those who are continuous learners will be able to keep pace. Nurses will have to be continuous learners if they expect to have a place in the new health care paradigm.

Historically, nurses have cared for the sick. In the new paradigm, nurses will focus on wellness and prevention. The nurse will be the primary person who works to help individuals stay well and do things that promote health. Nurses will have to increase their knowledge base about nutrition, exercise, vitamin replacement, and the effects of cigarette smoking and the use of alcohol. As "models of good health," some nurses will have to adopt healthier behaviors and lifestyles. They will also have to keep abreast of the most recent research in the prevention and treatment of cancer, AIDS, and other infections.

Nurses will also need to take an active role in preparing healthy citizens for the future by teaching children about exercise, nutrition, safety, and other habits for healthy living, at a time when lifelong habits are learned. Teaching children about sex, sexually transmitted diseases, alcohol, and drug abuse will also be a challenge. Pressures from parents and organized religion have made it difficult to offer sex education in public and private schools. Nurses must be advocates for children and actively work to see that sex education becomes part of the school curriculum.

PAST LESSONS THAT CAN HELP NURSES IN THE FUTURE

From what has happened in health care, nurses can learn many lessons that may help them deal with the future.

1. The health care delivery system in the United States is remarkably flexible. Since the 1800s, the U.S. health care system has responded quickly to changes in technology, scientific discoveries, and new health threats. Medical science has undergone several revolutionary redefinitions; many infectious diseases have been conquered, and new ones have taken their place; more of the population has been able to survive to old age; the hospital has been redefined from a place for the poor to die to a place for anyone to be restored to health. For those who do die, the causes of death have changed. One hundred years ago, the leading killers were polio and infectious diseases. Today's leading killers are heart disease, tobacco, AIDS, and violence. Health insurance, which was instituted in the early part of the century to support personal payment, now has become the main source of payment for health care.

2. Changes in the health care system have always occurred rapidly and sometimes without warning. Most of the changes outlined above took place quickly, and many of the advancements in medicine were unexpected or the result of war. Government and society did not set out to initiate Medicare or to institute diagnosis-related groups (DRGs) or, for that matter, to turn to managed care. These developments happened quickly as a way to solve an immediate problem. Clearly, the system is not driven by tradition or "cast in stone."

3. No one entity is in control of the health care system. Only a brief scan of any newspaper will reveal that no one body—neither physicians, federal or state governments, insurers or payers—controls the system, as President Clinton discovered when he tried to reform the system in the mid-1990s. Consumers are becoming more interested in how the system works and how to change it because it is their tax dollars that support it.

4. Health care providers, especially nurses, have made major strides each time the system changed. These most recent changes have clearly presented great opportunities for nurses and other nonphysician caregivers. New roles, roles most appropriately played by providers with an interest and preparation in prevention, are waiting to be filled by nurses.

As soon as one understands these lessons, the possibilities for the future become apparent. For example, it is possible for anyone to influence the development of tomorrow's health care system. Modifications will undoubtedly occur quickly and repeatedly as nations seek ways to provide quality health care for all. Control of the system will shift from one source to another. Because control has thus far resided with government, professionals, and insurance companies, it seems likely that consumers may be the next group to want and assume control (Bower, 1997).

VISIONS OF TOMORROW

Throughout this chapter several themes have emerged that provide the framework for a vision of tomorrow.

Health care will be provided mostly in the community. Whereas acute and critical phases of illness will be attended to in hospitals, most health care will be delivered within the community. During the 1960s, the number of hospitals grew rapidly because funding was available and because it was believed that the best care could be provided there. It has since been learned that hospital care is very costly, disrupts the family, and focuses on cure, not prevention. In the 2000s, care will be delivered primarily outside the hospital. Schools, churches, the workplace, home clinics, skilled nursing facilities, and nursing homes will be the sites for care.

Care is already provided in clinics, in nursing homes, in the home, and at skilled nursing facilities. More health care will be also provided in schools and in the workplace. The rise of alcohol and drug abuse in the young, the increasing incidence of HIV in adolescents and young adults, and the increasing number of teenage pregnancies will require more preventive care in the school setting. The same is true of the workplace: Occupational health care is growing because prevention is less costly than illness care. Reducing absenteeism and tardiness increases productivity. Also, employees will avail themselves of services that are easy to access; accessing care on the job is often preferable to taking time from work to visit a clinic.

Churches and other faith communities are natural places for health care, especially if there is a holistic approach. Much of what ails people is tied into their sense of self and how they cope. For many people, religious and spiritual resources can be integral to their ability to cope with illness or the threat of a health condition. Parish nursing is a new but growing field of nursing and has been particularly helpful in rural regions.

Healthmobiles will bring primary health care and dental services and screening to special locations, such as farmworkers' camps, retirement communities, and inner-city neighborhoods. Education to prevent problems will be a major focus for the homebound and the poor.

As the population grows older, Americans will receive more long-term care at home. Electronic monitoring equipment will be attached to telephones to allow those who are homebound to relay medical information to clinics or home health agencies. More and more follow-up will be done by telephone as reimbursement systems switch from fee-for-service to managed care and capitation.

Independent nonphysician providers, particularly nurses, will deliver a significant proportion of the nation's primary care. Because advanced nurse practitioners have responded so well to the country's need for more primary care providers, they will deliver a significant portion of the nation's primary care. Advanced nurse practitioners educated as family, pediatric, and geriatric care practitioners will complement physician family practitioners as the backbone of the nation's health care system. This linking will occur both in nurse-only practices and in collaborative practice arrangements with physicians. Nurse-midwives will take over many of the primary care functions of obstetricians/gynecologists, including the management of low-risk pregnancies. Physicians will continue to do what they have been doing, but there will be much more collaborative practice with nurses and other nonphysician providers. The clinical nurse specialist role and the nurse practitioner role will continue to blur as advanced-practice nurses provide care in communities as specialists in health promotion.

In the world of tomorrow, nurses will work collaboratively with physicians and other nonphysician providers. These groups of providers will offer their services in retail locations as small businesses (a major reason why all nurses will need a business education). Health "stores" will vary in size from small basic care operations located in shopping malls to free-standing buildings with huge clinics offering everything from dentistry and family medical care to physical therapy and life-saving emergency services.

The new providers (nurses, physicians, and other nonphysicians) will be much more attuned to what the consumer wants. The hours of service will change so the consumer can access the services in the evenings and on weekends. The larger locations will offer comprehensive wellness programs promoting healthy lifestyles, provide facilities for weight control and exercise, and offer programs about nutrition and exercise. Illness care will be available, but the major emphasis will be on health promotion.

Nurses will take the lead in the development of these "health centers" because the framework for nursing throughout its history has been holistic and comprehensive. Nurses have always promoted health and focused on the prevention of illness. Moreover, nurses can lead the way to better health and cut costs by helping the public assume responsibility for their lives as healthy individuals.

Physicians will assume roles as coproviders, specialty-care providers, and consultants. Although many physicians may express serious concern about what is happening and will happen in the future, nurses and consumers can expect that many physicians will quietly lead the way into the new system. Many physicians will remain as specialty care providers because there will still be a need for physicians who are prepared to care for specific health care problems, such as oncologists, orthopedists, neurologists, psychiatrists, cardiologists, and so on. Other physicians will join collaborative practices with advanced nurse practitioners to provide comprehensive basic care. Some physicians will seize the opportunity to enter entrepreneurial businesses. There will be plenty to do in the new system, but everyone will need to change their expectations and responsibilities.

Physician activity will affect nursing as nurses seize opportunities for collaborative practice. Advanced-practice nurses will need physician consultation in their independent practices, especially for their clients with more complex problems. Over time, physicians and nurses will work together in more ways and in better ways as it becomes more clear how the new system will unfold.

Informed consumers will become more self-directed and assume more responsibility for their health. One of the most exciting advances in the future will be one-stop diagnostic centers. Like a full-service gas station, these diagnostic centers will provide informed consumers access to urinalysis, blood tests, throat cultures, and even some radiographic tests. These diagnostic centers will be electronically linked to large, fully equipped laboratories for confirmation of diagnoses and to health databases that store consumer records. Educational services will also be available through interactive computer programs and video libraries.

Computer terminals in pharmacies will help consumers find answers to questions regarding health and illness. Pharmacists will be able to diagnose such common ailments as throat infections and skin rashes with the help of computer protocols and over-the-counter diagnostic tools. Women already can diagnose pregnancy at home using a simple diagnostic package purchased at a supermarket, pharmacy, or discount store.

For easy access, diagnostic centers will be located in health care clinics, supermarkets, shopping malls, and department stores. Consumers will also be able to authorize a pharmacist to access their personal medical records in order to check for allergies to prescrip-

tive drugs or other medications. It is easy to see that consumers will have much more control, involvement, and accountability in their health care. This is perhaps the most exciting aspect of the new system.

Access to health care/consultation will resemble the market for other services and products. Because health care/consultation will be easy to access, it will resemble other kinds of services the consumer uses. The clinics, pharmacies, and diagnostic centers will remain open nights and weekends; some may even remain open 24 hours a day. Clearly, tomorrow's health care agencies will be much more attuned to the needs of the customer. Larger agencies will offer comprehensive wellness programs that promote healthy lifestyles, including good nutrition and proper exercise.

Education and prevention will be the major product lines of the retail health and medical stores of the future. The focus of the new clinics will be on keeping people healthy as well as diagnosing and treating people who are ill. The dream of comprehensive care will finally become a reality.

Education for nurses will reflect the changes in the health care delivery system and the application of new educational technologies. Nurses' education, consistent with these many changes, will also change and will use virtual reality, simulators, and web-based/enhanced classes. The focus of the programs (regardless of the level) will be on the community and on prevention. Nurses will continue to teach how to care for the sick, but the major emphasis will be how to keep people well. Teaching, consulting, and learning referral skills will be essential for the nurses of the future, therefore much more time will be spent on helping students learn these skills.

Group work and a focus on working with aggregates will supersede the time spent on individual care. Since nurses will be in the community and focusing on prevention, it will be imperative that they can work with groups. Being able to work with parents, abused women, persons with AIDS, people with cardiovascular problems, and any number of other groups will be necessary if the nurse is to use time efficiently and spend it with the individuals who need the care. This means that the educational program must devote more time to developing nurses' group process skills.

Nursing students and nurses will also need computer skills. They will need not only word processing and spreadsheet skills but also the ability to use virtual reality equipment. Computer competence will probably become a prerequisite for admission to a nursing program in the future.

An important new focus for nursing education at

all levels will be on the *community*. Although students live in a community and read about communities, until they understand that a community is more than a geographic boundary, they will not be prepared for the health care of tomorrow. Much more time will be spent on the study of community and its impact on the health of the citizens. Nurses will also need to become more aware of the global community and become more geographically knowledgeable and culturally competent.

As geographic barriers become more passable, immigrants and refugees will move from areas with limited resources to areas with more opportunity. These immigrants will bring beliefs and practices about health care that are culturally driven; they also will bring illnesses that may be unique to their race or geographic homeland. Nurses will need to become more aware of global health problems and their impact on nursing practice. Through advances in technology, nurses have greater ability to communicate or travel to other countries and continents and are better able to network with the global nursing community.

Through technology, students will probably learn more at home than at the college or university. Student access to technology at home and the use of virtual reality will also change faculty behavior. Faculty will need to know how to manage distance education and keep abreast of ever-changing computer and video technology and the broadening concepts of community, prevention, health promotion, and the globalization of America.

An important and imperative looming change is a decision on the basic preparation of nurses. The ANA, NLN, and other specialty nursing organizations will

Bookshelf

Reich, R. B. 2001. *The future of success.* **New York: Alfred A. Knopf.**

The former secretary of labor under President Clinton presents the notion that technological advances and innovations are why Americans are working longer hours than ever before. He examines what success has come to mean and offers options to reestablish balance.

Schwartz, P. 1996. *The art of the long view: Planning for the future in an uncertain world.* **New York: Doubleday and Company, Inc.**

This book discusses the ability to visualize different kinds of futures incorporating what the authors refers to as "the intangibles": our hopes and fears, our beliefs and dreams. Stories and scenarios are used to present the ideas.

Research Box

Antrobus, S. M., and Kitson, A. D. 1999. Nursing leadership: Influencing and shaping health policy and nursing practice. *Journal of Advanced Nursing* **29(3): 746–753.**

The purpose of this study was to examine contemporary nursing leadership in the United Kingdom within the context of health policy. A qualitative, ethnographic design was applied using informal semistructured interviews with a purposive sample of 24 people recognized for their effectiveness in leading nursing. The interviews began by asking each of the leaders to locate himself or herself within a framework of four quadrants: political, executive, academic, or clinical, with leadership positioned at the center and spanning all four quadrants. An interview schedule was followed, but themes were developed with subsequent participants as they emerged from the data. Findings indicated that nursing and nursing leadership are shaped by the impact of policy and politics, and contemporary leadership has both an internal and an external focus. Effective nursing leadership is the vehicle through which both nursing practice and health policy are influenced and shaped. Five recommendations are made:

1. Continual investment in clinical leadership should occur to influence and shape policy and practice.
2. Establishing a national policy unit for the development of nursing should be considered.
3. Nursing leaders should be conversant in health, social policy, management, and research.
4. Career pathways integrate political, managerial, academic, and clinical domains.
5. A program of research into nursing leadership should be developed.

take the lead and determine the basic preparation of professional nurses. This action will not only help correct the confusion for potential students, but also lay the foundation for advanced practice. Legislators, other professional groups, and the public will finally know the scope of basic professional nursing practice. Statutes will be more clear, and regulations governing practice will be consistent. Nothing the profession can do will be as important or as necessary as this action.

The world of tomorrow is exciting. Health promotion, rather than medical care, will finally be the focus. With these changes will come a challenge for nursing. Nursing will need to grasp the opportunity and become the leader in the movement toward providing care that creates a better life for each citizen. Clearly there will be a need for more nurses prepared at the baccalaureate and master's levels to meet the demands of a community-based consumer population. New technologies will be available for nurses' use. The system is now ready and able to respond to the need, and the public is ready for the new ways. Nursing education and practice must seize the opportunity to make the necessary changes (Bower, 1997).

Consider . . .

- your own vision for the future of health care and nursing in your community, your nation, and the world. Is it consistent with the author's vision? Do you see different or additional changes that have not been discussed here? If yes, what are they?

Research Box

Wright, S. 1998. An eye to the future. *Nursing Standard* 12(48): 20–22.
This is a brief report of a project from the Royal College of Nursing in London. Nurses' views of the future were qualitatively examined for common themes. Some of these were that envisioning the future should be a continuous process built into the day-to-day work of the profession. Change overload has promoted feelings of powerlessness, highlighting a lack of involvement in decision making. The concept of equality in the multidisciplinary team is a myth because the physician emerges as the team leader. The positive aspects of expanding nursing roles were seen as being counterbalanced by the perceived loss of attention to the core of nursing. Nurses' concerns tended to focus on issues of practice development, organizational barriers, "good nursing", and quality of care. The rise of nursing research was seen as a positive change but identified that too little research reaches the practice arena. The falling number of qualified nurses and the dilution of skill mix was cited as compromising quality of care.

SELECTED REFERENCES

Aiken, L. H., Lake, E. T., Semaan, S., Lehman, H. P., O'Hare, P. A., Cole, C. S., Dunbar, D., and Frank, I. 1993, Fall. Nurse practitioner managed care for persons with HIV infection. *Image: The Journal of Nursing Scholarship* 25(3): 172–177.

Antrobus, S. M., and A. D. Kitson. 1999. Nursing leadership: Influencing and shaping health policy and nursing practice. *Journal of Advanced Nursing* 29(3): 746–753.

Bauer, J. 1994. *Not what the doctor ordered.* Chicago: Probus.

Benner, P. 2000. Shaping the future of nursing. *Nursing Management* 7(1): 31–35.

Bower, F. 1997. *Looking into the future.* In *Professional Nursing Practice: Concepts and Perspectives,* 3d ed. by B. Kozier, G. Erb, and K. Blais. Menlo Park, Calif: Addison Wesley Longman, Inc.

Heller, B., Oros, M. T., and Durney-Crowley, J. 2000. The future of nursing education: 10 trends to watch. *Nursing and Health Care Perspectives* 21(1): 9–13.

Jenkins, R. 1997. Superhighway for the future of nursing: Signposts. *Nurse Educator* 22(3): 44.

Jones, C. H. 1998. The future of nursing and complementary alternative health-care. *New Mexico Nurse* 43(3): 17.

Justice, D. 1999. Virtual nursing. *Nursing Standard* 14(8): 14–15.

Koplan, J. P., and Fleming, D. W. 2000. Current and future public health challenges. *Journal of the American Medical Association* 284(13): 1696–1698.

Mailer, S. S., Charles, J., Piper, S., Hunt-McCool, J., Wilborne-Davis, P., and Baigis, J. 2000. Analysis of the nursing work force compared with national trends. *Journal of Nursing Administration* **30**(10): 482–489.

Mundinger, M. O. 1995. Advanced practice nursing is the answer . . . what is the question? *N & H C Perspectives on Community* **16**(5): 254–259.

National League for Nursing. 1994. *Nursing data review.* New York: NLN.

Pew Health Professions Commission. 1995. *Licensure and regulation of health care providers.* San Francisco: UCSF Center for the Health Professions.

Robertson, K. A. 2000. Clinical major option: A model for implementing critical care nursing into baccalaureate preparation. *Canadian Critical Care Nurse* **11**(3): 22–24.

Wright, S. 1998. An eye to the future. *Nursing Standard* **12**(48): 20–22.

Index